Handbook of Diagnosis and Treatment of Bipolar Disorders

Handbook of Diagnosis and Treatment of Bipolar Disorders

Edited by

Terence A. Ketter, M.D.

Professor of Psychiatry and Behavioral Sciences
Department of Psychiatry and Behavioral Sciences;
Chief, Bipolar Disorders Clinic
Stanford University School of Medicine
Stanford, California

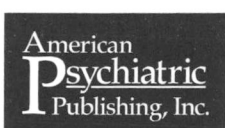

American Psychiatric Publishing, Inc.

Washington, DC
London, England

MONTREAL GENERAL HOSPITAL
MEDICAL LIBRARY

If you would like to buy between 25 and 99 copies of this or any other APPI title, you are eligible for a 20% discount; please contact APPI Customer Service at appi@psych.org or 800-368-5777. If you wish to buy 100 or more copies of the same title, please e-mail us at bulksales@psych.org for a price quote.

Copyright © 2010 American Psychiatric Publishing, Inc.
ALL RIGHTS RESERVED

Manufactured in the United States of America on acid-free paper
13   12   11   10   09   5   4   3   2   1
First Edition

Typeset in Adobe AGaramond and Formata.

American Psychiatric Publishing, Inc.
1000 Wilson Boulevard
Arlington, VA 22209-3901
www.appi.org

Library of Congress Cataloging-in-Publication Data
Handbook of diagnosis and treatment of bipolar disorders / edited by Terence A. Ketter. — 1st ed.
    p. ; cm.
   Includes bibliographical references and index.
   ISBN 978-1-58562-313-6 (alk. paper)

   1. Manic-depressive illness—Handbooks, manuals, etc. I. Ketter, Terence A.
[DNLM: 1. Bipolar Disorder—diagnosis—Handbooks. 2. Bipolar Disorder—therapy—Handbooks. WM 34 H2368 2009]
   RC516.H357 2009
   616.89'5—dc22

                                                                                          2009011729

British Library Cataloguing in Publication Data
A CIP record is available from the British Library.

Contents

Appendices

Contributors

John O. Brooks III, Ph.D., M.D.
Associate Professor in Residence and Director, Consultation & Liaison Psychiatry, Semel Institute for Neuroscience and Human Behavior, David Geffen School of Medicine at UCLA, Los Angeles, California

Kiki D. Chang, M.D.
Associate Professor of Psychiatry and Behavioral Sciences, Department of Psychiatry and Behavioral Sciences; and Director, Pediatric Bipolar Disorders Program, Stanford University School of Medicine, Stanford, California

Jenifer L. Culver, Ph.D.
Clinical Assistant Professor, Department of Psychiatry and Behavioral Sciences, Stanford University School of Medicine, Stanford, California

Meghan Howe, M.S.W.
Clinical Research Manager, Department of Psychiatry and Behavioral Sciences, Pediatric Bipolar Disorders Program, Stanford University School of Medicine, Stanford, California

Terence A. Ketter, M.D.
Professor of Psychiatry and Behavioral Sciences, Department of Psychiatry and Behavioral Sciences; and Chief, Bipolar Disorders Clinic, Stanford University School of Medicine, Stanford, California

Laura C. Pratchett, M.S.
Psychology Intern, Montefiore Medical Center; and Doctoral Candidate, Pacific Graduate School of Psychology–Stanford Psy.D. Consortium, Redwood City, California

Natalie L. Rasgon, M.D., Ph.D.
Professor of Psychiatry and Behavioral Sciences, Department of Psychiatry and Behavioral Sciences; and Director, Women's Wellness Clinic, Stanford University School of Medicine, Stanford, California

Manpreet K. Singh, M.D., M.S.
Instructor and Postdoctoral Fellow, Department of Psychiatry and Behavioral Sciences, Pediatric Bipolar Disorders Program, Stanford University School of Medicine, Stanford, California

Barbara R. Sommer, M.D.
Associate Professor of Psychiatry and Behavioral Sciences, and Director, Geriatric Psychiatry Program, Department of Psychiatry and Behavioral Sciences, Stanford University School of Medicine, Stanford, California

Po W. Wang, M.D.
Clinical Associate Professor, Department of Psychiatry and Behavioral Sciences, Stanford University School of Medicine, Stanford, California

Laurel N. Zappert, Psy.D.
Staff Psychologist, Counseling and Psychological Services, Vaden Health Center, Stanford University, Stanford, California

Disclosure of Competing Interests

The following contributors to this book have indicated a financial interest in or other affiliation with a commercial supporter, a manufacturer of a commercial product, a provider of a commercial service, a nongovernmental organization, and/or a government agency, as listed below:

John O. Brooks III, Ph.D., M.D.—*Speaker's bureau:* AstraZeneca, Eli Lilly, Pfizer

Kiki D. Chang, M.D.—*Research support:* AstraZeneca, Eli Lilly, GlaxoSmithKline, National Institute of Mental Health, NARSAD; *Consultant:* Eli Lilly, GlaxoSmithKline, Otsuka America; *Speaker's bureau:* AstraZeneca, Bristol Myers-Squibb, Eli Lilly

Terence A. Ketter, M.D.—*Grant/Research support:* Abbott, AstraZeneca, Bristol-Myers Squibb, Cephalon, Eli Lilly, GlaxoSmithKline, Pfizer, Repligen, Wyeth; *Consultant:* Abbott, AstraZeneca, Bristol-Myers Squibb, Dainippon Sumitomo, Eli Lilly, GlaxoSmithKline, Janssen, Jazz, Novartis, Organon, Solvay, Valeant, Vanda, Wyeth, XenoPort; *Lecture honoraria:* Abbott, AstraZeneca, Bristol-Myers Squibb, Eli Lilly, GlaxoSmithKline, Noven, Otsuka, Pfizer; *Employee* (Nzeera Ketter, M.D., spouse): Johnson & Johnson

Natalie L. Rasgon, M.D., Ph.D.—*Has received grant or research support and/or has been a consultant and /or received lecture honoraria from the following:* Wyeth-Ayerst; Abbott (past grant support); Bristol Myers-Squibb (past speaker); Forest, GlaxoSmithKline (past research support); Pfizer (past research support and past speaker)

Manpreet K. Singh, M.D., M.S.—*Grant/Research support:* American Psychiatric Association/AstraZeneca Young Minds in Psychiatry Award, Klingenstein Third Generation Foundation, NARSAD, National Institute of Mental Health, Stanford Child Health Research Program

Barbara R. Sommer, M.D.—*Stockholder (have held shares in):* Celgene Corporation, Genzyme Corporation, Johnson & Johnson, Thermo Fisher Scientific, Teva Pharmaceuticals

Po W. Wang, M.D.—*Grant/Research support:* None as principal investigator; *Consultant:* Abbott, Corcept Therapeutics, Pfizer, Sanofi-Aventis; *Lecture honoraria:* Abbott, AstraZeneca, Bristol-Myers Squibb, Eli Lilly, GlaxoSmithKline, Pfizer, Sanofi-Aventis

The following authors have no competing interests to report:

Jenifer L. Culver, Ph.D.
Meghan Howe, M.S.W.
Laura C. Pratchett, M.S.
Laurel N. Zappert, Psy.D.

Preface

This handbook of diagnosis and treatment of bipolar disorders is a readable, timely guide to the assessment and management of bipolar disorder. The field has seen dramatic and rapid advances in recent years, making it challenging for clinicians to keep abreast of the most recent research and integrate it into their practice.

The accelerating movement toward providing evidence-based care makes appreciating the quality of data supporting interventions increasingly important. Thus, recent controlled studies and U.S. Food and Drug Administration (FDA) approvals are emphasized. However, emphasis in this volume is also placed on translating such data into clinical practice because substantial differences are seen between the types of patients and interventions encountered in controlled trials and those encountered in real-world clinical practice. This manual provides clinicians with the necessary information to balance benefit (using number needed to treat analyses) and risk (using number needed to harm analyses) to provide individualized state-of-the-art evidence-based care. In this regard, plentiful figures, and summary tables, and appendices with key information serve as guides for clinicians, and case studies provide clinical immediacy to the content.

The content of this manual is based not only on controlled trials and FDA approvals but also on more than a decade of clinical research and clinical treatment experience by clinicians at Stanford University. As such, the manual offers an intermingling of evidence-based medicine and extensive personal clinical experiences to reflect the latest thinking about the diagnosis and management of bipolar disorder. Because this field is rapidly advancing, readers are encouraged to cross-reference our recommendations with other sources, particularly the latest edition of the *Physicians' Desk Reference* for medication information.

I would like to thank many individuals involved in writing this volume. My wife, Nzeera, has been patient and understanding regarding the need to spend time on this volume. The chapter authors and coauthors—Po Wang, Jenifer Culver, Laura Pratchett, Laurel Zappert, Natalie Rasgon, Kiki Chang, Manpreet Singh, Meghan Howe, John Brooks, and Barbara Sommer—deserve particular appreciation. The editorial staff at American Psychiatric Publishing, Inc. (APPI)—in particular, John McDuffie—deserve credit for their support, critical reading, and technical skill. The APPI leadership—in particular, Robert Hales—deserve thanks for their confidence. Our colleagues and trainees at Stanford deserve appreciation for their insights. Finally, but by no means least, we owe a great debt to patients and their families, who consistently prove that every one of them can teach us about bipolar disorder and its treatment on a daily basis.

We hope readers will find this volume helpful, and we look forward to their feedback.

Terence A. Ketter, M.D.

CHAPTER 1

Principles of Assessment and Treatment of Bipolar Disorders

Terence A. Ketter, M.D.

Advances in the diagnosis and treatment of bipolar disorders have been emerging at an accelerating pace. Unfortunately, our diagnostic system has not kept pace because the last substantial revision of diagnostic criteria for bipolar disorders was in 1994, when DSM-IV was published (American Psychiatric Association 1994), and DSM-IV-TR (American Psychiatric Association 2000) did not update the diagnostic criteria for bipolar disorders. Thus the diagnostic system is more than a decade old. Even more recent efforts to summarize treatment options for clinicians, such as the 2002 revision of the American Psychiatric Association's "Practice Guideline for the Treatment of Patients With Bipolar Disorder" (American Psychiatric Association 2002), have quickly become outdated. In this volume, we review recent developments, including advances in diagnosis and interventions supported by controlled studies. The emphasis is on the practical clinical applications of these advances.

Principles of Assessment of Bipolar Disorders

The diagnosis of bipolar disorders continues to rely on clinical information. Thus, as in general psychiatric practice, a comprehensive biopsychosocial assessment is crucial for effective management. In this section, I discuss assessment from this perspective. The presence of a significant other to provide collateral information may greatly enhance the accuracy of evaluation.

Chief Complaint

Individuals with bipolar disorder commonly present as outpatients, complaining of (often treatment-resistant) depressive symptoms, making the distinction of bipolar depression from unipolar major depressive disorder crucial. The prominent depressive symptoms of mixed episodes also make distinction of such episodes from agitated unipolar major depression crucial. Presentations of mood elevation can vary in severity from mildly to moderately irritable hypomania in outpatients, and thus risk being undetected, to severe psychotic manic or mixed episodes in inpatients, and thus risk being diagnosed as a psychotic disorder. Patients not in an acute mood episode at the time of presentation may be either euthymic or experiencing (and sometimes failing to notice) subsyndromal symptoms of depression or mood elevation.

The common occurrence of comorbid psychiatric (particularly anxiety and substance use) disorders, particularly if prominent, may on occasion draw attention away from a concurrent bipolar disorder. Patients may present complaining primarily of relationship or occupational problems, which on careful examination may be related to bipolar disorder and comorbid conditions.

History of the Current Illness

Careful characterization of the current clinical status of a syndromal manic, hypomanic, mixed, or major depressive episode compared with subsyndromal symptoms or euthymia is necessary to provide illness phase–appropriate treatment. Attention must be paid to the presence and absence of symptoms of not only mood elevation and depression but also comorbid psychiatric and medical disorders. Biological, psychological, and social stressors; relation to symptoms; and variations thereof over time require careful assessment.

In view of the risk of suicide or self-harm (and, less commonly, violence toward others), careful assessment of suicidal or self-harm (or homicidal) thoughts, fantasies, religious beliefs, specific methods considered (as well as access to firearms, medications, or other methods), impulses, and recent actions taken is necessary. Prior attempts, hopelessness, impulsiveness, anhedonia, panic attacks, anxiety and substance use disorders, psychosis (especially with command hallucinations), and absence of reasons for living and plans for the future are all ominous and indicate the need for aggressive interventions, including, if necessary, involuntary hospitalization to preserve life.

Current somatic and psychological treatment and adherence, as well as therapeutic and adverse effects, need to be assessed because current treatments may be attenuating or exacerbating symptoms, and responses will crucially affect treatment planning.

Psychiatric History

Precipitants, prodromes, onset, duration, frequency, and symptoms of episodes of mood elevation and depression, as well as comorbid psychiatric disorders, need to be characterized. Currently depressed patients may have difficulty recalling and identifying previous episodes of mood elevation; collateral history from a significant other can greatly enhance accuracy. Some patients with chronic illness may have difficulty recalling and identifying discrete episodes. Recall and identification of episodes may be facilitated by considering periods of decreased or increased function, important life events, and, for mood elevation, times immediately before and after depressive episodes. Previous therapeutic and adverse effects of (as well as adherence to) treatments (including hospitalizations) for mood, anxiety, substance use, and other disorders should be assessed. Evaluation should include detailed assessment of previous suicide attempts, aborted suicide attempts, and other self-harming behaviors.

Medical History

A detailed description of current and previous medical (particularly neurological and endocrine) disorders and treatments, including surgeries and hospitalizations, is necessary because these can yield secondary psychiatric disorders, exacerbate primary psychiatric disorders, and influence choice of psychiatric interventions.

Family History

A detailed family psychiatric, substance use, and medical history, with particular emphasis on first-degree relatives and including individuals with (suspected or actual) diagnosis and treatment (including hospitalization) of psychosis, suicide, suicide attempts, self-harm, or harm to others, is indicated. Therapeutic and adverse effects of psychiatric treatments in first-degree relatives may affect treatment planning.

Social History

The social and developmental history should include assessment of marital and employment status, living situation (including presence of vulnerable individuals in the home), external supports (including family), cultural and religious beliefs, and acute and chronic psychosocial stressors (including interpersonal, financial, and family problems; domestic violence; and sexual or physical abuse or neglect). All of these may affect psychiatric illness and treatment.

Mental Status Examination

Attire may be disheveled or drab during depression and flamboyant or bizarre during mood elevation. Psychomotor retardation and slow, low-volume speech suggest depression, whereas psychomotor agitation and rapid, high-volume speech may indicate hypomanic, manic, or mixed symptoms. Similarly, depressed or anhedonic mood with blunted affect may indicate depression, whereas euphoric, expansive, or irritable mood with labile affect suggests mood elevation. Ultradian (within a day) mood shifts may be seen in mixed episodes. Suicidal thoughts are seen primarily during depressive and mixed episodes, whereas psychotic symptoms and cognitive deficits can occur during either mood elevation or depression.

Multiaxial Diagnosis

Axis I diagnoses include disorder, subtype, and illness phase, as described in Chapter 2 of this volume, "DSM-IV-TR Diagnosis of Bipolar Disorders." A thorough understanding of DSM-IV-TR is necessary for clinicians to be able not only to provide reliable diagnoses according to the current system but also to offer care that integrates information from clinical studies and regulatory agencies. Although the DSM-IV-TR approach has notable strengths, it has important limitations. An understanding of the latter provides a basis for understanding how to address current diagnostic challenges. Ketter and Wang, in Chapter 3 in this volume, "Addressing Clinical Diagnostic Challenges in Bipolar Disorders," address clinical diagnostic challenges in bipolar disorders by providing strategies initially within the confines of the DSM-IV nosology and subsequently by using additional important information. Although the latter methods are not included in DSM-IV-TR, they are of sufficient validity that they arguably should be integrated into clinical practice to begin to address the important diagnostic challenges faced by clinicians striving to manage bipolar disorders in patients.

Axis II includes personality disorders, of which the dramatic cluster (Cluster B) may be viewed as personality analogues of the Axis I mood disorders. Axis III includes comorbid medical disorders, which are common in patients with bipolar disorders. Axis IV includes psychosocial stressors, which may trigger episodes to a greater extent early in bipolar disorder and to a lesser degree later in the course of the illness. Axis V includes a global assessment of function, which is typically decreased during mood episodes and may only very slowly improve after euthymic mood is achieved.

Not surprisingly, comorbid Axis I, II, and III disorders; concurrent Axis IV stressors; and poor Axis V function are all associated with greater complexity of treatment and poorer outcomes (American Psychiatric Association 2000).

Principles of Treatment of Bipolar Disorders

As with diagnosis, effective treatment of bipolar disorder relies on a biopsychosocial approach. Indeed, as described by Culver and Pratchett in Chapter 15 ("Adjunctive Psychosocial Interventions in the Management of Bipolar Disorders") in this volume, not only adjunctive psychosocial interventions but also comprehensive case management programs that incorporate psychoeducation, evidence-based pharmacotherapy, and increased access to care appear to yield better outcomes in bipolar disorder (Bauer et al. 2006a, 2006b; Simon et al. 2006).

Because bipolar disorder is a chronic, recurrent disorder, management involves aspects of models of the treatment of chronic disease; thus, therapy strives not only to rapidly control acute illness exacerbations but also in the longer term to prevent further episodes and optimize function. In Chapter 4 in this volume, "Multiphase Treatment Strategy for Bipolar Disorders," Ketter and colleagues describe crucial illness transition points and how these have been integrated with mood disorder illness phase knowledge to devise the multiphase treatment strategy. The latter is a systematic approach to the acute, continuation, and maintenance treatment phases of management of bipolar disorders.

Keck and McElroy (2004) have proposed treatment principles for bipolar disorder (Table 1–1), applying to bipolar disorder an approach to strategies (broad objectives) and tactics (specific aims) suggested by Rush (1999) for the management of unipolar major depressive disorder. Such principles need to be kept in mind as a broad conceptual framework when engaged in the detail-ridden implementation of specific interventions.

Specifics of Treatment of Bipolar Disorders

In addition to the concise broad principles in the previous section that provide a conceptual framework, an extraordinary amount of detailed specific information is necessary for the optimal management of bipolar disorders. In this volume,

TABLE 1–1.   Treatment principles for bipolar disorder

- Individually tailor guidelines.
- Use proven treatments first.
- Select best medication that is
  – Safe and tolerable
  – Easiest to use (for the patient)
  – Easiest to manage (for the physician)
- Aim for symptom remission, not just response.
- Measure symptomatic outcome.
- Remember that no medication is a panacea.
- Do not give up.
- Note that psychosocial restoration follows symptom relief.
- Also use family, educational, and social rhythm–targeted psychotherapies.
- Recognize that more chronic illness may respond more slowly.

Source. Reprinted with permission from Keck PE Jr, McElroy SL: "Treatment of Bipolar Disorder," in *The American Psychiatric Publishing Textbook of Psychopharmacology,* 3rd Edition. Edited by Schatzberg AF, Nemeroff CB. Washington, DC, American Psychiatric Publishing, 2004, pp. 865–883.

following the chapters on diagnosis and the multiphase treatment strategy, a series of chapters on the details of therapeutics are provided.

In Chapter 5, "Overview of Pharmacotherapy for Bipolar Disorders," Ketter and Wang provide a summary of recent developments, including the multiple new medications that have been approved for the treatment of bipolar disorders, that have fostered the emergence of evidence-based pharmacotherapy for bipolar disorders. This chapter also provides an overview of number needed to treat and number needed to harm analyses to facilitate evidence-based personalized benefit-to-risk assessments, as well as effectiveness studies that promise to permit more clinically relevant evidence-based information for clinicians treating bipolar disorders.

In Chapter 6, "Management of Acute Manic and Mixed Episodes in Bipolar Disorders," Ketter and Wang describe the substantial recent advances in this area. The evidence supporting the approvals of multiple new agents, including many second-generation antipsychotics, is reviewed, and practical applications of this information are offered.

Wang and Ketter consider recent developments in the treatment of the most pervasive illness phase with the fewest approved treatments in Chapter 7, "Management of Acute Major Depressive Episodes in Bipolar Disorders." Therapeutic options beyond mood stabilizers are needed; as for lithium, divalproex, and carbamazepine, efficacy in acute bipolar depression appears more modest than in acute mania. Certain second-generation antipsychotics, as well as other medications, and adjunctive psychosocial interventions are providing important new options for this phase of bipolar disorder.

Chapter 8, "Longer-Term Management of Bipolar Disorders," explores recent advances in the continuation and maintenance treatment phases of bipolar disorder. Controlled trials of recently approved longer-term pharmacotherapies such as lamotrigine and certain second-generation antipsychotics and emerging controlled data suggesting the efficacy of adjunctive psychosocial therapies are providing important new longer-term treatment options for patients with bipolar disorders. Longer-term compared with acute treatment provides distinctive opportunities and challenges with respect to managing medication adverse effects and maintaining the therapeutic alliance, treatment adherence, and involvement of significant others to enhance outcomes.

In Chapter 9, "Management of Rapid-Cycling Bipolar Disorders," Ketter and Wang describe recent developments in this area. To date, no treatment has received U.S. Food and Drug Administration approval for patients with bipolar disorder who have this illness course. However, results of controlled trials are beginning to provide clinically relevant insights into addressing the substantial therapeutic challenges encountered in the management of patients with rapid cycling.

In Chapter 10, "Management of Bipolar Disorders in Children and Adolescents," Chang and colleagues describe recent advances in the diagnosis and treatment of this challenging subgroup of patients. Emerging research has important management implications regarding the utility of mood stabilizers, second-generation antipsychotics, adjunctive psychotherapy, and combination treatments in children and adolescents with bipolar disorders. Therapeutic challenges include devising optimal interventions to manage comorbid disruptive behavior disorders, anxiety disorders, and substance use disorders and perhaps in the future to prevent the development of syndromal illness in individuals at risk, such as offspring of parents with bipolar disorders.

In Chapter 11, "Management of Bipolar Disorders in Women," Zappert and Rasgon describe recent advances in the treatment of bipolar disorder in this subgroup of patients who historically have been inadequately studied. Controlled data in this area remain limited, but recent research is yielding information with substantive clinical implications. Thus, important gender differences in the phenomenology and management of bipolar disorders in women compared with men are beginning to be understood, and emerging data are starting to clarify relations between the menstrual cycle and mood disturbance that can significantly affect illness course. Specific treatment considerations for women with bipolar disorders include pharmacological management of bipolar disorder during pregnancy and postpartum, management of medication-induced effects on reproductive function, and evaluation of mood effects of hormonal contraceptives.

In Chapter 12, "Management of Bipolar Disorders in Older Adults," Brooks and colleagues describe recent advances in the diagnosis and treatment of yet another subgroup of patients who historically have been inadequately studied. Once again, controlled data in this area remain limited. However, research in older adults with bipolar disorders and other psychiatric disorders is beginning to yield information about the safety and, to a more limited degree, the efficacy of interventions for bipolar disorders.

In Chapter 13, "Mood Stabilizers and Antipsychotics," Ketter and Wang describe the complex and varying pharmacology, adverse effects, and drug interactions of these medications. Although the mood stabilizers lithium, carbamazepine, valproate, and lamotrigine can be considered the foundational agents for the treatment of bipolar disorders, antipsychotics (particularly second-generation agents) are increasingly combined with mood stabilizers in clinical settings.

In Chapter 14, "Antidepressants, Anxiolytics/Hypnotics, and Other Medications," Ketter and Wang describe the even more complex and varying pharmacology, adverse effects, and drug interactions of these medications, which are commonly used adjuncts in the management of bipolar disorders. A sound knowledge of the information in this and the preceding chapter is necessary to permit clinicians to integrate these data with efficacy spectra described elsewhere in this volume in efforts to provide safe, effective, state-of-the-art pharmacotherapy for bipolar disorders.

In Chapter 15, "Adjunctive Psychosocial Interventions in the Management of Bipolar Disorders," Culver and Pratchett describe the remarkable recent advances in the application of randomized controlled trials methodology to systematic psychotherapeutic interventions for patients with bipolar disorders. The consistent effects reported in clinical trials suggest that the translation of these techniques to clinical settings described in this chapter should offer providers much-needed effective adjuncts to the pharmacotherapies described elsewhere in this volume.

Conclusion

Bipolar disorders are common, serious, but treatable psychiatric illnesses. Effective management begins with careful assessment and relies on evidence-based interventions to yield optimal outcomes. Emphasis in this volume is placed on translating research data into clinical practice. In this regard, case studies are provided at the end of several chapters to lend clinical immediacy to the content. Finally, appendices offer clinicians straightforward treatment guidelines (Appendix A), quick reference medication facts (Appendix B), and quick reference resources and readings (Appendix C).

References

American Psychiatric Association: Diagnostic and Statistical Manual of Mental Disorders, 4th Edition. Washington, DC, American Psychiatric Association, 1994

American Psychiatric Association: Diagnostic and Statistical Manual of Mental Disorders, 4th Edition, Text Revision. Washington, DC, American Psychiatric Association, 2000

American Psychiatric Association: Practice guideline for the treatment of patients with bipolar disorder (revision). Am J Psychiatry 159:1–50, 2002

Bauer MS, McBride L, Williford WO, et al: Collaborative care for bipolar disorder, part I: intervention and implementation in a randomized effectiveness trial. Psychiatr Serv 57:927–936, 2006a

Bauer MS, McBride L, Williford WO, et al: Collaborative care for bipolar disorder, part II: impact on clinical outcome, function, and costs. Psychiatr Serv 57:937–945, 2006b

Keck PE Jr, McElroy SL: Treatment of bipolar disorder, in The American Psychiatric Publishing Textbook of Psychopharmacology, 3rd Edition. Edited by Schatzberg AF, Nemeroff CB. Washington, DC, American Psychiatric Publishing, 2004, pp 865–883

Rush AJ: Strategies and tactics in the management of maintenance treatment for depressed patients. J Clin Psychiatry 60:21–26, 1999

Simon GE, Ludman EJ, Bauer MS, et al: Long-term effectiveness and cost of a systematic care program for bipolar disorder. Arch Gen Psychiatry 63:500–508, 2006

CHAPTER 2

DSM-IV-TR Diagnosis of Bipolar Disorders

Terence A. Ketter, M.D.

Po W. Wang, M.D.

In the past, manic-depressive illness was considered to be composed of heterogeneous mood disorders distinguished from schizophrenia by an episodic rather than a chronic course and characterized more by episode recurrence than by polarity (Kraepelin 1921). However, with time, more emphasis was placed on polarity and differences rather than similarities between bipolar disorders and (unipolar) depressive disorders. Some authors have seen this development as being unfortunate, reminding us of the important similarities between bipolar disorders and recurrent depressive disorders (Goodwin and Jamison 2007). Indeed, in most instances, patients with bipolar disorders spend far more time struggling with depressive symptoms than with mood elevation symptoms (Judd et al. 2002, 2003).

Nevertheless, important diagnostic and therapeutic differences are seen between bipolar disorders and depressive disorders. DSM-IV-TR emphasizes a clear categorical distinction between bipolar disorders and depressive disorders, in that the former but not the latter entail episodes of mood elevation (American Psychiatric Association 2000). Thus, DSM-IV-TR mood disorders include three distinct clusters, with two based on polarity (depressive disorders and bipolar disorders) and one being a residual group (other mood disorders) (Table 2–1).

TABLE 2–1.   DSM-IV-TR mood disorders

Depressive disorders

296.xx	Major depressive disorder
300.4	Dysthymic disorder
311	Depressive disorder not otherwise specified

Bipolar disorders

296.xx	Bipolar I disorder
296.89	Bipolar II disorder
301.13	Cyclothymic disorder
296.80	Bipolar disorder not otherwise specified

Other mood disorders

293.83	Mood disorder due to…[indicate the general medical condition]
29x.xx	Substance-induced mood disorder
296.90	Mood disorder not otherwise specified

DSM-IV-TR Mood Episode or State Nosology

DSM-IV-TR builds its mood disorder nosology by first specifying different types of mood episodes, which include syndromal manic, hypomanic, depressive, and mixed episodes. In addition, DSM-IV-TR provides specifiers of episode severity and psychosis and additional episode features. DSM-IV-TR uses specifiers of episode remission to denote additional (nonsyndromal) mood states characterized by varying degrees of remission of mood symptoms.

DSM-IV-TR Manic and Hypomanic Episodes

Manic episodes are characterized by the presence of significant euphoria, expansiveness, or irritability accompanied by at least three (four, if the mood is only irritable) additional symptoms for at least 1 week (or a briefer time if resulting in hospitalization) (Table 2–2). These additional symptoms include inflated self-esteem, decreased need for sleep, overtalkativeness, flight of ideas, distractibility (overly rapid shifting of focus), excessive goal-directed activity or psychomotor agitation, and impulsivity. Manic episodes are by definition severe, entailing psychosis, hospitalization, or severe impairment of occupational or psychosocial function. *Hypomanic episodes* are defined similarly to manic episodes, with the important difference that they are not severe; that is, they do not entail psychosis, hospitalization, or severe impairment (Table 2–3). Indeed, function may be enhanced. In addition, the minimum duration for hypomanic compared with manic episodes is briefer: 4, rather than 7, days. Criteria for both manic and hypomanic episodes require that symptoms be primary (due to a mood disorder) rather than secondary (due to effects of substances or general medical conditions) and stipulate that manic- and hypomanic-like episodes caused by somatic antidepressant treatments do not count toward a diagnosis of bipolar I disorder or bipolar II disorder, respectively.

DSM-IV-TR Major Depressive Episodes

Major depressive episodes are characterized by the presence of sadness or anhedonia (absence of positive emotion) accompanied by additional symptoms to yield a total of at least five pervasive (most of the day, nearly every day) symptoms for at least 2 weeks (Table 2–4). Curiously, in children and adolescents, the mood may be irritable, creating overlap with the criteria for mood elevation episodes. The specific additional symptoms include poor concentration (inability to focus), loss of energy, poor self-esteem or guilt, suicidality, sleep disturbance, weight change, and psychomotor disturbance. The latter three problems are heterogeneous, including increased or decreased sleep, increased or decreased weight, and psychomotor retardation or agitation. For major depressive episodes (as for manic, hypomanic, and mixed episodes), symptoms must be primary (due to a mood disorder) rather than secondary (due to effects of substances or general medical conditions). Also, the symptoms are not better accounted for by bereavement (i.e., after the loss of a loved one), in that they persist for longer than 2 months; or the symptoms are characterized by marked functional impairment, morbid preoccupation with worthlessness, suicidal ideation, psychotic symptoms, or psychomotor retardation. Major depressive episodes have a relatively low severity threshold; the criteria stipulate merely that symptoms must yield clinically significant distress or impairment in psychosocial or occupational function, and no criteria require psychosis or hospitalization. Thus, the degree of impairment and symptom severity in major depressive episodes can vary considerably (ranging from mild to moderate to marked). Hence major depressive episodes may be associated with psychosis, hospitalization, or marked impairment (as is required for manic and mixed episodes) or may not be associated with such phenomena (as is required for hypomanic episodes).

The criteria for major depressive episodes are identical for patients with bipolar disorders and patients with depressive disorders. However, some data suggest tendencies toward differential profiles of depressive symptoms in bipolar disorders as compared with depressive disorders.

TABLE 2–2.   DSM-IV-TR criteria for manic episode

A.   A distinct period of *abnormally and* persistently elevated, expansive, or irritable mood, lasting *at least 1 week (or any duration if hospitalization is necessary).*

B.   During the period of mood disturbance, three (or more) of the following symptoms have persisted (four if the mood is only irritable) and have been present to a significant degree:

(1)   inflated self-esteem or grandiosity

(2)   decreased need for sleep (e.g., feels rested after only 3 hours of sleep)

(3)   more talkative than usual or pressure to keep talking

(4)   flight of ideas or subjective experience that thoughts are racing

(5)   distractibility (i.e., attention too easily drawn to unimportant or irrelevant external stimuli)

(6)   increase in goal-directed activity (either socially, at work or school, or sexually) or psychomotor agitation

(7)   excessive involvement in pleasurable activities that have a high potential for painful consequences (e.g., engaging in unrestrained buying sprees, sexual indiscretions, or foolish business investments)

C.   *The symptoms do not meet criteria for a mixed episode (see Table 2–5).*

D.   *The mood disturbance is sufficiently severe to cause marked impairment in occupational functioning or in usual social activities or relationships with others, or to necessitate hospitalization to prevent harm to self or others, or there are psychotic features.*

E.   The symptoms are not due to the direct physiological effects of a substance (e.g., a drug of abuse, a medication, or other treatment) or a general medical condition (e.g., hyperthyroidism).

Note: Manic-like episodes that are clearly caused by somatic antidepressant treatment (e.g., medication, electroconvulsive therapy, light therapy) should not count toward a diagnosis of bipolar I disorder.

Note.   Text set in boldface and italic type indicates a difference from criteria for a hypomanic episode.
Source.   Modified from American Psychiatric Association: *Diagnostic and Statistical Manual of Mental Disorders,* 4th Edition, Text Revision. Washington, DC, American Psychiatric Association, 2000, p. 362. Used with permission.

DSM-IV-TR Mixed Episodes

Mixed episodes in DSM-IV-TR are characterized by meeting criteria for both a manic episode and a major depressive episode for at least 1 week (Table 2–5). Like manic episodes, mixed episodes are by definition severe (entailing psychosis, hospitalization, or severe impairment of occupational or psychosocial function) and occur in bipolar I disorder and not in bipolar II disorder. For mixed epi-

TABLE 2–3. DSM-IV-TR criteria for hypomanic episode

A. A distinct period of persistently elevated, expansive, or irritable mood, lasting *throughout at least 4 days, that is clearly different from the usual nondepressed mood.*

B. During the period of mood disturbance, three (or more) of the following symptoms have persisted (four if the mood is only irritable) and have been present to a significant degree:

   (1) inflated self-esteem or grandiosity

   (2) decreased need for sleep (e.g., feels rested after only 3 hours of sleep)

   (3) more talkative than usual or pressure to keep talking

   (4) flight of ideas or subjective experience that thoughts are racing

   (5) distractibility (i.e., attention too easily drawn to unimportant or irrelevant external stimuli)

   (6) increase in goal-directed activity (either socially, at work or school, or sexually) or psychomotor agitation

   (7) excessive involvement in pleasurable activities that have a high potential for painful consequences (e.g., the person engages in unrestrained buying sprees, sexual indiscretions, or foolish business investments)

C. *The episode is associated with an unequivocal change in functioning that is uncharacteristic of the person when not symptomatic.*

D. *The disturbance in mood and the change in functioning are observable by others.*

E. *The episode is not severe enough to cause marked impairment in social or occupational functioning, or to necessitate hospitalization, and there are no psychotic features.*

F. The symptoms are not due to the direct physiological effects of a substance (e.g., a drug of abuse, a medication, or other treatment) or a general medical condition (e.g., hyperthyroidism).

   Note: Hypomanic-like episodes that are clearly caused by somatic antidepressant treatment (e.g., medication, electroconvulsive therapy, light therapy) should not count toward a diagnosis of bipolar II disorder.

Note. Text set in boldface and italic type indicates a difference from criteria for a manic episode.
Source. Modified from American Psychiatric Association: *Diagnostic and Statistical Manual of Mental Disorders,* 4th Edition, Text Revision. Washington, DC, American Psychiatric Association, 2000, p. 368. Used with permission.

sodes (as for manic and hypomanic episodes), symptoms must be primary (due to a mood disorder) rather than secondary (due to effects of substances or general medical conditions), and the criteria specify that mixed-like episodes caused by somatic antidepressant treatments should not count toward a diagnosis of bipolar I disorder.

TABLE 2–4. DSM-IV-TR criteria for major depressive episode

A. Five (or more) of the following symptoms have been present during the same 2-week period and represent a change from previous functioning; at least one of the symptoms is either (1) depressed mood or (2) loss of interest or pleasure.

  Note: Do not include symptoms that are clearly due to a general medical condition, or mood-incongruent delusions or hallucinations.

  (1) depressed mood most of the day, nearly every day, as indicated by either subjective report (e.g., feels sad or empty) or observation made by others (e.g., appears tearful). **Note:** In children and adolescents, can be irritable mood.

  (2) markedly diminished interest or pleasure in all, or almost all, activities most of the day, nearly every day (as indicated by either subjective account or observation made by others)

  (3) significant weight loss when not dieting or weight gain (e.g., a change of more than 5% of body weight in a month), or decrease or increase in appetite nearly every day. **Note:** In children, consider failure to make expected weight gains.

  (4) insomnia or hypersomnia nearly every day

  (5) psychomotor agitation or retardation nearly every day (observable by others, not merely subjective feelings of restlessness or being slowed down)

  (6) fatigue or loss of energy nearly every day

  (7) feelings of worthlessness or excessive or inappropriate guilt (which may be delusional) nearly every day (not merely self-reproach or guilt about being sick)

  (8) diminished ability to think or concentrate, or indecisiveness, nearly every day (either by subjective account or as observed by others)

  (9) recurrent thoughts of death (not just fear of dying), recurrent suicidal ideation without a specific plan, or a suicide attempt or a specific plan for committing suicide

B. The symptoms do not meet criteria for a mixed episode (see Table 2–5).

C. The symptoms cause clinically significant distress or impairment in social, occupational, or other important areas of functioning.

D. The symptoms are not due to the direct physiological effects of a substance (e.g., a drug of abuse, a medication) or a general medical condition (e.g., hypothyroidism).

E. The symptoms are not better accounted for by bereavement, i.e., after the loss of a loved one, the symptoms persist for longer than 2 months or are characterized by marked functional impairment, morbid preoccupation with worthlessness, suicidal ideation, psychotic symptoms, or psychomotor retardation.

Source.   Reprinted from American Psychiatric Association: *Diagnostic and Statistical Manual of Mental Disorders,* 4th Edition, Text Revision. Washington, DC, American Psychiatric Association, 2000, p. 356. Used with permission.

TABLE 2–5.   DSM-IV-TR criteria for mixed episode

A.   The criteria are met both for a manic episode (see Table 2–2) and for a major depressive episode (see Table 2–4) (except for duration) nearly every day during at least a 1-week period.

B.   The mood disturbance is sufficiently severe to cause marked impairment in occupational functioning or in usual social activities or relationships with others, or to necessitate hospitalization to prevent harm to self or others, or there are psychotic features.

C.   The symptoms are not due to the direct physiological effects of a substance (e.g., a drug of abuse, a medication, or other treatment) or a general medical condition (e.g., hyperthyroidism).

Note: Mixed-like episodes that are clearly caused by somatic antidepressant treatment (e.g., medication, electroconvulsive therapy, light therapy) should not count toward a diagnosis of bipolar I disorder.

Source.   Reprinted from American Psychiatric Association: *Diagnostic and Statistical Manual of Mental Disorders,* 4th Edition, Text Revision. Washington, DC, American Psychiatric Association, 2000, p. 365. Used with permission.

The criteria for manic episode and major depressive episode specify that symptoms do not meet criteria for a mixed episode, reflecting the need to diagnose a mixed episode rather than simultaneously diagnose a manic episode and a major depressive episode. This approach suggests that a mixed episode represents a unique syndrome. However, mixed episodes also could be thought to represent other constructs, including 1) a combined syndrome, 2) ultra-ultra rapid cycling, 3) a transitional state, and 4) particularly severe mania (McElroy et al. 1992). Thus, consistent with construct 1, in some patients, mixed episodes may be characterized by simultaneous ("overlapping") depressive and manic symptoms. However, consistent with construct 2, in other patients, mixed episodes may be characterized by ultradian (within a day) cycling, with depressive symptoms most of the time (commonly earlier in the day) but also with manic symptoms to a significant degree each day (commonly later in the day). Thus, patients can experience different symptoms at different times of day. In occasional patients, consistent with construct 3, mixed episodes may predominantly arise during transitions between mood states (often during the switch from a manic episode to a major depressive episode). Finally, consistent with construct 4, in some patients, manic episodes may escalate in severity into mixed episodes.

Dysphoric Manic and Dysphoric Hypomanic Episodes (Non-DSM-IV-TR)

Clinicians frequently encounter patients with manic episodes or hypomanic episodes who are experiencing concurrent depressive symptoms that fall short of meeting criteria for a major depressive episode. Although DSM-IV-TR lacks terminology for such states, a substantial body of clinically relevant literature on this issue is available. Thus, the non-DSM-IV-TR terms *dysphoric mania* and *dysphoric hypomania* are found in the literature, and operational criteria for these states have been proposed (McElroy et al. 1992). Dysphoric mania or dysphoric hypomania requires a full manic episode or hypomanic episode accompanied by "nonoverlapping" depressive symptoms (Table 2–6). At least three such symptoms are required for a definite diagnosis.

DSM-IV-TR Clinical Status (Severity, Psychosis) Specifiers for Current or Most Recent Episode

For patients with bipolar I disorder, bipolar II disorder, or major depressive disorder, DSM-IV-TR also provides clinical status specifiers of severity and psychosis for current (or most recent) manic, mixed, and major depressive (but not hypomanic) episodes. For bipolar I disorder and major depressive disorder, these specifiers are recorded in the diagnostic code fifth digit; a value of 0 indi-

TABLE 2–6.   Dysphoric mania or hypomania (non-DSM-IV-TR)

"Nonoverlapping" depressive symptoms (included for dysphoric mania or hypomania)	"Overlapping" depressive symptoms (excluded for dysphoric mania or hypomania)
Increased appetite and weight	Decreased appetite and weight
Hypersomnia	Insomnia
Psychomotor retardation	Psychomotor agitation
Helplessness or hopelessness[a]	Poor concentration
Depressed mood	
Anhedonia	
Fatigue	
Worthlessness or guilt	
Suicidality	

Note.   Definite=three "nonoverlapping" symptoms; probable=two "nonoverlapping" symptoms; possible=one "nonoverlapping" symptom.
[a]Not a DSM-IV-TR depressive symptom.
Source.   Adapted from McElroy et al. 1992.

cates *unspecified* (Table 2–7). *Mild* episodes (diagnostic code fifth digit 1) entail few, if any, symptoms in excess of those required to make the diagnosis; for major depressive episodes, only minor occupational or psychosocial impairment occurs. In contrast, severe major depressive episodes entail several symptoms in excess of those required to make the diagnosis and marked occupational or psychosocial impairment, whereas severe manic episodes or mixed episodes require almost continual supervision to prevent physical harm to oneself or others. *Moderate* episodes (diagnostic code fifth digit 2) entail symptoms or functional impairment intermediate between that seen in mild and severe episodes. Severe episodes lacking and those having delusions or hallucinations are further subclassified as *severe without psychotic features* (diagnostic code fifth digit 3) and *severe with psychotic features* (diagnostic code fifth digit 4), respectively. Severe episodes with psychotic features are subclassified according to content (but all have the diagnostic code fifth digit 4). *Mood-congruent psychotic features* have content consistent with typical manic (inflated worth, power, knowledge, identity, or special relationship to a deity or famous person) or depressive (personal inadequacy, guilt, disease, death, nihilism, or deserved punishment) themes. *Mood-incongruent psychotic features* lack such themes and include symptoms such as persecutory delusions (not directly related to depressive or manic themes), thought insertion, thought broadcasting, and delusions of control. As described in the following subsection, the fifth-digit codes are also used to indicate degree of remission of symptoms for patients who are not currently experiencing syndromal mood episodes.

TABLE 2–7. DSM-IV-TR clinical status (severity/psychosis/remission) specifiers for current (or most recent) mood episodes (with fifth-digit codes for bipolar I disorder and major depressive disorder)

.x1—Mild

.x2—Moderate

.x3—Severe without psychotic features

.x4—Severe with psychotic features (mood-congruent psychotic features, mood-incongruent psychotic features)

.x5—In partial remission

.x6—In full remission

.x0—Unspecified

Note. Criteria for specifiers vary with episode types as described in the text.

Source. Adapted from American Psychiatric Association: *Diagnostic and Statistical Manual of Mental Disorders,* 4th Edition, Text Revision. Washington, DC, American Psychiatric Association, 2000. Used with permission.

The DSM-IV-TR episode severity or psychosis schema has some limitations worth noting. Understandably, major depressive episodes with psychosis or marked psychosocial or occupational impairment are considered severe. Curiously, despite a requirement of psychosis, hospitalization, or marked psychosocial or occupational impairment for manic episodes or mixed episodes, the DSM-IV-TR schema permits some such episodes to be considered mild or moderate, reserving the severe specifier for episodes requiring almost continual supervision (e.g., hospitalization) to prevent physical harm to self or others. Thus, in the DSM-IV-TR schema, manic episodes and mixed episodes compared with major depressive episodes are graded with different severity scales. For patients with bipolar I disorder, there is a provision for coding hypomanic episodes (diagnostic code 296.40), which commonly (but not always) escalate into full manic episodes or mixed episodes. Unfortunately, this provision is ambiguous because 296.40 also could be construed to represent bipolar I disorder, manic episode, with unspecified severity.

The DSM-IV-TR episode schema in patients with bipolar II disorder does not provide severity specifiers or fifth-digit diagnostic codes for hypomanic episodes or fifth-digit diagnostic codes for major depressive episodes because the diagnostic code fifth digit is already assigned (bipolar II disorder has code 296.89). Thus, in patients with bipolar II disorder and a current or recent major depressive episode, severity, psychosis, and remission specifiers may be applied, but fifth-digit codes cannot be used. An additional limitation for bipolar II disorder patients is the inability to code even the polarity of the current (or most recent) episode because the diagnostic code fourth digit is also already assigned.

DSM-IV-TR Clinical Status (Remission) Specifiers for Current or Most Recent Episode

DSM-IV-TR rounds out its mood episode or state nosology by specifying additional mood states that do not meet criteria for syndromal manic, hypomanic, mixed, or major depressive episodes. These states are incorporated, for patients with bipolar I disorder, into the specifiers of degree of remission for current (or most recent) manic, mixed, and major depressive episodes that are recorded in the diagnostic code fifth digit. Thus, patients with bipolar I disorder in whom symptoms of a mood episode are present but full criteria are not met or who have a period without any significant symptoms of a mood episode lasting less than 2 months following the end of the mood episode are considered to be *in partial remission* (diagnostic code fifth digit 5). In contrast, patients with bipolar I disorder in whom during the past 2 months no significant signs or symptoms of mood disturbance were present are considered to be *in full remission* (diagnostic code fifth digit 6). In patients with bipolar II disorder, with a recent major depressive episode (but not a recent hypomanic episode), the in partial remission or in full remission specifier may be applied, but again, no coding provision exists because the fifth digit is not available.

DSM-IV-TR Current or Most Recent Episode Features Specifiers

DSM-IV-TR provides specifiers describing features of the current or most recent episode. The specifier *with catatonic features* may be applied to major depressive episodes, manic episodes, or mixed episodes dominated by at least two of the following: 1) motoric immobility; 2) excessive motor activity; 3) extreme negativism or mutism; 4) bizarre posturing, stereotypy, mannerisms, or grimacing; or 5) echolalia or echopraxia.

The specifier *with melancholic features* may be applied to major depressive episodes with predominant anhedonia accompanied by at least three of the following: 1) distinct quality of depressed mood; 2) depression regularly worse in the morning; 3) early-morning awakening; 4) marked psychomotor disturbance; 5) significant anorexia or weight loss; or 6) excessive guilt.

The specifier *with atypical features* may be applied to major depressive episodes with predominant mood reactivity accompanied by at least two of the following: 1) significant weight gain or increased appetite, 2) hypersomnia, 3) heavy, leaden feelings in arms or legs, or 4) chronic interpersonal rejection sensitivity. For major depressive episodes with atypical features, an additional requirement is that criteria not be met for with melancholic features or with catatonic features during the same episode because these take precedence over with atypical features.

The specifier *chronic* may be applied to major depressive episodes that have lasted 2 years.

The specifier *with postpartum onset* may be applied to major depressive episodes, manic episodes, mixed episodes, or bipolar II disorder with onset within 4 weeks postpartum.

Beyond the DSM-IV-TR Mood Episode or State Nosology

Although DSM-IV-TR includes four types of mood episodes (manic, hypomanic, mixed, and major depressive) and two additional mood states (in full remission, in partial remission), these do not specify all possible combinations of varying levels and durations of symptoms of mood elevation and depression.

Episodes meeting criteria for mania that are either free of or accompanied by subsyndromal depressive symptoms, although identically classified as manic episodes in DSM-IV-TR, are termed *pure mania* and *dysphoric mania*, respectively, by some authors. Similarly, DSM-IV-TR does not distinguish between episodes meeting criteria for hypomania that are either free of or accompanied by subsyndromal depressive symptoms. In addition, episodes characterized by meeting criteria for both hypomanic episode and major depressive episode are not specified in DSM-IV-TR, which does not prohibit simultaneously diagnosing hypomanic episode and major depressive episode. Some authors advocate the use of the term *dysphoric hypomania* for such episodes. Episodes meeting criteria for major depression that are either free of or accompanied by subsyndromal mood elevation symptoms, although identically classified as major depressive episodes in DSM-IV-TR, are termed *pure depression* and *mixed depression*, respectively, by some authors. The most useful approach for episodes meeting criteria for major depression that also include subsyndromal mood elevation symptoms is the subject of spirited controversy. Such states could arguably be considered to be either within the bipolar spectrum or merely agitated (unipolar) major depression.

Patients in mood states characterized by subsyndromal levels of mood elevation and/or depression are considered to be in partial remission in DSM-IV-TR, but depending on the symptoms present, such mood states could be further subclassified as subsyndromal hypomania, subsyndromal depression, or subsyndromal mixed episode. In addition, in such instances, there may be merit in specifying whether the most recent mood state was a syndromal mood episode or sustained wellness. Thus, in the Systematic Treatment Enhancement Program for Bipolar Disorder (STEP-BD), subsyndromal symptoms following syndromal mood episodes and following sustained wellness were termed *continued symptoms* and *roughening*, respectively.

In DSM-IV-TR, patients lacking significant signs or symptoms of mood disturbance for at least 2 months are considered to be in full remission and tend to be at lower risk for reemergence of mood symptoms than are patients with less-sustained wellness, who are considered to be in partial remission. DSM-IV-TR fails to distinguish the latter from patients with subsyndromal symptoms.

DSM-IV-TR Mood Disorder Nosology

DSM-IV-TR mood disorders include three distinct clusters, with two based on polarity (bipolar disorders and depressive disorders) and one a residual group (other mood disorders). DSM-IV-TR constructs its nosology for bipolar disorders and depressive disorders by specifying conditions according to the presence or absence of different types of mood episodes.

DSM-IV-TR Bipolar Disorders

Patients with bipolar I disorder have experienced at least one manic episode or mixed episode (Table 2–8). Although the vast majority of patients with bipolar I disorder also have major depressive episodes, such episodes are not required for the diagnosis of bipolar I disorder. Although only a limited (up to 10%) proportion of patients with bipolar I disorder experience a single manic episode (with no other manic, mixed, or major depressive episodes), DSM-IV-TR includes this as a specific subtype (bipolar I disorder, single manic episode), with diagnostic code 296.0x. For the vast majority of patients with bipolar I disorder whose illness is characterized by recurrent episodes, DSM-IV-TR provides diagnoses (and diagnostic codes) according to whether the current or most recent episode is or was hypomanic (296.40), manic (296.4x), major depressive (296.5x), mixed (296.6x), or unspecified (296.7). Patients with bipolar II disorder (296.89) have experienced at least one hypomanic episode and at least one major depressive episode but no manic or mixed episode. For patients with bipolar II disorder, DSM-IV-TR notes that the most recent episode type can be specified, but the same diagnostic code (296.89) is used regardless of whether the most recent episode was hypomanic or major depressive.

Cyclothymic disorder (301.13) is a chronic disorder with a duration of at least 2 years (1 year for children and adolescents) without a 2-month interruption, and a pattern of subsyndromal mood elevation and depressive symptoms. No major depressive episode, manic episode, or mixed episode is permitted during the first 2 years of the disturbance (1 year for children and adolescents); cyclothymic disorder is not diagnosed if any of these episodes occur during this time because the chronic subsyndromal mood swings may be considered to be residual symptoms of bipolar I or II disorder. However, "after the initial 2 years (1 year in children and adolescents) of cyclothymic disorder, there may be superimposed manic or mixed episodes (in which case both bipolar I disorder and cyclothymic disorder may be diagnosed) or major depressive episodes (in which case both bipolar II disorder and cyclothymic disorder may be diagnosed)"

TABLE 2–8. DSM-IV-TR bipolar disorders and coding conventions

Code	Diagnosis	Current (or recent) episode	Prior manic or mixed episode(s)	Prior major depressive episode(s)	Prior hypomanic episode(s)
296.0x	Bipolar I disorder, single manic episode	Manic or mixed	1[a]	0	—
296.40	Bipolar I disorder, most recent episode hypomanic	Hypomanic	≥1	—	—
296.4x	Bipolar I disorder, most recent episode manic	Manic	≥1	—	—
296.5x	Bipolar I disorder, most recent episode depressed	Major depressive	≥1	—	—
296.6x	Bipolar I disorder, most recent episode mixed	Mixed	≥1	—	—
296.7	Bipolar I disorder, most recent episode unspecified	Subsyndromal by duration; manic, hypomanic, mixed, or major depressive	≥1	—	—
296.80	Bipolar disorder not otherwise specified	—	—	—	—
296.89	Bipolar II disorder	Hypomanic or major depressive	0	≥1[a]	≥1[a]
301.13	Cyclothymic disorder	—	0 in first 2 years	0 in first 2 years	0 in first 2 years

Note. —=not specified.
[a]Including current episode.

(American Psychiatric Association 2000, p. 400). Such instances might be considered as cyclothymic disorders that have progressed to situations in which syndromal mood episodes occur in addition to baseline chronic subsyndromal mood instability. Cyclothymic disorder may be considered to be a bipolar analogue of unipolar dysthymic disorder, with each of these representing affective temperaments that may or may not ultimately yield disorders that include syndromal mood episodes.

Patients with bipolar disorder not otherwise specified (296.80) experience significant symptoms of mood elevation, but these are insufficient to meet criteria for a specific bipolar disorder. Examples of such conditions cited in DSM-IV-TR are provided in Table 2–9.

DSM-IV-TR Depressive Disorders

Although not the focus of this volume, for comparison and completeness, a similar schema for the DSM-IV-TR depressive disorders is presented in Table 2–10. A substantial (up to 50%) proportion of patients with major depressive disorder experience only a single major depressive episode (with no manic, hypomanic, mixed, or other major depressive episodes), and DSM-IV-TR thus includes this as a specific subtype (major depressive disorder, single episode), with diagnostic code 296.2x. For the other approximately 50% of patients with major depressive disorder, whose illness is characterized by recurrent major depressive episodes, DSM-IV-TR provides the diagnosis major depressive disorder, recurrent (296.3x). Some authors consider highly recurrent forms of major depressive disorder to be related to bipolar disorders. Dysthymic disorder (300.4), as noted earlier, may be considered the depressive disorder analogue of cyclothymic disorder. Depressive disorder not otherwise specified (311) includes a wide variety of disorders with depressive features that do not meet criteria for other specific disor-

TABLE 2–9. Examples of bipolar disorder not otherwise specified

1. Very rapid alternation between subsyndromal by duration manic symptoms and depressive symptoms
2. Recurrent hypomanic episodes without intercurrent depressive symptoms
3. A manic episode or mixed episode superimposed on delusional disorder, residual schizophrenia, or psychotic disorder not otherwise specified
4. Hypomanic episodes, alternating with chronic depressive symptoms, that are too infrequent to qualify for cyclothymic disorder
5. Situations in which a bipolar disorder is present but it is unclear whether the disorder is primary or due to a general medical condition or substance use

TABLE 2–10. DSM-IV-TR depressive disorders and coding conventions

Code	Diagnosis	Current (or recent) episode	Prior manic or mixed episode(s)	Prior major depressive episode(s)	Prior hypomanic episode(s)
296.2x	Major depressive disorder, single episode	—	0	1	0
296.3x	Major depressive disorder, recurrent	—	0	≥2	0
300.4	Dysthymic disorder	—	0	0 in first 2 years	0
311	Depressive disorder not otherwise specified	—	—	—	—

Note. —=not specified.

ders such as major depressive disorder, dysthymic disorder, adjustment disorder with depressed mood, or adjustment disorder with mixed anxiety and depressed mood.

DSM-IV-TR Specifiers for Course of Recurrent Episodes

For recurrent major depressive disorder, bipolar I disorder, and bipolar II disorder, the course of recurrent episode specifiers *with full interepisode recovery* and *without full interepisode recovery* can be applied if full remission is or is not attained between the two most recent mood episodes, respectively. The specifier *with seasonal pattern* can be applied to these disorders if there is a pattern of major depressive episodes with the following criteria: 1) a regular temporal relationship between the onset and a particular time of the year (e.g., in fall or winter); 2) full remissions or changes from depression to mania or hypomania also at a particular time of the year (e.g., spring); 3) two major depressive episodes in the last 2 years with the seasonal relationships defined in the first two criteria and no nonseasonal major depressive episodes; and 4) substantially higher number of lifetime seasonal compared with nonseasonal major depressive episodes.

For recurrent bipolar I disorder and bipolar II disorder, the specifier *with rapid cycling* can be applied if at least four syndromal major depressive, manic, mixed, or hypomanic episodes have occurred in the previous 12 months. Such episodes are demarcated by either partial or full remission for at least 2 months or a switch to an episode of opposite polarity.

Other DSM-IV-TR Mood Disorders

The cluster of other mood disorders in DSM-IV-TR is a heterogeneous group that includes mood disorders that are secondary to (i.e., direct physiological consequences of) general medical conditions or substances. These conditions are in contrast to bipolar disorders and depressive disorders, which are primary in that they are not the direct consequences of general medical conditions or substances. Secondary mood disorders are more common in patients with mixed features, patients with frequent episodes, and the elderly (the latter two are discussed in this volume by Ketter and Wang in Chapter 9, "Management of Rapid-Cycling Bipolar Disorders," and by Brooks and colleagues in Chapter 12, "Management of Bipolar Disorders in Older Adults"). This cluster also includes the broad residual category mood disorder not otherwise specified.

Mood disorder due to a general medical condition (293.83) includes diverse conditions with prominent and persistent depressive (depression or anhedonia) and/or mood elevation (euphoria, expansiveness, or irritability) symptoms that are suggested by history, physical examination, or laboratory evidence to be direct physiological consequences of general medical conditions. A list of selected endocrine, infectious, and neurological conditions implicated in causing such problems is provided in Table 2–11. The mood disturbance must cause significant distress or psychosocial or occupational impairment and is not better accounted for by other primary mental disorders or delirium. These disorders may be further specified as being *with depressive features* (predominant subsyndromal depression), *with major depressive–like episode* (predominant syndromal depression), *with manic features* (predominant euphoria, expansiveness, or irritability), or *with mixed features* (manic and depressive symptoms, with neither predominating).

Substance-induced mood disorder (29x.xx) includes diverse conditions with prominent and persistent depressive (depression or anhedonia) and/or mood elevation (euphoria, expansiveness, or irritability) symptoms that by historical, physical examination, or laboratory evidence appear to have developed during, or within a month of, substance intoxication or withdrawal or to be etiologically related to medication use. A list of selected substances and treatments implicated in causing such problems is provided in Table 2–12. The mood disturbance must cause significant distress or psychosocial or occupational impairment and is not better accounted for by other primary mental disorders or delirium. These disorders may be further specified as being *with depressive features* (predominant depression), *with manic features* (predominant euphoria, expansiveness, or irritability), or *with mixed features* (manic and depressive symptoms, with neither predominating). DSM-IV-TR provides codes for mood disorders induced by alcohol (291.89) and other substances (292.84), with the latter including amphetamines (or amphetamine-like substances); cocaine; hallucinogens; inhalants; opioids; phencyclidine (or phencyclidine-like substances); sedatives, hypnotics, or anxiolytics; and other (or unknown) substances.

TABLE 2–11. Selected general medical conditions associated with secondary mood disorders

Endocrine—hypercortisolism (Cushing's disease/syndrome), hypocortisolism (Addison's disease), hyperthyroidism, hypothyroidism

Infectious—acquired immunodeficiency syndrome (AIDS), human immunodeficiency virus (HIV) infection, infectious mononucleosis, influenza, tertiary syphilis (general paresis), toxoplasmosis, viral hepatitis

Neurological—cerebral trauma, cerebral tumor, cerebrovascular infarction, dementia, epilepsy, multiple sclerosis, Parkinson's disease

TABLE 2–12. Selected substances and treatments associated with secondary mood disorders

Substances

Alcohol

Illicit substances—amphetamines, cocaine, hallucinogens, inhalants, opioids, phencyclidine (PCP)

Psychiatric treatments

Anxiolytics, sedative-hypnotics—barbiturates, benzodiazepines

Antidepressants—SNRIs, SSRIs, MAOIs, tricyclics

Stimulants—methylphenidate

Typical antipsychotics—haloperidol

Other somatic therapies—electroconvulsive therapy, light therapy

General medications

Analgesics—indomethacin, opiates

Anti-infectives—interferon, isoniazid, zidovudine

Antineoplastics—vincristine, vinblastine

Cardiac—hydralazine, propranolol, reserpine

Endocrine—corticosteroids, hormonal contraceptives

Neurological—anticholinergics, baclofen, levodopa

Note. MAOI=monoamine oxidase inhibitor; SNRI=serotonin-norepinephrine reuptake inhibitor; SSRI=selective serotonin reuptake inhibitor.

The final residual category of mood disorder not otherwise specified (296.90) includes disorders with mood symptoms that do not meet criteria for any specific mood disorder and in which it is difficult to choose between bipolar disorder not otherwise specified and depressive disorder not otherwise specified (e.g., acute agitation).

DSM-IV-TR Mood Disorders: Case Examples With Schematics

To integrate the previous description of the DSM-IV-TR mood disorder nosology, and show clinical applications, four case examples with schematics are provided. As noted in Chapter 3, "Addressing Clinical Diagnostic Challenges in Bipolar Disorders," in the "Distinguishing Bipolar Disorder Subtypes From One Another" section on prospective longitudinal mood charting, graphic representation of the longitudinal course of bipolar disorders can be a useful tool to

confirm diagnosis prospectively. Such an approach also can have utility in identifying features of the DSM-IV-TR nosology or of individual cases.

The cases and schematics in this section involve selected DSM-IV-TR mood
disorders, with the schematics incorporating the most elementary features of mood
charting. The horizontal axis represents time. The vertical axis represents degree of mood disturbance, with mood elevation and depression above and below the horizontal axis, respectively. The white areas above and black areas below
the horizontal axis represent occurrences of mood elevation and depression
symptoms, respectively. Note that diagnoses are dynamic, changing as episodes
emerge and resolve.

Evolution of Bipolar I Disorder

Figure 2–1 illustrates a case in which an index manic episode is followed by a
major depressive episode, which is followed initially by brief wellness, which ultimately becomes sustained wellness. The most recent episode specifiers and
associated fourth-digit codes and the clinical status of most recent episode specifiers and associated fifth-digit codes change as the illness evolves, with these
names and codes indicating an index manic episode, followed by a major depressive episode, followed by partial remission, which ultimately becomes full
remission.

The sinusoidal waveform (manic episode then major depressive episode) in
this case, which is on occasion referred to as a mania-depression-interval pattern, is considered to be a "classic" presentation for bipolar I disorder and may
even be associated with better responses to lithium. Some individuals have their
major depressive episodes only after manic episodes, suggesting that the former
may even be a consequence of the latter, at least in some instances. Postmania
major depressive episodes compared with prior manic episodes tend to be
longer (perhaps as much as twice as long). In the past, manic episodes were frequently treated with typical antipsychotics, and concerns were periodically raised
that such agents could induce subsequent dysphoria or even major depressive
episodes. However, the mania-depression-interval pattern is sufficiently common (even in the absence of any treatment) that it is challenging to implicate
treatments for manic episodes as causing subsequent major depressive episodes.
Thus, DSM-IV-TR does not even mention the possibility of encountering entities
such as antipsychotic-induced mood disorder with depressive features or lithium-
induced mood disorder with depressive features.

Evolution of Bipolar II Disorder

Figure 2–2 shows a case in which an index major depressive episode is followed
by a hypomanic episode, which is followed initially by brief wellness, which ulti-

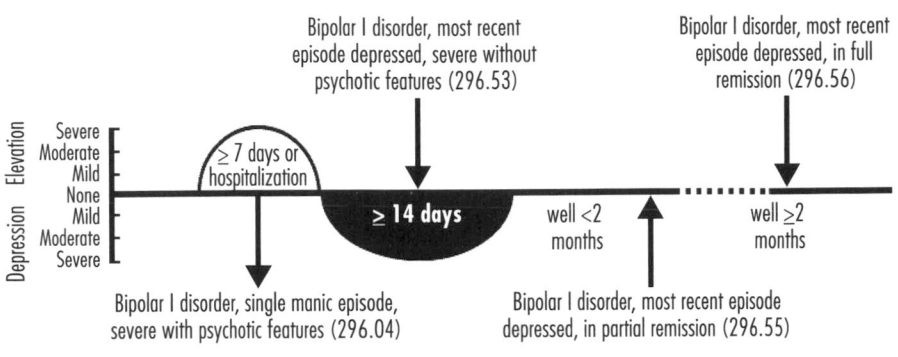

FIGURE 2–1.   Evolution of bipolar I disorder.

mately becomes sustained wellness. This case confirms some of the limitations of the DSM-IV-TR mood disorder nosology because the index major depressive episode is initially interpreted to represent major depressive disorder, only to have the diagnosis change to bipolar II disorder on emergence of the first hypomanic episode. Note that the hypomanic episode and the subsequent brief wellness, as well as the ultimate sustained wellness, all lack clinical status of most recent episode specifiers because these apply only to major depressive episodes. Also note the static bipolar II disorder fourth- and fifth-digit codes. Thus, the names and codes are unchanged (bipolar II disorder, most recent episode hypomanic, 296.89) as the illness further evolves, failing to distinguish a hypomanic episode, brief wellness, and the ultimate sustained wellness. In contrast, had the most recent episode been a major depressive episode, the clinical status of most recent episode specifiers would apply, permitting the names (but not codes) to describe the severity of a major depressive episode and to distinguish it from the initial partial remission, as well as the subsequent full remission.

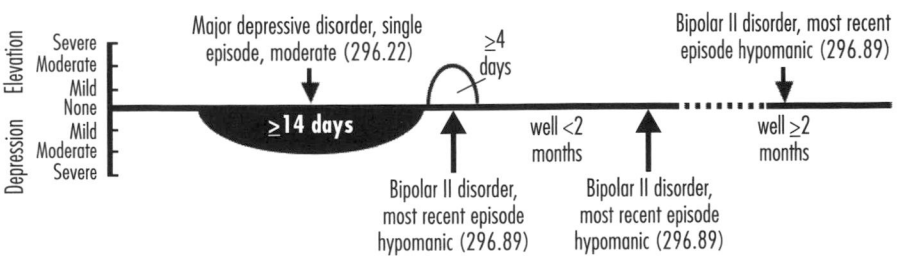

FIGURE 2–2.   Evolution of bipolar II disorder.

Course of Cyclothymic Disorder

Figure 2–3 illustrates a case of cyclothymic disorder, which is characterized by frequent instances of subsyndromal depressive and mood elevation symptoms. Note that the mood disturbance need not be continuous but needs to be present for more than 50% of the time for at least 2 years (1 year in children and adolescents), with any interruption lasting less than 2 months. No major depressive episode, manic episode, or mixed episode is permitted during the first 2 years of the disturbance.

Course of Major Depressive Disorder, Single Episode, and Antidepressant-Induced Mood Disorder With Manic Features

Figure 2–4 shows a case of major depressive disorder, single episode, and antidepressant-induced mood disorder with manic features. As in the second case on the evolution of bipolar II disorder earlier in this chapter, this case indicates some of the limitations of DSM-IV-TR. In this case, an index major depressive episode was ultimately treated with antidepressant medication, and this intervention was soon followed by the emergence of a severe manic-like episode. Note that the index major depressive episode yields a diagnosis of major depressive disorder, single episode, which does change as the subsequent severe manic-like episode is interpreted as induced by antidepressant therapy. The diagnosis of antidepressant-induced mood disorder with manic features permits designation of the polarity but not the severity of the manic-like episode, which must entail prominent and persistent (albeit unspecified duration) euphoria, expansiveness, or irritability but may include the presence or absence of a wide range of additional symptoms of mood elevation with variable severity and duration. Such symptoms may range from mere brief subsyndromal hypomanic-like symptoms that could even yield mildly enhanced function and go unnoticed by the patient to meeting full syndromal criteria for a sustained psychotic manic-like episode resulting in severe psychosocial and occupational impairment and even hospitalization.

By the end of this challenging pair of events, the patient's diagnosis is major depressive disorder, single episode, and antidepressant-induced mood disorder with manic features. There is controversy regarding this rather cumbersome approach to a condition that in many instances may yield later spontaneous (i.e., not antidepressant-induced) manic episodes or hypomanic episodes (and thus a subsequent diagnosis of bipolar I disorder or bipolar II disorder). Thus, some authors prefer non-DSM-IV-TR designators such as "bipolar spectrum disorder" or "bipolar III disorder." This issue is discussed further in the section "Use of Non-DSM-IV-TR Information" in Chapter 3.

The sinusoidal waveform (major depressive episode then manic episode) in this case, which may be referred to as a *depression-mania-interval pattern,* is en-

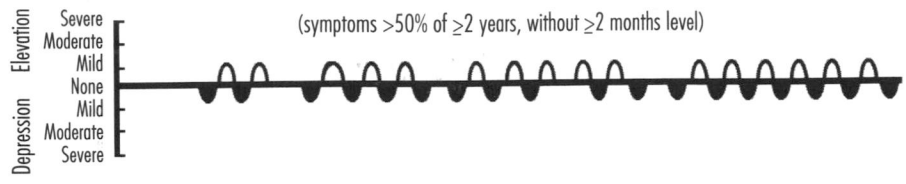

FIGURE 2–3.   Course of cyclothymic disorder (301.13).

countered on occasion in patients with bipolar I disorder and might be associated with poorer responses to lithium. A few individuals have their manic episodes only after major depressive episodes, suggesting that manic episodes may even be a consequence of the major depressive episodes, at least in a few instances. Although the depression-mania-interval pattern may be seen even in the absence of any treatment, this phenomenon appears to be not common enough to have had a substantive effect on the DSM-IV-TR approach to the nosology of manic-like episodes soon after the administration of an antidepressant for a major depressive episode. Hence the diagnosis of the second episode in this case is antidepressant-induced mood disorder with manic features. Had the episode sequence in Figure 2–4 occurred in the absence of any somatic treatment for depression (e.g., with psychotherapeutic treatment or no treatment), the diagnosis would have changed to bipolar I disorder, most recent episode manic.

Conclusion

The DSM-IV-TR mood disorder nosology presented in this chapter has notable strengths and limitations. The latter have contributed occasionally to a spirited controversy regarding the most appropriate approach for clinicians to embrace.

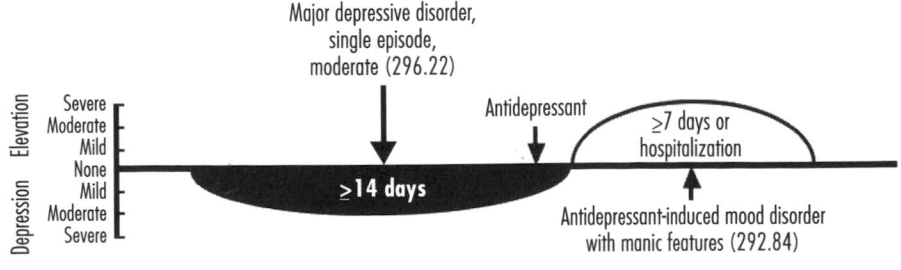

FIGURE 2–4.   Major depressive disorder, single episode, and antidepressant-induced mood disorder with manic features.

Strengths of DSM-IV-TR Mood Disorder Nosology

The DSM-IV-TR mood disorder nosology has the strength of being an established approach that is familiar to major stakeholders such as advocacy groups, clinicians, regulatory agencies, and third-party payers. The categorical nature of the system is amenable to its use in genetic, neurobiological, epidemiological, phenomenological, and therapeutic studies. In particular, this categorical approach can yield reliable diagnoses, which facilitate not only randomized controlled trials of interventions but also similar characterization of patients by those of their providers who are interested in applying the findings of such studies in clinical settings.

Limitations of DSM-IV-TR Mood Disorder Nosology

The DSM-IV-TR mood disorder nosology is substantially limited by being a complex yet not comprehensive system that 1) relies on only a limited subset of mood symptom phenomenology (e.g., a subset of symptoms of mood episodes and limited course of illness information); 2) neglects other important aspects of mood symptom phenomenology and course of illness information (e.g., onset age, patterns of episode onset and offset, comorbidity); 3) neglects treatment effects; 4) neglects family history and genetics; and 5) attempts to distinguish bipolar from unipolar episodes and disorders in a categorical rather than dimensional fashion. An example of one aspect of the first and second points is described earlier in this text, in that the categorical DSM-IV-TR mood episode nosology fails to reflect the rich diversity of combinations of symptoms of mood elevation and depression that are encountered clinically. Other limitations are described in the following paragraphs and can be found in a recently published report of the Task Force for Diagnostic Guidelines of the International Society for Bipolar Disorders (Ghaemi et al. 2008), and methods to begin to address such limitations are described in Chapter 3.

A crucial limitation of the DSM-IV-TR mood disorder nosology is its use of a categorical rather than a dimensional approach or hybrid approach. Bipolar disorder and major depressive disorder have characteristics such as genetics, phenomenology, biology, therapeutic response, and brain imaging findings that suggest both commonalities with and dissociations from each other. Taken together, these characteristics are in some instances more consistent with a dimensional view, with bipolar disorders being on a continuum with depressive disorders, especially for patients with highly recurrent, treatment-resistant forms of the latter (Akiskal and Pinto 1999; Ghaemi et al. 2004) (Table 2–13). Similarly, bipolar disorders may be considered to be on a continuum with psychotic dis-

TABLE 2–13. Diagnostic spectra—a dimensional approach to bipolar disorders

Mood disorders[a,b]

    BPI—BPII—BPNOS—BPIII—MDD

Psychotic disorders[c]

    BPII—BPI—SABT—SPT—SUT

Personality disorders[d]

    BPI—BPII—BPNOS—Borderline

Note. Borderline=borderline personality disorder; BPI=bipolar I disorder; BPII=bipolar II disorder; BPIII (non-DSM)=antidepressant-associated hypomania or mania; BPNOS=bipolar disorder not otherwise specified; MDD=major depressive disorder; SABT=schizoaffective disorder, bipolar type; SPT=schizophrenia, paranoid type; SUT=schizophrenia, undifferentiated type.
[a]Akiskal and Pinto 1999.
[b]Ghaemi et al. 2004.
[c]Ketter et al. 2004.
[d]Akiskal et al. 1985.

orders such as schizoaffective disorder and schizophrenia (Ketter et al. 2004) and personality disorders such as borderline personality disorder (Akiskal et al. 1985) (Table 2–13). Nevertheless, in some instances, a categorical approach still appears useful. Although more research is clearly necessary to address the dimensional versus categorical controversy, it is feasible that at least in the interim, a hybrid dimensional and categorical approach could provide additional insights into pathophysiology and management options, which would not be available if only one of these models were used.

Some patients are particularly focused on obtaining a definitive categorical diagnosis of either bipolar disorder or a depressive disorder and are distressed by any ambiguity. In instances in which the patient's diagnosis appears to be at the boundary of a category, a dimensional approach emphasizing commonalities across categories may prove useful. For example, in patients with frequently recurring major depressive disorder who have subthreshold mood elevation symptoms and antidepressant resistance, intervention with mood stabilizers may yield benefit.

For clinicians, a key challenge is determining when to think categorically, as in DSM-IV-TR, and when to think dimensionally, with a non-DSM-IV-TR approach. We hope that this challenge will be addressed in future schemas such as DSM-V, which is in the planning stage. In the meantime, clinicians are faced with integrating a lively debate regarding this issue. One topical approach emphasizes the importance of temperament and bipolar features when assessing patients with mood disorders and advocates the concept of a broad bipolar spectrum (Akiskal et al. 1989). This approach emphasizes the importance of not only cyclothymic (chronic alternating subsyndromal mood elevation and depressive symptoms) and dysthymic (chronic subsyndromal depressive symptoms) temperaments that are accounted for by cyclothymic disorder and dysthymic disorder, respectively, in DSM-IV-TR but also hyperthymic (chronic subsyndromal mood elevation symptoms) and irritable temperaments as non-DSM-IV-TR components of the mood disorder nosology.

The last three decades have already seen a substantial broadening of the concept of bipolar disorders to include not only classical forms of the disorder, characterized by euphoric mania, infrequent episodes, and excellent lithium responses, but also forms with mixed mania, rapid cycling, and poor responses to lithium. To date, this degree of broadening has appeared useful because mood-stabilizing anticonvulsants (such as divalproex, carbamazepine, and lamotrigine) and atypical antipsychotics (such as olanzapine, risperidone, quetiapine, ziprasidone, and aripiprazole) may have utility in such lithium-resistant, nonclassical forms of bipolar disorders.

However, spirited controversy exists regarding the advisability of further expansion of bipolar disorders to include the broad bipolar spectrum concept. Critics of the bipolar spectrum approach may argue that it entails potential overdiagnosis of bipolar disorder (at the expense of other disorders such as major depressive disorder and borderline personality disorder), leading to overuse of mood stabilizers and underuse of other potentially effective medical and psychotherapeutic interventions.

In Chapter 3, Ketter and Wang describe methods to begin to address diagnostic challenges facing clinicians that may be in part related to the limitations of the DSM-IV-TR mood disorder nosology noted earlier in this chapter.

References

Akiskal HS, Pinto O: The evolving bipolar spectrum: prototypes I, II, III, and IV. Psychiatr Clin North Am 22:517–534, vii, 1999

Akiskal HS, Chen SE, Davis GC, et al: Borderline: an adjective in search of a noun. J Clin Psychiatry 46:41–48, 1985

Akiskal HS, Cassano GB, Musetti L, et al: Psychopathology, temperament, and past course in primary major depressions, 1: review of evidence for a bipolar spectrum. Psychopathology 22:268–277, 1989

American Psychiatric Association: Diagnostic and Statistical Manual of Mental Disorders, 4th Edition, Text Revision. Washington, DC, American Psychiatric Association, 2000

Ghaemi SN, Hsu DJ, Ko JY, et al: Bipolar spectrum disorder: a pilot study. Psychopathology 37:222–226, 2004

Ghaemi SN, Bauer M, Cassidy F, et al: Diagnostic guidelines for bipolar disorder: a summary of the International Society for Bipolar Disorders Diagnostic Guidelines Task Force Report. Bipolar Disord 10:117–128, 2008

Goodwin FR, Jamison K: Manic-Depressive Illness: Bipolar Disorders and Recurrent Depression, 2nd Edition. New York, Oxford University Press, 2007

Judd LL, Akiskal HS, Schettler PJ, et al: The long-term natural history of the weekly symptomatic status of bipolar I disorder. Arch Gen Psychiatry 59:530–537, 2002

Judd LL, Akiskal HS, Schettler PJ, et al: A prospective investigation of the natural history of the long-term weekly symptomatic status of bipolar II disorder. Arch Gen Psychiatry 60:261–269, 2003

Ketter TA, Wang PW, Becker OV, et al: Psychotic bipolar disorders: dimensionally similar to or categorically different from schizophrenia? J Psychiatr Res 38:47–61, 2004

Kraepelin E: Manic-Depressive Insanity and Paranoia. Salem, NH, Ayer Company, 1921

McElroy SL, Keck PE Jr, Pope HG Jr, et al: Clinical and research implications of the diagnosis of dysphoric or mixed mania or hypomania. Am J Psychiatry 149:1633–1644, 1992

Addressing Clinical Diagnostic Challenges in Bipolar Disorders

Terence A. Ketter, M.D.

Po W. Wang, M.D.

The DSM-IV-TR (American Psychiatric Association 2000) approach to the diagnosis of bipolar disorders is complex yet not comprehensive and, along with its noteworthy strengths and limitations, is described in the preceding chapter. We begin this chapter by outlining some important challenges in the clinical diagnosis of bipolar disorders. We then describe methods to begin to address these challenges, initially within the confines of the DSM-IV-TR nosology and subsequently by using additional important information. Although the latter methods are not included in DSM-IV-TR, they are of sufficient validity that they arguably should be integrated into clinical practice to begin to address the important diagnostic challenges faced by clinicians striving to manage patients with bipolar disorders. For example, the recently published summary of the report of the Task Force on Diagnostic Guidelines of the International Society for Bipolar Disorders outlines limitations of the DSM-IV-TR mood disorder nosology and proposes definitions that may lead to enhanced clinical diagnosis (Ghaemi et al. 2008).

Challenges in the Clinical Diagnosis of Bipolar Disorders

The average patient with bipolar disorder may endure as long as a decade of affective symptoms before appropriate diagnosis and treatment (Hirschfeld et al. 2003; Lish et al. 1994). The most common incorrect initial diagnosis is major depressive disorder (Ghaemi et al. 1999, 2000). This unfortunate situation is most likely related to multiple causes, including 1) the complex, variable phenomenology of bipolar disorder, including different subtypes, mood states, and illness courses, as well as age-dependent presentations (e.g., disruptive behavior disorders in youths); 2) the pervasiveness of depressive symptoms, which makes major depressive disorder crucial in the differential diagnosis; and 3) the complex and confounding comorbidities encountered, which include disruptive behavior disorders (attention-deficit/hyperactivity disorder [ADHD], oppositional defiant disorder, conduct disorder), substance use disorders, anxiety disorders, and Cluster B personality disorders.

The diagnosis of bipolar I disorder (compared with bipolar II disorder) may be considered more straightforward because of the requirement that manic episodes or mixed episodes that occur in bipolar I disorder be severe, entailing psychosis, hospitalization, or severe impairment of occupational or psychosocial function. In contrast, hypomanic episodes that occur in bipolar II disorder must *not* be severe; that is, they must *not* entail psychosis, hospitalization, or severe impairment of occupational or psychosocial function. Indeed, function may be enhanced during hypomania, making it more challenging to recognize or distinguish hypomanic episodes from euthymia.

Nevertheless, diagnostic challenges occur in patients with bipolar I disorder because patients (who frequently present during major depressive episodes) may not recall previous manic or mixed episodes or may not be able to distinguish them from major depressive episodes, raising the risk that they may receive an incorrect diagnosis of major depressive disorder. Also, approximately half of the patients with bipolar disorders have an index major depressive episode rather than an index mood elevation episode, initially suggesting a major depressive disorder, only later to have a mood elevation episode that indicates a bipolar disorder (e.g., "Evolution of Bipolar II Disorder" case example in Chapter 2, "DSM-IV-TR Diagnosis of Bipolar Disorders"). In addition, the severity of mood elevation episodes may be inconclusive, making it unclear whether the patient has bipolar I or II disorder. Another challenge is the phenomenon of treatment-emergent affective switch with antidepressant medications, which can yield manic- or mixed-like episodes in patients with bipolar II disorder, bipolar disorder not otherwise specified, major depressive disorder (e.g., "Course of Major Depressive Disorder, Single Episode, and Antidepressant-Induced Mood Disorder With Manic Features" case example in Chapter 2), or even nonaffective illnesses (e.g., anxiety disorders or eating disorders). Although DSM-IV-TR does not permit treatment-emergent affective switch to count toward diagnoses of bipolar disorders, patients with treatment-emergent affective switch are at risk for future spontaneous mood elevation and need to be treated with considerable caution, often in a fashion similar to that for patients with bipolar disorders.

Prominent psychotic symptoms in patients with bipolar I disorder may suggest a diagnosis of schizoaffective disorder or even schizophrenia, particularly early in the illness, when the longitudinal course characteristics (e.g., recurrent vs. chronic) remain to be established. Also, slower resolution of psychotic compared with mood symptoms after intervention with mood stabilizers could lead clinicians to consider a diagnosis of schizoaffective disorder. Despite Kraepelin's formulation categorically differentiating bipolar disorder (then *manic-depressive psychosis*) and schizophrenia (then *dementia praecox*), emerging evidence supports the existence of a continuum between these disorders, with schizoaffective disorder being an intermediate condition, but more research is needed in this area (Ketter et al. 2004).

Comorbid conditions may confound the diagnosis of bipolar disorder. Alcohol and substance (particularly stimulants and cocaine) use disorders, particularly in younger patients, or medical disorders (particularly certain neurological and endocrine disorders), or their treatments (e.g., steroids), particularly in older patients, may cause or exacerbate mood elevation symptoms, making the diagnosis of bipolar disorder more challenging.

Symptoms of other concurrent psychiatric disorders (e.g., anxiety disorders, disruptive behavior disorders, eating disorders, and Cluster B personality disorders) may contribute prominently to complaints of patients and their families at the time of initial presentation to clinicians. This can yield distractions that delay the diagnosis of a bipolar disorder.

Patients with early-onset mood disorders can present considerable diagnostic challenges. Almost half of prepubertal patients with major depressive episodes may ultimately receive a bipolar disorder diagnosis (Geller et al. 2001). Moreover, approximately 40% of patients with severe major depressive episodes in adolescence or emerging adulthood (ages 18–25 years) ultimately receive a bipolar disorder diagnosis (Goldberg et al. 2001).

Pediatric patients may present with disruptive behavior disorders that may have considerable symptom overlap with bipolar disorder. In such instances, the presence of a family history of bipolar disorder (particularly in a parent) may provide an important indicator of risk for a bipolar outcome (Chang et al. 2000). In juveniles with symptoms of ADHD, missing a diagnosis of bipolar disorder could lead to administration of stimulant medication in the absence of antimanic agents, potentially yielding mood destabilization. These considerations may have contributed to a recent rapid increase in the diagnosis of pediatric bipolar disorder, which has resulted in the need for clinical epidemiological reliability studies to determine the accuracy of clinical diagnoses of child and adolescent bipolar disorder in community practice (Moreno et al. 2007). The diagnosis and treatment of pediatric bipolar disorder are discussed in Chapter 10 in this volume, "Management of Bipolar Disorders in Children and Adolescents."

At the other end of the age spectrum, elderly patients may present diagnostic challenges related to general medical conditions or their treatments that raise the possibility of a secondary bipolar disorder. This topic is discussed further in Chapter 12 in this volume, "Management of Bipolar Disorders in Older Adults."

Beginning to Address Diagnostic Challenges in Bipolar Disorder

Fortunately, clinicians have options to begin to address the diagnostic challenges described in the previous section. These include 1) routine use of collateral information from family members and/or significant others; 2) skillful use of the DSM-IV-TR diagnostic system (including the use of a diagnostic screening instrument); and 3) use of additional (non-DSM-IV-TR) information.

Routine Use of Collateral Information

Routinely using collateral information from family members and/or significant others when diagnosing mood disorders is crucial to enhance diagnostic accuracy. Patients themselves are often sensitive reporters of depressive symptoms. Indeed, patients' statements of presenting problems often involve descriptions of depressive symptoms. However, collateral sources are commonly more sensitive reporters of mood elevation symptoms. This is particularly important in patients with bipolar II disorder or bipolar disorder not otherwise specified, who may be unable to distinguish hypomanic episodes or subsyndromal hypomanic symptoms from their normal mood. The DSM-IV-TR criteria for hypomania implicitly suggest the need for collateral information to make the diagnosis because they include the stipulation that the disturbance in mood and the change in functioning be observable by others.

Skillful Use of DSM-IV-TR

In view of the overlapping symptoms of DSM-IV-TR bipolar disorders, depressive disorders, and other mood disorders described in Chapter 2, it is understandable that distinguishing bipolar disorders from depressive disorders, from other mood disorders, and from one another raises crucial diagnostic challenges. Methods to address these challenges are described in the following subsections and summarized in Table 3–1.

Distinguishing Bipolar Disorders From Depressive Disorders

Arguably, the most common and clinically crucial diagnostic challenge in the management of bipolar disorders is distinguishing them from depressive disorders. This differential diagnostic challenge is common because the lifetime prevalence of major depressive disorder (13.2%) (Hasin et al. 2005) is approximately three times that of bipolar disorders (4.4%) (Merikangas et al. 2007), and patients with bipolar disorders commonly present with major depressive episodes (e.g., "Evolution of Bipolar II Disorder" case example in Chapter 2). This differential diagnostic challenge is clinically crucial because misdiagnosing bipolar disorders as depressive disorders suggests treatment with antidepressants rather than mood stabilizers, which may yield inadequate relief of depressive symptoms or trigger mood elevation symptoms in patients with bipolar disorders. Misdiagnosing depressive disorders as bipolar disorders suggests treatment with mood stabilizers rather than antidepressants, which may yield inadequate relief of depressive symptoms or cause more somatic adverse effects in patients with depressive disorders.

Mood Disorder Questionnaire. Use of the Mood Disorder Questionnaire (MDQ) to evaluate any new patient with a suspected mood disorder can help distinguish patients with bipolar disorders from those with depressive disorders. This survey, which is presented in Figure 3–1 and is also available at http://www.dbsalliance.org/, consists of 13 questions about lifetime history of symptoms of mood elevation (Hirschfeld et al. 2000). Respondents who endorse more than half (i.e., seven or more "yes" answers), acknowledge that several symptoms have happened concurrently, and report at least moderate occupational, interpersonal, or financial problems, are considered to have a positive

TABLE 3–1. Distinguishing bipolar disorders from depressive disorders, from other mood disorders, and from one another

Diagnostic challenge	Approach
Distinguishing bipolar disorders from depressive disorders	
Bipolar disorders vs. major depressive disorder	Using the Mood Disorder Questionnaire
	Distinguishing mixed episodes or dysphoric hypomanic episodes from major depressive episodes with prominent irritability or agitation
	Prudent use of the diagnosis bipolar disorder not otherwise specified
	"Rounding up toward bipolarity" (?)
Distinguishing bipolar disorders from other mood disorders	
Bipolar disorders vs. mood disorders due to medical conditions	Assessing temporal relations between general medical conditions and mood symptoms
	Assessing whether the general medical condition of concern has been implicated in yielding mood symptoms in the medical literature
	Prudent use of the diagnosis bipolar disorder not otherwise specified
Bipolar disorders vs. substance-induced mood disorders	Assessing temporal relations between substance or medication exposure and mood symptoms
	Assessing whether the substance or medication of concern has been implicated in yielding mood symptoms in the medical literature
	Prudent use of the diagnosis bipolar disorder not otherwise specified
Distinguishing bipolar disorder subtypes from one another	
Bipolar I disorder vs. bipolar II disorder	Systematic assessment of psychosocial or occupational impairment and its relation to mood elevation
	Prospective longitudinal mood charting integrating collateral information
	"Rounding up toward bipolarity" (?)
Bipolar II disorder vs. bipolar disorder not otherwise specified	Prospective longitudinal mood charting integrating collateral information
	"Rounding up toward bipolarity" (?)

Note. (?) = controversial approach.

Has there ever been a period of time when you were not your usual self and...

1) ...you felt so good or so hyper that other people thought you were not your normal self or you were so hyper that you got into trouble? — Yes No

2) ...you were so irritable that you shouted at people or started fights or arguments? — Yes No

3) ...you felt much more self-confident than usual? — Yes No

4) ...you got much less sleep than usual and found you didn't really miss it? — Yes No

5) ...you were much more talkative or spoke much faster than usual? — Yes No

6) ...thoughts raced through your head or you couldn't slow your mind down? — Yes No

7) ...you were so easily distracted by things around you that you had trouble concentrating or staying on track? — Yes No

8) ...you had much more energy than usual? — Yes No

9) ...you were much more active or did many more things than usual? — Yes No

10) ...you were much more social or outgoing than usual, for example, you telephoned friends in the middle of the night? — Yes No

11) ...you were much more interested in sex than usual? — Yes No

12) ...you did things that were unusual for you or that other people might have thought were excessive, foolish, or risky? — Yes No

13) ...spending money got you or your family into trouble? — Yes No

14) If you checked Yes to more than one of the above, have several of these ever happened during the same period of time? — Yes No

15) How much of a problem did any of these cause you — like being unable to work; having family, money or legal troubles; getting into arguments or fights? — No Problem Minor Problem Moderate Problem Serious Problem

FIGURE 3–1. Mood disorder questionnaire.

Source. Reprinted from Hirschfeld RM, Williams JB, Spitzer RL, et al.: "Development and Validation of a Screening Instrument for Bipolar Spectrum Disorder: The Mood Disorder Questionnaire." *American Journal of Psychiatry* 157:1873–1875, 2000. Used with permission.

MDQ screen. In outpatient clinics that primarily treated mood disorders, the MDQ had very good specificity because 90% of the patients with a positive MDQ screen had bipolar disorders according to the Structured Clinical Interview for DSM-IV (SCID; First et al. 1997) and good sensitivity because 73% of the patients with bipolar disorder by the SCID had a positive MDQ screen (Hirschfeld et al. 2000). Although this issue has not been studied formally, clinical experience suggests that sensitivity may be enhanced by integrating additional information from an MDQ rating of the patient obtained from a collateral source.

Distinguishing mixed episodes or dysphoric hypomanic episodes from major depressive episodes with prominent irritability or agitation.   Distinguishing mixed episodes or dysphoric hypomanic episodes from major depressive episodes with prominent irritability or agitation can be crucial for the accurate diagnosis of bipolar disorders as compared with depressive disorders. The presence of decreased need for sleep (rather than mere insomnia), increased goal-directed activity (rather than mere psychomotor agitation), distractibility (rather than mere decreased concentration), and impulsivity suggests the possibility of a mixed episode or a dysphoric hypomanic episode (hypomanic episode with a concurrent major depressive episode) rather than a mere agitated major depressive episode. In patients presenting with "depression with agitation" (with psychomotor agitation, insomnia, and weight loss, which may overlap with depression with melancholic features) or with "depression with retardation" (with psychomotor retardation, hypersomnia, and weight gain, which may overlap with depression with atypical features), asking about prior episodes with the opposite type of depression can be instructive. Thus, the presence of both depression with agitation and depression with retardation in the same individual may suggest a bipolar disorder rather than a depressive disorder. In such instances, careful questioning including collateral sources may determine that depression with agitation represents in fact a mixed episode or a dysphoric hypomanic episode.

Prudent use of the diagnosis bipolar disorder not otherwise specified. Prudent use of the diagnosis bipolar disorder not otherwise specified can be a helpful way to indicate a degree of lack of diagnostic certainty if all of the above still yields an inconclusive assessment. The diagnosis of bipolar disorder not otherwise specified is particularly useful in this regard because it is applicable to a wide range of conditions with sufficient bipolar features to raise clinical concern yet insufficient to meet criteria for a specific bipolar disorder, sometimes referred to as *bipolar spectrum disorders.* The bipolar disorder not otherwise specified diagnosis can acknowledge the evidence of bipolarity in such instances yet preserve the integrity of the specific bipolar disorder constructs (bipolar I disorder, bipolar II disorder, and cyclothymic disorder). When bipolarity is even less certain, a diagnosis of mood disorder not otherwise specified may be applied.

Rounding up toward bipolarity.   "Rounding up toward bipolarity" is a controversial option to consider when information yields an inconclusive assessment. Thus, a convention of "rounding upward" from major depressive disorder to bipolar disorder not otherwise specified, or bipolar II disorder, may be advocated by some individuals. Such "erring on the side of bipolarity" would be expected to yield interventions that decrease the risk of iatrogenic illness exacerbation by administration of unopposed (in the absence of antimanic counterbalance) or inadequately opposed antidepressant therapy.

Distinguishing Bipolar Disorders From Other Mood Disorders

In view of the frequent general medical disorder and substance use disorder comorbidities seen in patients with bipolar disorders, and the common occurrence of general medical conditions and treatments thereof and illicit substances yielding affective symptoms, distinguishing bipolar disorders from other mood disorders (i.e., secondary mood disorders) is a common clinical challenge.

Assessing temporal relations between general medical conditions and mood symptoms.   Assessing temporal relations between general medical conditions and mood symptoms can help determine whether the former caused the latter. Thus, in mood disorder due to a general medical condition, the general medical condition precedes the onset of the mood disturbance. However, this may not be obvious for general medical conditions with either subtle or nonspecific early symptoms that may overlap with those of mood disorders (e.g., disturbance of sleep, appetite, energy, or concentration). In some instances, resolution of the general medical condition that results in resolution of the mood disturbance can help confirm the causal role of the general medical condition. In bipolar disorders with a comorbid general medical condition, the mood disturbance precedes the general medical condition and persists even after resolution of the general medical condition. In some instances, symptoms of a primary bipolar disorder may be exacerbated by a subtle general medical condition (e.g., lithium-induced hypothyroidism yielding depressive-like symptoms), and mood symptoms may tend to covary with symptoms of the general medical condition, making assessment of causal relations and accurate diagnosis complex.

Assessing whether the general medical condition of concern has been implicated in yielding mood symptoms in the medical literature.   Assessing whether the general medical condition of concern has been implicated in yielding mood symptoms in the medical literature can help determine whether the former is a plausible cause of the latter. For example, cerebrovascular infarctions yielding mood elevation have been reported frequently in the medical literature; thus, these conditions are plausible causes of mood elevation. Table 2–11 in Chapter 2 includes a list of selected general medical conditions associated with secondary mood disorders.

Assessing temporal relations between substance or medication exposure and mood symptoms.   Assessing temporal relations between substance or medication exposure and mood symptoms can help determine whether the former caused the latter. Thus, in substance-induced mood disorders, the substance or medication exposure precedes the onset of the mood disturbance. In addition, termination of substance or medication exposure resulting in resolution of the mood disturbance can help confirm the causal role of the substance or medication exposure. DSM-IV-TR acknowledges that clinical judgment is essential to determine whether the substance or medication of concern is truly causal or whether a primary mood episode just happened to have its onset during exposure. For example, a patient with presumptive major depressive disorder who developed a manic-like episode within a month of starting nortriptyline would continue to be regarded as having major depressive disorder and would receive the additional diagnosis of nortriptyline-induced mood disorder with manic features (as in "Course of Major Depressive Disorder, Single Episode, and Antidepressant-Induced Mood Disorder With Manic Features" case example in Chapter 2). However, if such a manic-like episode emerged only after a decade of nortriptyline therapy, nortriptyline would not be considered causal, so the major depressive disorder diagnosis would be changed to bipolar I disorder, and the diagnosis of nortriptyline-induced mood disorder with manic features, would *not* be applied. DSM-IV-TR does not specify a maximum duration of antidepressant treatment in order for it to be considered causal in inducing a subsequent manic episode. In the Systematic Treatment Enhancement Program for Bipolar Disorder (STEP-BD), treatment-emergent affective switch was diagnosed only if the antidepressant had been started or increased within 3 months before the onset of mood elevation.

In bipolar disorder with comorbid substance or medication exposure, the mood disturbance precedes the substance or medication exposure and persists even after termination of the substance or medication exposure. In some instances, substance use disorders can covary with symptoms of bipolar disorder (e.g., patients attempting to attenuate or intensify mood symptoms with substances), making assessment of temporal relations more challenging.

Assessing whether the substance or medication has been implicated in yielding mood symptoms in the medical literature. Assessing whether the substance or medication of concern has been implicated in yielding mood symptoms in the medical literature can help in determining whether the former is a plausible cause of the latter. For example, exposure to antidepressants (particularly in the absence of antimanic agents) yielding mood elevation has been reported frequently in the medical literature; thus, such agents are plausible causes of mood elevation (e.g., "Course of Major Depressive Disorder, Single Episode, and Antidepressant-Induced Mood Disorder With Manic Features" case example in Chapter 2). Indeed, this phenomenon is sufficiently frequent that DSM-IV-TR specifically addresses it. The DSM-IV-TR approach does not permit episodes with symptoms of mood elevation that are clearly caused by somatic antidepressant treatment (e.g., medication, electroconvulsive therapy, light therapy) to count toward a diagnosis of bipolar disorder. For example, a patient with major depressive disorder who developed a manic-like episode after treatment with nortriptyline would receive the diagnosis of major depressive disorder and nortriptyline-induced mood disorder with manic features (in a fashion similar to that of the case example in "Course of Major Depressive Disorder, Single Episode, and Antidepressant-Induced Mood Disorder With Manic Features" in Chapter 2). Table 2–12 in Chapter 2 includes a list of selected substances and treatments associated with secondary mood disorders.

Prudent use of the diagnosis bipolar disorder not otherwise specified. Prudent use of the diagnosis bipolar disorder not otherwise specified can be a helpful way to indicate a degree of lack of certainty whether a bipolar disorder is primary or secondary if all of the above assessments yield an inconclusive diagnosis.

Distinguishing Bipolar Disorder Subtypes From One Another

Systematic assessment of psychosocial or occupational impairment and its relation to mood elevation. Systematic assessment of psychosocial or occupational impairment and its relation to mood elevation can help address an important limitation of the DSM-IV-TR distinction between hypomanic and manic or mixed episodes—the lack of an operationalized approach to quantifying the degree of psychosocial or occupational impairment and attributing causality of such impairment to mood elevation episodes. For accurate diagnosis of hypomanic as compared with manic or mixed episodes, it is crucial to quantify whether the degree of impairment is severe (as required for manic and mixed episodes) or merely mild to moderate (as required for hypomanic episodes). Systematically inquiring about any history of bankruptcy, violence, arrests, incarceration, other legal problems, multiple relationship failures, and multiple employment terminations can provide evidence of severe psychosocial or occupational impairment. Once such problems have been detected, carefully assessing the degree to which they have been related to episodes of mood elevation as opposed to other causes (e.g., episodes of depression, comorbid Axis I and Axis II psychiatric disorders, comorbid medical disorders, or environmental factors) can be crucial in distinguishing hypomanic from manic or mixed episodes. In patients, denial and other factors may lead to underestimating the degree of dysfunction or the relation of dysfunction to episodes of mood elevation. Collateral observers can provide crucial additional information to aid in assessing these factors.

Prospective longitudinal mood charting integrating collateral information. Prospective longitudinal mood charting integrating collateral information to confirm whether syndromal hypomanic, manic, or mixed episodes occur can help determine whether a diagnosis of bipolar I disorder rather than bipolar II disorder applies or if a diagnosis of bipolar II disorder rather than bipolar disorder not otherwise specified applies. Mood charting dates back more than a century to the time of Emil Kraepelin (Livianos-Aldana and Rojo-Moreno 2006) and can document valuable data regarding illness course. The cases presented in Chapter 2 are accompanied by schematics (Figures 2–1 through 2–4) that include elementary features of mood charting, such as the horizontal axis representing time and areas above and below the horizontal axis representing mood elevation and depression, respectively. The National Institute of Mental Health–Life Chart Method (NIMH-LCM) is a more detailed and rigorous, as well as validated, prospective longitudinal monitoring tool (Denicoff et al. 2000). The NIMH-LCM Patient Self-Rated Prospective Form (LCM-S/P), which is presented in Figure 3–2, is also available (along with its accompanying manual and other versions of life-charting materials) at http://www.bipolarnews. org/.

Distinguishing Bipolar Disorders From Psychiatric Disorders Other Than Mood Disorders

Although the most common diagnostic challenges encountered in the management of bipolar disorders entail distinguishing them from one another, from depressive disorders, and from other mood disorders, as described earlier in this section, there are additional important considerations in the differential diagnosis of bipolar disorders. For example, because psychotic symptoms may be prominent, it is important to distinguish bipolar disorders from psychotic disorders such as schizophrenia and schizoaffective disorder. In addition, affective lability may be dramatic, so it is important to distinguish bipolar disorders from other disorders with this phenomenon such as Cluster B personality disorders in general and borderline personality disorder in particular. Also, hyperactivity, inattention, and impulsivity may be prominent, so it is important to distinguish bipolar disorders from other disorders with such features such as disruptive behavior disorders in general and ADHD in particular.

Methods to address these challenges are described in the following subsections and summarized in Table 3–2.

Determining the presence and chronicity of symptoms characteristic of schizophrenia and their duration compared with any mood episodes. Determining the presence and chronicity of symptoms characteristic of schizophrenia and the duration of these symptoms compared with any mood episodes can facilitate distinguishing schizophrenia from bipolar disorders. In schizophrenia, at least two characteristic symptoms (psychosis, disorganized speech or behavior, or negative symptoms) are present for a significant portion of 1 month (or less if successfully treated), accompanied by marked deterioration of psychosocial or occupational function, and continuous signs of disturbance are present for at least 6 months, with any mood episodes accounting for only a relatively brief portion of the total illness duration.

Detecting the presence and duration of psychotic symptoms in the absence of syndromal mood episodes. Detecting the presence and duration of psychotic symptoms in the absence of syndromal mood episodes can facilitate distinguishing schizoaffective disorder from bipolar disorders. In schizoaffective disorder, at least subchronic (at least 2 weeks' duration) psychotic symptoms are present in the absence of prominent mood symptoms, yet mood episodes account for a substantial portion of total illness duration.

NIMH-LCM™ Self/PROSPECTIVE Ratings: The LCM-S/P™

Name _____ Month _____ Year _____

LCM-SPTM Version 2-32

Days of Month

| 1 | 2 | 3 | 4 | 5 | 6 | 7 | 8 | 9 | 10 | 11 | 12 | 13 | 14 | 15 | 16 | 17 | 18 | 19 | 20 | 21 | 22 | 23 | 24 | 25 | 26 | 27 | 28 | 29 | 30 | 31 |

Enter Total # of tablets TAKEN per day

Please track all medications that you are currently taking.

Medication Name	DOSE per tablet	UNIT (mg, mcg, gm)
Lithium		
Tegretol		
Depakote		

Days of Month

| 1 | 2 | 3 | 4 | 5 | 6 | 7 | 8 | 9 | 10 | 11 | 12 | 13 | 14 | 15 | 16 | 17 | 18 | 19 | 20 | 21 | 22 | 23 | 24 | 25 | 26 | 27 | 28 | 29 | 30 | 31 |

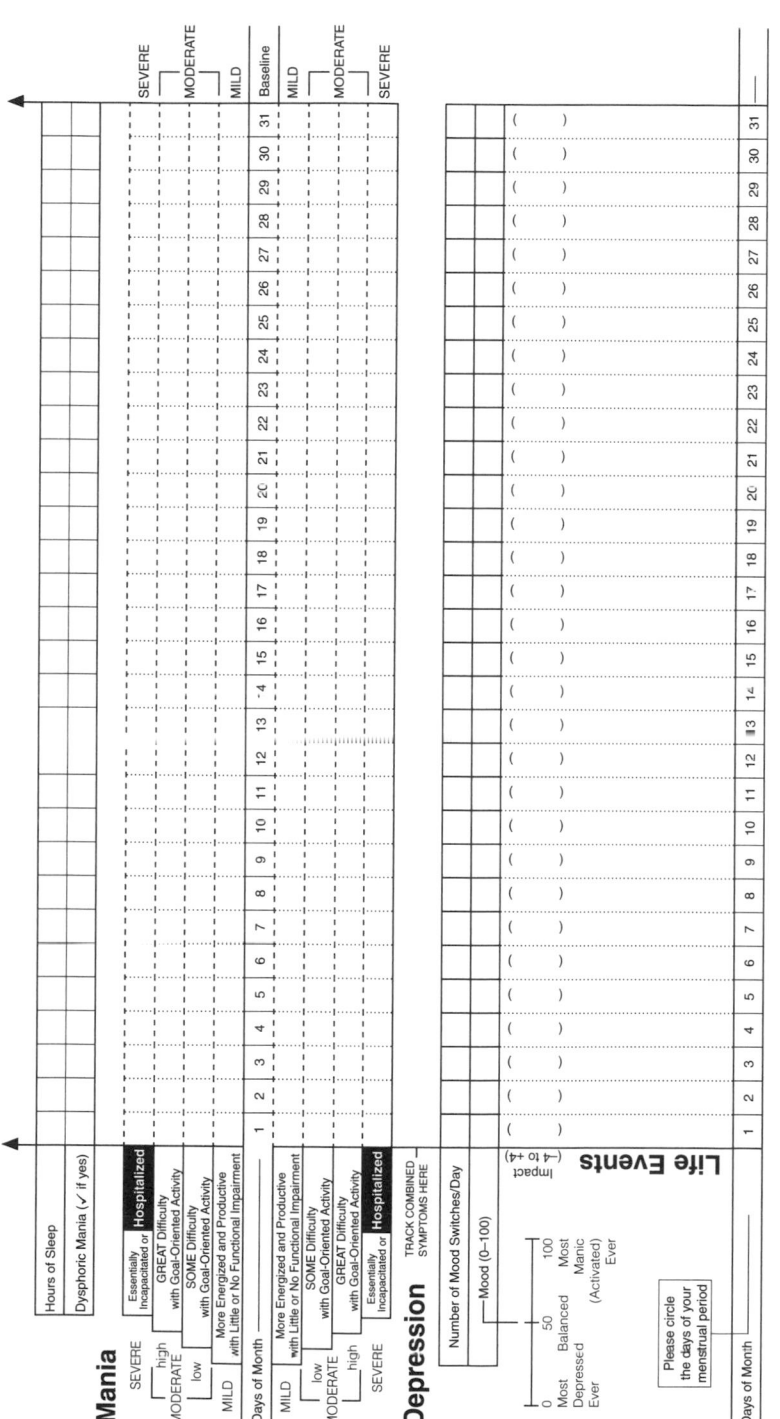

FIGURE 3–2. **National Institute of Mental Health—Life Chart Method (NIMH-LCM) Patient Self-Rated Prospective Form (LCM-S/P).**

Source. Reprinted from Denicoff et al. 2000.

TABLE 3–2.　Distinguishing bipolar disorders from psychiatric disorders other than mood disorders

Diagnostic challenge	Approach
Bipolar disorders vs. schizophrenia	Determining the presence and chronicity of symptoms characteristic of schizophrenia, and the duration of these symptoms, compared with any mood episodes
	Prudent use of the diagnosis psychotic disorder not otherwise specified
Bipolar disorders vs. schizoaffective disorder	Detecting the presence and duration of psychotic symptoms in the absence of syndromal mood episodes
	Prudent use of the diagnosis psychotic disorder not otherwise specified
Bipolar disorders vs. borderline personality disorder	Distinguishing mixed or dysphoric hypomanic episodes from affective lability
	Assessing whether borderline personality disorder–like symptoms resolve
Bipolar disorders vs. attention-deficit/ hyperactivity disorder	Assessing onset age, chronicity, and the presence or absence of euphoria, expansiveness, and psychosis

Prudent use of the diagnosis psychotic disorder not otherwise specified. Prudent use of the diagnosis psychotic disorder not otherwise specified can be a helpful way to indicate a lack of certainty whether a psychotic episode represents schizophrenia or schizoaffective disorder as opposed to bipolar disorder if all of the above recommendations yield an inconclusive assessment. Such ambiguity may be encountered early in the course of illness or in the setting of very limited historical information.

Distinguishing mixed or dysphoric hypomanic episodes from affective lability. Distinguishing mixed or dysphoric hypomanic episodes from affective lability can be crucial for accurate diagnosis of bipolar disorders as compared with borderline personality disorder. This is most likely to pose a challenge when patients are experiencing ultradian (within a day) mood cycling. Such patients may present with sadness or anhedonia in the morning and afternoon, followed by irritability or even euphoria in the evening.

Perhaps even more challenging are patients who report mood changes several times per day. If patients experience sadness or anhedonia most of the day nearly every day (key features of depression), yet on a daily basis also experience significant irritability or euphoria (key features of mood elevation), careful assessment (with collateral information) may identify sufficient symptoms to diagnose a mixed or dysphoric hypomanic episode.

Assessing whether borderline personality disorder–like symptoms resolve. Assessing whether borderline personality disorder–like symptoms resolve can help determine whether such phenomena were merely related to mood episodes, as in bipolar disorders, or are pervasive, as in borderline personality disorder. For example, although during hypomanic, manic, or mixed episodes patients with bipolar disorders may show borderline personality disorder–like interpersonal maneuvers (Janowsky et al. 1970), resolution of such difficulties with euthymia suggests a diagnosis of a bipolar disorder rather than a borderline personality disorder. Early-onset, chronic problems with symptoms of irritability, unstable intense interpersonal relationships, unstable self-image, paranoia, impulsivity, and recurrent suicidal behaviors that are not all confined to mood episodes are suggestive of borderline personality disorder. These disorders are not mutually exclusive. Indeed, borderline personality disorder and bipolar disorders are commonly comorbid, with the presence of one increasing the risk of the other.

Assessing onset age, chronicity, and the presence or absence of euphoria, expansiveness, and psychosis. Assessing onset age, chronicity, and the presence or absence of euphoria, expansiveness, and psychosis can help distinguish bipolar disorders from ADHD. The latter has an onset before age 7 years; is chronic rather than episodic; and lacks euphoria, expansiveness, and psychosis. These disorders are not mutually exclusive. Indeed, they are commonly comorbid, with early-onset bipolar disorders increasing the risk of ADHD. This challenging and at times controversial topic is discussed in more detail in Chapter 10.

Use of Non-DSM-IV-TR Information

Emerging data indicate that the time for clinicians to begin to use non-DSM-IV-TR information to better inform the diagnosis of bipolar disorders is rapidly approaching, if it has not already arrived. This contention is supported by evidence that 1) the limitations of the DSM-IV-TR mood disorder nosology are significantly problematic; 2) the clinical need for enhanced bipolar disorders diagnosis is great; and 3) the utility of invoking additional non-DSM-IV-TR information is sufficiently promising. The first two items have been discussed earlier in this chapter and in the preceding chapter. In this section, we discuss the third item with respect to incorporating information about additional symptomatology, course of illness, family history, and probabilistic (dimensional) components.

Additional Symptomatology

Although not included in DSM-IV-TR, several additional aspects of symptomatology, as well as course of illness and family history information, appear useful in distinguishing bipolar disorders from depressive disorders. A recently published report from the bipolar depression subgroup of the Task Force on Diagnostic Guidelines of the International Society for Bipolar Disorders reviews the evidence base in detail and provides suggestions for integrating this information into a probabilistic approach to the diagnosis of bipolar depression (Mitchell et al. 2008).

Atypical depressive symptoms.   Atypical depressive symptoms may be markers of increased risk of bipolarity (Benazzi 2003; Mitchell et al. 2001; Serretti et al. 2002). Thus, increased sleep (Andreasen et al. 1988; Benazzi 2006) may suggest increased risk of bipolarity, whereas initial insomnia (Brockington et al. 1982; Mitchell et al. 2001) and decreased sleep (Perlis et al. 2006) may be markers of increased risk of unipolar illness. Similarly, increased eating (Andreasen et al. 1988; Benazzi 2006) and weight gain (Benazzi 2006) may indicate increased risk of bipolarity, whereas decreased appetite (Papadimitriou et al. 2002) and weight loss (Abrams and Taylor 1980) may suggest increased risk of unipolar illness. Psychomotor retardation is a replicated marker of increased risk of bipolarity (Andreasen et al. 1988; Dunner et al. 1976; Mitchell et al. 2001; Parker et al. 2000), although there have been some negative study results (Benazzi 2002; Katz et al. 1982; Kuhs and Reschke 1992; Mitchell et al. 1992; Perris 1966; Popescu et al. 1991).

Mood elevation symptoms.   Mood elevation symptoms (Abrams and Taylor 1980), such as irritability (Benazzi 2006), mood lability (Akiskal et al. 1995; Brockington et al. 1982), racing thoughts (Benazzi 2006), overtalkativeness (Benazzi 2006), impulsivity, and increased goal-directed activity (Benazzi 2006) are, perhaps not surprisingly, suggestive of increased risk of bipolarity.

Psychotic features.   Psychotic features have indicated increased risk of bipolarity in multiple studies (Akiskal et al. 1983; Andreasen et al. 1988; Coryell et al. 1995; Endicott et al. 1985; Goldberg et al. 2001; Guze et al. 1975; Mitchell et al. 2001; Othmer et al. 2007; Strober and Carlson 1982), although there have been some negative reports (Beigel and Murphy 1971; Black and Nasrallah 1989). Thus, in the Collaborative Program on the Psychobiology of Depression, psychosis was seen in 22% of the patients with bipolar I disorder, compared with only 8% of the patients with unipolar major depressive disorder (Solomon et al. 2006).

Comorbid disorders. Comorbid disorders such as a current alcohol use disorder (Olfson et al. 2005) and panic disorder or generalized anxiety disorder (Simon et al. 2003) appear to be markers of increased risk for bipolarity. Some of the highest comorbidity rates for any disorder occur in patients with bipolar disorders. For example, in the Epidemiologic Catchment Area program, more than 61% of the participants with bipolar disorders had any substance use disorder, the highest such comorbidity rate seen in any Axis I disorder (Regier et al. 1990). In the National Comorbidity Survey Replication, participants with bipolar disorders were almost 10-fold more likely to have alcohol dependence and 8-fold more likely to have any other substance use disorder compared with the general population (Kessler et al. 2005). In that study, comorbidities that were numerically more common in patients with bipolar disorders compared with depressive disorders included not only substance use disorders (alcohol abuse, alcohol dependence, and substance abuse) and anxiety disorders (panic disorder, social anxiety disorder) but also disruptive behavior disorders (ADHD, oppositional defiant disorder, and conduct disorder) and intermittent explosive disorder (Kessler et al. 2005).

Course of Illness

Earlier onset of depression. Earlier onset of depression may be a marker of increased risk of bipolarity (Andreasen et al. 1988; Othmer et al. 2007; Solomon et al. 2006). Indeed, in the Collaborative Program on the Psychobiology of Depression, the mean age at onset in participants with bipolar I disorder (23.0 years) was almost a decade earlier than that in unipolar major depressive disorder (32.7 years) (Solomon et al. 2006). Among patients with bipolar disorders, earlier onset is commonly accompanied by having an affected first-degree relative and appears to have important associations with other illness features. For example, in the STEP-BD, earlier onset was associated with greater rates of comorbid anxiety disorders and substance abuse, more recurrences, shorter periods of euthymia, greater likelihood of suicide attempts and violence, and greater likelihood of being in a mood episode at study entry (Perlis et al. 2004). Prepubertal-onset depression is of particular significance because almost 50% of the patients will meet criteria for a bipolar disorder within a decade (Figure 3–3, left) (Geller

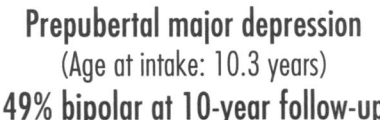

Prepubertal major depression
(Age at intake: 10.3 years)
49% bipolar at 10-year follow-up

Adolescents / Young adults
hospitalized for major depression
(Age at intake: 23.0 years)
41% bipolar at 15-year follow-up

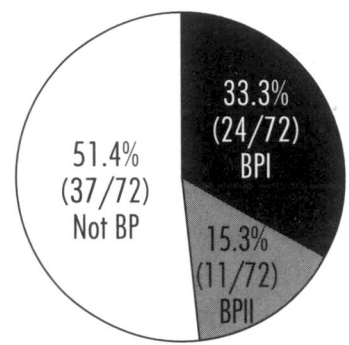

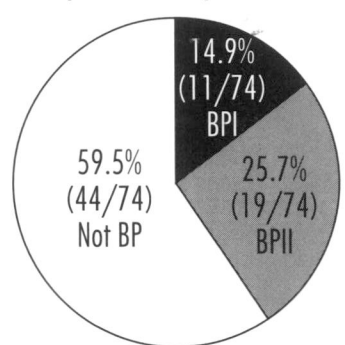

FIGURE 3–3.   High bipolarity risk in prepubertal and severe adolescent or early-adulthood major depression.

Early-onset depression is a risk marker for bipolar outcome in children and, if depression is severe, in adolescents and young adults as well. BP=bipolar; BPI=bipolar I disorder; BPII=bipolar II disorder.

Source.   Data from Geller et al. 2001 (*left*) and Goldberg et al. 2001 (*right*).

et al. 2001). Similarly, among individuals with late-adolescent or early-adulthood depressions severe enough to warrant hospitalization, more than 40% of the patients will meet criteria for a bipolar disorder within 15 years (Figure 3–3, right) (Goldberg et al. 2001).

More prior depressive episodes.   More prior depressive episodes may be a marker of increased risk of bipolarity (Andreasen et al. 1988; Solomon et al. 2006). As noted in Chapter 2, approximately 90% of patients with bipolar I disorder have recurrent episodes, compared with only approximately 50% of patients with unipolar major depressive disorder. Indeed, in the Collaborative Program on the Psychobiology of Depression, a history of recurrent depressions was seen in 96% of the participants with bipolar I disorder, compared with 59% of the participants with unipolar major depressive disorder (Solomon et al. 2006). Moreover, a history of three or more prior episodes of depression was evident in 78% of the participants with bipolar I disorder, compared with only 23% of the participants with unipolar major depressive disorder.

Family History

Bipolar family history is a consistent marker of increased risk for bipolarity (Akiskal et al. 1983; Andreasen et al. 1988; Coryell et al. 1995; Othmer et al. 2007; Solomon et al. 2006; Strober and Carlson 1982). This is not surprising because bipolar disorders are among the most familial of psychiatric disorders—having one affected first-degree relative may carry a 20% risk, whereas having an affected identical twin or two affected parents may increase the risk to approximately 70%.

Probabilistic (Dimensional) Components

The above-mentioned risk factors for bipolar disorders in depressed patients, although in some instances related to one another, nevertheless appear to be additive. For example, among outpatients with a history of a major depressive episode, also having a history of psychosis or early-onset depression or a family history of bipolar disorder was associated with double to triple the risk of having bipolar I disorder (Othmer et al. 2007). Also, having none, one, two, or three of these risk factors was associated with 15%, 19%, 49%, and 67% risks of having bipolar I disorder, respectively (Figure 3–4).

The recently published report from the bipolar depression subgroup of the International Society for Bipolar Disorders Task Force on Diagnostic Guidelines provides suggestions for integrating the above information into a probabilistic approach to the diagnosis of bipolar depression (Mitchell et al. 2008). The subgroup suggests that among depressed patients, having at least five of the above-mentioned risk factors is associated with a more likely bipolar disorder, whereas having at least four of the (generally opposite) unipolar risk factors is associated with a more likely (unipolar) major depressive disorder (Table 3–3). Such a schema could allow clinicians to quantify the degree of likelihood of a bipolar disorder as compared with a depressive disorder. This could then be integrated with the degree of risk tolerance of the patient and provider in the process of individualized treatment planning.

Another potential dimensional approach is the Bipolarity Index, an instrument devised by Dr. Gary Sachs (2004) at Massachusetts General Hospital and used in the STEP-BD. The Bipolarity Index is a five-item scale, with each of five domains (episode characteristics, age at onset, illness course/associated features, response to treatment, and family history) contributing up to 20 points, with a maximum total score of 100 points. Thus, the Bipolarity Index score has a component based on episode characteristics derived from the DSM-IV-TR approach of using cross-sectional symptomatic criteria and episode types to define

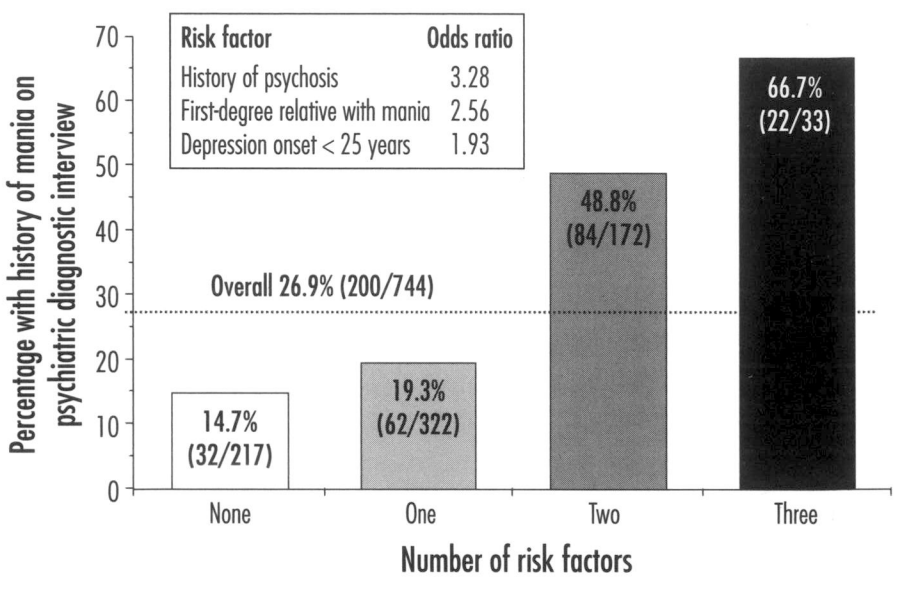

FIGURE 3–4.   Additive effects of history of psychosis, family history of bipolar disorder, and early-onset depression on risk of bipolar I disorder.

Mean age of patients was 37.5 years. Patients were assessed with the Psychiatric Diagnostic Interview (Othmer et al. 1981). $P<0.001$.
Source.   Data from Othmer et al. 2007.

bipolar disorders (Table 3–4). However, the Bipolarity Index also includes additional important (non-DSM-IV-TR) data regarding age at onset, illness course/associated features, response to treatment, and family history to provide a more comprehensive illness metric.

Thus, an age at onset of 19 years or younger results in a higher Bipolarity Index score. Similarly, the presence of illness course/associated features, such as a high recurrence rate of episodes, affective psychosis, comorbid substance abuse, and legal problems related to impulsivity, increases the score. With respect to response to treatment, the presence of either poor outcomes (mood destabilization or inefficacy) with antidepressants or good outcomes with mood stabilizers increases scores. In addition, a positive family history of bipolar disorders or recurrent major depressive disorder increases the score. Among researchers, there is consensus regarding the validity and potential utility of four of these five domains, with the sole exception being response to treatment (Ghaemi et al. 2008; Mitchell et al. 2008).

TABLE 3–3. **Probabilistic approach to bipolar depression proposed by the Task Force on Diagnostic Guidelines of the International Society for Bipolar Disorders**

Bipolar I depression more likely if ≥ 5:	Unipolar depression more likely if ≥ 4:
Symptomatology	
Hypersomnia	Insomnia
Hyperphagia	Decreased appetite
Psychomotor retardation	Psychomotor agitation
Other "atypical" symptoms	
Psychosis and/or pathological guilt	Somatic complaints
Mood lability or manic symptoms	
Course of illness	
Earlier onset (<25 years)	Later onset (>25 years)
Multiple depressions (≥5 episodes)	Long current depression (>6 months)
Family history	
Bipolar disorder	No bipolar disorder

Note. Confirmation of specific numbers requires further study.
Source. Adapted from Mitchell et al. 2008.

TABLE 3–4. **The Bipolarity Index: five bipolarity domains**

I. Episode characteristics (DSM-IV-TR)
   Mania; hypomania; cyclothymia
II. Age at onset (non-DSM)
   Especially 15–19 years
III. Illness course/associated features (non-DSM)
   Recurrence and remission; comorbidity
IV. Response to treatment (non-DSM)
   Mood stabilizers—effective
   Antidepressants—ineffective; adverse effects
V. Family history (non-DSM)
   Bipolar; recurrent unipolar

Source. Adapted from Sachs 2004.

Although the exact psychometrics of this instrument remain to be established, certain properties are beginning to emerge. Thus, factor analysis of this five-item scale identified two factors, with the first consisting of the episode characteristics, illness course/associated features, and response to treatment items and the second consisting of the age at onset and family history items (Del Debbo et al. 2007).

Much further research, including comparing scores in patients with bipolar disorders and major depressive disorders, needs to be performed with probabilistic or dimensional instruments. Nevertheless, some preliminary speculations may give readers a sense of potential directions and possible clinical applications. If proven valid and reliable, such instruments might be considered to provide approximate estimates of the "percentile of bipolarity" of an individual's mood disorder. This would change the clinical question from "Does this patient have a bipolar disorder or a depressive disorder?" to "What is the degree of bipolarity of this patient's mood disorder?"

To show some of the potential of this kind of work, assume for a moment that a five-domain Bipolarity Index–like scale ultimately proves to yield scores that are very high (80–100) in bipolar I disorder, moderately high (60–80) in bipolar II disorder, intermediate (40–60) in bipolar disorder not otherwise specified, low (20–40) in highly recurrent treatment-resistant major depressive disorder, and very low in minimally recurrent treatment-responsive major depressive disorder. Such an instrument could perhaps then be used in tandem with a hybrid categorical-dimensional mood disorders schema as illustrated in Figure 3–5. This could lead to novel illness constructs such as having inclusive (type II) and exclusive (type I) phenotypes for both bipolar disorders and depressive disorders. Such a hybrid approach might ultimately permit patients and providers to integrate this hybrid diagnostic information with their degree of risk tolerance in individualized treatment planning. Although such a scenario is currently merely a provocative speculation, current diagnostic research trends, if successful, could begin to facilitate movement in such a direction.

Other Future Directions in Diagnosis

The recently published report of the Task Force on Diagnostic Guidelines of the International Society for Bipolar Disorders proposes, in addition to the suggestions for bipolar depression discussed earlier, revisions to the DSM-IV-TR mood disorder nosology (Ghaemi et al. 2008). Although detailed discussion of these is beyond the scope of this chapter, selected revisions are listed in Table 3–5.

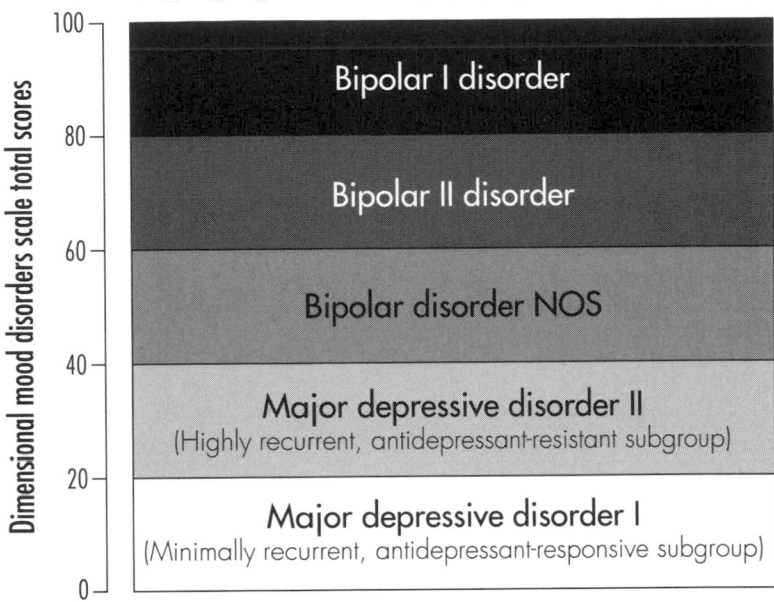

FIGURE 3-5. Possible categorical dimensional mood disorders schema.

Speculative demonstration of potential utility of a theoretical dimensional mood disorders scale in a hybrid (categorical-dimensional) approach to the diagnosis of mood disorders. Total scores on a five-domain bipolar-unipolar dimensional mood scale, similar to the Bipolarity Index (Sachs 2004), could be used to assign various diagnoses, depending on the degree of bipolarity. I=exclusive phenotype; II=inclusive phenotype; NOS=not otherwise specified.

TABLE 3–5.   Selected revisions to DSM-IV-TR proposed by the International Society for Bipolar Disorders Diagnostic Guidelines Task Force

Hypomanic episode—revision:

1. Decrease minimum duration from 4 to 2 days.

2. Permit mild-to-moderate depressive symptoms (mixed hypomania).

3. Permit the presence of medication, substance intake, or physical illness not clearly etiologically related to symptoms.

Bipolar II disorder—add:

1. Depressive symptoms must cause clinically significant distress or psychosocial impairment.

2. Hypomanic symptoms do not necessarily cause clinically significant distress or psychosocial impairment.

3. Course specifier: with hypomanic or depressive predominant polarity.

Bipolar disorder not otherwise specified—add examples:

1. Subthreshold hypomanic episodes in the context of multiple other signs of bipolarity.*

2. Multiple signs of bipolarity without hypomanic or manic episodes (also known as *bipolar spectrum disorder*).*

   *Clinicians should specify precisely which such signs are present and include this list in their assessment statement, as follows:

  a. Family history (bipolar diagnoses; multigenerational mental illness; alcohol and other substance use; suicides)

  b. Depressive symptom phenomenology (atypical, seasonal, psychomotor slowing, psychosis)

  c. Course of illness (early age at onset, short duration of episodes, greater number of episodes)

Pediatric bipolar disorder—add:

1. An acute manic, hypomanic, or mixed episode (by adult criteria) plus depressed episodes occur before age 18 years.

2. In acute manic, hypomanic, or mixed episodes, if mood is merely irritable (and not euphoric), documented spontaneously episodic fluctuations in mood elevation symptoms are required.

Schizoaffective disorder—drop diagnostic category altogether and replace with:

1. Additional specifiers for chronic psychosis in mood disorders.

2. New specifiers for mood episodes in schizophrenia.

Source.   Adapted from Ghaemi et al. 2008.

References

Abrams R, Taylor MA: A comparison of unipolar and bipolar depressive illness. Am J Psychiatry 137:1084–1087, 1980

Akiskal HS, Walker P, Puzantian VR, et al: Bipolar outcome in the course of depressive illness: phenomenologic, familial, and pharmacologic predictors. J Affect Disord 5:115–128, 1983

Akiskal HS, Maser JD, Zeller PJ, et al: Switching from 'unipolar' to bipolar II: an 11-year prospective study of clinical and temperamental predictors in 559 patients. Arch Gen Psychiatry 52:114–123, 1995

American Psychiatric Association: Diagnostic and Statistical Manual of Mental Disorders, 4th Edition, Text Revision. Washington, DC, American Psychiatric Association, 2000

Andreasen NC, Grove WM, Endicott J, et al: The phenomenology of depression. Psychiatry and Psychobiology 3:1–10, 1988

Beigel A, Murphy DL: Unipolar and bipolar affective illness: differences in clinical characteristics accompanying depression. Arch Gen Psychiatry 24:215–220, 1971

Benazzi F: Psychomotor changes in melancholic and atypical depression: unipolar and bipolar-II subtypes. Psychiatry Res 112:211–220, 2002

Benazzi F: Clinical differences between bipolar II depression and unipolar major depressive disorder: lack of an effect of age. J Affect Disord 75:191–195, 2003

Benazzi F: Symptoms of depression as possible markers of bipolar II disorder. Prog Neuropsychopharmacol Biol Psychiatry 30:471–477, 2006

Black DW, Nasrallah A: Hallucinations and delusions in 1,715 patients with unipolar and bipolar affective disorders. Psychopathology 22:28–34, 1989

Brockington IF, Altman E, Hillier V, et al: The clinical picture of bipolar affective disorder in its depressed phase: a report from London and Chicago. Br J Psychiatry 141:558–562, 1982

Chang KD, Steiner H, Ketter TA: Psychiatric phenomenology of child and adolescent bipolar offspring. J Am Acad Child Adolesc Psychiatry 39:453–460, 2000

Coryell W, Endicott J, Maser JD, et al: Long-term stability of polarity distinctions in the affective disorders. Am J Psychiatry 152:385–390, 1995

Del Debbo A, Blais MA, Nierenberg AA, et al: Psychometric properties of the Bipolarity Index Rating System (Abstract P55). Presentation at the Seventh International Conference on Bipolar Disorder. Pittsburgh, PA, June 7–9, 2007

Denicoff KD, Leverich GS, Nolen WA, et al: Validation of the prospective NIMH-Life-Chart Method (NIMH-LCM-p) for longitudinal assessment of bipolar illness. Psychol Med 30:1391–1397, 2000

Dunner DL, Dwyer T, Fieve RR: Depressive symptoms in patients with unipolar and bipolar affective disorder. Compr Psychiatry 17:447–451, 1976

Endicott J, Nee J, Andreasen N, et al: Bipolar II: combine or keep separate? J Affect Disord 8:17–28, 1985

First MB, Spitzer RL, Gibbon M, et al: Structured Clinical Interview for DSM-IV Axis I Disorders, Research Version, Patient Edition (SCID-I/P). New York, Biometrics Research, New York State Psychiatric Institute, 1997

Geller B, Zimerman B, Williams M, et al: Bipolar disorder at prospective follow-up of adults who had prepubertal major depressive disorder. Am J Psychiatry 158:125–127, 2001

Ghaemi SN, Sachs GS, Chiou AM, et al: Is bipolar disorder still underdiagnosed? Are antidepressants overutilized? J Affect Disord 52:135–144, 1999

Ghaemi SN, Boiman EE, Goodwin FK: Diagnosing bipolar disorder and the effect of antidepressants: a naturalistic study. J Clin Psychiatry 61:804–808; quiz 809, 2000

Ghaemi SN, Bauer M, Cassidy F, et al: Diagnostic guidelines for bipolar disorder: a summary of the International Society for Bipolar Disorders Diagnostic Guidelines Task Force Report. Bipolar Disord 10:117–128, 2008

Goldberg JF, Harrow M, Whiteside JE: Risk for bipolar illness in patients initially hospitalized for unipolar depression. Am J Psychiatry 158:1265–1270, 2001

Guze SB, Woodruff RA Jr, Clayton PJ: The significance of psychotic affective disorders. Arch Gen Psychiatry 32:1147–1150, 1975

Hasin DS, Goodwin RD, Stinson FS, et al: Epidemiology of major depressive disorder: results from the National Epidemiologic Survey on Alcoholism and Related Conditions. Arch Gen Psychiatry 62:1097–1106, 2005

Hirschfeld RM, Williams JB, Spitzer RL, et al: Development and validation of a screening instrument for bipolar spectrum disorder: the Mood Disorder Questionnaire. Am J Psychiatry 157:1873–1875, 2000

Hirschfeld RM, Lewis L, Vornik LA: Perceptions and impact of bipolar disorder: how far have we really come? Results of the National Depressive and Manic-Depressive Association 2000 Survey of Individuals With Bipolar Disorder. J Clin Psychiatry 64:161–174, 2003

Janowsky DS, Leff M, Epstein RS: Playing the manic game: interpersonal maneuvers of the acutely manic patient. Arch Gen Psychiatry 22:252–261, 1970

Katz MM, Robins E, Croughan J, et al: Behavioural measurement and drug response characteristics of unipolar and bipolar depression. Psychol Med 12:25–36, 1982

Kessler RC, Chiu WT, Demler O, et al: Prevalence, severity, and comorbidity of 12-month DSM-IV disorders in the National Comorbidity Survey Replication. Arch Gen Psychiatry 62:617–627, 2005

Ketter TA, Wang PW, Becker OV, et al: Psychotic bipolar disorders: dimensionally similar to or categorically different from schizophrenia? J Psychiatr Res 38:47–61, 2004

Kuhs H, Reschke D: Psychomotor activity in unipolar and bipolar depressive patients. Psychopathology 25:109–116, 1992

Lish JD, Dime-Meenan S, Whybrow PC, et al: The National Depressive and Manic-Depressive Association (DMDA) survey of bipolar members. J Affect Disord 31:281–294, 1994

Livianos-Aldana L, Rojo-Moreno L: Life-chart methodology: a long past and a short history. Bipolar Disord 8:200–202, 2006

Merikangas KR, Akiskal HS, Angst J, et al: Lifetime and 12-month prevalence of bipolar spectrum disorder in the National Comorbidity Survey Replication. Arch Gen Psychiatry 64:543–552, 2007

Mitchell P, Parker G, Jamieson K, et al: Are there any differences between bipolar and unipolar melancholia? J Affect Disord 25:97–105, 1992

Mitchell PB, Wilhelm K, Parker G, et al: The clinical features of bipolar depression: a comparison with matched major depressive disorder patients. J Clin Psychiatry 62:212–216; quiz 217, 2001

Mitchell PB, Goodwin GM, Johnson GF, et al: Diagnostic guidelines for bipolar depression: a probabilistic approach. Bipolar Disord 10:144–152, 2008

Moreno C, Laje G, Blanco C, et al: National trends in the outpatient diagnosis and treatment of bipolar disorder in youth. Arch Gen Psychiatry 64:1032–1039, 2007

Olfson M, Das AK, Gameroff MJ, et al: Bipolar depression in a low-income primary care clinic. Am J Psychiatry 162:2146–2151, 2005

Othmer E, Penick EC, Powell BJ: The Psychiatric Diagnostic Interview (PDI). Los Angeles, CA, Western Psychological Services, 1981

Othmer E, Desouza CM, Penick EC, et al: Indicators of mania in depressed outpatients: a retrospective analysis of data from the Kansas 1500 study. J Clin Psychiatry 68:47–51, 2007

Papadimitriou GN, Dikeos DG, Daskalopoulou EG, et al: Co-occurrence of disturbed sleep and appetite loss differentiates between unipolar and bipolar depressive episodes. Prog Neuropsychopharmacol Biol Psychiatry 26:1041–1045, 2002

Parker G, Roy K, Wilhelm K, et al: The nature of bipolar depression: implications for the definition of melancholia. J Affect Disord 59:217–224, 2000

Perlis RH, Miyahara S, Marangell LB, et al: Long-term implications of early onset in bipolar disorder: data from the first 1000 participants in the Systematic Treatment Enhancement Program for Bipolar Disorder (STEP-BD). Biol Psychiatry 55:875–881, 2004

Perlis RH, Brown E, Baker RW, et al: Clinical features of bipolar depression versus major depressive disorder in large multicenter trials. Am J Psychiatry 163:225–231, 2006

Perris C: A study of bipolar (manic-depressive) and unipolar recurrent depressive psychoses. Acta Psychiatr Scand Suppl 194:1–189, 1966

Popescu C, Ionescu R, Jipescu I, et al: Psychomotor functioning in unipolar and bipolar affective disorders. Rom J Neurol Psychiatry 29:17–33, 1991

Regier DA, Farmer ME, Rae DS, et al: Comorbidity of mental disorders with alcohol and other drug abuse: results from the Epidemiologic Catchment Area (ECA) study. JAMA 264:2511–2518, 1990

Sachs GS: Strategies for improving treatment of bipolar disorder: integration of measurement and management. Acta Psychiatr Scand Suppl 422:7–17, 2004

Serretti A, Mandelli L, Lattuada E, et al: Clinical and demographic features of mood disorder subtypes. Psychiatry Res 112:195–210, 2002

Simon NM, Smoller JW, Fava M, et al: Comparing anxiety disorders and anxiety-related traits in bipolar disorder and unipolar depression. J Psychiatr Res 37:187–192, 2003

Solomon DA, Leon AC, Maser JD, et al: Distinguishing bipolar major depression from unipolar major depression with the Screening Assessment of Depression-Polarity (SAD-P). J Clin Psychiatry 67:434–442, 2006

Strober M, Carlson G: Bipolar illness in adolescents with major depression: clinical, genetic, and psychopharmacologic predictors in a three- to four-year prospective follow-up investigation. Arch Gen Psychiatry 39:549–555, 1982

CHAPTER 4

Multiphase Treatment Strategy for Bipolar Disorders

Terence A. Ketter, M.D.
Po W. Wang, M.D.
Jenifer L. Culver, Ph.D.

The treatment of bipolar disorders is challenging for multiple reasons. As described in the preceding chapters, bipolar disorders constitute a heterogeneous group of illnesses with varying mood symptoms, courses of illness, and comorbid conditions and thus are inherently complex. Nevertheless, efforts to conceptualize how to manage these conditions have met with some success. Bipolar disorder subtype and current phase of illness, described in the preceding chapters, are crucial determinants of appropriate treatment. In this chapter, we first consider illness transition points and then consider how these have been integrated with mood disorder illness phase knowledge to devise the multiphase treatment strategy, a systematic approach to the treatment of mood disorders in general and bipolar disorders in particular.

Illness Transition Points (The Five R's)

Since the 1990s, there have been substantial efforts to define illness transition points (i.e., crucial junctures during the course of mood disorders) to provide researchers and clinicians with the concepts and terms necessary to approach treatment in a comprehensive, systematic fashion (Frank et al. 1991; Kupfer 1991; Rush et al. 2006; Sachs et al. 2002). Five particularly crucial illness transition points have emerged—namely, response, remission, recovery, relapse, and recurrence (Table 4–1). The effort needed to master these terms is well spent because it provides one with a lexicon not only to better understand published clinical trials but also to provide a foundation for the systematic clinical management of bipolar disorders in individual patients.

Response is defined as the emergence of clinically significant improvement on administration of an intervention (Table 4–1; Figure 4–1). Response is most often defined in relative terms, such as attaining a 50% or greater decrease in mania or depression ratings. The *response rate* (percentage of patients achieving response) is commonly used in clinical trials as a secondary outcome measure that has greater clinical relevance (but less statistical power) than the most common primary outcome measure of change in mania or depression ratings from before to after treatment. If response is attained and tolerability is adequate, then the intervention is considered to be sufficiently beneficial to continue its administration, although additional interventions still may be necessary. Response is commonly, but not always, associated with a sufficient decrease in symptoms so that the patient no longer meets criteria for a syndromal mood episode (Figure 4–1).

TABLE 4–1.   Mood disorder illness transition points (the five R's)

Response

Clinically significant (e.g., ≥50%) improvement

Partially suppressed index episode still present

Remission

Virtual absence of symptoms<2 months

Fully suppressed index episode still present

Recovery

Virtual absence of symptoms≥2 months

Index episode ended (i.e., no episode present)

Relapse

Index episode returns after response or remission

Recurrence

New episode emerges after recovery

Source.   Adapted from Frank et al. 1991; Kupfer 1991; Rush et al. 2006; Sachs et al. 2002.

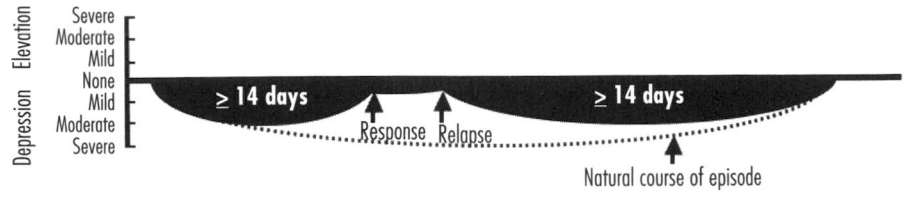

FIGURE 4–1. Response, then relapse.

Unfortunately, in many instances, despite a response being attained, subsyndromal symptoms remain. Persistence of such symptoms can undermine function and quality of life and constitute a risk factor for *relapse;* that is, a reemergence of syndromal symptoms that is thought to represent a return of the original syndromal episode that has persisted, albeit partially suppressed by treatment (Table 4–1; Figure 4–1). Discontinuation of treatment as soon as response has been attained carries a very high risk of relapse, related to the original episode persisting in an attenuated but still viable fashion because it was only briefly and incompletely suppressed.

Remission is defined as the emergence of a virtual absence of symptoms on administration of an intervention (Table 4–1; Figure 4–2). Remission is generally defined in absolute terms, such as decreasing Young Mania Rating Scale scores to less than 9 (Gopal et al. 2005) or Montgomery-Åsberg Depression Rating Scale scores to less than 11 (Zimmerman et al. 2004), consistent with euthymia (i.e., normal or very nearly normal mood). The *remission rate* (percentage of patients achieving remission) is increasingly used in clinical trials as a secondary outcome measure with even greater clinical relevance than the response rate. Understandably, remission rates in such trials are commonly lower than response rates. If remission is attained and tolerability is adequate, then the intervention is considered to be sufficiently beneficial not only to continue its administration but also to obviate, most likely, the need for additional intervention(s). Remission is associated with a sufficient decrease in symptoms so that the patient no longer meets criteria for a syndromal mood episode and virtually lacks even subsyndromal symptoms that, as noted earlier, can undermine function and quality of life and constitute a risk factor for relapse. Thus, with remission compared with response, there appears to be less psychosocial or occupational impairment and better quality of life (Miller et al. 1998), as well as lower risk of relapse (Judd et al. 2000; Paykel et al. 1995; Thase et al. 1992).

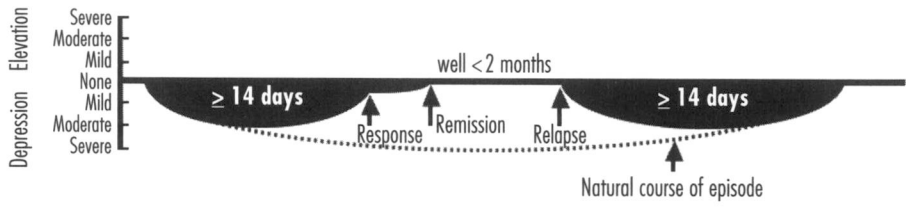

FIGURE 4–2.   Response, then remission, then relapse.

Despite the virtual absence of mood symptoms, discontinuation of treatment as soon as remission has been attained carries a risk of relapse, related to the completely suppressed original episode persisting in a covert but still viable fashion because it was only briefly suppressed (Figure 4–2).

Recovery is defined as the persistence of the virtual absence of symptoms for a time exceeding the natural duration of an episode, which in DSM-IV-TR (American Psychiatric Association 2000) is defined to be at least 2 months (Table 4–1; Figure 4–3). The *recovery rate* (percentage of patients achieving recovery) is occasionally used in clinical trials as an outcome measure, with arguably even greater clinical relevance than the response rate or remission rate (Nierenberg et al. 2006; Sachs et al. 2007). Understandably, recovery rates are commonly lower than remission rates, which are lower than response rates. If recovery is attained and tolerability is adequate, then the intervention is considered to be very beneficial and, in many instances, worthy of being considered as a long-term treatment option. Recovery is associated with a sufficiently persistent and comprehensive suppression of symptoms that the patient can ideally return to baseline function and quality of life. Indeed, the assumption is that the index episode is not simply suppressed but has ended, so no viable covert episode would emerge if treatment were discontinued. Thus, discontinuation of treatment as soon as

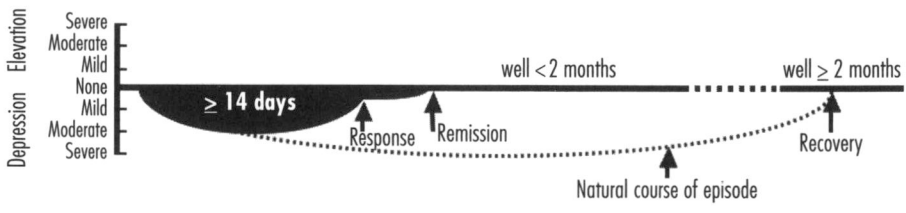

FIGURE 4–3.   Response, then remission, then recovery (ideal).

recovery is attained carries only a modest risk of early *recurrence;* that is, an emergence of syndromal symptoms that is thought to represent a new syndromal episode because the original episode is no longer thought to be present. However, because of the recurrent nature of bipolar disorders, over the long term, patients are at risk for recurrence, and this risk is only partially mitigated because of the efficacy limitations of treatments and challenges with adherence.

Multiphase Treatment Strategy

The multiphase treatment strategy is a systematic approach to the management of mood disorders, based on modification of treatment related to the current illness phase. The foundation of this approach is the notion that there are important differences in therapeutic strategies across three treatment phases: 1) acute treatment, 2) continuation treatment, and 3) maintenance treatment (Table 4–2). The version of the multiphase treatment strategy described in this chapter is based on and extends a substantial body of work by multiple researchers (Keller 2004; Sachs 1996, 2003; Swann 2005). Applications of this approach are found in subsequent chapters in this volume describing the management of acute manic

TABLE 4–2. **Multiphase treatment strategy**

	Acute	**Continuation**	**Maintenance**
Duration	3–8 weeks	2–6 months	Indefinite
Symptoms	Syndromal	Subsyndromal or absent	Absent or subsyndromal
Episode	Overt	±Overt or covert (partially or fully suppressed)	Absent or ±overt
Goals	Response; remission (ideally)	Recovery; relapse prevention; improved function	Recurrence prevention; full function
Priority	Efficacy	Efficacy–tolerability balance	Tolerability
Medications	Increase; add	Continue; ±decrease; ±increase	Optimize; address prodromes
Psychosocial	Support/structure; education; involve family	Adherence; cognitive, behavioral, family; institute monitoring	Adherence; optimize adaptation; anticipate prodromes

Source. Adapted from Keller 2004; Sachs 1996, 2003; Swann 2005.

and mixed episodes and major depressive episodes and the long-term treatment of bipolar disorders.

Acute Treatment Phase

The acute treatment phase is often invoked when patients are first encountered because they commonly present during syndromal mood episodes. However, this phase is also invoked in patients who have experienced illness exacerbation during ongoing treatment. This phase starts with either relapse (into a prior episode after response or remission) or recurrence (of a new episode after a period of recovery). During this phase, an overt (syndromal) mood episode is present. The duration of this phase is the time needed to attain response or remission, which is often 3–8 weeks (common durations of acute mania and acute depression trials) but could be shorter or longer. For example, in bipolar disorders, the acute phase can last for years in patients with bipolar disorders who have chronic treatment-resistant major depressive episodes.

The therapeutic goals of the acute phase include attaining rapid control of mood symptoms sufficient to yield response or, ideally, remission. Medication strategies focus on efficacy and include increasing mood stabilizer(s) to effective or full doses as tolerated and adding or increasing phase-appropriate adjuncts as tolerated. Such adjuncts may include antipsychotics (often second-generation agents) and anxiolytics and, during major depressive episodes, antidepressants or novel agents. Phase-inappropriate adjuncts (such as antidepressants, or stimulants during manic, hypomanic, and mixed episodes) are discontinued because they not only are unnecessary at this point but also can exacerbate the current episode. Additional interventions commonly include structured psychotherapy, including outpatient interventions (such as frequent visits, telephone contacts, and partial hospitalization), as well as inpatient hospitalization, if necessary.

Psychoeducation is an important component of this phase of treatment and includes enhancing the patient's and family's knowledge of bipolar disorders, their treatment, and available resources. Family involvement is crucial to obtain essential collateral information that the patient may not have insight into because of the severity of acute illness. Family members can monitor and, if necessary, administer medications to promote adherence. In view of the risk of intentional or unintentional self-harm, family members may even need to maintain control of medications or other potentially dangerous items in the home. Ideally, the duration of the acute treatment phase is brief, and remission is attained, but improvement may be slow and limited to response.

Continuation Treatment Phase

The continuation treatment phase provides a crucial bridge between the acute treatment phase and the maintenance treatment phase and shares some characteristics with each. This phase starts with either response or (ideally) remission, so that subsyndromal symptoms may be present or absent, respectively. Thus, overt or covert (partially or fully suppressed) mood symptoms are considered to be present. This phase ideally ends with recovery (Figure 4–3), but unfortunately may end with relapse (Figures 4–1 and 4–2).

The duration of the continuation treatment phase is the time needed to exceed the natural episode duration (Prien and Kupfer 1986), which is commonly considered to be 2–6 months in patients with bipolar disorders (as opposed to 6–12 months for major depressive disorder) but could be shorter or longer. For example, if a patient with response (rather than remission) has a very rapid relapse, the continuation treatment phase might last only a few days. In view of the cyclic nature of bipolar disorders, it is not uncommon for patients to oscillate between syndromal and subsyndromal depression, frequently crossing the threshold between the acute treatment phase and the continuation treatment phase. Also, patients experiencing a switch from a manic episode to a major depressive episode may have a brief intervening period of subsyndromal symptoms and hence brief continuation phase treatment. Duration estimates for this phase may be individualized, according to the patient's previous episode durations, but in other instances may not be individualized (i.e., be based on the manic and depressive episode durations seen in populations, with the former being shorter than the latter).

Of the three treatment phases, the continuation treatment phase is the most poorly understood and the least studied (Prien and Kupfer 1986). Although the continuation treatment phase and the maintenance treatment phase are considered categorically different in theory, the distinction is commonly blurred in clinical research and clinical practice (Quitkin et al. 1976). For example, for the second-generation antipsychotics olanzapine and aripiprazole, which are approved as monotherapy by the U.S. Food and Drug Administration for longer-term treatment of bipolar I disorder, the prescribing information appears to resemble more approvals for the continuation treatment phase than for the maintenance treatment phase. In contrast, for the second-generation antipsychotics quetiapine and quetiapine extended release, which are approved as adjunctive (added to lithium or divalproex) therapies for longer-term treatment of bipolar I disorder, the prescribing information resembles that for the maintenance treatment phase. Continuation treatment phase information also may be embedded in studies aiming to obtain approval from European regulatory authorities for the acute treatment phase.

The continuation treatment phase is commonly invoked in the ongoing care of patients receiving treatment for acute episodes as they improve. However, this phase may on occasion be invoked when patients are first encountered (e.g., when a new patient is seen immediately after hospitalization).

The therapeutic goals of this phase include attaining sufficient and persistent enough relief of mood symptoms to yield recovery, and preventing relapse. Medication strategies focus on balancing the dual, and at times conflicting, needs for efficacy and tolerability. These strategies primarily include striving to continue full doses of mood stabilizer(s) and adjuncts that yielded remission, as tolerated. However, it may be necessary to decrease doses to relieve adverse effects, or to increase doses to relieve subsyndromal symptoms.

During continuation phase treatment, the illness and its treatment can be in a considerable state of fluctuation. For example, patients recently discharged from the hospital for acute manic episodes frequently have received aggressive treatment with mood stabilizers and second-generation antipsychotics that have yielded substantial hypersomnolence and sedation. These adverse effects may have been tolerated during hospitalization, but they tend to become increasingly problematic as patients strive to function outside of the hospital. Moreover, as patients' biology gradually normalizes (as the now covert manic episode resolves), their ability to tolerate these agents lessens. Thus, clinicians may strive to decrease medication(s) gradually to relieve adverse effects, only to see these same problems worsen. The optimal rate to taper such agents is highly individualized. Tapering too slowly interferes with return of function, whereas tapering too quickly runs the risk of relapse back into the index manic episode.

Psychosocial approaches during the continuation treatment phase commonly include cognitive, behavioral, and family interventions overlapping those used in both acute phase treatment and maintenance phase treatment. Adherence may be undermined by patients and families interpreting symptomatic improvement as an indication that treatment is no longer necessary. Vigorous psychoeducational efforts to instill a healthy degree of respect for the risk of relapse may help address this problem. As patients become more functional, they may take on a more active role in self-monitoring their mood and responsibility for taking medications. Ideally, the duration of the continuation treatment phase is relatively brief and recovery is attained, although, not uncommonly, improvement may be slow and relapse may occur.

Maintenance Treatment Phase

Although the maintenance treatment phase has some commonalities with the continuation treatment phase, it varies markedly from the acute treatment phase. The maintenance treatment phase starts with recovery, so that at least initially, even subsyndromal symptoms are absent, and no underlying current episode is present. Ideally, this phase represents the vast majority of time spent in treatment, but unfortunately, recurrences are common in bipolar disorders, marking an end to this phase and a return to the acute treatment phase. The duration of the maintenance treatment phase is indefinite. North American guidelines recommend preventive treatment after the first manic episode (American Psychiatric Association 2002; Keck et al. 2004; Suppes et al. 2005), whereas European guidelines are more conservative (Goodwin 2003; Grunze et al. 2002), with some tending to recommend preventive treatment after the second or even third manic episode.

The therapeutic goals of the maintenance treatment phase include maintaining stable mood, preventing recurrence, and facilitating a return to full function. Medication strategies focus on tolerability and include efforts to decrease medication burden by tapering off adjuncts that may no longer be necessary. Thus, antidepressants are commonly discontinued but may be necessary in some patients to prevent depression, and this is an area of lively controversy, as described in Chapter 8 in this volume, "Longer-Term Management of Bipolar Disorders." It is important that any medication decreases be gradual to limit the risk of recurrence. For example, rapid (less than 2 weeks) as compared with gradual (more than 2 weeks) discontinuation of lithium has been associated with more rapid and more frequent recurrence (Baldessarini et al. 1997; Faedda et al. 1993; Suppes et al. 1991).

Medication adjustments may be necessary to address prodromal symptoms, which were referred to as *roughening* in the Systematic Treatment Enhancement Program for Bipolar Disorders (described in Chapter 2 in this volume, "DSM-IV-TR Diagnosis of Bipolar Disorders") (Sachs et al. 2002). Such efforts may decrease the risk of subsyndromal symptoms progressing to a full syndromal episode (i.e., recurrence). For example, in patients with bipolar I disorder, without additional intervention within 1 month, hypomanic episodes may progress to manic episodes in more than 75% of patients, and subsyndromal depressive symptoms may progress to major depressive episodes in almost 40% of patients (Keller et al. 1992).

Psychosocial interventions during the maintenance treatment phase are an important component of preventing recurrence (Colom et al. 2003). These interventions include striving to enhance adherence, which, in view of the prolonged absence of symptoms, may be an even greater problem than during the continuation treatment phase. Providing psychoeducation to patients and families during periods of mood stability may confer important benefits because both patients and families may be better equipped to use such information more effectively in the absence of acute mood symptoms. With sufficient education, patient and family monitoring of psychiatric, medical, social, and occupational changes can help detect warning signs of impending episodes earlier and thus facilitate more timely intervention. Increasing patients' and families' awareness of individual patient characteristics such as seasonality, stress sensitivity, and patterns of symptom emergence can help facilitate early detection of emerging symptoms, which can improve outcomes (Lam et al. 2001). Furthermore, during the maintenance treatment phase, interventions may address ongoing self-stigma and effects of the illness on interpersonal relationships (e.g., increased family stress as a result of role changes) and occupational functioning (e.g., decreased confidence at work). Unfortunately, as with pharmacotherapy, adherence to psychosocial interventions may decline in the absence of mood symptoms. Further educating patients and families about the benefits of psychosocial interventions during the maintenance treatment phase appears to be an important component of recurrence prevention.

Summary of the Multiphase Treatment Strategy

The multiphase treatment strategy described in this section is based on the notion that three fundamental phases of treatment (acute, continuation, and maintenance) are related to five crucial illness transition points (response, remission, recovery, relapse, and recurrence). The relations among these components are illustrated in Figure 4–4. Treatment decisions at any given time will be influenced not only by the diagnosis (e.g., bipolar I disorder vs. bipolar II disorder) but also by the current clinical status and treatment phase. In Chapter 5, "Overview of Pharmacotherapy for Bipolar Disorders," Ketter and Wang begin to show the relevance of this schema to therapeutics, a topic expanded on in subsequent chapters in this volume.

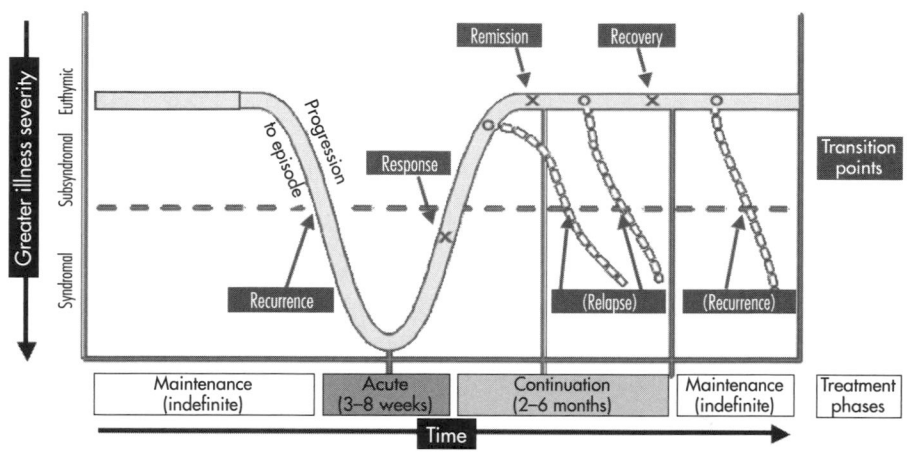

FIGURE 4–4.   Treatment phases and illness transition points for bipolar disorder.

Source. Adapted from Frank et al. 1991; Kupfer 1991; Rush et al. 2006; Sachs et al. 2002.

References

American Psychiatric Association: Diagnostic and Statistical Manual of Mental Disorders, 4th Edition, Text Revision. Washington, DC, American Psychiatric Association, 2000

American Psychiatric Association: Practice guideline for the treatment of patients with bipolar disorder (revision). Am J Psychiatry 159:1–50, 2002

Baldessarini RJ, Tondo L, Floris G, et al: Reduced morbidity after gradual discontinuation of lithium treatment for bipolar I and II disorders: a replication study. Am J Psychiatry 154:551–553, 1997

Colom F, Vieta E, Martinez-Aran A, et al: A randomized trial on the efficacy of group psychoeducation in the prophylaxis of recurrences in bipolar patients whose disease is in remission. Arch Gen Psychiatry 60:402–407, 2003

Faedda GL, Tondo L, Baldessarini RJ, et al: Outcome after rapid vs gradual discontinuation of lithium treatment in bipolar disorders. Arch Gen Psychiatry 50:448–455, 1993

Frank E, Prien RF, Jarrett RB, et al: Conceptualization and rationale for consensus definitions of terms in major depressive disorder: remission, recovery, relapse, and recurrence. Arch Gen Psychiatry 48:851–855, 1991

Goodwin GM: Evidence-based guidelines for treating bipolar disorder: recommendations from the British Association for Psychopharmacology. J Psychopharmacol 17:149–173; discussion 147, 2003

Gopal S, Steffens DC, Kramer ML, et al: Symptomatic remission in patients with bipolar mania: results from a double-blind, placebo-controlled trial of risperidone monotherapy. J Clin Psychiatry 66:1016–1020, 2005

Grunze H, Kasper S, Goodwin G, et al: World Federation of Societies of Biological Psychiatry (WFSBP) guidelines for biological treatment of bipolar disorders, part I: treatment of bipolar depression. World J Biol Psychiatry 3:115–124, 2002

Judd LL, Paulus MJ, Schettler PJ, et al: Does incomplete recovery from first lifetime major depressive episode herald a chronic course of illness? Am J Psychiatry 157:1501–1504, 2000

Keck PE Jr, Perlis RH, Otto MW, et al: The expert consensus guideline series: medication treatment of bipolar disorder 2004. Postgrad Med Spec No:1–120, 2004

Keller MB: Improving the course of illness and promoting continuation of treatment of bipolar disorder. J Clin Psychiatry 65 (suppl 15):10–14, 2004

Keller MB, Lavori PW, Kane JM, et al: Subsyndromal symptoms in bipolar disorder: a comparison of standard and low serum levels of lithium. Arch Gen Psychiatry 49:371–376, 1992

Kupfer DJ: Long-term treatment of depression. J Clin Psychiatry 52:28–34, 1991

Lam D, Wong G, Sham P: Prodromes, coping strategies and course of illness in bipolar affective disorder—a naturalistic study. Psychol Med 31:1397–1402, 2001

Miller IW, Keitner GI, Schatzberg AF, et al: The treatment of chronic depression, part 3: psychosocial functioning before and after treatment with sertraline or imipramine. J Clin Psychiatry 59:608–619, 1998

Nierenberg AA, Ostacher MJ, Calabrese JR, et al: Treatment-resistant bipolar depression: a STEP-BD equipoise randomized effectiveness trial of antidepressant augmentation with lamotrigine, inositol, or risperidone. Am J Psychiatry 163:210–216, 2006

Paykel ES, Ramana R, Cooper Z, et al: Residual symptoms after partial remission: an important outcome in depression. Psychol Med 25:1171–1180, 1995

Prien RF, Kupfer DJ: Continuation drug therapy for major depressive episodes: how long should it be maintained? Am J Psychiatry 143:18–23, 1986

Quitkin F, Rifkin A, Klein DF: Prophylaxis of affective disorders: current status of knowledge. Arch Gen Psychiatry 33:337–341, 1976

Rush AJ, Kraemer HC, Sackeim HA, et al: Report by the ACNP Task Force on response and remission in major depressive disorder. Neuropsychopharmacology 31:1841–1853, 2006

Sachs GS: Bipolar mood disorder: practical strategies for acute and maintenance phase treatment. J Clin Psychopharmacol 16:32S–47S, 1996

Sachs GS: Decision tree for the treatment of bipolar disorder. J Clin Psychiatry 64 (suppl 8):35–40, 2003

Sachs GS, Guille C, McMurrich SL: A clinical monitoring form for mood disorders. Bipolar Disord 4:323–327, 2002

Sachs GS, Nierenberg AA, Calabrese JR, et al: Effectiveness of adjunctive antidepressant treatment for bipolar depression. N Engl J Med 356:1711–1722, 2007

Suppes T, Baldessarini RJ, Faedda GL, et al: Risk of recurrence following discontinuation of lithium treatment in bipolar disorder. Arch Gen Psychiatry 48:1082–1088, 1991

Suppes T, Dennehy EB, Hirschfeld RM, et al: The Texas Implementation of Medication Algorithms: update to the algorithms for treatment of bipolar I disorder. J Clin Psychiatry 66:870–886, 2005

Swann AC: Long-term treatment in bipolar disorder. J Clin Psychiatry 66 (suppl 1):7–12, 2005

Thase ME, Simons AD, McGeary J, et al: Relapse after cognitive behavior therapy of depression: potential implications for longer courses of treatment. Am J Psychiatry 149:1046–1052, 1992

Zimmerman M, Posternak MA, Chelminski I: Derivation of a definition of remission on the Montgomery-Asberg Depression Rating Scale corresponding to the definition of remission on the Hamilton Rating Scale for Depression. J Psychiatr Res 38:577–582, 2004

CHAPTER 5

Overview of Pharmacotherapy for Bipolar Disorders

Terence A. Ketter, M.D.

Po W. Wang, M.D.

Pharmacotherapies for bipolar disorders are emerging at an accelerating rate. Lithium was reported to be effective in acute mania in 1949 and saw widespread use in Europe by the 1960s but was only approved for the treatment of acute mania by the U.S. Food and Drug Administration (FDA) in 1970. Chlorpromazine was approved by the FDA for the treatment of acute mania in the United States in 1973. The following year, lithium received a maintenance therapy indication for the treatment of bipolar disorders. The anticonvulsants carbamazepine and valproate were increasingly used off-label for bipolar disorders in the 1980s and 1990s, respectively. The divalproex formulation of the latter was approved by the FDA for the treatment of acute mania in the United States in 1994. Since 2000, there has been rapid further evolution of the field, with multiple potential new medications and adjunctive psychosocial interventions being assessed for utility in the treatment of bipolar disorders. In this chapter, we provide an overview of recent developments, including the emergence of evidence-based pharmacotherapy in the management of bipolar disorders.

Pharmacotherapy Indications for Bipolar Disorders

The FDA has provided pharmacotherapy indications for 11 treatments for the management of bipolar disorders (Table 5–1). These indications are related to treatment phases. The most indications are for the acute treatment phase, with 9 monotherapy and 4 adjunctive therapy approvals for acute manic episodes and 1 monotherapy and 1 combination therapy approval for acute major depressive episodes. The approvals for longer-term treatment include 4 monotherapy indications and 1 adjunctive therapy indication. With the exception of the approval of quetiapine for acute major depressive episodes in patients with bipolar I or bipolar II disorder, all the indications in Table 5–1 are exclusively for patients with bipolar I disorder.

Although the schema in Table 5–1 is broadly consistent with the multiphase treatment strategy described in Chapter 4, "Multiphase Treatment Strategy for Bipolar Disorders," there are some inconsistencies, primarily related to the continuation treatment phase and the maintenance treatment phase, which in Table 5–1 are combined under the category of longer-term treatment. There are several reasons for this, not the least of which are the challenges of distinguishing these two treatment phases from each other and reconciling such differences to the methodology of contemporary longer-term treatment trials.

As described in Chapter 8 in this volume, "Longer-Term Management of Bipolar Disorders," because of the limited duration of stability prior to randomization (in some instances as little as 2 weeks), controlled trials aiming to obtain longer-term treatment indications commonly appear to best resemble assessments of the efficacy of interventions in continuation/maintenance treatment (Bowden et al. 2000, 2003; Calabrese et al. 2003; Keck et al. 2006; Tohen et al. 2006). In such longer-term treatment indication registration studies, the open stabilization stage and the early part of the randomized controlled stage reflect the continuation treatment phase, whereas the later part of the randomized controlled stage reflects the maintenance treatment phase. Thus, these studies, and to some extent the related FDA indications for some agents, blur the distinction between the continuation treatment phase and the maintenance treatment phase.

In addition, studies aiming to obtain European regulatory approval for the acute treatment phase can include continuation treatment phase information. Specifically, European regulatory authorities require that efficacy studies of treatments for acute manic episodes not only have an initial 3-week, randomized, controlled acute treatment phase component but also have, for patients attaining response, an additional 9-week continuation treatment phase component, which

TABLE 5–1. Evidence-based treatment of bipolar disorders

	Acute mania (monotherapy)	Acute mania (adjunctive)	Acute depression	Longer-term treatment
Mood stabilizers				
Lithium	1970			1974
Divalproex, divalproex ER	1994, 2005			
Carbamazepine ER	2004			
Lamotrigine			+	2003
Typical antipsychotics				
Chlorpromazine	1973			
Haloperidol	+	+		
Atypical antipsychotics				
Olanzapine	2000	2003	+	2004
Risperidone	2003	2003		
Quetiapine, quetiapine XR	2004, 2008	2004, 2008	2006, 2008	2008, 2008 (adjunct)
Ziprasidone	2004			
Aripiprazole	2004	2008		2005
Asenapine	+			
Other				
Olanzapine+fluoxetine			2003	

Note. Years indicate U.S. Food and Drug Administration approval dates. += Unapproved treatments supported by controlled trials. ER, XR=extended release.

is, unfortunately, referred to by the confusing term *maintenance of effect* (Bowden et al. 2004, 2005; McIntyre et al. 2005; Smulevich et al. 2005; Tohen et al. 2003; Vieta et al. 2005). This approach is not used by the FDA, which maintains a clear distinction between the acute treatment phase and longer-term treatment.

The wording of FDA longer-term treatment indications for the treatment of bipolar disorders is variable, more resembling that of the maintenance treatment phase for the mood stabilizers lithium ("maintenance therapy") and lamotrigine ("maintenance treatment"), and, in contrast, more resembling that of the continuation treatment phase for the second-generation antipsychotic olanzapine ("maintaining bipolar patients…after achieving a responder status for an average duration of two weeks"), with the prescribing information also including the caveat "The physician who elects to use [olanzapine] for extended periods should periodically reevaluate the long-term risks and benefits of the drug for the individual patient." Although the FDA longer-term treatment indication for aripiprazole appears more consistent with use in the maintenance treatment phase ("maintenance treatment of manic and mixed episodes"), the prescribing information includes the caveat "Physicians who elect to use [aripiprazole] for extended periods, that is, longer than 6 weeks, should periodically reevaluate the long-term usefulness of the drug for the individual patient." In contrast, the FDA longer-term treatment indication for adjunctive quetiapine appears consistent with use in the maintenance treatment phase ("maintenance of bipolar I disorder as adjunct therapy to lithium or divalproex"). The variability in wording of FDA longer-term treatment indications may be due to, in addition to the brief open stabilization stages in some trials, a tradition of considering mood stabilizers as foundational for all phases of bipolar disorders management (including the maintenance treatment phase) and antipsychotics as being used primarily for the acute treatment phase (especially for manic episodes) but having some utility during the continuation treatment phase.

Four of the five medications with longer-term treatment indications also have acute treatment phase indications, but one (lamotrigine) lacks an acute treatment phase indication. This challenges a basic premise of the multiphase treatment strategy—namely, that maintenance treatment phase interventions arise from continuing to administer therapies that were successful in the acute treatment phase and the continuation treatment phase.

The information in this section suggests that although FDA pharmacotherapy indications for the management of bipolar disorders are broadly consistent with the multiphase treatment strategy, some inconsistencies need to be addressed, particularly with respect to longer-term treatment.

Evidence-Based Pharmacotherapy for Bipolar Disorders

Evidence-based medicine entails "integrating individual clinical expertise with the best available external clinical evidence from systematic research" (Sackett et al. 1996, p. 71). The rapid pace of research in bipolar disorders provides clinicians with not only opportunities but also challenges in integrating the sheer volume of new findings into clinical practice. Multiple (nine) treatments are indicated for acute mania, but only a few (five) have been approved for longer-term therapy, and only two are indicated for acute bipolar depression (Table 5–1). The rapid rate of progress is evident in that more than two-thirds of all 21 indications were obtained since 2000. Because FDA approval generally requires (commonly at least two) adequately sized, multicenter, randomized, double-blind, placebo-controlled trials showing efficacy and safety, indicated medications are typically considered the most well-established management options. However, because of the amount of time required to obtain FDA indications, this list may not include treatment options that already have comparable (two adequately sized, multicenter, randomized, double-blind, placebo-controlled trials) or emerging (one adequately sized, multicenter, randomized, double-blind, placebo-controlled trial) substantial evidence of efficacy and tolerability. Despite the growing number of approved therapies, important limitations still remain in the number of approved treatment options for longer-term treatment, for acute bipolar depression, and for the diverse combinations of medications commonly encountered in clinical practice.

FDA-Approved Pharmacotherapies

Acute manic or mixed episode treatment options with FDA approvals have proliferated in recent years. Lithium monotherapy was the first treatment to receive an acute mania indication, in 1970, followed by chlorpromazine monotherapy in 1973 and divalproex monotherapy in 1994. Since 2000, five second-generation antipsychotics (olanzapine, risperidone, quetiapine, ziprasidone, and aripiprazole) have received monotherapy indications and four (olanzapine, risperidone, quetiapine, and aripiprazole) received adjunctive therapy (added to lithium or divalproex) indications for acute mania. In 2004 a proprietary beaded, extended-release capsule formulation of carbamazepine, and in 2005 an extended-release formulation of divalproex, received a monotherapy indication for acute mania. Some, but not all, of the agents approved for acute manic episodes are also approved for acute mixed episodes, with the most notable exceptions being lithium because of attenuated efficacy in mixed episodes compared with manic episodes and quetiapine immediate-release formulation because of the absence of patients with mixed episodes in the registration trials. For details, please refer to Chapter 6, "Management of Acute Manic and Mixed Episodes in Bipolar Disorders."

Acute bipolar depression treatment options with FDA approvals are substantially fewer. In 2003, the first treatment (olanzapine plus fluoxetine combination) received FDA approval for major depressive episodes in patients with bipolar I disorder. In 2006, quetiapine monotherapy received FDA approval for the treatment of major depressive episodes not only in patients with bipolar I disorder but also in patients with bipolar II disorder. For details, please refer to Chapter 7, "Management of Acute Major Depressive Episodes in Bipolar Disorders."

Longer-term treatment options with FDA approvals are also few. In 2003, lamotrigine monotherapy became the first new treatment in 29 years to receive FDA approval for this indication, and in the following 5 years, olanzapine monotherapy, aripiprazole monotherapy, and quetiapine adjunctive therapy also were approved. Lithium remains an important longer-term treatment option. For details, please refer to Chapter 8 in this volume.

Non-FDA-Approved Pharmacotherapies

Clinical needs commonly exceed the management options supported by FDA indications. In such instances, the next best-established treatments are those supported by at least one adequately sized randomized controlled trial. Table 5–2 provides a schema regarding the quality of evidence supporting the use of various medications for acute mania and acute bipolar depression in adults. In this schema, treatments that have evidence from at least one adequately sized (at least 40 patients receiving the active treatment considered) randomized, double-blind, placebo-controlled trial are considered "effective" (if positive) or "ineffective" (if negative); medications with less compelling controlled data (most often because of sample size limitations) are described as having "inadequate data"; and treatments with "no controlled data" are also listed.

Table 5–2 shows that although 11 treatments have adequate controlled data supporting efficacy for acute mania, only 7 have such data indicating efficacy for acute bipolar depression. Importantly, many treatments have either inadequate or no controlled data, particularly with respect to efficacy in acute bipolar depression.

Acute manic and mixed episode treatment options with controlled data suggesting efficacy include not only the nine agents with FDA approvals (Table 5–1)

TABLE 5–2. Treatment studies of acute manic episodes and acute major depressive episodes in bipolar disorders

	Effective[a]	Inadequate data	No controlled data	Ineffective
Acute mania studies	Aripiprazole[b] Asenapine Carbamazepine[b] Chlorpromazine[b] Divalproex[b] Haloperidol Lithium[b] Olanzapine[b,c] Quetiapine[b,c] Risperidone[b,c] Ziprasidone[b,c]	Electroconvulsive therapy Oxcarbazepine Phenytoin	Clozapine Levetiracetam Tiagabine[d] Zonisamide	Gabapentin Lamotrigine Topiramate
Acute depression studies	Carbamazepine Lamotrigine (small effect) Lithium Modafinil Olanzapine (small effect) Olanzapine+fluoxetine[b] Quetiapine[b]	Antidepressants[e] Divalproex Electroconvulsive therapy Gabapentin Mifepristone Pramipexole T_3, T_4 Topiramate Tranylcypromine	Chlorpromazine Clozapine Haloperidol Levetiracetam Oxcarbazepine Phenytoin Risperidone Tiagabine Ziprasidone Zonisamide	Aripiprazole Bupropion Paroxetine Ziprasidone

Note. T_3 = triiodothyronine; T_4 = thyroxine. [a] Active treatment, $N > 40$. [b] Treatments with FDA indications. [c] Adjunctive (with lithium or divalproex) as well as monotherapy. [d] Negative small open trial. [e] Adjunctive, other than olanzapine plus fluoxetine combination, bupropion, paroxetine.

but also asenapine and haloperidol (Table 5–2). For details, please refer to Chapter 6 of this volume.

Acute bipolar depression treatment options with controlled data suggesting efficacy include not only the two with FDA approvals (Table 5–1) but also carbamazepine, lamotrigine (small effect), lithium, modafinil, and olanzapine (small effect) (Table 5–2). Although lamotrigine monotherapy and olanzapine monotherapy did not receive approval for the treatment of acute bipolar depression, data from large randomized controlled trials (including a meta-analysis of five lamotrigine trials) suggest that these agents may have modest efficacy. Single adequately powered controlled trials have suggested that carbamazepine monotherapy and adjunctive modafinil have efficacy, and it is hoped that adequate controlled trials for additional agents will occur in the future. Although adjunctive antidepressants are commonly used in acute bipolar depression, the evidence supporting this practice is less compelling, and more research is clearly needed. For details, please refer to Chapter 7 of this volume.

Longer-term treatment options with controlled data suggesting efficacy include not only the five with FDA approvals (Table 5–1) but also carbamazepine and divalproex. For details, please refer to Chapter 8 of this volume.

The two main categories of potential new medication treatment options for bipolar disorders are second-generation antipsychotics and newer anticonvulsants. Second-generation antipsychotics generally appear effective for acute mania, and emerging data suggest potential utility for at least some of these agents in maintenance treatment and acute bipolar depression (Table 5–3).

In contrast, newer anticonvulsants appear to have diverse psychotropic profiles but are not (with the possible exception of oxcarbazepine) generally effective for acute mania (Table 5–4). However, controlled trials to date suggest that newer anticonvulsants may have utility for other aspects of bipolar disorders (such as lamotrigine for maintenance treatment or possibly acute bipolar depression) or comorbid conditions (such as gabapentin for anxiety and pain; pregabalin for anxiety, pain, and fibromyalgia; topiramate for obesity, eating disorders, migraine prevention, and alcohol dependence; and zonisamide for obesity).

Special Populations of Patients With Bipolar Disorders

With the exception of a limited number of recent indications for the treatment of bipolar disorders in children and adolescents, all of the FDA indications to date are for adults with bipolar disorders, and none are for special populations of patients with bipolar disorders. These are briefly described below and covered in detail in separate chapters in this volume.

TABLE 5–3.   Emerging diverse roles of second-generation antipsychotics in patients with bipolar disorders

As primary therapies

Aripiprazole—mania, longer-term

Asenapine—mania

Olanzapine—mania, longer-term, depression (combined with fluoxetine)

Quetiapine—mania, depression

Risperidone—mania

Ziprasidone—mania

As adjuncts

Aripiprazole—mania

Clozapine—treatment-resistant

Olanzapine—mania

Quetiapine—mania, longer-term

Risperidone—mania

Rapid-cycling bipolar disorders constitute an important treatment-resistant subtype of bipolar disorders that lack any FDA-indicated treatment. However, results of controlled trials are beginning to provide clinically relevant insights into the management of rapid cycling. Although older data suggested that divalproex and carbamazepine may be more effective than lithium in bipolar disorder with rapid cycling, more recent data indicate that this illness course may be generally resistant to such treatments, even when combinations of medica-

TABLE 5–4.   Emerging diverse roles of anticonvulsants in patients with bipolar disorders

As primary therapies

Carbamazepine—mania, ±longer-term, ±rapid cycling

Divalproex—mania, ±longer-term, ±rapid cycling

Lamotrigine—longer-term, ±depression, ±rapid cycling

Oxcarbazepine—±mania

As adjuncts for comorbid conditions

Benzodiazepines—anxiety, insomnia, agitation

Gabapentin—anxiety, insomnia, pain

Pregabalin—anxiety, pain, fibromyalgia

Topiramate—obesity, eating disorders, migraine, alcoholism

Zonisamide—±obesity, ±eating disorders

tions are used. Controlled data support the efficacy of lamotrigine among bipolar II patients with rapid cycling and risperidone long-acting injectable formulation in bipolar disorders associated with frequent relapse. More limited evidence suggests that the potential efficacy of other second-generation antipsychotics such as olanzapine, aripiprazole, and quetiapine in patients with rapid cycling is worth systematically exploring. For details, please refer to Chapter 9 of this volume, "Management of Rapid-Cycling Bipolar Disorders."

Children and adolescents with bipolar disorders constitute an important special population. To date, few treatments have received FDA approval for children and adolescents with bipolar disorder, and controlled data are limited. Lithium was the first agent approved for the treatment of mania in adolescents (age 12 years and older). Risperidone monotherapy, aripiprazole monotherapy, and adjunctive therapy have been approved for the treatment of acute manic episodes in this population. Additional controlled data suggest that olanzapine, quetiapine, and ziprasidone monotherapy have efficacy in acute mania as well. Research is advancing in this area. For details, please refer to Chapter 10, "Management Bipolar Disorders in Children and Adolescents."

Women with bipolar disorders constitute another subgroup of patients who lack specific FDA-indicated treatments and historically have been inadequately studied. Controlled data in this area remain limited, but recent research is yielding information about therapeutic implications of the female reproductive cycle with substantive clinical implications. For details, please refer Chapter 11, "Management of Bipolar Disorders in Women."

Older adults with bipolar disorders constitute yet another subgroup of patients who lack specific FDA-indicated treatments and historically have been inadequately studied. Controlled data in this area are sparse, but research in older adults with bipolar disorders and other psychiatric disorders is beginning to yield information about the safety and to a more limited degree the efficacy of interventions. For details, please refer to Chapter 12, "Management of Bipolar Disorders in Older Adults."

Clinical Interpretation of Pharmacotherapy Trials Data

A crucial step in providing evidence-based care is the translation of data from clinical trials to real-world clinical settings. Industry-sponsored efficacy studies conducted to obtain FDA approval routinely use primary outcome measures that are continuous variables. Such measures provide robust statistical power to facilitate confirmation of benefits superior to placebo.

In acute treatment studies, primary outcome measures most often involve assessment of change in mood disturbance (e.g., mania or depression) ratings from baseline (immediately before randomization to active drug or placebo) to end point (completion of participation in the study). Such data are commonly depicted in graphs with the vertical axis representing mood ratings and the horizontal axis representing time, with lines (one for each treatment group) starting at the point of randomization and connecting the weekly mood ratings. With the passage of time, the lines descend (reflecting decreased mood disturbance) and separate (reflecting differences in abilities of the interventions to decrease mood disturbance).

In longer-term treatment studies, primary outcome measures commonly involve time to relapse or recurrence. Such data are commonly depicted in "survival" graphs, with the vertical axis representing the percentage of subjects still well and the horizontal axis representing time, with lines (one for each treatment group) starting at the point of randomization (with 100% of patients still well) and connecting the weekly percentages of patients still well. With the passage of time, the lines descend (reflecting decreased percentages of patients still well) and separate (reflecting differences in abilities of the interventions to prevent relapse or recurrence).

Week-by-week observations in such studies are commonly reported in two different formats: 1) observed cases and 2) last observation carried forward. Observed cases analyses include week-by-week data only for participants still in the study. Thus, as participants discontinue, the sample size decreases each week. Observed cases analyses can be meaningful to clinicians because they reflect "best-case scenarios"; that is, what happens in individuals who experience sufficient efficacy and tolerability to continue receiving the intervention. However, observed cases analyses are biased and therefore do not provide realistic assessments of efficacy and tolerability limitations of treatments and thus are not used as primary analyses for registration studies. Last observation carried forward analyses include week-by-week data for all participants randomized in the study by using the last observation before discontinuation for all subsequent weeks of the study. Thus, even as participants discontinue, the sample size remains the same week-by-week. Last observation carried forward analyses also can be meaningful to clinicians because they reflect "worst-case scenarios"; that is, what happens over time in all individuals, with an ongoing penalty (i.e., repeating the last observation) applied for participants who discontinue because of poor efficacy or tolerability. Because last observation carried forward analyses may provide more conservative assessments of efficacy and tolerability limitations of treatments, they are commonly used as primary analyses for registration studies.

Response, Remission, and Relapse or Recurrence Rate Analyses: More Clinically Meaningful Benefit Assessment

Unfortunately, the continuous variables described earlier have only limited direct clinical relevance. Thus, registration studies commonly also include categorical secondary outcome measures, which provide less statistical power but more clinical relevance. In acute treatment studies, the most common such secondary outcome measure is the *response rate,* which is the rate of clinically significant improvement (e.g., percentage of patients with a 50% or more decrease in mood disturbance ratings). However, the *remission rate,* which is the percentage of individuals with a virtual absence of symptoms, is increasingly used in clinical trials as a secondary outcome measure with even greater clinical relevance than the response rate.

In longer-term treatment studies, the most common such secondary outcome measure is the *relapse or recurrence rate,* which is the percentage of patients who experience the emergence of syndromal symptoms, which are thought to represent either the return of the index episode (relapse) or the onset of a new episode (recurrence).

Clinical interpretation of such data involves assessing not only the rates but also the differences in rates for the intervention and the control condition. If a statistically significant difference is found in the response rate, then the study is "positive," and one intervention appears to have better efficacy than the other (e.g., drug A is superior to drug B). However, if the size of the statistically significant difference is small (e.g., less than 10%), as can happen with very large samples, then this may lack clinical significance. Thus, clinicians need to beware of "overpowered" positive studies (e.g., with several hundred participants in each group). In addition, "underpowered" (i.e., small sample size; e.g., 10 in each group) positive studies raise concern with respect to their greater likelihood to be published compared with underpowered "negative" studies, risking overly optimistic perceptions of efficacy on the basis of the literature. Also, underpowered studies, whether positive or negative, have inadequate ability to detect low-frequency adverse effects, risking overly optimistic perceptions of tolerability.

If no statistically significant difference is seen in the response rate, then one intervention appears to have similar efficacy to the other (e.g., drug A is similar to placebo, or drug B is similar to drug C), provided the sample was sufficiently large to detect differences (i.e., had adequate power). Thus, clinicians need to beware of underpowered (e.g., fewer than 100 participants in each group) negative studies that may appear to indicate that treatments are equivalent. There is an understandable bias against publishing such data. However, because adverse effect differences are commonly more consistent than efficacy differences, articles with limited sample sizes suggesting that two active treatments have similar efficacy but that one has better tolerability may be published. Specifically, underpowered negative studies comparing two active drugs may suggest equivalent efficacy, but one intervention actually may be superior, and those comparing active drug with placebo may indicate that a potentially useful drug lacks benefit.

Study designs that include not only a study drug and placebo but also an active comparator that has prior evidence of efficacy may mitigate some of the above problems by confirming the validity (or lack thereof) of the study on the basis of whether the active comparator separates from placebo, thus facilitating interpretation. Hence if a putative new antimanic agent does not separate from placebo but lithium does, then the study is valid and thus may be considered a "negative" study with respect to the efficacy of the study drug. Such was the case for acute mania studies in which topiramate failed to separate from placebo, but lithium did (Kushner et al. 2006). On the contrary, if both a putative new antimanic agent and lithium separate from placebo, then the study may be considered "positive" with respect to the efficacy of the study drug, as well as valid (because lithium separated from placebo). Such was the case in an acute mania study in which both divalproex and lithium separated from placebo (Bowden et al. 1994). Finally, if both a putative new agent and lithium fail to separate from placebo, then the study is not valid (because lithium failed to separate from placebo) and thus may be considered a "failed" study with respect to attempting to assess the efficacy of the study drug. Such was the case in a study in which both divalproex and lithium failed to separate from placebo in relapse and recurrence prevention (Bowden et al. 2000). Although the direct clinical relevance of "failed" studies may be less evident, there may be important methodological implications and, if considered carefully, some worthwhile clinical implications, as noted with respect to this particular study in Chapter 8 in this volume on the longer-term management of bipolar disorders.

In subsequent chapters in this volume, preference has been given to reporting results of trials in terms of categorical secondary outcome measures, such as response, remission, and relapse or recurrence rates, rather than in terms of continuous primary outcome measures, such as changes in mood ratings or time to relapse or recurrence, to enhance the clinical meaning of the findings.

On occasion (but fortunately not often), because of the reduced statistical power of such an approach, there may be no significant difference in such categorical secondary outcome measures across groups, even though there was a significant difference in the continuous primary outcome measures across groups. In such instances, this is noted in the text.

Number Needed to Treat Analyses: Even More Clinically Meaningful Benefit Assessment

In recent years, there has been increasing interest in providing even more clinically meaningful benefit assessment. Thus, studies are increasingly reporting number needed to treat (NNT) analyses. The NNT is the expected number of patients who would need to be treated to yield one additional good outcome (e.g., response, remission, or prevention of relapse or recurrence) compared with a control intervention (Laupacis et al. 1988). For example, the NNT for response is calculated by assessing the reciprocal of the absolute risk reduction (difference in the response rates for a treatment and a control intervention). Thus, if a medication and placebo had response rates of 50% and 25%, respectively, then the NNT for response would be $1/(0.50-0.25)=1/0.25=4$. That is, four patients would need to be treated to expect to obtain one more responder compared with placebo. Perhaps a more straightforward way to calculate the NNT is to use percentages rather than fractions. With this approach, the previous NNT would be $100\%/(50\%-25\%)=100\%/25\%=4$. Figure 5–1 provides a schema for the clinical implications of such an NNT.

There is a convention to "round up" the NNT to the next higher integer. Thus, if a medication and placebo had response rates of 75% and 28%, respectively, then the NNT for response would be $100\%/(75\%-28\%)=100\%/47\%=2.1 \rightarrow 3$ (rounded up). Lower NNTs represent better outcomes, with (preferably low) single digits representing adequate outcomes in bipolar disorders.

Figure 5–2 provides a schema for the clinical implications of various NNTs. Unfortunately, very low NNTs (e.g., 1 or 2) remain unattained goals. NNTs of 3, 4, and 9 represent large, medium, and small effect sizes, respectively (Citrome 2008). FDA-approved treatments for bipolar disorders have single-digit NNTs. Alternative treatments worth considering may have NNTs as high as the low teens in the setting of good tolerability and a lack of well-tolerated agents with lower NNTs. Even in the setting of excellent tolerability, NNTs of 20 or more represent options that are unlikely to help.

Example of NNT for response

Assume: drug response rate = 50%; placebo response rate = 25%

$$NNT = \frac{100}{(\text{drug response rate} - \text{placebo response rate})} = \frac{100}{(50 - 25)} = \frac{100}{25} = \boxed{4}$$

	Response rate	Expected outcome in four patients			
Drug	50%	R	(R)	NR	NR
Placebo	25%	R	NR	NR	NR

FIGURE 5–1. Envisioning clinical implications of number needed to treat (NNT).

With a drug response rate of 50% and a placebo response rate of 25%, the absolute risk reduction is 25%, and the NNT is 4. NR = nonresponder; R = responder.

NNT	Advantage (%)	Clinical implications
1	100	Unattained goals
2	50	
3	33	**FDA-approved bipolar treatments**
4	25	
5	20	
6	17	
7	14	
8	13	
9	11	
10	10	Alternatives
15	7	
≥ 20	≤ 5	Unlikely to help

FIGURE 5–2. Clinical implications of number needed to treat (NNT) in bipolar disorders.

Advantage = absolute risk reduction (e.g., drug response rate – placebo response rate). FDA = U.S. Food and Drug Administration.

Number Needed to Harm Analyses: Clinically Meaningful Risk Assessment

Treatments yield not only potential benefits but also risks of adverse effects. In clinical trials, safety and tolerability are commonly reported in terms of rates of individual adverse effects for active treatments (e.g., lamotrigine yields an approximately 10% risk of benign rash and approximately 0.1% risk of serious rash) compared with placebo or with other active treatments.

In a fashion similar to NNT, the number needed to harm (NNH) is the number of patients who would have to be treated before one additional patient would be expected to experience an adverse effect compared with a control intervention. The NNH for an adverse effect is calculated by assessing the reciprocal of the absolute risk increase (difference in the adverse effect rates for a treatment and a control intervention). Thus, if a medication and placebo had sedation rates of 40% and 20%, respectively, then the NNH for sedation would be 100%/(40%−20%)=100%/20%=5. That is, five patients would need to be treated to expect to encounter one more with sedation compared with placebo. Figure 5–3 provides a schema for the clinical implications of such an NNH. There is a convention to "round up" the NNH to the next higher integer. Higher NNHs represent better outcomes, with double digits representing adequate outcomes, depending on the degree of severity of the poor outcome. Because treatments more

Example of NNH for sedation
Assume: drug sedation rate = 40%; placebo sedation rate = 20%

$$NNH = \frac{100}{(\text{drug sedation rate} - \text{placebo sedation rate})} = \frac{100}{(40 - 20)} = \frac{100}{20} = \boxed{5}$$

	Sedation rate (%)	Expected outcome in five patients				
Drug	40	S	(S)	NS	NS	NS
Placebo	20	S	NS	NS	NS	NS

FIGURE 5–3.   **Envisioning clinical implications of number needed to harm (NNH).**

With a drug sedation rate of 40% and a placebo sedation rate of 20%, the absolute risk increase is 20%, and the NNH is 5. NS = no sedation; S = sedation.

likely to help rather than harm are preferred, we strive for interventions with a lower NNT than NNH.

Interpreting Number Needed to Treat Analyses in Bipolar Disorders

In the subsequent chapters, in addition to response, remission, and relapse or recurrence rate analyses, NNT analyses are reported for treatments for bipolar disorders. Figure 5–4 provides sample NNT calculations for bipolar disorder treatments. For example, as described by Ketter and Wang in greater detail in Chapter 6, on the management of acute manic and mixed episodes in bipolar disorders, data from contemporary registration trials of agents approved for acute manic and mixed episodes indicate that the pooled response rate for all approved treatments is 51.0% and for placebo is 29.5%. This yields an NNT for response of 5 (Figure 5–4, top). Thus, clinicians who administer an approved medication for acute manic and mixed episodes can expect to need to treat five patients to yield one more response compared with that expected with placebo.

Similarly, as described by Ketter and Wang in greater detail in Chapter 8, on the longer-term management of bipolar disorders, data from contemporary registration trials of agents approved for longer-term monotherapy treatment indicate that the pooled relapse or recurrence rate for all approved treatments is 44.9% and for placebo is 63.9%. This yields an NNT for prevention of relapse or recurrence of 6 (Figure 5–4, bottom). Thus, clinicians who administer an approved medication for longer-term treatment can expect to need to treat six pa-

Acute mania monotherapy with approved drug
NNT for response

$$NNT = \frac{100}{(\text{drug response rate} - \text{placebo response rate})} = \frac{100}{(51.0 - 29.5)} = \frac{100}{21.5} = 4.7 \rightarrow \boxed{5}$$

Maintenance monotherapy with approved drug
NNT for relapse prevention

$$NNT = \frac{100}{(\text{placebo relapse rate} - \text{drug relapse rate})} = \frac{100}{(63.9 - 44.9)} = \frac{100}{19.0} = 5.3 \rightarrow \boxed{6}$$

FIGURE 5–4. Number needed to treat (NNT) calculations for bipolar disorder treatments.

tients to yield one less relapse or recurrence compared with that expected with placebo.

Such NNTs reflect the clinical reality of treating bipolar disorders, which commonly entails multiple trials of different medications alone and in combination in efforts to provide effective, well-tolerated individualized therapy. In clinical practice, monotherapy is the exception rather than the rule, and patients are commonly taking multiple medications. However, participants in the registration clinical trials underlying the NNTs provided may have had more challenging illness and treatment resistance than do those encountered in community settings. Thus, in community practice, providers may experience more encouraging results (i.e., lower NNTs). However, as described later in this chapter in the section "Efficacy-Effectiveness Gap," the strict entry criteria for registration clinical trials (e.g., patients have minimal psychiatric and medical comorbidity) may yield findings that fail to translate to more complex clinical environments. Thus, in community practice, providers treating complex psychiatric and medical comorbidities may experience less encouraging results (i.e., higher NNTs).

Figure 5–5 and Table 5–5 provide NNTs in bipolar disorders according to data from contemporary registration trials of agents approved for the treatment of different phases of bipolar disorders. Data for selected unapproved medications with multicenter, randomized, double-blind, placebo-controlled trials are also included in Table 5–5. Note that approved treatments (as well as some unapproved treatments) have single-digit NNTs. On occasion, if only a few approved treatments exist that entail substantive risks of adverse effects (e.g., in acute bipolar depression), use of an unapproved agent with a slightly higher NNT but substantive tolerability advantages (e.g., lamotrigine for bipolar depression, NNT=12) may be considered. Options with much higher NNTs (e.g., aripiprazole for bipolar depression, NNT=44) would be unlikely to yield benefit.

Likelihood to Be Helped or Harmed Analyses: Clinically Meaningful Benefit-to-Risk Ratio Assessment

Making optimal clinical management decisions entails considering not only NNTs but also NNHs, as well as diagnosis, illness phase, and individual patient characteristics and preferences. Thus, in the treatment of acute severe illness, as in the acute treatment phase of a manic episode, a lower NNT (i.e., greater efficacy) may mitigate a lower NNH (i.e., more adverse effect risk). For example, olanzapine in acute mania (NNT=5) may be chosen despite the risks of sedation and weight gain. However, in longer-term treatment of relatively stable

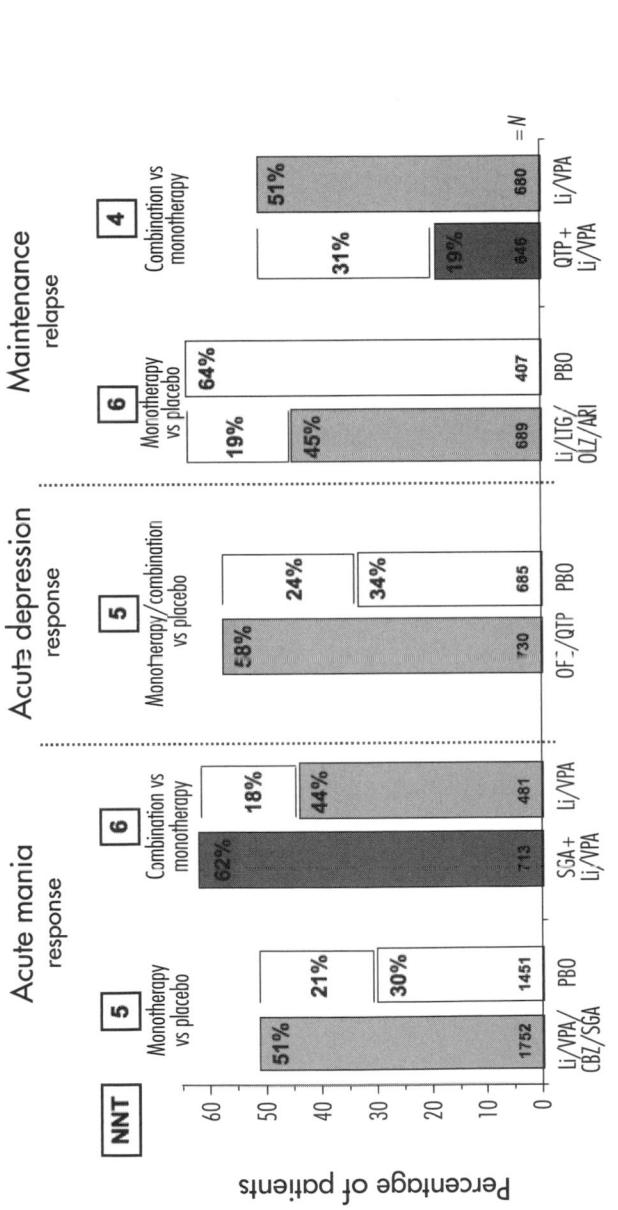

FIGURE 5–5. Overview of bipolar disorder registration studies.

Numbers needed to treat (NNTs) for response and relapse prevention; and response and relapse rates and differences used to calculate NNTs. ARI=aripiprazole; CBZ=carbamazepine; Li=lithium; LTG=lamotrigine; OFC=olanzapine plus fluoxetine combination; OLZ=olanzapine; PBO=placebo; QTP=quetiapine; SGA=second-generation antipsychotics; VPA=valproate.

TABLE 5–5. Numbers needed to treat (NNTs) in bipolar disorders

	Acute mania (monotherapy)	Acute mania (adjunctive)	Acute depression	Longer-term treatment
Mood stabilizers				
Lithium[a]	4[a]			7[a]
Divalproex, divalproex ER[a]	7[a]			8
Carbamazepine ER[a]	4[a]			
Lamotrigine[a]			12	9[a]
Typical antipsychotics				
Chlorpromazine[a]				
Haloperidol	5	6		
Atypical antipsychotics				
Olanzapine[a]	5[a]	5[a]	12	3[a]
Risperidone[a]	4[a]	6[a]		
Quetiapine[a]	6[a]	8[a]	6[a]	4 (adjunctive)[a]
Ziprasidone[a]	7[a]	7[a]		
Aripiprazole[a]	5[a]		44	6[a]
Asenapine	8			
Other				
Olanzapine+fluoxetine[a]			4[a]	

[a]Drug name and NNTs for approved treatments.

illness, as in the maintenance treatment phase, a higher NNT (i.e., less efficacy) may be mitigated by a higher NNH (i.e., less adverse effect risk). For example, lamotrigine in maintenance treatment (NNT=9) may be chosen because of the low risks of sedation and weight gain.

The likelihood to be helped or harmed (LHH) is a metric that represents the benefit-to-risk ratio (Straus 2002). The LHH is the ratio of the absolute risk reduction (1/NNT) to the absolute risk increase (1/NNH); that is, (1/NNT)/ (1/NNH)=NNH/NNT. Thus, if a medication had an NNT for response of 5 and an NNH for weight gain of 10, then the LHH would be 10/5=2. That is, the likelihood of being helped (i.e., responding) is twice that of the likelihood of being harmed (i.e., experiencing weight gain). Higher LHHs represent better outcomes, with values greater than 1 representing being more likely to be helped than harmed and values less than 1 (before rounding) representing being more likely to be harmed than helped. LHH values representing adequate outcomes will depend on individual patient characteristics and be determined by patient and clinician consensus of balancing severity of illness and severity of adverse effects.

Efficacy-Effectiveness Gap

The industry-sponsored efficacy studies conducted to obtain FDA approval report that simplified interventions (e.g., monotherapies vs. placebo) work under simplified conditions (e.g., patients with minimal psychiatric and medical comorbidity), and thus their findings can fail to translate to more complex clinical environments (Institute of Medicine 1985; March et al. 2005; Wells 1999). For example, such studies commonly do not assess the use of complex therapies; rate of, timing of, and reason for treatment discontinuation; patterns of subsequent additional interventions; and utility in longer-term treatment and in patients with comorbid disorders.

Thus, scant data are available regarding the utility of medications in the heterogeneous groups of bipolar disorder patients with complex psychiatric and medical comorbidities who are already receiving complex combination therapies that are commonly encountered in clinical practice. Indeed, there appear to be substantial challenges in generalizing findings from efficacy studies in research populations to more complex "real world" patients. Effectiveness studies attempt to bridge this gap (Table 5–6) by involving more heterogeneous clinical samples, more complex treatment regimens, and more clinically relevant outcome measures such as recovery (Nierenberg et al. 2006; Sachs et al.

TABLE 5–6.   Comparison of efficacy and effectiveness trials

Factor	Efficacy trials	Effectiveness trials
Inclusion criteria	Restrictive	Broad
Intervention(s)	Simple (e.g., one drug vs. placebo)	Complex (e.g., combination therapies)
Outcomes	Theoretical (e.g., rating scales)	Practical (e.g., recovery)
End points	One	Commonly more than one
Clinical relevance	Less	More
Validity	Internal	External (generalizability, applicability)

Source.   Adapted from Gartlehner et al. 2006; Meyer 2007; Nasrallah 2007.

2007) or all-cause discontinuation (Lieberman et al. 2005). The National Institute of Mental Health has sponsored several such studies, including the Systematic Treatment Enhancement Program for Bipolar Disorder (Sachs et al. 2003).

The subsequent chapters describing pharmacotherapy for bipolar disorders integrate information from the numerous efficacy studies to date with emerging data from an increasing number of effectiveness studies to provide clinicians with the knowledge necessary to offer state-of-the-art evidence-based care. Florida Best Practice Medication Guidelines are provided in Appendix A, and Quick Reference Medication Facts are provided in Appendix B to assist in this endeavor.

References

Bowden CL, Brugger AM, Swann AC, et al: Efficacy of divalproex vs lithium and placebo in the treatment of mania. The Depakote Mania Study Group. JAMA 271:918–924, 1994

Bowden CL, Calabrese JR, McElroy SL, et al: A randomized, placebo-controlled 12-month trial of divalproex and lithium in treatment of outpatients with bipolar I disorder. Divalproex Maintenance Study Group. Arch Gen Psychiatry 57:481–489, 2000

Bowden CL, Calabrese JR, Sachs G, et al: A placebo-controlled 18-month trial of lamotrigine and lithium maintenance treatment in recently manic or hypomanic patients with bipolar I disorder. Arch Gen Psychiatry 60:392–400, 2003

Bowden CL, Myers JE, Grossman F, et al: Risperidone in combination with mood stabilizers: a 10-week continuation phase study in bipolar I disorder. J Clin Psychiatry 65:707–714, 2004

Bowden CL, Grunze H, Mullen J, et al: A randomized, double-blind, placebo-controlled efficacy and safety study of quetiapine or lithium as monotherapy for mania in bipolar disorder. J Clin Psychiatry 66:111–121, 2005

Calabrese JR, Bowden CL, Sachs G, et al: A placebo-controlled 18-month trial of lamotrigine and lithium maintenance treatment in recently depressed patients with bipolar I disorder. J Clin Psychiatry 64:1013–1024, 2003

Citrome L: Compelling or irrelevant? Using number needed to treat can help decide. Acta Psychiatr Scand 117:412–419, 2008

Gartlehner G, Hansen RA, Nissman D, et al: A simple and valid tool distinguished efficacy from effectiveness studies. J Clin Epidemiol 59:1040–1048, 2006

Institute of Medicine: Assessing Medical Technologies. Washington, DC, National Academy Press, 1985

Keck PE Jr, Calabrese JR, McQuade RD, et al: A randomized, double-blind, placebo-controlled 26-week trial of aripiprazole in recently manic patients with bipolar I disorder. J Clin Psychiatry 67:626–637, 2006

Kushner SF, Khan A, Lane R, et al: Topiramate monotherapy in the management of acute mania: results of four double-blind placebo-controlled trials. Bipolar Disord 8:15–27, 2006

Laupacis A, Sackett DL, Roberts RS: An assessment of clinically useful measures of the consequences of treatment. N Engl J Med 318:1728–1733, 1988

Lieberman JA, Stroup TS, McEvoy JP, et al: Effectiveness of antipsychotic drugs in patients with chronic schizophrenia. N Engl J Med 353:1209–1223, 2005

March JS, Silva SG, Compton S, et al: The case for practical clinical trials in psychiatry. Am J Psychiatry 162:836–846, 2005

McIntyre RS, Brecher M, Paulsson B, et al: Quetiapine or haloperidol as monotherapy for bipolar mania—a 12-week, double-blind, randomised, parallel-group, placebo-controlled trial. Eur Neuropsychopharmacol 15:573–585, 2005

Meyer JM: Strategies for the long-term treatment of schizophrenia: real-world lessons from the CATIE trial. J Clin Psychiatry 68 (suppl 1):28–33, 2007

Nasrallah HA: The roles of efficacy, safety, and tolerability in antipsychotic effectiveness: practical implications of the CATIE schizophrenia trial. J Clin Psychiatry 68 (suppl 1):5–11, 2007

Nierenberg AA, Ostacher MJ, Calabrese JR, et al: Treatment-resistant bipolar depression: a STEP-BD equipoise randomized effectiveness trial of antidepressant augmentation with lamotrigine, inositol, or risperidone. Am J Psychiatry 163:210–216, 2006

Sachs GS, Thase ME, Otto MW, et al: Rationale, design, and methods of the Systematic Treatment Enhancement Program for Bipolar Disorder (STEP-BD). Biol Psychiatry 53:1028–1042, 2003

Sachs GS, Nierenberg AA, Calabrese JR, et al: Effectiveness of adjunctive antidepressant treatment for bipolar depression. N Engl J Med 356:1711–1722, 2007

Sackett DL, Rosenberg WM, Gray JA, et al: Evidence based medicine: what it is and what it isn't. BMJ 312:71–72, 1996

Smulevich AB, Khanna S, Eerdekens M, et al: Acute and continuation risperidone monotherapy in bipolar mania: a 3-week placebo-controlled trial followed by a 9-week double-blind trial of risperidone and haloperidol. Eur Neuropsychopharmacol 15:75–84, 2005

Straus SE: Individualizing treatment decisions: the likelihood of being helped or harmed. Eval Health Prof 25:210–224, 2002

Tohen M, Goldberg JF, Gonzalez-Pinto Arrillaga AM, et al: A 12-week, double-blind comparison of olanzapine vs haloperidol in the treatment of acute mania. Arch Gen Psychiatry 60:1218–1226, 2003

Tohen M, Calabrese JR, Sachs GS, et al: Randomized, placebo-controlled trial of olanzapine as maintenance therapy in patients with bipolar I disorder responding to acute treatment with olanzapine. Am J Psychiatry 163:247–256, 2006

Vieta E, Bourin M, Sanchez R, et al: Effectiveness of aripiprazole v. haloperidol in acute bipolar mania: double-blind, randomised, comparative 12-week trial. Br J Psychiatry 187:235–242, 2005

Wells KB: Treatment research at the crossroads: the scientific interface of clinical trials and effectiveness research. Am J Psychiatry 156:5–10, 1999

CHAPTER 6

Management of Acute Manic and Mixed Episodes in Bipolar Disorders

Terence A. Ketter, M.D.

Po W. Wang, M.D.

Over a period of 24 years, the U.S. Food and Drug Administration (FDA) approved the first three agents for monotherapy treatment of acute mania—lithium in 1970, chlorpromazine in 1973, and divalproex (a proprietary formulation of valproate) in 1994 (Table 6–1). For much of the 1970s and 1980s, lithium and first-generation antipsychotics were the main treatments for acute mania, but this changed as the efficacy limitations of lithium and tolerability limitations of first-generation antipsychotics became more evident, and new treatment options emerged. By the late 1990s, divalproex had overtaken lithium, and in the 2000s, second-generation antipsychotics overtook first-generation antipsychotics. Thus, since 2000, five second-generation antipsychotics (olanzapine, risperidone, quetiapine, ziprasidone, and aripiprazole) have received monotherapy indications for acute mania, and four (olanzapine, risperidone, quetiapine, and aripiprazole) received adjunctive indications for acute mania. In 2004 a proprietary beaded, extended-release capsule formulation of carbamazepine, and in 2005 an extended-release formulation of divalproex (divalproex ER), received a monotherapy indication for acute mania. In

TABLE 6–1. Evidence-based treatment of acute manic and mixed episodes

	Manic episodes	Mixed episodes	With or without psychotic features	Agitation associated with bipolar disorder
Mood stabilizers				
Lithium[a]	1970	–	+	
Divalproex[a]	1994		+	
Divalproex extended-release formulation[a]	2005	2005	2005	
Carbamazepine extended-release capsule[a]	2004	2004		
Typical antipsychotics				
Chlorpromazine[a]	1973			
Haloperidol	+	+	+	
Atypical antipsychotics				
Olanzapine[a]	2000, 2003[b]	2000, 2003[b]	+	2004
Risperidone[a]	2003, 2003[b]	2003, 2003[b]	+	
Quetiapine[a]	2004[b,c]		+	
Quetiapine extended-release formulation[a]	2008[b,c]	2008[b,c]	+	
Ziprasidone[a]	2004	2004	2004	[d]
Aripiprazole[a]	2004,[b] 2008[b]	2004, 2008[b]	2004	2006
Asenapine	+	+		

Note. Dates signify year of initial approval in the United States. + = effective; – = not effective in multicenter, randomized, double-blind, placebo-controlled trials.

[a] U.S. Food and Drug Administration–approved treatments.

[b] When added to lithium or valproate, increases antimanic efficacy.

[c] Up to 3 months as monotherapy.

[d] Agitation associated with schizophrenia only (2002).

2008, an extended-release formulation of quetiapine (quetiapine XR) received monotherapy and adjunctive indications for acute mania. Thus, by the late 2000s, clinicians had a substantial armamentarium of approved treatments for acute manic and mixed episodes.

The FDA indications vary somewhat, commonly in relation to the types of patients participating in the registration trials. Thus, some of the agents approved for acute manic episodes are also approved for acute mixed episodes (Table 6–1), with the most notable exceptions being lithium (because of attenuated efficacy in mixed episodes compared with manic episodes) and quetiapine immediate-release formulation (because of the absence of patients with mixed episodes in the registration trials). For some medications, the indications also include a specification for with and without psychotic features (Table 6–1), although some medications lacking such specifications have controlled data supporting their use in both types of patients. In addition to the approved agents, the first-generation antipsychotic haloperidol and the second-generation antipsychotic asenapine have multicenter, randomized, double-blind, placebo- and active-comparator-controlled clinical trials supporting their use in acute mania.

The FDA-approved treatments are generally supported by at least two multicenter, randomized, double-blind, placebo-controlled clinical trials In most instances, these are 3-week inpatient studies of monotherapy in patients with very limited psychiatric and medical comorbidities. In these trials, in aggregate, the previously mentioned agents with FDA indications for the monotherapy treatment of acute mania have yielded response (at least 50% improvement in mania ratings) rates of approximately 50%, as compared with approximately 30% with placebo, thus representing about a 20% increase in response rate (Figure 6–1, left side). Patients receiving either active treatment or placebo also received additional substantial psychosocial (acute psychiatric hospitalization) and modest pharmacotherapy (as-needed benzodiazepine for approximately 1 week) interventions, accounting for a portion of both the active drug and the placebo responses. Similarly, in aggregate, the response rates for two-drug combination therapy (with olanzapine, risperidone, quetiapine, or aripiprazole added to lithium or divalproex) exceeded those for monotherapy (with lithium or divalproex) by almost 20% (Figure 6–1, right side).

Treatment of Acute Mania: Balancing Benefits and Risks

Comparisons suggest that monotherapy response rates are more similar than different across individual approved agents and across mood stabilizers compared with atypical antipsychotics (Figure 6–2). However, as noted earlier, some

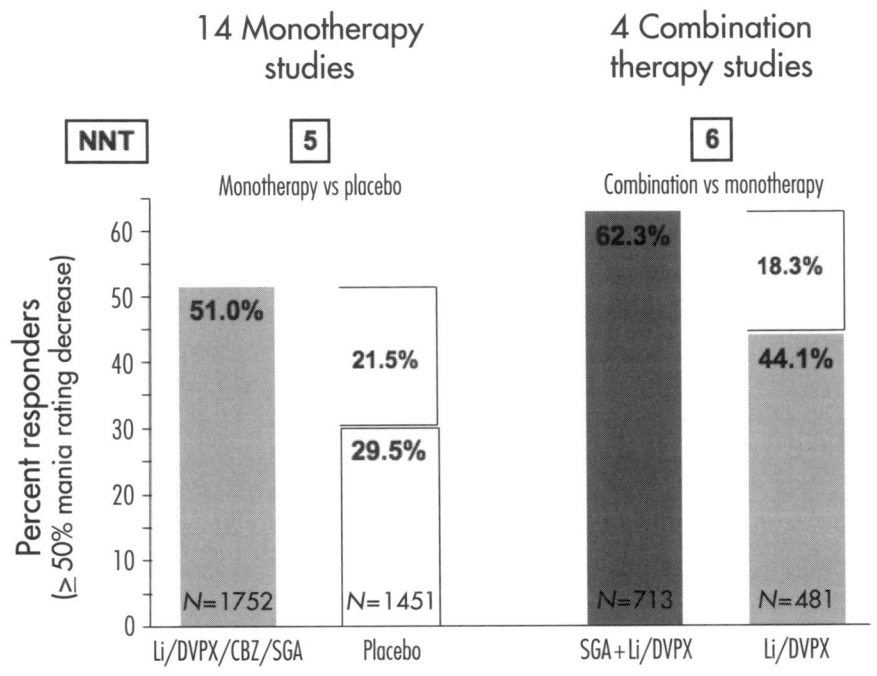

FIGURE 6–1. **Overview of 18 acute mania studies, with pooled response rates and numbers needed to treat (NNTs) for response.**

Pooled data from 14 recent monotherapy (*left;* see Figure 6–2 legend for citations) and 4 recent combination (second-generation antipsychotic [SGA] plus lithium [Li] or divalproex [DVPX]) therapy (*right;* Sachs et al. 2002; Tohen et al. 2002b; Vieta et al. 2008a; Yatham et al. 2004) acute mania studies. Monotherapy yielded approximately a 21% increase in pooled response rate compared with placebo (approximately 51% vs. 30%). Active drug and placebo rates are in part related to both groups also having acute hospitalization and a few days of rescue benzodiazepine. Monotherapy compared with placebo had an NNT for response of 5 (i.e., 100/21.5=4.7→5, rounded up). Combination therapy yielded about a 20% increase in pooled response rate compared with monotherapy (approximately 62% vs. 44%) and an NNT for response of 6 (i.e., 100/18.3=5.5→6, rounded up). CBZ=carbamazepine.

differences are seen in the established efficacy profiles of the approved agents (Table 6–1). Nevertheless, adverse effect differences among individual agents appear to be more noteworthy and are noted later in this chapter and described in detail in Chapter 13, "Mood Stabilizers and Antipsychotics," and Chapter 14, "Antidepressants, Anxiolytics/Hypnotics, and Other Medications," of this handbook.

In addition to data regarding mood stabilizers and atypical antipsychotics, there have been multiple controlled trials of other anticonvulsants in acute mania; however, as discussed later in this chapter, to date, only divalproex and carbamazepine and possibly oxcarbazepine appear effective.

In this chapter, we review the treatment of acute mania, emphasizing findings of recent controlled studies. Such work is helping us to refine our knowledge about lithium, divalproex, and carbamazepine; to appreciate the utility of second-generation antipsychotics; and to understand the limitations of other anticonvulsants in acute mania. Thus, in addition to the mood stabilizers lithium, divalproex, and carbamazepine, we consider two main categories of potential new treatment options for acute mania: second-generation antipsychotics and other anticonvulsants. Second-generation antipsychotics generally appear effective for acute mania (Table 6–1). In contrast, other anticonvulsants appear to have diverse psychotropic profiles, and although (with the possible exception of oxcarbazepine) they are not effective for acute mania, they may have utility for other aspects of bipolar disorders or comorbid conditions.

A Four-Tier Approach

Interventions for the treatment of acute mania are reviewed using the four-tier system presented in Table 6–2. This system is a hybrid approach, combining evidence-based medical information about efficacy and tolerability with more empirical constructs such as familiarity and patient acceptability to prioritize treatments in a fashion broadly consistent with North American clinical practice and treatment guidelines.

Tier I treatment options have FDA approval for acute mania and are supported by the most compelling evidence of efficacy. However, tolerability limitations (particularly in the longer term) of at least some Tier I treatments may lead clinicians and patients, after comparing the risks and benefits, to consider other treatments.

The Tier II treatment option (asenapine) lacks FDA approval for the treatment of acute mania but has compelling evidence of efficacy and tolerability advantages that might make it attractive for a substantial number of patients once it receives approval.

Tier III treatment options in most instances lack FDA approval for the treatment of acute mania and have substantive tolerability (i.e., side effect) limitations and/or less compelling evidence of efficacy than do Tier I or II options. In general, treatment guidelines do not consider these modalities to be first-line interventions but cite them as intermediate priority options. However, some Tier III options have mitigating advantages that might make them attractive

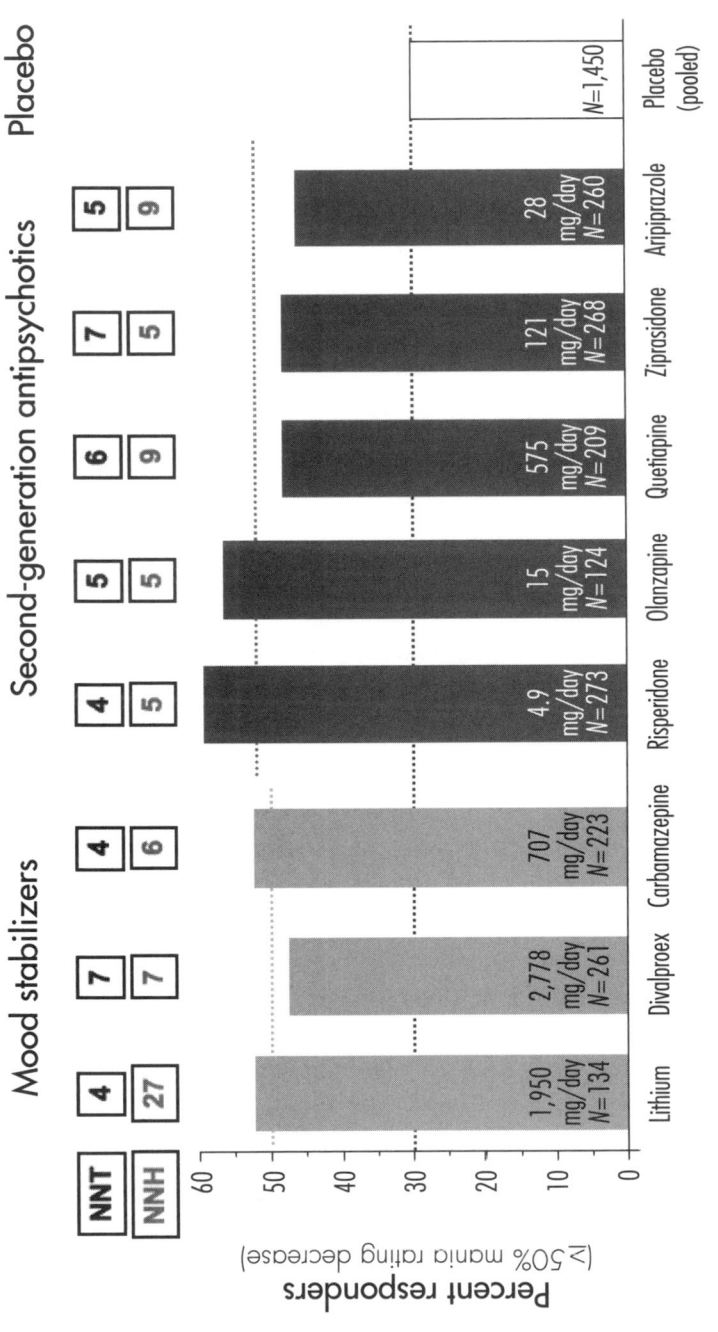

FIGURE 6–2.   Overview of 14 acute mania monotherapy registration studies, with numbers needed to treat (NNTs) for response, numbers needed to harm (NNHs) for sedation, and response rates.

Pooled data from controlled trials of the mood stabilizers lithium (Bowden et al. 1994, 2005), divalproex (Bowden et al. 1994, 2006), and carbamazepine (Weisler et al. 2004a, 2005) and the second-generation antipsychotics olanzapine (Tohen et al. 1999, 2000), risperidone (Hirschfeld et al. 2004; Khanna et al. 2005), quetiapine (Bowden et al. 2005; McIntyre et al. 2005), ziprasidone (Keck et al. 2003b; Potkin et al. 2005), and aripiprazole (Keck et al. 2003a; Sachs et al. 2006), as well as placebo (Bowden et al. 1994, 2005, 2006; Hirschfeld et al. 2004; Keck et al. 2003a, 2003b; Khanna et al. 2005; McIntyre et al. 2005; Potkin et al. 2005; Sachs et al. 2006; Tohen et al. 1999, 2000; Weisler et al. 2004a, 2005). NNTs for response for individual agents ranged from 4 to 7, related to differences in response rates for active drugs and placebo across studies. Pooled studies of mood stabilizer monotherapies compared with placebo yielded response rates of approximately 50% and 28%, respectively, and a pooled NNT for response of 5 ($100/22.3 = 4.5 \rightarrow 5$, rounded up). Pooled studies of second-generation antipsychotics and placebo yielded response rates of approximately 51% and 35%, respectively, and an NNT for response of 7 ($100/16.3 = 6.1 \rightarrow 7$, rounded up). Thus, a somewhat higher pooled placebo response rate in studies of second-generation antipsychotics compared with mood stabilizers yielded a somewhat higher pooled NNT for response for the former, despite similar response rates for active drugs. Aside from lithium, NNHs for sedation are comparable to NNTs for response, reflecting the sedative actions of approved treatments when dosed aggressively as in acute mania. Context of effects is crucial—sedation of extremely agitated patients early in the treatment of acute mania may not yield prohibitive problems but may become increasingly unacceptable as mania resolves and discharge approaches.

TABLE 6–2.   Four-tier approach to the management of acute mania

Tier	Priority	Name	Treatment options
I	High	Approved	Mood stabilizers: lithium, divalproex
			Second-generation antipsychotics: olanzapine, risperidone, quetiapine, ziprasidone, aripiprazole
II	High	High-priority unapproved	Other second-generation antipsychotics: asenapine
III	Intermediate	Other	Other mood stabilizers: carbamazepine
			First-generation antipsychotics: chlorpromazine, thioridazine, thiothixene, pimozide, haloperidol
			Other second-generation antipsychotics: clozapine
			Adjunctive benzodiazepines
			Electroconvulsive therapy
IV	Low	Novel adjuncts	Other mood stabilizers: lamotrigine[a]
			Other anticonvulsants: oxcarbazepine, gabapentin,[a] topiramate,[a] tiagabine,[b] levetiracetam,[b] zonisamide[b]
			Adjunctive psychotherapy

[a]Ineffective in controlled acute mania trials.
[b]Not assessed in controlled acute mania trials, as of early 2009.

for selected patients, and in certain circumstances, some of these interventions may be considered early on (e.g., electroconvulsive therapy [ECT] in pregnant women).

Tier IV treatment options lack FDA approval for the treatment of acute mania and have even more limited evidence of efficacy than do Tier I, II, or III options. Indeed, some of these interventions have been proven to be ineffective in acute mania but may have utility for comorbid conditions. In general, treatment guidelines consider these modalities to be low-priority interventions.

Tier I: Approved Acute Mania Treatment Options for Bipolar Disorder

The approved acute mania treatments include three mood stabilizers (lithium, divalproex, and carbamazepine), five second-generation antipsychotics (olanzapine, risperidone, quetiapine, ziprasidone, and aripiprazole), and the first-generation antipsychotic chlorpromazine. Because of complexity of use and tolerability limitations, carbamazepine and chlorpromazine are assigned to Tier III. As noted earlier and described in greater detail in this section, Tier I options have favorable efficacy (single-digit NNTs; Figure 6–2), although some also may have safety or tolerability challenges. Thus, tolerability limitations of some Tier I treatments may lead clinicians and patients, after comparing the risks and benefits, to consider other treatments.

Mood Stabilizers

Mood stabilizers are considered foundational treatments for bipolar disorders, and three of these agents (lithium, divalproex, and carbamazepine) have indications for the treatment of acute mania. The first-line acute mania treatment options—lithium and divalprocx—are discussed in this section, whereas the alternative treatment carbamazepine is discussed in the section on Tier III treatments. The other mood stabilizer, lamotrigine, as discussed in the section on Tier IV treatments, is ineffective in acute mania.

Lithium.   Lithium was first reported to have efficacy in acute mania by John Cade (1949), was widely used for the treatment of mania in Europe in the 1960s, and received FDA approval as monotherapy for manic episodes of manic-depressive illness in 1970 and as maintenance therapy to prevent or diminish the intensity of subsequent episodes in those manic-depressive patients with a history of mania in 1974. In the 1970s and 1980s, lithium and first-generation antipsychotics were the primary agents used in the treatment of mania. As noted in Chapter 10 of this volume, "Management of Bipolar Disorders in Children and Adolescents," lithium was the first agent approved for the treatment of mania in adolescents (age 12 years and older). However, with the emergence of divalproex and atypical antipsychotics, this changed dramatically in the late 1990s and early 2000s. However, lithium continued to be commonly used, particularly in combination with other agents. Indeed, between 2003 and 2008, four second-generation antipsychotics (olanzapine, risperidone, quetiapine, and aripiprazole) were approved for use in combination with lithium (or divalproex) for acute mania.

Early placebo-controlled studies of lithium in acute mania had randomized (Maggs 1963; Schou et al. 1954) and nonrandomized (Goodwin et al. 1969; Stokes et al. 1971) crossover designs. Despite methodological differences and limitations, these studies consistently found that approximately 80% of the patients with acute mania responded to lithium (Goodwin and Zis 1979).

Individual early studies found that lithium compared with first-generation antipsychotics tended to have comparable overall efficacy, with advantages later in treatment with lithium for achieving remission of the full manic syndrome sufficient to permit discharge but disadvantages early in treatment with lithium with respect to rapid control of agitation in highly active patients (Garfinkel et al. 1980; Johnson et al. 1968, 1971; Prien et al. 1972; Shopsin et al. 1975). However, a meta-analysis of five controlled acute mania trials (Johnson et al. 1968, 1971; Shopsin et al. 1975; Spring et al. 1970; Takahashi et al. 1975) found the pooled response rate with lithium (89%) superior to that with neuroleptics (38%) (Janicak et al. 1992). In some studies, combining first-generation antipsychotics with lithium appeared to yield enhanced therapeutic effects (Garfinkel et al. 1980; Small et al. 1995).

With time, it became evident that although lithium provided impressive benefits in classic (pure) mania, it had substantial efficacy limitations in mixed episodes (Freeman et al. 1992; Keller et al. 1986; Secunda et al. 1985), dysphoric mania (Swann et al. 2002), secondary mania (Krauthammer and Klerman 1978), and rapid-cycling bipolar disorder (Kukopulos et al. 1980).

Contemporary multicenter, randomized double-blind, placebo-controlled trials of other medications, in which lithium was an active comparator, have confirmed lithium's efficacy in acute mania (Bowden et al. 1994, 2000, 2005; Niufan et al. 2008), albeit at times with somewhat lower response rates than in early studies.

Randomized double-blind, placebo-controlled acute mania studies have indicated efficacy when lithium (or divalproex) was augmented with olanzapine (Tohen et al. 2002b), risperidone (Sachs et al. 2002; Yatham et al. 2003), quetiapine (Sachs et al. 2004; Yatham et al. 2004), or aripiprazole (Vieta et al. 2008a). In these studies, mean serum lithium concentrations ranged between 0.7 and 0.8 mEq/L, and as described later in this chapter (see subsection "Second-Generation Antipsychotics"), addition of a second-generation antipsychotic tended to yield more adverse effects. In view of these combination therapy studies, the 2002 revision of the American Psychiatric Association (2002) "Practice Guideline for the Treatment of Patients With Bipolar Disorder" recommended combinations of antipsychotics and mood stabilizers as first-line interventions for the treatment of severe cases of acute mania.

The U.S. prescribing information for lithium recommends targeting serum lithium concentrations for acute mania therapy of 1.0–1.5 mEq/L, which usually are achieved with divided dosages of 1,800 mg/day. To limit early adverse effects, lithium for acute mania is commonly introduced at lower (600–900 mg/day) dosages and gradually increased to higher dosages until therapeutic efficacy is adequate, adverse effects supervene, or serum concentrations exceed 1.2 mEq/L. Clinicians and patients commonly endeavor to have most of or, if possible, the entire lithium dose taken at bedtime to enhance convenience and to have peak lithium serum concentrations, and hence the major burden of adverse effects, during sleep. Euthymic or depressed compared with manic patients tend to be less able to tolerate adverse effects and thus may require even more gradual initiation and lower final dosages. Response with adequate tolerability of lithium in acute mania tends to occur with serum concentrations between 0.8 and 1.2 mEq/L. Serum concentrations greater than 1.2 mEq/L yield increasingly problematic adverse effects, so that clinically it is uncommon to exceed 1.2 mEq/L, despite 1.5 mEq/L being the recommended maximum dosage in the prescribing information.

Lithium limitations include common adverse effects such as tremor, polyuria, and polydipsia that can occur when serum concentrations are within the therapeutic range (0.8–1.2 mEq/L). Increasingly problematic diarrhea, vomiting, drowsiness, muscular weakness, and incoordination can occur with higher levels, and severe adverse effects involving multiple organ systems emerge at concentrations greater than 2.0 mEq/L. Lithium dosages less than 1,000 mg/day are usually well tolerated, whereas dosages greater than 2,000 mg/day commonly yield side effects, but adverse effects are more closely related to serum lithium concentrations than to dosage. Thus, the U.S. prescribing information includes a boxed warning that lithium toxicity is closely related to serum lithium concentrations and can occur at doses yielding close to therapeutic serum concentrations. The prescribing information also includes a warning to avoid lithium in patients with significant renal or cardiovascular disease, severe debilitation or dehydration, or sodium depletion because the risk of lithium toxicity is very high. Other warnings in the prescribing information include the risks of renal adverse effects, including nephrogenic diabetes insipidus, risks of glomerular and interstitial fibrosis with chronic lithium therapy, and reports of cases of encephalopathic syndrome (weakness; lethargy; fever; tremulousness; confusion; extrapyramidal symptoms; leukocytosis; and elevated serum enzymes, serum urea nitrogen, and fasting blood sugar) followed by irreversible brain damage when lithium was combined with neuroleptics—most notably, haloperidol. This issue is considered in greater detail in the section on lithium in Chapter 13 of this volume.

Extended-compared with immediate-release lithium formulations may attenuate adverse effects in general by yielding lower peak serum concentrations and fewer upper gastrointestinal adverse effects (nausea and vomiting) by delaying absorption but can exacerbate lower gastrointestinal problems (such as diarrhea) as a result of delayed absorption. Laboratory monitoring of not only serum lithium concentrations but also thyroid and renal function is necessary because thyroid and renal adverse effects also can occur. As discussed in Chapter 11 of this volume, "Management of Bipolar Disorders in Women," lithium is also teratogenic (FDA pregnancy category D because of cardiac malformations in approximately 1%).

Physiological conditions, medical disorders, and drug interactions can increase serum lithium concentrations, potentially yielding toxicity. Thus, serum lithium concentrations rise with dehydration; sodium depletion; advanced age; renal disease; and concomitant administration of angiotensin-converting enzyme inhibitors, metronidazole, thiazide diuretics, and nonsteroidal anti-inflammatory drugs.

In summary, lithium is a traditional treatment for acute mania. Despite lithium's tolerability limitations and the emergence of multiple new treatment options, lithium remains a foundational treatment for bipolar disorder. As discussed in Chapter 8 of this volume, "Longer-Term Management of Bipolar Disorders," lithium also has a longer-term bipolar treatment indication and is considered a high-priority maintenance therapy by multiple treatment guidelines. Thus, patients with acute antimanic responses also may be good candidates for longer-term lithium therapy.

Divalproex. The anticonvulsant divalproex has been available for the treatment of epilepsy in the United States since 1978. Divalproex received FDA approval as monotherapy for manic episodes associated with bipolar disorder in 1994 (Bowden et al. 1994). By the late 1990s, divalproex had overtaken lithium as the most common treatment for acute mania, in part because of enhanced tolerability and in part because of a broader spectrum of efficacy. Between 2003 and 2008, four second-generation antipsychotics (olanzapine, risperidone, quetiapine, and aripiprazole) were approved for use in combination with divalproex (or lithium) for acute mania. In 2005, a divalproex extended-release formulation (divalproex ER) received a monotherapy indication for the treatment of acute manic and mixed episodes (Bowden et al. 2006).

Divalproex appears to have a broader spectrum of efficacy than does lithium, yielding benefit in patients with histories of lithium failure (Bowden et al. 1994; Pope et al. 1991) and lithium-resistant illness subtypes, such as patients with dysphoric manic (Freeman et al. 1992; Swann et al. 1997) and multiple prior (Swann et al. 2000) episodes.

Two multicenter, randomized, double-blind, active-comparator studies suggested that for divalproex compared with olanzapine in acute mania, divalproex had a modest tolerability (less sedation and weight gain) advantage and olanzapine had a slight efficacy advantage (Tohen et al. 2002a; Zajecka et al. 2002).

Randomized, double-blind, placebo-controlled acute mania studies have indicated efficacy when divalproex (or lithium) was augmented with olanzapine (Tohen et al. 2002b), risperidone (Sachs et al. 2002; Yatham et al. 2003), quetiapine (DelBello et al. 2002; Sachs et al. 2004; Yatham et al. 2004), aripiprazole (Vieta et al. 2008a). In these studies, mean serum valproate concentrations ranged between 64 and 104 μg/mL, and as described later in this chapter (see subsection "Second-Generation Antipsychotics"), addition of a second-generation antipsychotic tended to yield somewhat more adverse effects.

In another multicenter, randomized, double-blind, placebo-controlled study, valproate combined with antipsychotics (primarily haloperidol and/or perazine) was significantly more effective than placebo plus antipsychotics (Muller-Oerlinghausen et al. 2000). In this study, cotherapy with valproate was associated with lower antipsychotic doses and was generally well tolerated, with asthenia as the only adverse effect more common with combination therapy and a low rate of discontinuation for adverse events (2.9% vs. 3.0% with monotherapy).

In view of the combination therapy studies described earlier in this section, the 2002 revision of the American Psychiatric Association (2002) "Practice Guideline for the Treatment of Patients With Bipolar Disorder" recommended combinations of antipsychotics and mood stabilizers as first-line interventions for the treatment of severe cases of acute mania.

Recent studies are helping to refine further our knowledge of the clinical utility of divalproex in bipolar disorders. Thus, divalproex oral loading (initiating at 20–30 mg/kg/day for 2 days and then 20 mg/kg/day) rapidly yielded therapeutic (50–125 μg/mL) blood concentrations and appeared to be rapidly effective and well tolerated in acute mania (Hirschfeld et al. 2003).

A large multicenter, randomized, double-blind, placebo-controlled 3-week trial in patients with acute manic episodes and mixed episodes, with and without psychosis, found divalproex ER to be effective from day 5 onward (Bowden et al. 2006). Divalproex ER was administered once daily in the morning, starting at 25 mg/kg, increasing by 500 mg on day 3, and adjusting to serum valproate concentrations of 85–125 μg/mL. Mean serum valproate concentrations greater than 105 μg/mL were associated with more frequent gastrointestinal adverse effects. The authors concluded that serum valproate concentrations generally should not exceed 100 µg/mL for manic patients with adequate clinical improvement. Clinically significant weight gain (at least 7% increase) was more common with divalproex ER (9%) than with placebo (3%).

Divalproex tends to be somewhat better tolerated than lithium or carbamazepine, with central nervous system and gastrointestinal problems being the most common adverse effects. The prescribing information in the United States has been revised to add rare pancreatitis to the prior boxed warnings of teratogenicity (FDA pregnancy category D, due to spina bifida in approximately 1%–2%) and rare hepatotoxicity. As noted in Chapter 11 of this volume, recent data suggest that rates of malformations with divalproex could be higher compared with rates with lamotrigine or compared with rates with no anticonvulsant exposure (Alsdorf et al. 2004; Cunnington 2004; Vajda et al. 2004). Other warnings in the prescribing information include the risks of hyperammonemic encephalopathy in patients with rare urea cycle disorders, increased somnolence in the elderly, and thrombocytopenia.

In 2008, the FDA released an alert regarding increased risk of suicidality (suicidal behavior or ideation) in patients with epilepsy and psychiatric disorders for 11 anticonvulsants (including divalproex). In the FDA's analysis, anticonvulsants compared with placebo yielded approximately twice the risk of suicidality (0.43% vs. 0.22%). The relative risk for suicidality was higher in the patients with epilepsy than in those with psychiatric disorders.

As noted in Chapter 11 of this volume, for more than a decade there have been varying reports regarding a possible association between valproate therapy and polycystic ovary syndrome in women with epilepsy (Isojarvi et al. 1993; Rasgon 2004). Two recent studies in patients with bipolar disorder reported the possibility of a 8%–10% risk of polycystic ovary syndrome in women with bipolar disorder treated with valproate (Joffe et al. 2006; Rasgon et al. 2005) and have indicated the need for prospective trials to assess this issue systematically.

Valproate has some drug interactions; it can inhibit metabolism of other drugs, including lamotrigine and the active carbamazepine epoxide metabolite. Moreover, valproate is susceptible to enzyme inducers, so that carbamazepine decreases valproate serum concentrations. Additional information about valproate is provided in Chapter 13 of this volume.

In summary, divalproex is an important treatment option for acute mania that may have efficacy and tolerability advantages over lithium. As discussed in Chapter 8 of this volume, although lacking an FDA longer-term treatment indication, divalproex has sufficient evidence of efficacy to be considered a high-priority maintenance therapy by multiple treatment guidelines, so that patients with acute antimanic responses also may be good candidates for longer-term divalproex therapy.

Second-Generation Antipsychotics

In 1994, the second-generation antipsychotic risperidone was approved for the treatment of schizophrenia. In the late 1990s and the early 2000s, second-generation antipsychotics overtook first-generation antipsychotics in treatment of schizophrenia and then acute mania, primarily because of tolerability concerns regarding the older agents and the impressive efficacy evidence base accumulated for the newer drugs. The use of second-generation antipsychotics in mania is described in the following subsections, with additional information about newer antipsychotics provided in Chapter 13 of this volume.

Olanzapine.   Olanzapine received FDA approval for the treatment of schizophrenia in 1997, for acute manic or mixed episodes associated with bipolar disorder as monotherapy in adults in 2000, and as combination therapy (with lithium or valproate) in adults in 2003. Despite controlled evidence of efficacy as monotherapy for acute manic or mixed episodes associated with bipolar disorder in adolescents ages 13–17 years (Tohen et al. 2007), this use has not yet been approved by the FDA. This issue is discussed in Chapter 10 of this volume. A rapid-acting intramuscular formulation of olanzapine was indicated for the treatment of agitation associated with schizophrenia and bipolar I mania in adults in 2004.

Controlled trials also indicated that olanzapine had utility in other phases of bipolar disorders. As noted in Chapter 8 of this volume, olanzapine received an indication for longer-term monotherapy for bipolar disorder in 2004. Also, as described in Chapter 7 of this volume, "Management of Acute Major Depressive Episodes in Bipolar Disorders," in late 2003, the combination of olanzapine with fluoxetine became the first treatment approved for acute bipolar depression.

Substantial evidence supports the efficacy of olanzapine in acute manic and mixed episodes. Multicenter, randomized, double-blind, placebo-controlled trials indicate that olanzapine is effective in acute manic and mixed episodes both as monotherapy (Tohen et al. 1999, 2000) and as adjunctive treatment (added to lithium or valproate) (Tohen et al. 2002b).

As noted earlier, two multicenter, randomized, double-blind, active-comparator trials suggested that in acute manic and mixed episodes, olanzapine compared with divalproex was slightly more effective but had slightly more adverse effects (Tohen et al. 2002a; Zajecka et al. 2002). Olanzapine also has been assessed in head-to-head comparisons with lithium and haloperidol in acute mania. Compared with lithium, olanzapine was somewhat more effective but yielded more weight gain (Niufan et al. 2008). Olanzapine compared with haloperidol yielded similar efficacy and fewer extrapyramidal adverse effects but more weight gain (Tohen et al. 2003).

Also, a multicenter, randomized, double-blind, active-comparator trial suggested that in inpatients with acute manic and mixed episodes, olanzapine compared with risperidone had similar antimanic efficacy but an advantage with respect to depressive symptoms and somewhat different adverse effects (Perlis et al. 2006). Olanzapine compared with risperidone yielded significantly more weight gain but significantly less hyperprolactinemia and sexual dysfunction.

Adjunctive olanzapine (added to lithium or divalproex) was effective in acute mania trials and was approved by the FDA for this indication. However, with combination therapy compared with monotherapy, the efficacy benefit was accompanied by tolerability limitations such as somnolence, dry mouth, tremor, and slurred speech; increased appetite; weight gain; and discontinuation because of adverse events.

In contrast, adjunctive olanzapine (added to carbamazepine) was no better than adjunctive placebo added to carbamazepine in patients with manic and mixed episodes but yielded more weight gain and higher serum triglyceride concentrations (Tohen et al. 2008).

Olanzapine is available in an intramuscular formulation that is indicated for the treatment of agitation associated with schizophrenia and bipolar I mania in adults (Meehan et al. 2001).

In acute manic and mixed episodes in adults, oral olanzapine as monotherapy is started at 10–15 mg once daily and titrated as high as 20 mg/day; when combined with lithium or divalproex, olanzapine is started at 10 mg once daily and titrated to 5–20 mg/day. The recommended intramuscular olanzapine dose is 10 mg (lower doses may be considered as clinically indicated) and, as necessary and tolerated, can be repeated after 2 hours, and repeated again after 4 more hours, for a maximum dosage of 30 mg/day. The most common adverse effects with oral olanzapine are somnolence, dry mouth, dizziness, asthenia, constipation, dyspepsia, increased appetite, and tremor. Somnolence is the most common adverse effect with intramuscular olanzapine. Maximal dosing of intramuscular olanzapine may yield substantial orthostatic hypotension, so that administration of additional doses to patients with clinically significant postural changes in systolic blood pressure is not recommended.

The U.S. prescribing information for olanzapine includes a boxed warning regarding the increased risk of mortality (primarily cardiovascular or infectious) in elderly patients with dementia-related psychosis (an antipsychotic class warning). The FDA has stipulated changes in the olanzapine U.S. prescribing information to reflect the risk of hyperglycemia and diabetes mellitus, and the report of a recent consensus development conference suggested that the risks of obesity, diabetes, and hyperlipidemia with this agent (and clozapine) are greater than with other second-generation antipsychotics (*Physicians' Desk Reference* 2008). Thus, clinical and (as indicated) laboratory monitoring for obesity, diabetes, and hyperlipidemia appears prudent for patients receiving olanzapine. Other warnings in the prescribing information include the risks of cerebrovascular adverse events, including stroke, in elderly patients with dementia; neuroleptic malignant syndrome; and tardive dyskinesia. To date, olanzapine has not been associated with congenital malformations in humans (FDA pregnancy category C).

Olanzapine has some drug-drug interactions because certain enzyme inducers such as carbamazepine and tobacco smoking can decrease serum olanzapine concentrations. Indeed, in a combination therapy study, carbamazepine yielded lower than expected blood olanzapine concentrations, and even though this was addressed in part by more aggressive olanzapine dosing, the efficacy of the olanzapine plus carbamazepine combination was still not significantly better than that of carbamazepine monotherapy in the treatment of acute mania (Tohen et al. 2008). Also, tobacco smoking was associated with poorer olanzapine response in a post hoc analysis of three olanzapine acute mania studies (Berk et al. 2008). In contrast, some enzyme inhibitors such as fluvoxamine may increase serum olanzapine concentrations. Concerns have been raised regarding the risks of excessive sedation and cardiorespiratory depression with concomitant administration of intramuscular olanzapine and benzodiazepines.

In summary, olanzapine, as both monotherapy and adjunctive therapy, is effective for acute mania. Moreover, olanzapine has a longer-term bipolar treatment indication, so that patients with acute antimanic responses also may be good candidates for longer-term olanzapine therapy. However, sedation, weight gain, and metabolic problems may limit the utility of this agent, particularly in longer-term treatment.

Risperidone.   Risperidone received FDA approval for the treatment of schizophrenia in 1994, for acute manic or mixed episodes associated with bipolar I disorder in adults as monotherapy as well as in combination with lithium or valproate in 2003, and for acute manic or mixed episodes associated with bipolar I disorder as monotherapy in children and adolescents ages 10–17 years in 2007 (*Physicians' Desk Reference* 2008; http://www.fda.gov/bbs/topics/NEWS/2007/NEW01686.html). The latter is described in Chapter 10 of this volume. Risperidone also received an indication for irritability and behavior problems associated with autistic disorder in children and adolescents ages 5–16 years in 2006 (McCracken et al. 2002). A long-acting injectable formulation of risperidone was approved for the treatment of schizophrenia (but not bipolar disorder as of early 2009) in 2003. The active metabolite of risperidone (paliperidone) was approved for the treatment of schizophrenia (but not bipolar disorder as of early 2009) in 2006.

Multicenter, double-blind, placebo-controlled trials established the efficacy of risperidone monotherapy in acute mania (Hirschfeld et al. 2004; Khanna et al. 2005).

As noted earlier in this chapter, a multicenter, randomized, double-blind, active-comparator trial suggested that in inpatients with acute manic and mixed episodes, olanzapine compared with risperidone had similar antimanic efficacy but an advantage with respect to depressive symptoms and somewhat different adverse effects (Perlis et al. 2006).

In addition, two multicenter, randomized, double-blind, placebo-controlled studies confirmed the efficacy of adjunctive (added to lithium or divalproex) risperidone in acute mania (Sachs et al. 2002; Yatham et al. 2003).

In acute mania in adults, risperidone is started at 2–3 mg once daily and adjusted by 1 mg/day as necessary and tolerated, within a range of 1–6 mg/day. The most common risperidone adverse effects with monotherapy are somnolence, dystonia, akathisia, dyspepsia, nausea, parkinsonism, blurred vision, and increased salivation and with adjunctive therapy are somnolence, dizziness, parkinsonism, increased salivation, akathisia, abdominal pain, and urinary incontinence. Risperidone also causes hyperprolactinemia, so assessment of serum prolactin may prove useful in patients who have menstrual irregularities, galactorrhea, or difficulties with sexual desire and function.

The U.S. prescribing information for risperidone includes a boxed warning regarding the increased risk of mortality (primarily cardiovascular or infectious) in elderly patients with dementia-related psychosis (an antipsychotic class warning). The FDA has stipulated changes in the risperidone U.S. prescribing information to reflect the risks of hyperglycemia and diabetes mellitus, and the report of a recent consensus development conference suggested that the risks of obesity, diabetes, and hyperlipidemia with this agent are intermediate, being less than with clozapine and olanzapine but more than with ziprasidone and aripiprazole (*Physicians' Desk Reference* 2008). Thus, clinical and (as indicated) laboratory monitoring for obesity, diabetes, and hyperlipidemia appears prudent for patients receiving risperidone. Other warnings in the prescribing information include the risks of cerebrovascular adverse events, including stroke, in elderly patients with dementia; neuroleptic malignant syndrome; and tardive dyskinesia. To date, risperidone has not been associated with congenital malformations in humans (FDA pregnancy category C).

Risperidone has some drug-drug interactions because certain enzyme inducers such as carbamazepine can decrease serum risperidone concentrations.

In summary, risperidone is effective for acute mania, both as monotherapy and as adjunctive therapy, but lacks a longer-term bipolar treatment indication. Sedation, weight gain, and metabolic problems may limit the utility of this agent, particularly in longer-term treatment.

Quetiapine.   Quetiapine received FDA approval for the treatment of schizophrenia in 1997 and for the treatment of acute manic episodes associated with bipolar disorder, either as monotherapy or as adjunctive therapy to lithium or divalproex, in 2004. Patients with rapid cycling and mixed episodes were not included in the original acute mania studies. Recent controlled evidence suggests efficacy as monotherapy for acute manic episodes associated with bipolar disorder in children and adolescents ages 10–17 years (DelBello et al. 2007), but this use has not yet been approved by the FDA. This issue is discussed in Chapter 10 of this volume. In 2006, quetiapine was approved for the treatment of bipolar depression (Calabrese et al. 2005; Thase et al. 2006), as described in Chapter 7 of this volume. In addition, in 2008, quetiapine added to lithium or valproate was approved for the longer-term treatment of bipolar I disorder (Suppes et al. 2009; Vieta et al. 2008b), as described in Chapter 8 of this volume. An extended-release formulation of quetiapine (quetiapine XR) was approved for the treatment of schizophrenia in 2007 and in late 2008 received indications for monotherapy or adjunctive therapy of acute manic or mixed episodes, monotherapy treatment of bipolar depression, and adjunctive bipolar maintenance treatment.

Multicenter, double-blind, placebo-controlled trials established the efficacy of quetiapine monotherapy in acute mania and quetiapine XR monotherapy in acute manic or mixed episodes (Bowden et al. 2005; McIntyre et al. 2005).

In addition, multicenter, randomized, double-blind, placebo-controlled studies confirmed the efficacy of adjunctive (added to lithium or divalproex) quetiapine in acute mania (Sachs et al. 2004; Yatham et al. 2004).

In controlled clinical studies, the quetiapine dosage most often was 100 mg on day 1, 200 mg on day 2, 300 mg on day 3, 400 mg on day 4, up to 600 mg on day 5, and up to 800 mg thereafter, and the mean final quetiapine dosages in responders were approximately 430–500 mg/day for monotherapy and approximately 430–575 mg/day for adjunctive therapy. This approach is thus the recommended regimen in the U.S. prescribing information. Quetiapine XR was started at 300 mg at bedtime, increased to 600 mg at bedtime on day 2, and subsequently dosed between 400 and 800 mg at bedtime.

The most common adverse events with quetiapine are somnolence, dizziness (postural hypotension), dry mouth, constipation, increased alanine transaminase, weight gain, and dyspepsia.

The U.S. prescribing information for quetiapine includes boxed warnings regarding the increased risks of 1) mortality (primarily cardiovascular or infectious) in elderly patients with dementia-related psychosis (an antipsychotic class warning) and 2) suicidality (related to use of antidepressant drugs in patients younger than age 24 years and based on an antidepressant class warning). The FDA has stipulated changes in the quetiapine prescribing information to reflect the risks of hyperglycemia and diabetes mellitus, and the report of a recent consensus development conference suggested that the risks of obesity, diabetes, and hyperlipidemia with this agent are intermediate, being less than with clozapine and olanzapine but more than with ziprasidone and aripiprazole (*Physicians' Desk Reference* 2008). Thus, clinical and (as indicated) laboratory monitoring for obesity, diabetes, and hyperlipidemia appears prudent for patients receiving quetiapine. Other warnings in the prescribing information include the risks of neuroleptic malignant syndrome, tardive dyskinesia, leukopenia, neutropenia, and agranulocytosis. To date, quetiapine has not been associated with congenital malformations in humans (FDA pregnancy category C).

Quetiapine has some drug-drug interactions because certain enzyme inducers such as carbamazepine can decrease serum quetiapine concentrations and some enzyme inhibitors such as macrolide antibiotics may increase serum quetiapine concentrations. In addition, combining quetiapine with antiarrhythmic medications is not recommended because of the concerns about the potential for additive cardiac conduction delays.

In summary, quetiapine is effective for acute mania, both as monotherapy and as adjunctive therapy. As described in Chapter 8 of this volume, adjunctive quetiapine and quetiapine XR (added to lithium or divalproex) have indications for bipolar maintenance treatment, so that patients with acute antimanic adjunctive responses also may be good candidates for longer-term adjunctive therapy. However, sedation, weight gain, and metabolic problems may limit the utility of this agent, particularly in longer-term treatment.

Ziprasidone.   Ziprasidone received FDA approval for the treatment of schizophrenia in 2001 and for the treatment of acute manic or mixed episodes associated with bipolar disorder, with or without psychotic features, as monotherapy in 2004. Recent controlled evidence suggests efficacy as monotherapy for acute manic episodes associated with bipolar disorder in children and adolescents ages 10–17 years (DelBello et al. 2008), but this use has not yet been approved by the FDA. A rapid-acting intramuscular formulation of ziprasidone was approved for the treatment of acute agitation in schizophrenic patients in 2002 but not in patients with bipolar disorder.

Multicenter, double-blind, placebo-controlled trials established the efficacy of ziprasidone monotherapy in acute mania (Keck et al. 2003b; Potkin et al. 2005).

In a pooled analysis of the two pivotal acute mania studies, ziprasidone monotherapy appeared to have a broad spectrum of efficacy, showing comparable benefits in patients with manic or mixed episodes and with or without psychotic symptoms (Potkin et al. 2004; Warrington et al. 2007). In the subset of patients with dysphoric mania, compared with placebo, ziprasidone yielded greater decreases in depression ratings (Stahl et al. 2005; Warrington et al. 2007).

In addition, controlled trials have assessed ziprasidone monotherapy compared with haloperidol monotherapy and adjunctive ziprasidone (added to lithium) in acute mania. Ziprasidone monotherapy was superior to placebo at week 3; in the continuation phase, ziprasidone was comparable to haloperidol at week 12 but yielded less frequent extrapyramidal adverse effects (Ramey et al. 2005; Warrington et al. 2007). Ziprasidone combined with open lithium compared with placebo combined with open lithium yielded a significantly greater mean mania rating decrease at day 4 but was only numerically superior at days 7, 14, and 21 (Warrington et al. 2007; Weisler et al. 2004b). The authors suggested that combining ziprasidone with lithium in acute mania might accelerate response. Ziprasidone plus lithium compared with lithium monotherapy yielded more somnolence, extrapyramidal symptoms, dizziness, agitation, and discontinuations because of adverse events.

Ziprasidone is available in a rapid-acting intramuscular formulation that is indicated for the treatment of acute agitation in schizophrenic patients for whom treatment with ziprasidone is appropriate and who need intramuscular antipsychotic medication for rapid control of agitation, but intramuscular ziprasidone has not been approved for the treatment of bipolar disorder. However, intramuscular ziprasidone appeared to yield benefit at 10–20 mg (up to four doses in 24 hours) in psychotic agitated patients with bipolar disorder (manic or mixed episodes with psychotic features) or schizoaffective disorder, bipolar type, in a subgroup analysis of two similarly designed small, 24-hour, randomized, double-blind, fixed-dose studies (Daniel et al. 2004).

In acute mania studies, oral ziprasidone was started at 40 mg twice per day with food, increased to 60 or 80 mg twice per day with food on the second day, and subsequently adjusted as needed and tolerated within the range of 40–80 mg twice per day with food. Intramuscular ziprasidone has a recommended dosage for agitation in schizophrenia of 10 mg every 2 hours (or 20 mg every 4 hours) as needed up to 40 mg/day. In clinical practice, lower (e.g., <80 mg/day) compared with higher (e.g., at least 80 mg/day) oral ziprasidone dosages may increase the risk of akathisia (Oral et al. 2006), so that optimal titration of this agent may involve avoiding lower dosages to prevent akathisia or abruptly increasing to higher dosages if akathisia develops at lower dosages. Adjunctive lorazepam used in clinical trials may have decreased problems with akathisia.

The most common adverse events associated with discontinuation of ziprasidone in acute mania were akathisia, anxiety, depression, dizziness, dystonia, rash, and vomiting. The most common adverse events with intramuscular ziprasidone in schizophrenic patients were headache, nausea, and somnolence.

The U.S. prescribing information for ziprasidone includes a boxed warning regarding the increased risk of mortality (primarily cardiovascular or infectious) in elderly patients with dementia-related psychosis (an antipsychotic class warning). The FDA has stipulated that the ziprasidone U.S. prescribing information include the risks of hyperglycemia and diabetes mellitus, but the report of a recent consensus development conference suggested that the risks of obesity, diabetes, and hyperlipidemia with this agent were similar to those with aripiprazole and were less than with other second-generation antipsychotics (*Physicians' Desk Reference* 2008). Thus, clinical and (as indicated) laboratory monitoring for obesity, diabetes, and hyperlipidemia may be prudent for patients receiving ziprasidone. Other warnings in the prescribing information include the risks of neuroleptic malignant syndrome, tardive dyskinesia, QT prolongation, and sudden death. In a recent epidemiological study, current use of first- and second-generation antipsychotics was associated with dose-related increases in rates of sudden cardiac death (1.99 and 2.26, respectively) (Ray et al. 2009). Although premarketing studies suggested that ziprasidone yielded cardiac conduction delays, postmarketing experience to date has failed to indicate clinically significant problems with cardiac conduction. To date, ziprasidone has not been associated with congenital malformations in humans (FDA pregnancy category C).

Ziprasidone has some drug-drug interactions because certain enzyme inducers such as carbamazepine can decrease serum ziprasidone concentrations, and some enzyme inhibitors such as macrolide antibiotics may increase serum ziprasidone concentrations. The clinical significance of these interactions remains to be determined. In addition, combining ziprasidone with antiarrhythmic medications is not recommended because of concerns about the potential for additive cardiac conduction delays.

In summary, ziprasidone is effective for acute mania but lacks a longer-term bipolar treatment indication. Sedation, weight gain, and metabolic concerns appear to be much less problematic with ziprasidone compared with some other second-generation antipsychotics, although dosing complexity and akathisia may limit its utility in some patients.

Aripiprazole.   Aripiprazole received FDA approval for the treatment of schizophrenia in 2002; as monotherapy for the treatment of acute manic or mixed episodes associated with bipolar disorder in adults in 2004 and in children and adolescents ages 10–17 years in 2008; as adjunctive therapy (added to lithium or valproate) in adults, children, and adolescents in 2008; and as longer-term monotherapy treatment for bipolar I disorder in adults in 2005 and in children and adolescents in 2008. The use of aripiprazole for acute manic and mixed episodes in children and adolescents is described in Chapter 10 of this volume. Aripiprazole was approved as an adjunctive treatment to antidepressants for major depressive disorder in 2007. A rapid-acting intramuscular formulation of aripiprazole was indicated for the treatment of agitation associated with schizophrenia or bipolar disorder, manic or mixed episodes, in 2006.

Multicenter, double-blind, placebo-controlled trials established the efficacy of aripiprazole monotherapy in acute mania (Keck et al. 2003a; Sachs et al. 2006). In a pooled analysis of acute mania studies, aripiprazole monotherapy appeared to have a broad spectrum of efficacy (Suppes et al. 2008). Thus, aripiprazole had comparable benefits in patients with more severe (baseline Young Mania Rating Scale [YMRS] score≥28) or less severe (baseline YMRS score < 28) mania, with manic or mixed episodes, with or without psychotic symptoms, and with or without rapid cycling.

In addition, a multicenter, double-blind, placebo-controlled trial assessed aripiprazole compared with haloperidol monotherapy in acute mania (Vieta et al. 2005). Efficacy was comparable, but aripiprazole compared with haloperidol yielded fewer extrapyramidal symptoms and less akathisia. Other adverse events observed with both agents included tremor, headache, depression, and insomnia.

Two multicenter, double-blind, placebo- and active comparator–controlled trials indicated aripiprazole monotherapy compared with lithium monotherapy (Keck et al. 2007) and haloperidol monotherapy (Sanchez et al. 2008) in acute mania yielded comparable efficacy and tolerability, although haloperidol yielded more extrapyramidal symptoms.

A multicenter, double-blind, placebo-controlled trial indicated that adjunctive aripiprazole (added to lithium or valproate) was effective in acute mania (Vieta et al. 2008a).

A multicenter, double-blind, placebo-controlled study reported the efficacy of a rapid-acting intramuscular formulation of aripiprazole for the treatment of agitation associated with manic or mixed episodes (Zimbroff et al. 2007).

In early adult acute mania studies, oral aripiprazole was started at 30 mg/day and could be reduced to 15 mg/day for tolerability if needed, with mean final daily dosages being approximately 28 mg/day. However, in later adult acute mania studies, oral aripiprazole was started at 15 mg/day and could be increased to 30 mg/day for efficacy if needed. The U.S. prescribing information for the treatment of acute manic and mixed episodes in adults suggests starting oral aripiprazole at 15 mg/day, which was also the recommended dosage, but if necessary and tolerated, the dosage could be increased to as high as the maximum dosage of 30 mg/day. Because of concerns about adverse effects, and the lack of additional benefit with doses higher than 9.75 mg per injection in clinical trials, the U.S. prescribing information recommends administering intramuscular aripiprazole at a dose of 9.75 mg (rather than 15 mg) per injection, or 5.25 mg intramuscularly if clinically indicated, and repeating 9.75-mg (or 5.25-mg) intramuscular injections as often as every 2 hours as necessary and tolerated, with a maximum of 30 mg/day.

Perhaps because of partial agonist effects at dopamine receptors, nausea and vomiting can occur when aripiprazole is started. Tolerability may be enhanced in patients with gastrointestinal or other adverse effects if aripiprazole is initiated at 15 mg or lower in divided doses for a few days before being increased to as much as 30 mg/day. Adjunctive lorazepam used in clinical trials may have decreased problems with akathisia. Somnolence and constipation may be encountered with aripiprazole, but weight gain is less of a concern than with olanzapine, quetiapine, and risperidone.

The U.S. prescribing information for aripiprazole includes boxed warnings regarding the increased risks of 1) mortality (primarily cardiovascular or infectious) in elderly patients with dementia-related psychosis (an antipsychotic class warning) and 2) suicidality (related to use of antidepressant drugs in patients up to age 24 years and based on an antidepressant class warning). The FDA has stipulated that the aripiprazole U.S. prescribing information include the risks of hyperglycemia and diabetes mellitus, but the report of a recent consensus development conference suggested that the risks of obesity, diabetes, and hyperlipidemia with this agent were similar to those with ziprasidone and less than with other second-generation antipsychotics (*Physicians' Desk Reference* 2008). Thus, clinical and (as indicated) laboratory monitoring for obesity, diabetes, and hyperlipidemia may be prudent for patients receiving aripiprazole. Other warnings in the prescribing information include the risks of cerebrovascular adverse events, including stroke, in elderly patients with dementia; neuroleptic malignant syndrome; and tardive dyskinesia. To date, aripiprazole has not been associated with congenital malformations in humans (FDA pregnancy category C).

Aripiprazole has some drug-drug interactions because enzyme inducers such as carbamazepine can decrease serum aripiprazole concentrations and some enzyme inhibitors such as macrolide antibiotics may increase serum aripiprazole concentrations.

In summary, aripiprazole is effective for acute mania and has a longer-term bipolar treatment indication, so patients with acute antimanic responses also may be good candidates for longer-term aripiprazole therapy. Although sedation, weight gain, and metabolic concerns may be less problematic with aripiprazole than with some other second-generation antipsychotics, akathisia may limit its utility in some patients.

Tier II: High-Priority Unapproved Acute Mania Treatment Options

As noted earlier, safety and tolerability limitations (particularly in the longer term) of some Tier I approved medications for the treatment of acute mania may lead clinicians and patients to consider other options. When assessing alternative treatments, one approach is to consider potentially approvable medications, such as new second-generation antipsychotics. One such agent—asenapine—has not yet been approved by the FDA for the treatment of acute mania or schizophrenia, or marketed in the United States, because the pivotal trials described in this section are still under review. It is anticipated that in the near future, asenapine and possibly other new second-generation antipsychotics will be approved.

Two positive multicenter, randomized, double-blind, placebo-controlled trials suggested that asenapine may ultimately be approved for the treatment of acute manic and mixed episodes in patients with bipolar I disorder (McIntyre et al. 2008).

In a pooled analysis of the two pivotal studies, asenapine and olanzapine were both superior to placebo, yielding NNTs of 8 and 5, respectively (Figure 6–3, left side), but both also caused weight gain, yielding NNHs of 17 and 7, respectively (Figure 6–3, right side). Head-to-head comparisons indicated that olanzapine compared with asenapine was more efficacious (NNT=11; $P<0.01$) but yielded more weight gain (NNH=11; $P<0.001$). Thus, for olanzapine compared with asenapine, the efficacy advantage was offset by a comparable tolerability disadvantage. Thus, for olanzapine compared with asenapine, for every additional responder, one could expect an additional patient with clinically significant ($\geq7\%$ increase) weight gain.

Balancing benefits and risks is a crucial component of treatment selection. For some patients with very acute and very severe mania who lack substantive weight or metabolic problems, the efficacy advantage of olanzapine may make it more attractive. In contrast, for other patients with less acute and less severe mania who have substantive weight or metabolic problems, the tolerability advantage of asenapine may make it more attractive.

Tier III: Intermediate-Priority Other Acute Mania Treatment Options

The management of acute mania is sufficiently challenging that clinical need may outstrip the previously discussed evidence-based treatment options. In this section, we consider other (in most instances unapproved) treatment options with tolerability limitations and/or more limited evidence of efficacy compared with the Tier I and II treatments. These alternatives include other mood stabilizers (carbamazepine), first-generation antipsychotics (chlorpromazine, thioridazine, thiothixene, pimozide, and haloperidol), other second-generation antipsychotics (clozapine), adjunctive benzodiazepines, and ECT. In general, treatment guidelines do not consider these modalities to be first-line interventions but cite them as intermediate-priority options (American Psychiatric Association 2002; Goodwin 2003; Grunze et al. 2002; Keck et al. 2004; Suppes et al. 2005; Yatham et al. 2006). However, some Tier III options have mitigating advantages that might make them attractive for selected patients,

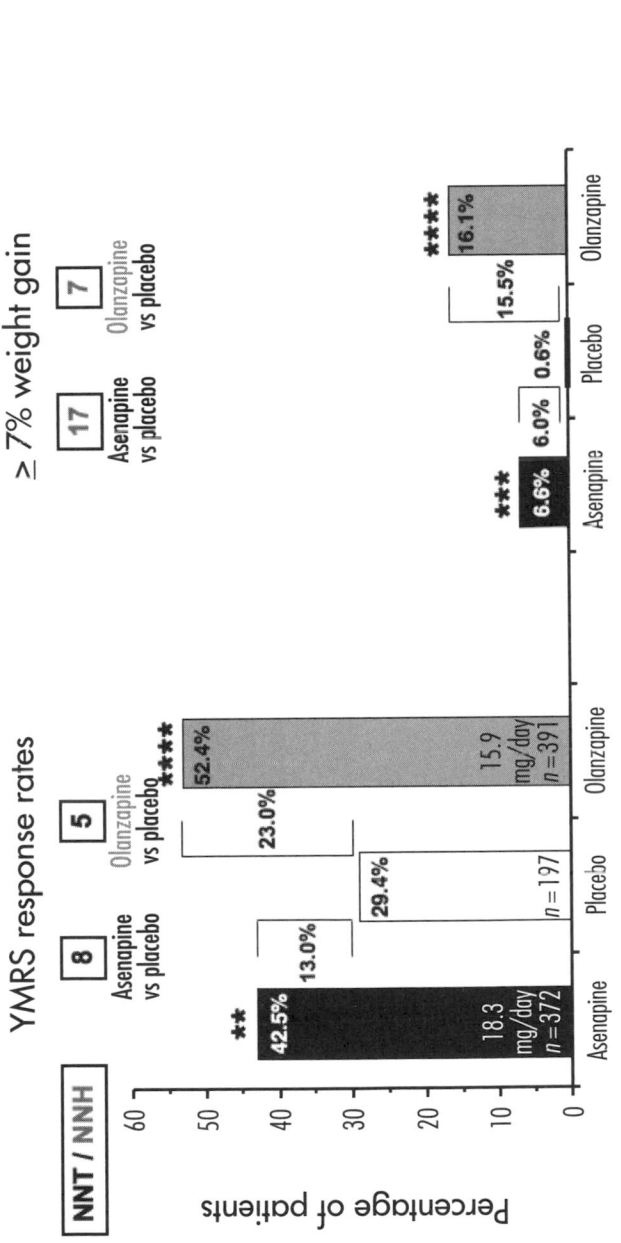

Figure 6–3.   Three-week double-blind asenapine monotherapy versus olanzapine monotherapy versus placebo in acute mania.

Number needed to treat (NNT), number needed to harm (NNH), and response and clinically significant (≥7% increase) weight gain rates are shown. Asenapine monotherapy (black bars) and olanzapine monotherapy (gray bars) compared with placebo monotherapy (white bars) had superior efficacy but yielded more clinically significant weight gain. For olanzapine compared with asenapine, the efficacy advantage was offset by a comparable tolerability disadvantage. YMRS=Young Mania Rating Scale. **$P<0.01$, ***$P<0.001$, ****$P<0.0001$ versus placebo.

Source.   Adapted from McIntyre et al. 2008.

and in certain circumstances, some of these interventions may be considered early on (e.g., ECT in pregnant women).

Other Mood Stabilizers: Carbamazepine

Despite carbamazepine's having approval for the treatment of acute mania, complexity of use related to drug interaction as well as tolerability limitations and less compelling evidence of maintenance efficacy led to this medication being considered as an alternative rather than a first-line antimanic agent. Nevertheless, selected patients who report inadequate efficacy and/or tolerability with Tier I or II options may find carbamazepine a worthwhile alternative.

The anticonvulsant carbamazepine has been available for the treatment of epilepsy in the United States since 1974. In the 1980s, controlled carbamazepine studies using active comparator and on-off-on designs provided preliminary evidence of efficacy in acute mania. Because of economic concerns such as patent protection limitations and the high cost of obtaining FDA approval, a carbamazepine indication in acute mania was not initially sought in the United States but was obtained from agencies in Canada, Japan, Australia, and several European countries. As noted above, the absence of an FDA indication and complexity of use led carbamazepine to be considered an alternative rather than a first-line intervention in acute mania (American Psychiatric Association 2002). However, eventually multicenter, randomized, double-blind, placebo-controlled trials confirmed the efficacy of a proprietary beaded, extended-release capsule formulation of carbamazepine in acute manic and mixed episodes (Weisler et al. 2004a, 2005), yielding an FDA indication for this formulation in late 2004.

Older studies suggested utility for carbamazepine combined with lithium (Kramlinger and Post 1989) or antipsychotics (Okuma et al. 1989) in the treatment of acute mania. However, carbamazepine can increase the hepatic metabolism of multiple other agents, potentially compromising the efficacy of combination therapies (Ketter et al. 1991a, 1991b). In a subsequent study that reemphasized this point, carbamazepine yielded substantial decreases in blood risperidone concentrations, compromising efficacy of the combination in the treatment of acute mania (Yatham et al. 2003). In another combination therapy study, carbamazepine yielded lower than expected blood olanzapine concentrations, and even though this was addressed in part by more aggressive olanzapine dosing, the efficacy of the olanzapine plus carbamazepine combination was still not significantly better than that of carbamazepine monotherapy in the treatment of acute mania (Tohen et al. 2008). However, olanzapine plus carbamazepine compared with carbamazepine monotherapy yielded higher triglyceride levels and more frequent clinically significant (≥7%) weight gain.

To limit early adverse effects, carbamazepine is commonly introduced at low (100–400 mg/day) dosages and gradually increased, until therapeutic efficacy is adequate, adverse effects supervene, or serum concentrations exceed 12 μg/mL. Euthymic or depressed compared with manic patients tend to be less able to tolerate adverse effects and thus may require more gradual initiation. Although response in bipolar disorder does not appear related to serum concentrations, the 4–12 μg/mL range from epilepsy may be considered as a broad target, and serum carbamazepine concentrations may be used as pharmacokinetic checks for extreme values.

Carbamazepine has several important limitations and has boxed warnings in the U.S. prescribing information regarding the risks of serious dermatological reactions and the HLA-B*1502 allele, as well as aplastic anemia and agranulocytosis. Carbamazepine is also associated with common benign leukopenia, which in rare instances may be an early indication of serious blood dyscrasia. Other warnings in the prescribing information include the risks of teratogenicity and increased intraocular pressure as a result of mild anticholinergic activity.

In 2008, the FDA released an alert regarding increased risk of suicidality (suicidal behavior or ideation) in patients with epilepsy as well as psychiatric disorders for 11 anticonvulsants (including carbamazepine). The relative risk for suicidality was higher in the patients with epilepsy compared with those with psychiatric disorders.

As discussed in Chapter 11 of this volume, carbamazepine has the potential for teratogenicity (FDA pregnancy category D), including craniofacial defects, fingernail hypoplasia, and developmental delay in approximately 11%–26% and spina bifida in approximately 3%. Carbamazepine is also associated with common benign rashes, which in rare instances may be harbingers of rare serious rashes. However, in occasional patients, carbamazepine may be better tolerated than other agents, and data continue to support the notion that one potential advantage of carbamazepine is the relatively low risk of clinically significant weight gain (Ketter et al. 2004).

Carbamazepine drug interactions can yield carbamazepine toxicity (e.g., when erythromycin or valproate is added to carbamazepine) and inefficacy of other medications (e.g., hormonal contraceptives and multiple psychotropic drugs, including several newer anticonvulsants and second-generation antipsychotics). Additional information about carbamazepine is provided in Chapter 13.

In summary, carbamazepine is an option for acute mania that has drug interaction and tolerability limitations. In addition, in contrast to lithium and divalproex, evidence supporting the use of carbamazepine in the longer-term management of bipolar disorders is limited. Thus, carbamazepine is considered an intermediate-priority acute mania therapy by multiple treatment guidelines. Nevertheless, selected patients, particularly those who are not taking multiple medications and report inadequate efficacy and/or tolerability with Tier I or II options, may find carbamazepine a useful treatment for acute mania.

First-Generation Antipsychotics

First-generation antipsychotics, also referred to as *typical antipsychotics,* figure importantly in the history of treatment of bipolar disorders but in recent years have been superseded by second-generation antipsychotics, primarily because the latter have more favorable adverse-effect profiles. Multiple first-generation antipsychotics were approved by the FDA for the treatment of schizophrenia in the 1950s, 1960s, and 1970s, but only one such agent, chlorpromazine, was eventually approved for acute mania.

Individual early studies found that first-generation antipsychotics compared with lithium tended to have comparable overall efficacy, with advantages early in treatment for rapid control of agitation in highly active patients but disadvantages later in treatment compared with lithium for achieving remission of the full manic syndrome sufficient to permit discharge (Garfinkel et al. 1980; Johnson et al. 1968, 1971; Prien et al. 1972; Shopsin et al. 1975). However, a meta-analysis of five controlled acute mania trials (Johnson et al. 1968, 1971; Shopsin et al. 1975; Spring et al. 1970; Takahashi et al. 1975) found the pooled response rate with lithium (89%) superior to that with neuroleptics (38%) (Janicak et al. 1992). In some studies, combining first-generation antipsychotics with lithium appeared to yield enhanced therapeutic effects (Garfinkel et al. 1980; Small et al. 1995).

In the 1970s and 1980s, American psychiatrists, perhaps more focused on the later advantages of lithium, tended to consider first-generation antipsychotics as adjuncts for acute mania, with lithium being the primary treatment for both acute mania and maintenance. In contrast, European psychiatrists, perhaps more focused on the earlier advantages of first-generation antipsychotics, tended to consider first-generation antipsychotics to be the primary treatments for acute mania and lithium as an adjunct in acute mania but the primary bipolar maintenance treatment. Hence first-generation antipsychotics were not thought to be foundational treatments for bipolar disorders but were considered to be primarily for acute mania, with unimodal activity attenuating manic symptoms, sometimes at the cost of exacerbating depressive symptoms. For example, these agents were implicated in yielding postmania depression in some (Kukopulos et al. 1980; Morgan 1972), but not all (Lucas et al. 1989), studies.

Nevertheless, first-generation antipsychotics were commonly used (often in combination with lithium) for the treatment of acute mania on both sides of the Atlantic in the 1970s and 1980s, but this changed as the tolerability limitations of first-generation antipsychotics became more evident and new treatment options emerged. Thus, the role of first-generation antipsychotics in the management of bipolar disorders became increasingly limited because of concerns about acute extrapyramidal symptoms (Nasrallah et al. 1988), tardive dyskinesia (Kane and Smith 1982), and induction of dysphoria (Ahlfors et al. 1981), problems that were much less of a concern with second-generation antipsychotics.

The rapid onset of action of first-generation antipsychotics was particularly evident with intramuscular administration. Indeed, intramuscular haloperidol (often combined with lorazepam to enhance efficacy and diphenhydramine to decrease extrapyramidal symptoms) persisted as an important treatment for acute agitation even into the era of second-generation antipsychotics, although this was eventually challenged by the availability of intramuscular formulations of agents such as olanzapine, ziprasidone, and aripiprazole.

The use of first-generation antipsychotics in acute mania, particularly haloperidol (in view of the large amount of data supporting its use), is described in the following subsections. Additional information about first-generation antipsychotics is provided in Chapter 13.

Chlorpromazine.   Chlorpromazine, the prototypical first-generation antipsychotic, was known to relieve acute agitation as early as 1952 (Delay et al. 1952; Lehmann and Hanrahan 1954) and was approved by the FDA for the treatment of schizophrenia in 1954 and to control the manifestations of the manic type of manic-depressive illness in 1973. Controlled trials established the efficacy of chlorpromazine in acute mania as monotherapy (Post et al. 1980; Prien et al. 1972; Shopsin et al. 1975) and in combination with lithium (Cookson et al. 1981; Janicak et al. 1988). However, the clinical utility of this low-potency first-generation antipsychotic was limited by prominent sedation and hypotension, which resulted in increased use of intermediate- and high-potency agents, particularly haloperidol.

Thioridazine, thiothixene, and pimozide.   Controlled trials also reported efficacy in acute mania for the low-potency agent thioridazine (Post et al. 1980) and the high-potency agents thiothixene (Janicak et al. 1988) and pimozide (Cookson et al. 1981; Post et al. 1980).

Haloperidol.   The high-potency first-generation antipsychotic haloperidol, compared with the low-potency agent chlorpromazine, yields substantially less sedation and hypotension but more frequent extrapyramidal adverse effects. Early trials suggested that haloperidol was effective in acute mania both as mono-therapy (Garfinkel et al. 1980; Shopsin et al. 1975) and as an adjunct to lithium (Garfinkel et al. 1980).

In acute agitation in schizophrenia or mania, intramuscular haloperidol, 5 mg, compared with intramuscular lorazepam, 2 mg, injections every 30–60 min-utes as needed appeared to have similar efficacy, although haloperidol yielded more extrapyramidal adverse effects (Bieniek et al. 1998; Foster et al. 1997). However, combining these agents appeared to yield more rapid benefit compared with either as monotherapy and perhaps even fewer extrapyramidal symptoms compared with haloperidol monotherapy (Battaglia et al. 1997).

Several contemporary multicenter, randomized, double-blind, acute ma-nia studies of second-generation antipsychotics have included haloperidol as an active comparator, providing a substantial amount of data supporting its ef-ficacy in the treatment of acute mania as monotherapy (McIntyre et al. 2005; Smulevich et al. 2005; Tohen et al. 2003; Vieta et al. 2005) and as an adjunct to lithium or valproate (Sachs et al. 2002).

Contemporary acute mania studies compared with early studies have used more consistent and conservative haloperidol dosages, with mean dosages rang-ing between 5 and 11 mg/day (minimum: 2–10 mg/day; maximum: 10–15 mg/ day) for monotherapy (Smulevich et al. 2005; Tohen et al. 2003; Vieta et al. 2005) and the mean dosage being 6.2 mg/day (minimum dosage = 2 mg/day; maximum dosage = 12 mg/day) for combination therapy (Sachs et al. 2002).

The U.S. prescribing information for haloperidol has been revised to in-clude a boxed warning (like other antipsychotics) indicating that it may increase mortality in elderly patients with dementia-related psychosis (Wang et al. 2005). Warnings in the haloperidol prescribing information include the risks of car-diovascular effects (sudden death, QTc prolongation, and torsades de pointes), tardive dyskinesia, neuroleptic malignant syndrome, teratogenicity, broncho-pneumonia, and an encephalopathic syndrome (weakness; lethargy; fever; tremulousness; confusion; extrapyramidal symptoms; leukocytosis; and ele-vated serum enzymes, serum urea nitrogen, and fasting blood sugar) followed by irreversible brain damage when combined with lithium. The latter issue is considered in greater detail by Ketter and Wang in the section on lithium in Chapter 13 of this volume. In a recent epidemiological study, current use of first- and second-generation antipsychotics was associated with dose-related increases in rates of sudden cardiac death (1.99 and 2.26, respectively) (Ray et al. 2009).

In summary, some first-generation antipsychotics (particularly chlorprom- azine and haloperidol) have evidence supporting their efficacy in acute mania, but safety/tolerability concerns commonly result in first-generation antipsy- chotics being held in reserve for patients with inadequate efficacy or tolerability with mood stabilizers and second-generation antipsychotics in Tiers I and II.

Other Second-Generation Antipsychotics: Clozapine

Clozapine is the only second-generation antipsychotic with an FDA schizo- phrenia indication that lacks an acute mania indication. Limited data support the effectiveness of this agent in bipolar disorders, but safety and tolerability considerations limit its utility.

After its introduction in clinical studies in the United States in the early 1970s, clozapine was withdrawn in 1974 because of the risk of agranulocytosis and was not approved for clinical use in the treatment of schizophrenia in the United States until 1990. Although clozapine lacks an FDA indication for acute mania, this medication was of interest not only because it was the prototypical atypical antipsychotic but also because it was the only agent approved for treatment- resistant schizophrenia and for decreasing suicidal behavior in patients with schizophrenia (Meltzer et al. 2003).

Uncontrolled reports (for reviews, see Frye et al. 1998; Zarate et al. 1995) and two controlled trials (Barbini et al. 1997; Suppes et al. 1999) suggested that clozapine might have efficacy in bipolar disorders. In published reports, mean clozapine dosages in patients with bipolar disorder ranged from approximately 125 to 550 mg/day.

However, clozapine generally has a challenging adverse-effect profile com- pared with other treatment options. The U.S. prescribing information for clozapine includes boxed warnings regarding the risks of 1) agranulocytosis, 2) seizures, 3) myocarditis, 4) other adverse cardiovascular and respiratory ef- fects, and 5) increased mortality (primarily cardiovascular or infectious) in elderly patients with dementia-related psychosis (an antipsychotic class warn- ing). Hence this agent tends to be held in reserve for patients with treatment- resistant bipolar disorders.

Increasing concerns have been raised regarding the risks of hyperglycemia and diabetes mellitus with clozapine and second-generation antipsychotics. Indeed, the FDA has stipulated changes in the prescribing information not only for clozapine but also for olanzapine, risperidone, quetiapine, ziprasidone, and aripiprazole to reflect these risks, suggesting a class effect for such problems. In contrast, the report of a recent consensus development conference on antipsychotics and obesity, diabetes, and hyperlipidemia emphasized differences among agents, with clozapine and olanzapine being the most, risperidone and quetiapine being less, and ziprasidone and aripiprazole being the least implicated (*Physicians' Desk Reference* 2008). Thus, clinical and (as indicated) laboratory monitoring for obesity, diabetes, and hyperlipidemia appears prudent for patients receiving clozapine. Other warnings in the prescribing information include the risks of eosinophilia and neuroleptic malignant syndrome. To date, clozapine has not been associated with congenital malformations in humans (FDA pregnancy category B).

Clozapine has some drug-drug interactions because certain enzyme inducers such as carbamazepine can decrease serum clozapine concentrations and some enzyme inhibitors such as macrolide antibiotics may increase serum clozapine concentrations. In addition, combining clozapine with bone marrow suppressants is not recommended because of concerns about the potential for increasing the risk of agranulocytosis. Finally, concerns have been raised regarding the risks of excessive sedation and cardiorespiratory depression with concomitant administration of clozapine and benzodiazepines.

In summary, safety and tolerability concerns and limited efficacy data commonly result in clozapine being held in reserve for patients with inadequate efficacy and/or tolerability with mood stabilizers and second-generation antipsychotics in Tiers I and II or first-generation antipsychotics in Tier III.

Adjunctive Benzodiazepines

Benzodiazepines (most commonly lorazepam) may have modest antimanic activity, particularly as adjuncts to control agitation early in treatment, and may be useful in the treatment of comorbid anxiety.

The utility of adding lorazepam to lithium (Lenox et al. 1992) or haloperidol (Battaglia et al. 1997) for acute agitation has been confirmed in controlled trials. In a small (24-patient) 2-week double-blind acute mania study, lorazepam and clonazepam monotherapy yielded response rates of 61% and 18%, respectively (Bradwejn et al. 1990).

The modest degree of antimanic benefit with benzodiazepines is documented by experience derived from their common use as adjunctive medications early in the randomized phase of controlled trials of other agents in acute mania. Typically, in such trials, an agent such as lorazepam is permitted as needed for insomnia, anxiety, or agitation, starting at approximately 4–6 mg/day and tapering to zero over approximately 1 week. Although this intervention may briefly attenuate some symptoms in patients with acute mania, it does not appear to attenuate the full manic syndrome or systematically interfere with the ability to separate approved treatments from placebo, consistent with adjunctive benzodiazepines having at most modest antimanic effects. Thus, in contemporary acute mania trials, the control intervention of as-needed lorazepam, psychiatric hospitalization, and placebo yields an overall response rate of approximately 30%, and adding an approved antimanic agent increases the overall response rate to approximately 50%.

The hypnotic (Andersen and Lingjaerde 1969) and anxiolytic (Ballenger et al. 1988) actions of benzodiazepines can prove clinically beneficial in patients with bipolar disorders because insomnia and anxiety are common symptoms. For example, up to 20% of patients with bipolar disorders also may have panic disorder (MacKinnon et al. 2002). Thus, like gabapentin and topiramate (which are described later in this chapter as Tier IV treatments), benzodiazepines do not appear to be effective as primary treatments for bipolar disorders, but they may yield adjunctive benefit in common comorbid problems (such as anxiety disorders and insomnia).

Benzodiazepines are generally well tolerated but can cause sedation and ataxia, especially when combined with other agents with such effects. Benzodiazepines appear to be associated with minor congenital malformations (FDA pregnancy category D). In addition, the utility of these agents is limited by their abuse potential (particularly in patients with histories of substance abuse) and the risk of disinhibition (particularly in children and adolescents and patients with Cluster B personality disorders).

Benzodiazepines have some noteworthy drug interactions. For example, concerns have been raised regarding the risks of excessive sedation and cardiorespiratory depression with concomitant administration of benzodiazepines and clozapine or intramuscular olanzapine. Additional information about benzodiazepines is provided in Chapter 14.

In summary, benzodiazepines appear to be useful adjuncts to control agitation early in the treatment of acute mania and for the treatment of comorbid anxiety disorders. Although benzodiazepines are generally well tolerated, care is indicated in patient selection because these agents have abuse potential and may yield disinhibition.

Electroconvulsive Therapy

Limited controlled evidence supports a role for ECT in the treatment of acute mania (Mukherjee et al. 1994).

Although case reports and case series suggested that ECT may be effective for mixed episodes (Gruber et al. 2000; Liang et al. 1988; Valenti et al. 2008), a review by Valenti and associates (2008) indicated that there are varying and few systematic data regarding this issue.

Despite the potential utility of ECT in acute mania, treatment-emergent affective switch in acute bipolar depression with ECT has been reported with variable incidence.

Concerns based on case reports regarding the risks of delirium, seizures, and prolonged apnea resulted in recommendations that lithium not be combined with ECT (Small and Milstein 1990).

In summary, although some evidence supports the efficacy of ECT in acute mania, it is generally held in reserve for patients intolerant of or refractory to pharmacotherapy because of the risk of cognitive adverse effects, stigma, consent challenges, or logistical concerns such as coordination of care and aftercare. Nevertheless, in certain circumstances, ECT may be considered early on (e.g., in pregnant women with acute mania).

Tier IV: Novel Adjunctive Treatments

Treatment resistance or intolerance and comorbid conditions are sufficiently common in patients with bipolar disorders that even the above-mentioned armamentarium may be insufficient to meet clinical needs of some patients. In this section, we describe novel adjunctive treatments with even more limited evidence of efficacy than the previously described treatments. These treatments include other mood stabilizers (lamotrigine), other anticonvulsants (oxcarbazepine, gabapentin, topiramate, tiagabine, levetiracetam, and zonisamide), and adjunctive psychotherapy. Very careful consideration of the specific role(s) of these agents in patients with bipolar disorders is warranted. For example, for some of these interventions, controlled trials indicate inefficacy in acute mania but potential efficacy for other phases of bipolar disorder (e.g., lamotrigine for longer-term treatment) or in the management of common comorbid conditions (e.g., gabapentin and topiramate for anxiety and alcohol use disorders, respectively). In general, treatment guidelines consider these modalities to be low-priority interventions or not recommended as interventions in the treatment of acute mania (American Psychiatric Association 2002; Goodwin 2003; Grunze et al. 2002; Keck et al. 2004; Suppes et al. 2005; Yatham et al. 2006). Nevertheless, some Tier IV options could prove to be worthwhile adjuncts for very carefully selected patients, after consideration of Tier I–III treatments (e.g., in patients with prominent comorbid conditions).

Other Mood Stabilizers: Lamotrigine

The anticonvulsant lamotrigine has a distinctive psychotropic profile compared with other mood stabilizers because it has a bipolar longer-term treatment indication but lacks an acute indication and appears more effective for depressive than for mood elevation symptoms. In the absence of an acute indication, clinicians may ponder the optimal timing of initiating lamotrigine therapy. In most instances, this will be during euthymia or syndromal or subsyndromal depression (on occasion, immediately after an acute manic episode) rather than during acute mania.

Lamotrigine was approved for the longer-term treatment of bipolar disorder in 2003. Lamotrigine, unlike the anticonvulsants divalproex and carbamazepine, does *not* appear effective in acute mania (Bowden et al. 2000; Goldsmith et al. 2003).

In contrast, double-blind, placebo-controlled studies found lamotrigine monotherapy effective in maintenance treatment (particularly for preventing depressive episodes) in bipolar I disorder (Bowden et al. 2003; Calabrese et al. 2003). Thus, as described in Chapter 8 of this volume, lamotrigine monotherapy received an FDA indication for maintenance treatment in bipolar I disorder to delay the time to occurrence of mood episodes (depression, mania, hypomania, mixed episodes) in patients receiving standard therapy for acute mood episodes. Also, as described in Chapter 7 of this volume, controlled data suggest that lamotrigine may yield modest benefits in acute bipolar depression (Calabrese et al. 1999, 2008), but lamotrigine does not have an FDA indication for this use. Finally, as noted in Chapter 9 of this volume, "Management of Rapid-Cycling Bipolar Disorders," controlled data suggest that lamotrigine may be effective in rapid-cycling bipolar II disorder (a depression-predominant subtype of bipolar II disorder) (Calabrese et al. 2000) and in treatment-resistant (primarily rapid-cycling bipolar) mood disorders (Frye et al. 2000).

Hence lamotrigine may "stabilize mood from below" in the sense that it may maximally affect depressive symptoms in bipolar disorders (Ketter and Calabrese 2002). In contrast, the older mood stabilizers (lithium, carbamazepine, and valproate) and at least some second-generation antipsychotics appear to "stabilize mood from above" in the sense that they may maximally affect manic or hypomanic symptoms in bipolar disorders.

Although lamotrigine does not have efficacy for acute mania, occasionally clinicians may consider adding lamotrigine as soon as standard therapy for acute mania has begun, with the goal of preventing or delaying a postmania depression. Although controlled data are limited, observations from the open stabilization phase of a maintenance trial in patients with bipolar I disorder who were currently or recently (within prior 2 months) manic or hypomanic are worth noting (Bowden et al. 2003). In this study, open addition of lamotrigine to standard therapies allowed 175 of 349 patients (50%) to stabilize sufficiently within 8–16 weeks (despite tapering off other medications) to be randomly assigned to the controlled maintenance trial. This intervention was generally well tolerated. This approach has the strength of achieving full dosage of lamotrigine sooner, which is particularly desirable given the gradual initial titration of lamotrigine. Limitations include potential adverse effects and drug interactions related to introduction of a medication not directly targeting mood elevation during acute mania. For example, concurrent valproate may increase the risk of the common (1 in 10) benign and rare (1 in 1,000) serious rashes associated with lamotrigine, and valproate doubles and carbamazepine halves serum lamotrigine concentrations, requiring lamotrigine dosage adjustments. In addition, some patients may experience activation with lamotrigine. However, in two controlled studies, similar percentages of patients had mania rating score increases for lamotrigine, lithium, and placebo (Bowden et al. 2000), suggesting that activation may be a sporadic occurrence, certainly of clinical significance in patients in whom it has been observed, but not a significant population-wide effect that generally would contraindicate introducing lamotrigine as soon as standard therapy for acute mania has commenced.

As noted earlier, in 2008, the FDA released an alert regarding increased risk of suicidality (suicidal behavior or ideation) in patients with epilepsy and psychiatric disorders for 11 anticonvulsants (including lamotrigine).

In summary, lamotrigine does not appear to be effective in acute mania and may have only modest efficacy in the prevention of mania. Thus, the strengths and limitations of adding lamotrigine as soon as standard therapy for acute mania has begun (e.g., to initiate prophylaxis as soon as possible) must be carefully considered on a patient-by-patient basis before embarking on such an intervention. Additional controlled trials would help to better inform clinicians about this issue.

Other Anticonvulsants

The efficacy and tolerability limitations of lithium and antipsychotics and the utility of valproate, carbamazepine, and lamotrigine in bipolar disorders resulted in the assessment of several other anticonvulsants in acute mania. These other anticonvulsants appear to have diverse psychotropic profiles. Although not generally effective for acute mania, with the possible exception of oxcarbazepine (Table 6–3), these medications may have utility for comorbid conditions (such as anxiety or alcohol use disorders or pain syndromes).

In 2008, the FDA released an alert regarding increased risk of suicidality (suicidal behavior or ideation) in patients with epilepsy and psychiatric disorders for 11 anticonvulsants (carbamazepine, felbamate, gabapentin, lamotrigine, levetiracetam, oxcarbazepine, pregabalin, tiagabine, topiramate, valproate, and zonisamide). In the FDA's analysis, anticonvulsants compared with placebo yielded approximately twice the risk of suicidality (0.43% vs. 0.22%). The relative risk for suicidality was higher in the patients with epilepsy than in those with psychiatric disorders. Additional information about other anticonvulsants is provided in Chapter 14.

Oxcarbazepine. Oxcarbazepine, a congener of carbamazepine, may differ from other newer anticonvulsants in that, like carbamazepine and valproate, it may have efficacy in acute mania. Oxcarbazepine's structural similarity to car-

TABLE 6–3. Benzodiazepines, lamotrigine, and other anticonvulsants not proven effective in acute mania

Drug	Evidence
Benzodiazepines	Underpowered active-comparator monotherapy study (Bradwejn et al. 1990)
	Common adjuncts that do not interfere with separation of active treatments from placebo
Lamotrigine	Negative placebo- and lithium-controlled adjunctive study (Bowden et al. 2000)
Oxcarbazepine	Underpowered active-comparator monotherapy studies (Emrich 1990)
	Negative trial in children and adolescents (Wagner et al. 2006)
Gabapentin	Negative placebo-controlled adjunctive study (Pande et al. 2000a)
Topiramate	Negative placebo- and lithium-controlled adult monotherapy studies (Kushner et al. 2006)
Tiagabine	Negative open adjunctive study (Grunze et al. 1999)
Levetiracetam	No controlled study
Zonisamide	No controlled study

bamazepine suggests that oxcarbazepine could have psychotropic effects that overlap those of carbamazepine, and as noted later in this subsection, it has more favorable adverse-effect and drug interaction profiles than does carbamazepine. Unfortunately, very little evidence (far less than for carbamazepine) indicates that oxcarbazepine has efficacy in bipolar disorders. Specifically, to date, no positive large double-blind, placebo-controlled trials of oxcarbazepine in bipolar disorders have been done.

On the basis of generally better tolerability and fewer drug interactions compared with carbamazepine, oxcarbazepine has been proposed as an alternative intervention for acute mania and maintenance treatment of bipolar disorders (American Psychiatric Association 2002). However, large double-blind, placebo-controlled studies are necessary to determine whether oxcarbazepine is effective in bipolar disorders.

Oxcarbazepine dosages are approximately 50% higher than those used with carbamazepine, often starting with 300–600 mg/day and increasing by 300 mg/day every few days as necessary and tolerated to maximum dosages ranging between 900 and 2,400 mg/day and serum concentrations ranging between 10 and 35 µg/mL. The latter values are derived from epilepsy studies, and oxcarbazepine is generally dosed clinically in bipolar disorders, titrating to desired effect as tolerated.

Oxcarbazepine appears to be generally better tolerated than carbamazepine, yielding less neurotoxicity and rash (Friis et al. 1993). Oxcarbazepine has not been associated with blood dyscrasias, lacks a boxed warning in the U.S. prescribing information, and does not appear to require hematological monitoring. Warnings in the prescribing information include the 25% chance of cross-hypersensitivity with carbamazepine and the risk of hyponatremia. As noted earlier, in 2008, the FDA released an alert regarding increased risk of suicidality (suicidal behavior or ideation) in patients with epilepsy and psychiatric disorders for 11 anticonvulsants (including oxcarbazepine).

Hyponatremia may be the main adverse effect that occurs more commonly with oxcarbazepine than with carbamazepine (Isojarvi et al. 2001). Oxcarbazepine, like carbamazepine, may yield transaminase elevations and gastrointestinal adverse effects but less weight gain than with valproate (Rattya et al. 1999). Oxcarbazepine, in contrast to carbamazepine, has not to date been associated with congenital malformations in humans (FDA pregnancy category C). However, this could be merely related to fewer oxcarbazepine exposures.

Oxcarbazepine has generally fewer drug interactions than does carbamazepine. Unlike carbamazepine, oxcarbazepine does not yield autoinduction of metabolism, and its metabolism is not susceptible to enzyme inhibitors. Thus, addition of other drugs does not tend to increase oxcarbazepine blood concentrations. Also, oxcarbazepine, compared with carbamazepine, appears to have weaker heteroinduction. Hence unlike with carbamazepine, dosage adjustment of some other medications such as lamotrigine or valproate in patients receiving oxcarbazepine is not recommended. However, oxcarbazepine appears to have a clinically significant interaction with hormonal contraceptives, decreasing contraceptive blood concentrations by up to 50% (Fattore et al. 1999).

In summary, in view of the sparse evidence of efficacy, oxcarbazepine should be held in reserve for patients who show inadequate tolerability or efficacy with the more established therapies in Tiers I–III.

Gabapentin.   Although early open reports of gabapentin in bipolar disorders were encouraging, later randomized, double-blind, placebo-controlled studies were discouraging (Frye et al. 2000; Pande et al. 2000a). In view of the absence of controlled data supporting efficacy in mania, gabapentin was not considered to be an important option in the management of mania in the 2002 revision of the American Psychiatric Association (2002) "Practice Guideline for the Treatment of Patients With Bipolar Disorder."

However, gabapentin appeared effective in several comorbid conditions seen in patients with bipolar disorders, with double-blind, placebo-controlled trials indicating efficacy in anxiety disorders, such as social phobia (Pande et al. 1999) and (in a post hoc analysis) moderate to severe panic disorder (Pande et al. 2000b), and in pain syndromes, such as neuropathic pain (Serpell 2002), chronic daily headache (Spira and Beran 2003), and postherpetic neuralgia (Rowbotham et al. 1998); gabapentin received an FDA indication for the latter.

In summary, gabapentin does not appear to be effective in acute mania but is generally well tolerated and may be worth considering as an adjunct for comorbid conditions in selected patients.

Topiramate.   Although early open reports of topiramate in bipolar disorders were encouraging, later multicenter, randomized, double-blind, placebo-controlled studies were discouraging. Thus, in several trials, topiramate proved no better or worse than placebo in adults with acute mania (Kushner et al. 2006). In view of the absence of controlled data supporting efficacy in mania, topiramate was not considered to be an important option in the management of mania in the 2002 revision of the American Psychiatric Association (2002) "Practice Guideline for the Treatment of Patients With Bipolar Disorder."

However, topiramate appeared effective in several comorbid conditions seen in patients with bipolar disorders, with randomized, double-blind, placebo-controlled trials reporting efficacy in eating disorders, such as obesity with or without diabetes mellitus (Bray et al. 2003; Rosenstock et al. 2007; Stenlof et al. 2007; Toplak et al. 2007; Tremblay et al. 2007), obesity with binge-eating disorder (Claudino et al. 2007; McElroy et al. 2003), obesity with bipolar disorder (McElroy et al. 2007), olanzapine-associated weight gain (Egger et al. 2007); bulimia (Hoopes et al. 2003); alcohol dependence (Johnson et al. 2003, 2007); essential tremor (Ondo et al. 2006); chronic low back pain (Muehlbacher et al. 2006); borderline personality disorder (Loew et al. 2006); and the prevention of migraine headaches (Brandes et al. 2004; Silberstein et al. 2007). Weight loss has been consistently observed in controlled trials with topiramate, not only in patients with eating disorders but also in patients with mania (Kushner et al. 2006) and in the depressive phase of bipolar disorders (McIntyre et al. 2002).

In summary, topiramate has tolerability limitations and does not appear to be effective in acute mania but may be worth considering as an adjunct for comorbid conditions in selected patients.

Tiagabine. No controlled studies of tiagabine in bipolar disorders are available. Although some experience with open low-dose tiagabine in bipolar disorders has been encouraging (Schaffer et al. 2002), other open reports have suggested problems with both efficacy and tolerability (Grunze et al. 1999; Suppes et al. 2002).

In contrast, a small controlled trial reported that low-dose (≤16 mg/day) tiagabine was generally well tolerated and yielded benefit in generalized anxiety disorder (Rosenthal 2003).

Like gabapentin and topiramate, tiagabine does not appear to be effective as a primary treatment for bipolar disorders but may yield benefit in comorbid problems (such as generalized anxiety disorder). However, reports of tolerability problems suggest that considerable caution should be exercised with tiagabine in patients with bipolar disorders.

Levetiracetam. To date, no controlled studies and only a few open reports regarding levetiracetam's effects in bipolar disorders are available (Goldberg and Burdick 2002; Grunze et al. 2003; Post et al. 2005).

Thus, levetiracetam may have adequate tolerability, but controlled studies are needed to assess its tolerability better as well as its potential roles in bipolar disorders and comorbid conditions.

Zonisamide. To date, no controlled studies and only a few open reports regarding zonisamide's effects in bipolar disorders are available (Ghaemi et al. 2006, 2008; Kanba et al. 1994; McElroy et al. 2005).

Emerging evidence suggests that zonisamide, like topiramate, may have utility in obesity and eating disorders. In a double-blind, placebo-controlled trial, zonisamide yielded weight loss in obesity patients as monotherapy (Gadde et al. 2003) or combined with bupropion (Gadde et al. 2007), and in an open trial (McElroy et al. 2004) and a small double-blind, placebo-controlled trial (McElroy et al. 2006), zonisamide offered benefit in binge-eating disorder with obesity. Another study suggested that open adjunctive zonisamide, starting with 100 mg/day at bedtime and increasing by 100 mg/day every 2 weeks as tolerated, targeting 300–600 mg/day (mean dosage of approximately 375 mg/day), might yield weight loss in obese euthymic medicated patients with bipolar disorder (Wang et al. 2008).

In summary, zonisamide has tolerability limitations, and controlled studies are needed to assess its potential roles in bipolar disorders and comorbid conditions.

Adjunctive Psychotherapy

Emerging data from controlled trials indicate the increasing importance of adjunctive psychosocial interventions in the management of bipolar disorders, as discussed in detail in Chapter 15 of this volume, "Adjunctive Psychosocial Interventions in the Management of Bipolar Disorders."

These treatments may have illness phase–specific features, with the optimal time of administration being during depression or euthymia as opposed to during mania (Swartz and Frank 2001), a mood state that entails such marked cognitive and behavioral disruptions that psychological interventions may not be feasible.

Although the theory and case studies of the application of psychotherapy to mania have been described (Kahn 1990; Mester 1986), it is not surprising that controlled studies of psychosocial interventions administered during acute manic and mixed episodes are lacking. Thus, multiple treatment guidelines that recommend adjunctive psychotherapy for the treatment of acute bipolar depression or maintenance treatment do *not* recommend this intervention for the treatment of acute manic or mixed episodes (American Psychiatric Association 2002; Goodwin 2003; Keck et al. 2004).

However, one guideline recommended psychotherapy plus medication for the treatment of hypomania in patients with bipolar II disorder (Keck et al.

2004). Although it may be argued in theory that cognitive-behavioral therapy should be well suited to address maladaptive false beliefs occurring during hypomania (Scott 1996), in a small (four bipolar patients) cognitive-behavioral therapy group, the individual who obtained the least benefit had the highest Internal State Scale activation score, suggesting hypomania (Palmer et al. 1995).

In summary, adjunctive psychotherapy, although useful in acute bipolar depression and bipolar maintenance treatment, lacks compelling evidence of utility in the acute treatment of mood elevation.

Conclusion

Recent clinical trials not only have helped us better understand the utility of older agents such as lithium, valproate, and carbamazepine but also have provided clinicians with additional options for the management of acute mania. Second-generation antipsychotics and other anticonvulsants are the two main groups of non–mood stabilizer agents that have been investigated and have important differences. Second-generation antipsychotics generally appear effective for acute mania but may differ from one another with respect to adverse effects. In contrast, other anticonvulsants have diverse psychotropic profiles and, although not generally effective for acute mania (with the possible exception of oxcarbazepine), may have utility for other aspects of bipolar disorders or comorbid conditions. Additional clinical studies of these second-generation antipsychotics and other anticonvulsants promise to yield further new insights into the pathophysiology and treatment of acute mania.

Case Study: Management of Acute Manic and Mixed Episodes

Mr. A, a 30-year-old single graduate student, had a 9-year history of bipolar I disorder, with two prior hospitalizations for psychotic mania at ages 21 and 28, with the latter followed by a major depressive episode that was managed on an outpatient basis. In the past, lithium had yielded partial response for acute mania with good tolerability, whereas divalproex, olanzapine, and quetiapine had yielded more consistent relief of acute mania but had not been tolerated in longer-term treatment because of weight gain and sedation. He had been given methylphenidate briefly for attention-deficit/hyperactivity disorder in childhood, but this was discontinued because of the development of increased agitation. He also had a history of occasional binge drinking. He had a paternal grandfather with possible bipolar disorder, but his family psychiatric history was otherwise negative.

When first seen in clinic, Mr. A was taking lithium, 1,200 mg/day, which yielded a serum concentration of 1.0 mEq/L, as well as quetiapine, 50 mg at bedtime, with the dose of lithium limited by tremor and the dose of quetiapine limited by sedation. He weighed 190 pounds on a 5-foot, 11-inch frame.

He did well for several months with this regimen, but the following spring during an academic conference in Europe, his mood rapidly escalated. Thus, he developed euphoria (laughing inappropriately, disrupting two scientific sessions at the conference), overtalkativeness (having to be escorted out of these two sessions), racing thoughts (journaling multiple scientific ideas around the clock), inflated self-esteem (believing that he was about to receive a major award at the conference), increased goal-directed activity (attending the conference all day and working on his dissertation all night), decreased need for sleep (feeling energetic despite only 1–2 hours' sleep per night), and impulsivity (becoming intoxicated at a party and having a sexual encounter with a woman he met there, who happened to be related to his thesis supervisor).

The day after his return home, Mr. A's live-in girlfriend of 10 months, who had remained at home during his trip to Europe, brought Mr. A to the emergency department because he had developed even more severe symptoms, including wandering naked in the street in the middle of the night and paranoid delusions (believing his food was being poisoned).

In the emergency department, Mr. A was disheveled, with psychomotor agitation (pacing about in the small interview room), pressured speech, and euphoric more than irritable mood. His affect was labile, and he admitted to paranoid delusions but denied hallucinations. He admitted to discontinuing quetiapine and only sporadic adherence to lithium during the prior week and had a serum lithium concentration of 0.4 mEq/L. His urine toxicology screen had negative results.

Mr. A was admitted to the hospital, and on hospital day 1, lithium was restarted at 600 mg twice per day, and lorazepam at 1 mg twice per day and risperidone at 2 mg at bedtime were added, and that night he slept 4 hours. Risperidone was administered because he refused divalproex, olanzapine, and quetiapine. By the next morning, on hospital day 2, he had some affective improvement but was still delusional, so risperidone was increased to 3 mg at bedtime, and he slept 5 hours. The following day, hospital day 3, he had additional affective improvement but still had residual delusional symptoms, so risperidone was increased to 4 mg at bedtime, and he slept 8 hours. The next day, hospital day 4, his mood improved further, and he denied psychotic symptoms but complained of muscle stiffness and had very mild cogwheel rigidity on physical examination. Thus, benztropine (1 mg twice a day) was added, and he slept 9 hours. The following day, hospital day 5, his mood was euthymic, he denied psychotic symptoms, and the muscle stiffness and cogwheel rigidity had resolved, but he complained of mild sedation in the morning, so lorazepam was decreased to 0.5 mg twice per day, and he slept 9 hours.

The following day, hospital day 6, his mood was euthymic, and he denied psychotic symptoms, muscle stiffness, and sedation. After a couple's meeting with Mr. A and his girlfriend, at which he agreed to participate in the partial hospitalization program and to have her monitor his medication adherence and mood, he was discharged taking lithium 600 mg twice per day, risperidone 4 mg at bedtime, lorazepam 0.5 mg twice per day, and benztropine 1 mg twice per day. His serum lithium concentration was 1.1 mEq/L. At this point, he weighed 192 pounds.

In summary, this man with bipolar I disorder and a history of partial response for acute mania with good tolerability with lithium, and more consistent relief of acute mania but longer-term tolerability problems (weight gain and sedation) with divalproex, olanzapine, and quetiapine, had a good acute response to lithium combined with risperidone, with adequate acute tolerability. Nonadherence to medications and international travel appeared to contribute to emergence of acute mania. Although acute response was achieved, substantial longer-term challenges remain with respect to optimizing medication dosages to limit adverse effects, determining an effective and well-tolerated maintenance treatment, and providing psychoeducation for the patient and his significant other with respect to the importance of vigilance for prodromal symptoms and adherence to medications.

References

Ahlfors UG, Baastrup PC, Dencker SJ, et al: Flupenthixol decanoate in recurrent manic-depressive illness: a comparison with lithium. Acta Psychiatr Scand 64:226–237, 1981

Alsdorf RM, Wyszynski DF, Holmes LB, et al: Evidence of increased birth defects in the offspring of women exposed to valproate during pregnancy: findings from the AED pregnancy registry (abstract). Birth Defects Res A Clin Mol Teratol 70:245, 2004

American Psychiatric Association: Practice guideline for the treatment of patients with bipolar disorder (revision). Am J Psychiatry 159:1–50, 2002

Andersen T, Lingjaerde O: Nitrazepam (Mogadon) as a sleep-inducing agent: an analysis based on a double-blind comparison with phenobarbitone. Br J Psychiatry 115:1393–1397, 1969

Ballenger JC, Burrows GD, DuPont RL Jr, et al: Alprazolam in panic disorder and agoraphobia: results from a multicenter trial, I: efficacy in short-term treatment. Arch Gen Psychiatry 45:413–422, 1988

Barbini B, Scherillo P, Benedetti F, et al: Response to clozapine in acute mania is more rapid than that of chlorpromazine. Int Clin Psychopharmacol 12:109–112, 1997

Battaglia J, Moss S, Rush J, et al: Haloperidol, lorazepam, or both for psychotic agitation? A multicenter, prospective, double-blind, emergency department study. Am J Emerg Med 15:335–340, 1997

Berk M, Ng F, Wang WV, et al: Going up in smoke: tobacco smoking is associated with worse treatment outcomes in mania. J Affect Disord 110:126–134, 2008

Bieniek SA, Ownby RL, Penalver A, et al: A double-blind study of lorazepam versus the combination of haloperidol and lorazepam in managing agitation. Pharmacotherapy 18:57–62, 1998

Bowden CL, Brugger AM, Swann AC, et al: Efficacy of divalproex vs lithium and placebo in the treatment of mania. The Depakote Mania Study Group. JAMA 271:918–924, 1994

Bowden C, Calabrese J, Ascher J, et al: Spectrum of efficacy of lamotrigine in bipolar disorder: overview of double-blind placebo-controlled studies. Abstract presented at the 39th annual meeting of the American College of Neuropsychopharmacology, San Juan, Puerto Rico, December 10–14, 2000, p 291

Bowden CL, Calabrese JR, Sachs G, et al: A placebo-controlled 18-month trial of lamotrigine and lithium maintenance treatment in recently manic or hypomanic patients with bipolar I disorder. Arch Gen Psychiatry 60:392–400, 2003

Bowden CL, Grunze H, Mullen J, et al: A randomized, double-blind, placebo-controlled efficacy and safety study of quetiapine or lithium as monotherapy for mania in bipolar disorder. J Clin Psychiatry 66:111–121, 2005

Bowden CL, Swann AC, Calabrese JR, et al: A randomized, placebo-controlled, multicenter study of divalproex sodium extended release in the treatment of acute mania. J Clin Psychiatry 67:1501–1510, 2006

Bradwejn J, Shriqui C, Koszycki D, et al: Double-blind comparison of the effects of clonazepam and lorazepam in acute mania. J Clin Psychopharmacol 10:403–408, 1990

Brandes JL, Saper JR, Diamond M, et al: Topiramate for migraine prevention: a randomized controlled trial. JAMA 291:965–973, 2004

Bray GA, Hollander P, Klein S, et al: A 6-month randomized, placebo-controlled, dose-ranging trial of topiramate for weight loss in obesity. Obes Res 11:722–733, 2003

Cade JF: Lithium salts in the treatment of psychotic excitement. Med J Aust 2:349–352, 1949

Calabrese JR, Bowden CL, Sachs GS, et al: A double-blind placebo-controlled study of lamotrigine monotherapy in outpatients with bipolar I depression. Lamictal 602 Study Group. J Clin Psychiatry 60:79–88, 1999

Calabrese JR, Suppes T, Bowden CL, et al: A double-blind, placebo-controlled, prophylaxis study of lamotrigine in rapid-cycling bipolar disorder. Lamictal 614 Study Group. J Clin Psychiatry 61:841–850, 2000

Calabrese JR, Bowden CL, Sachs G, et al: A placebo-controlled 18-month trial of lamotrigine and lithium maintenance treatment in recently depressed patients with bipolar I disorder. J Clin Psychiatry 64:1013–1024, 2003

Calabrese JR, Keck PE Jr, Macfadden W, et al: A randomized, double-blind, placebo-controlled trial of quetiapine in the treatment of bipolar I or II depression. Am J Psychiatry 162:1351–1360, 2005

Calabrese JR, Huffman RF, White RL, et al: Lamotrigine in the acute treatment of bipolar depression: results of five double-blind, placebo-controlled clinical trials. Bipolar Disord 10:323–333, 2008

Claudino AM, de Oliveira IR, Appolinario JC, et al: Double-blind, randomized, placebo-controlled trial of topiramate plus cognitive-behavior therapy in binge-eating disorder. J Clin Psychiatry 68:1324–1332, 2007

Cookson J, Silverstone T, Wells B: Double-blind comparative clinical trial of pimozide and chlorpromazine in mania: a test of the dopamine hypothesis. Acta Psychiatr Scand 64:381–397, 1981

Cunnington MC: The International Lamotrigine pregnancy registry update for the epilepsy foundation (letter). Epilepsia 45:1468, 2004

Daniel DG, Brook S, Warrington L, et al: Intramuscular ziprasidone in agitated psychotic patients (NR780), in 2004 New Research Program and Abstracts, American Psychiatric Association 157th Annual Meeting, New York, NY, May 1–6, 2004. Washington, DC, American Psychiatric Association, 2004, pp 293–294

Delay J, Deniker P, Harl JM: Utilisation en thérapeutique psychiatrique d'une phénothiazine d'action centrale élective (4560 RP). Ann Med Psychol (Paris) 110:112–117, 1952

DelBello MP, Schwiers ML, Rosenberg HL, et al: A double-blind, randomized, placebo-controlled study of quetiapine as adjunctive treatment for adolescent mania. J Am Acad Child Adolesc Psychiatry 41:1216–1223, 2002

DelBello MP, Findling RL, Earley WR, et al: Efficacy of quetiapine in children and adolescents with bipolar mania: a 3-week, double-blind, randomized, placebo-controlled trial. Abstract presented at the 46th annual meeting of the American College of Neuropsychopharmacology, Boca Raton, FL, December 9–13, 2007

DelBello M, Findling RL, Wang PP, et al: Safety and efficacy of ziprasidone in pediatric bipolar disorder. Biol Psychiatry 63(7S):283S, 2008

Egger C, Muehlbacher M, Schatz M, et al: Influence of topiramate on olanzapine-related weight gain in women: an 18-month follow-up observation. J Clin Psychopharmacol 27:475–478, 2007

Emrich HM: Studies with oxcarbazepine (Trileptal) in acute mania. Int Clin Psychopharmacol 5:83–88, 1990

Fattore C, Cipolla G, Gatti G, et al: Induction of ethinylestradiol and levonorgestrel metabolism by oxcarbazepine in healthy women. Epilepsia 40:783–787, 1999

Foster S, Kessel J, Berman ME, et al: Efficacy of lorazepam and haloperidol for rapid tranquilization in a psychiatric emergency room setting. Int Clin Psychopharmacol 12:175–179, 1997

Freeman TW, Clothier JL, Pazzaglia P, et al: A double-blind comparison of valproate and lithium in the treatment of acute mania. Am J Psychiatry 149:108–111, 1992

Friis ML, Kristensen O, Boas J, et al: Therapeutic experiences with 947 epileptic outpatients in oxcarbazepine treatment. Acta Neurol Scand 87:224–227, 1993

Frye MA, Ketter TA, Altshuler LL, et al: Clozapine in bipolar disorder: treatment implications for other atypical antipsychotics. J Affect Disord 48:91–104, 1998

Frye MA, Ketter TA, Kimbrell TA, et al: A placebo-controlled study of lamotrigine and gabapentin monotherapy in refractory mood disorders. J Clin Psychopharmacol 20:607–614, 2000

Gadde KM, Franciscy DM, Wagner HR 2nd, et al: Zonisamide for weight loss in obese adults: a randomized controlled trial. JAMA 289:1820–1825, 2003

Gadde KM, Yonish GM, Foust MS, et al: Combination therapy of zonisamide and bupropion for weight reduction in obese women: a preliminary, randomized, open-label study. J Clin Psychiatry 68:1226–1229, 2007

Garfinkel PE, Stancer HC, Persad E: A comparison of haloperidol, lithium carbonate and their combination in the treatment of mania. J Affect Disord 2:279–288, 1980

Ghaemi SN, Zablotsky B, Filkowski MM, et al: An open prospective study of zonisamide in acute bipolar depression. J Clin Psychopharmacol 26:385–388, 2006

Ghaemi SN, Shirzadi AA, Klugman J, et al: Is adjunctive open-label zonisamide effective for bipolar disorder? J Affect Disord 105:311–314, 2008

Goldberg JF, Burdick KE: Levetiracetam for acute mania (letter). Am J Psychiatry 159:148, 2002

Goldsmith DR, Wagstaff AJ, Ibbotson T, et al: Lamotrigine: a review of its use in bipolar disorder. Drugs 63:2029–2050, 2003

Goodwin FK, Zis AP: Lithium in the treatment of mania: comparisons with neuroleptics. Arch Gen Psychiatry 36:840–844, 1979

Goodwin FK, Murphy DL, Bunney WE Jr: Lithium-carbonate treatment in depression and mania: a longitudinal double-blind study. Arch Gen Psychiatry 21:486–496, 1969

Goodwin GM: Evidence-based guidelines for treating bipolar disorder: recommendations from the British Association for Psychopharmacology. J Psychopharmacol 17:149–173; discussion 147, 2003

Gruber NP, Dilsaver SC, Shoaib AM, et al: ECT in mixed affective states: a case series. J ECT 16:183–188, 2000

Grunze H, Erfurth A, Marcuse A, et al: Tiagabine appears not to be efficacious in the treatment of acute mania. J Clin Psychiatry 60:759–762, 1999

Grunze H, Kasper S, Goodwin G, et al: World Federation of Societies of Biological Psychiatry (WFSBP) guidelines for biological treatment of bipolar disorders, part I: treatment of bipolar depression. World J Biol Psychiatry 3:115–124, 2002

Grunze H, Langosch J, Born C, et al: Levetiracetam in the treatment of acute mania: an open add-on study with an on-off-on design. J Clin Psychiatry 64:781–784, 2003

Hirschfeld RM, Baker JD, Wozniak P, et al: The safety and early efficacy of oral-loaded divalproex versus standard-titration divalproex, lithium, olanzapine, and placebo in the treatment of acute mania associated with bipolar disorder. J Clin Psychiatry 64:841–846, 2003

Hirschfeld RM, Keck PE Jr, Kramer M, et al: Rapid antimanic effect of risperidone monotherapy: a 3-week multicenter, double-blind, placebo-controlled trial. Am J Psychiatry 161:1057–1065, 2004

Hoopes SP, Reimherr FW, Hedges DW, et al: Treatment of bulimia nervosa with topiramate in a randomized, double-blind, placebo-controlled trial, part 1: improvement in binge and purge measures. J Clin Psychiatry 64:1335–1341, 2003

Isojarvi JI, Laatikainen TJ, Pakarinen AJ, et al: Polycystic ovaries and hyperandrogenism in women taking valproate for epilepsy. N Engl J Med 329:1383–1388, 1993

Isojarvi JI, Huuskonen UE, Pakarinen AJ, et al: The regulation of serum sodium after replacing carbamazepine with oxcarbazepine. Epilepsia 42:741–745, 2001

Janicak PG, Bresnahan DB, Sharma R, et al: A comparison of thiothixene with chlorpromazine in the treatment of mania. J Clin Psychopharmacol 8:33–37, 1988

Janicak PG, Newman RH, Davis JM: Advances in the treatment of mania and related disorders. Psychiatr Ann 22:92–103, 1992

Joffe H, Cohen LS, Suppes T, et al: Valproate is associated with new-onset oligoamenorrhea with hyperandrogenism in women with bipolar disorder. Biol Psychiatry 59:1078–1086, 2006

Johnson BA, Ait-Daoud N, Bowden CL, et al: Oral topiramate for treatment of alcohol dependence: a randomised controlled trial. Lancet 361:1677–1685, 2003

Johnson BA, Rosenthal N, Capece JA, et al: Topiramate for treating alcohol dependence: a randomized controlled trial. JAMA 298:1641–1651, 2007

Johnson G, Gershon S, Hekimian LJ: Controlled evaluation of lithium and chlorpromazine in the treatment of manic states: an interim report. Compr Psychiatry 9:563–573, 1968

Johnson G, Gershon S, Burdock EI, et al: Comparative effects of lithium and chlorpromazine in the treatment of acute manic states. Br J Psychiatry 119:267–276, 1971

Kahn D: The psychotherapy of mania. Psychiatr Clin North Am 13:229–240, 1990

Kanba S, Yagi G, Kamijima K, et al: The first open study of zonisamide, a novel anticonvulsant, shows efficacy in mania. Prog Neuropsychopharmacol Biol Psychiatry 18:707–715, 1994

Kane JM, Smith JM: Tardive dyskinesia: prevalence and risk factors, 1959 to 1979. Arch Gen Psychiatry 39:473–481, 1982

Keck PE Jr, Marcus R, Tourkodimitris S, et al: A placebo-controlled, double-blind study of the efficacy and safety of aripiprazole in patients with acute bipolar mania. Am J Psychiatry 160:1651–1658, 2003a

Keck PE Jr, Versiani M, Potkin S, et al: Ziprasidone in the treatment of acute bipolar mania: a three-week, placebo-controlled, double-blind, randomized trial. Am J Psychiatry 160:741–748, 2003b

Keck PE Jr, Perlis RH, Otto MW, et al: The expert consensus guideline series: medication treatment of bipolar disorder 2004. Postgrad Med Spec No:1–120, 2004

Keck PE, Sanchez R, Torbeyns AF, et al: Aripiprazole monotherapy in the treatment of acute bipolar I mania: a randomized placebo- and lithium-controlled study (NR304), in 2007 New Research Program and Abstracts, American Psychiatric Association 160th Annual Meeting, San Diego, CA, May 19–24, 2007. Washington, DC, American Psychiatric Association, 2007

Keller MB, Lavori PW, Coryell W, et al: Differential outcome of pure manic, mixed/cycling, and pure depressive episodes in patients with bipolar illness. JAMA 255:3138–3142, 1986

Ketter TA, Calabrese JR: Stabilization of mood from below versus above baseline in bipolar disorder: a new nomenclature. J Clin Psychiatry 63:146–151, 2002

Ketter TA, Post RM, Worthington K: Principles of clinically important drug interactions with carbamazepine: part I. J Clin Psychopharmacol 11:198–203, 1991a

Ketter TA, Post RM, Worthington K: Principles of clinically important drug interactions with carbamazepine: part II. J Clin Psychopharmacol 11:306–313, 1991b

Ketter TA, Kalali AH, Weisler RH: A 6-month, multicenter, open-label evaluation of beaded, extended-release carbamazepine capsule monotherapy in bipolar disorder patients with manic or mixed episodes. J Clin Psychiatry 65:668–673, 2004

Khanna S, Vieta E, Lyons B, et al: Risperidone in the treatment of acute mania: double-blind, placebo-controlled study. Br J Psychiatry 187:229–234, 2005

Kramlinger KG, Post RM: Adding lithium carbonate to carbamazepine: antimanic efficacy in treatment-resistant mania. Acta Psychiatr Scand 79:378–385, 1989

Krauthammer C, Klerman GL: Secondary mania: manic syndromes associated with antecedent physical illness or drugs. Arch Gen Psychiatry 35:1333–1339, 1978

Kukopulos A, Reginaldi D, Laddomada P, et al: Course of the manic-depressive cycle and changes caused by treatment. Pharmakopsychiatr Neuropsychopharmakol 13:156–167, 1980

Kushner SF, Khan A, Lane R, et al: Topiramate monotherapy in the management of acute mania: results of four double-blind placebo-controlled trials. Bipolar Disord 8:15–27, 2006

Lehmann HE, Hanrahan GE: Chlorpromazine; new inhibiting agent for psychomotor excitement and manic states. AMA Arch Neurol Psychiatry 71:227–237, 1954

Lenox RH, Newhouse PA, Creelman WL, et al: Adjunctive treatment of manic agitation with lorazepam versus haloperidol: a double-blind study. J Clin Psychiatry 53:47–52, 1992

Liang RA, Lam RW, Ancill RJ: ECT in the treatment of mixed depression and dementia. Br J Psychiatry 152:281–284, 1988

Loew TH, Nickel MK, Muehlbacher M, et al: Topiramate treatment for women with borderline personality disorder: a double-blind, placebo-controlled study. J Clin Psychopharmacol 26:61–66, 2006

Lucas CP, Rigby JC, Lucas SB: The occurrence of depression following mania: a method of predicting vulnerable cases. Br J Psychiatry 154:705–708, 1989

MacKinnon DF, Zandi PP, Cooper J, et al: Comorbid bipolar disorder and panic disorder in families with a high prevalence of bipolar disorder. Am J Psychiatry 159:30–35, 2002

Maggs R: Treatment of manic illness with lithium carbonate. Br J Psychiatry 109:56–65, 1963

McCracken JT, McGough J, Shah B, et al: Risperidone in children with autism and serious behavioral problems. N Engl J Med 347:314–321, 2002

McElroy SL, Arnold LM, Shapira NA, et al: Topiramate in the treatment of binge eating disorder associated with obesity: a randomized, placebo-controlled trial. Am J Psychiatry 160:255–261, 2003

McElroy SL, Kotwal R, Hudson JI, et al: Zonisamide in the treatment of binge-eating disorder: an open-label, prospective trial. J Clin Psychiatry 65:50–56, 2004

McElroy SL, Suppes T, Keck PE Jr, et al: Open-label adjunctive zonisamide in the treatment of bipolar disorders: a prospective trial. J Clin Psychiatry 66:617–624, 2005

McElroy SL, Kotwal R, Guerdjikova AI, et al: Zonisamide in the treatment of binge eating disorder with obesity: a randomized controlled trial. J Clin Psychiatry 67:1897–1906, 2006

McElroy SL, Frye MA, Altshuler LL, et al: A 24-week, randomized, controlled trial of adjunctive sibutramine versus topiramate in the treatment of weight gain in overweight or obese patients with bipolar disorders. Bipolar Disord 9:426–434, 2007

McIntyre RS, Mancini DA, McCann S, et al: Topiramate versus bupropion SR when added to mood stabilizer therapy for the depressive phase of bipolar disorder: a preliminary single-blind study. Bipolar Disord 4:207–213, 2002

McIntyre RS, Brecher M, Paulsson B, et al: Quetiapine or haloperidol as monotherapy for bipolar mania—a 12-week, double-blind, randomised, parallel-group, placebo-controlled trial. Eur Neuropsychopharmacol 15:573–585, 2005

McIntyre R, Hirschfeld R, Alphs L, et al: Asenapine in the treatment of acute mania in bipolar I disorder: outcomes from two randomized placebo controlled trials (abstract). Bipolar Disord 10 (suppl 1):49, 2008

Meehan K, Zhang F, David S, et al: A double-blind, randomized comparison of the efficacy and safety of intramuscular injections of olanzapine, lorazepam, or placebo in treating acutely agitated patients diagnosed with bipolar mania. J Clin Psychopharmacol 21:389–397, 2001

Meltzer HY, Alphs L, Green AI, et al: Clozapine treatment for suicidality in schizophrenia: International Suicide Prevention Trial (InterSePT). Arch Gen Psychiatry 60:82–91, 2003

Mester R: The psychotherapy of mania. Br J Med Psychol 59 (pt 1):13–19, 1986

Morgan HG: The incidence of depressive symptoms during recovery from hypomania. Br J Psychiatry 120:537–539, 1972

Muehlbacher M, Nickel MK, Kettler C, et al: Topiramate in treatment of patients with chronic low back pain: a randomized, double-blind, placebo-controlled study. Clin J Pain 22:526–531, 2006

Mukherjee S, Sackeim HA, Schnur DB: Electroconvulsive therapy of acute manic episodes: a review of 50 years' experience. Am J Psychiatry 151:169–176, 1994

Muller-Oerlinghausen B, Retzow A, Henn FA, et al: Valproate as an adjunct to neuroleptic medication for the treatment of acute episodes of mania: a prospective, randomized, double-blind, placebo-controlled, multicenter study. European Valproate Mania Study Group. J Clin Psychopharmacol 20:195–203, 2000

Nasrallah HA, Churchill CM, Hamdan-Allan GA: Higher frequency of neuroleptic-induced dystonia in mania than in schizophrenia. Am J Psychiatry 145:1455–1456, 1988

Niufan G, Tohen M, Qiuqing A, et al: Olanzapine versus lithium in the acute treatment of bipolar mania: a double-blind, randomized, controlled trial. J Affect Disord 105:101–108, 2008

Okuma T, Yamashita I, Takahashi R, et al: Clinical efficacy of carbamazepine in affective, schizoaffective, and schizophrenic disorders. Pharmacopsychiatry 22:47–53, 1989

Ondo WG, Jankovic J, Connor GS, et al: Topiramate in essential tremor: a double-blind, placebo-controlled trial. Neurology 66:672–677, 2006

Oral ET, Altinbas K, Demirkiran S: Sudden akathisia after a ziprasidone dose reduction (letter). Am J Psychiatry 163:546, 2006

Palmer AG, Williams H, Adams M: CBT in a group format for bi-polar affective disorder. Behavioural and Cognitive Psychotherapy 23:153–168, 1995

Pande AC, Davidson JR, Jefferson JW, et al: Treatment of social phobia with gabapentin: a placebo-controlled study. J Clin Psychopharmacol 19:341–348, 1999

Pande AC, Crockatt J, Janney CA, et al: Gabapentin in bipolar disorder: a placebo-controlled trial of adjunctive therapy. Gabapentin Bipolar Disorder Study Group. Bipolar Disord 2:249–255, 2000a

Pande AC, Pollack MH, Crockatt J, et al: Placebo-controlled study of gabapentin treatment of panic disorder. J Clin Psychopharmacol 20:467–471, 2000b

Perlis RH, Baker RW, Zarate CA Jr, et al: Olanzapine versus risperidone in the treatment of manic or mixed states in bipolar I disorder: a randomized, double-blind trial. J Clin Psychiatry 67:1747–1753, 2006

Physicians' Desk Reference, 62nd Edition. Montvale, NJ, Thomson Healthcare, 2008

Pope HG Jr, McElroy SL, Keck PE Jr, et al: Valproate in the treatment of acute mania: a placebo-controlled study. Arch Gen Psychiatry 48:62–68, 1991

Post RM, Jimerson DC, Bunney WE Jr, et al: Dopamine and mania: behavioral and biochemical effects of the dopamine receptor blocker pimozide. Psychopharmacology (Berl) 67:297–305, 1980

Post RM, Altshuler LL, Frye MA, et al: Preliminary observations on the effectiveness of levetiracetam in the open adjunctive treatment of refractory bipolar disorder. J Clin Psychiatry 66:370–374, 2005

Potkin SG, Sprague R, Keck PE Jr, et al: Ziprasidone in bipolar mania: efficacy across patient subgroups (NR777), in 2004 New Research Program and Abstracts, American Psychiatric Association 157th Annual Meeting, New York, NY, May 1–6, 2004. Washington, DC, American Psychiatric Association, 2004, p 292

Potkin SG, Keck PE Jr, Segal S, et al: Ziprasidone in acute bipolar mania: a 21-day randomized, double-blind, placebo-controlled replication trial. J Clin Psychopharmacol 25:301–310, 2005

Prien RF, Caffey EM Jr, Klett CJ: Comparison of lithium carbonate and chlorpromazine in the treatment of mania: report of the Veterans Administration and National Institute of Mental Health Collaborative Study Group. Arch Gen Psychiatry 26:146–153, 1972

Ramey TS, Giller E Jr, English P, et al: Ziprasidone efficacy and safety in acute bipolar mania: 12-week study (NR317), in 2005 New Research Program and Abstracts, American Psychiatric Association 158th Annual Meeting, Atlanta, GA, May 21–26, 2005. Washington, DC, American Psychiatric Association, 2005, pp 117–118

Rasgon N: The relationship between polycystic ovary syndrome and antiepileptic drugs: a review of the evidence. J Clin Psychopharmacol 24:322–334, 2004

Rasgon NL, Altshuler LL, Fairbanks L, et al: Reproductive function and risk for PCOS in women treated for bipolar disorder. Bipolar Disord 7:246–259, 2005

Rattya J, Vainionpaa L, Knip M, et al: The effects of valproate, carbamazepine, and oxcarbazepine on growth and sexual maturation in girls with epilepsy. Pediatrics 103:588–593, 1999

Ray WA, Chung CP, Murray KT, et al: Atypical antipsychotic drugs and the risk of sudden cardiac death. N Engl J Med 360:225–235, 2009

Rosenstock J, Hollander P, Gadde KM, et al: A randomized, double-blind, placebo-controlled, multicenter study to assess the efficacy and safety of topiramate controlled release in the treatment of obese type 2 diabetic patients. Diabetes Care 30:1480–1486, 2007

Rosenthal M: Tiagabine for the treatment of generalized anxiety disorder: a randomized, open-label, clinical trial with paroxetine as a positive control. J Clin Psychiatry 64:1245–1249, 2003

Rowbotham M, Harden N, Stacey B, et al: Gabapentin for the treatment of postherpetic neuralgia: a randomized controlled trial. JAMA 280:1837–1842, 1998

Sachs GS, Grossman F, Ghaemi SN, et al: Combination of a mood stabilizer with risperidone or haloperidol for treatment of acute mania: a double-blind, placebo-controlled comparison of efficacy and safety. Am J Psychiatry 159:1146–1154, 2002

Sachs G, Chengappa KN, Suppes T, et al: Quetiapine with lithium or divalproex for the treatment of bipolar mania: a randomized, double-blind, placebo-controlled study. Bipolar Disord 6:213–223, 2004

Sachs G, Sanchez R, Marcus R, et al: Aripiprazole in the treatment of acute manic or mixed episodes in patients with bipolar I disorder: a 3-week placebo-controlled study. J Psychopharmacol 20:536–546, 2006

Sanchez R, Dillenschneider A, McQuade RD, et al: Aripiprazole monotherapy in acute bipolar I mania: a randomized placebo- and haloperidol-controlled study (NR3-100), in 2008 New Research Program and Abstracts, American Psychiatric Association 161st Annual Meeting, Washington, DC, May 3–8, 2008. Washington, DC, American Psychiatric Association, 2008

Schaffer LC, Schaffer CB, Howe J: An open case series on the utility of tiagabine as an augmentation in refractory bipolar outpatients. J Affect Disord 71:259–263, 2002

Schou M, Juel-Nielsen N, Strömgren E, et al: The treatment of manic psychosis by the administration of lithium salts. J Neurol Neurosurg Psychiatry 17:250–260, 1954

Scott J: Cognitive therapy for clients with bipolar disorders. Cogn Behav Pract 3:29–51, 1996

Secunda SK, Katz MM, Swann A, et al: Mania: diagnosis, state measurement and prediction of treatment response. J Affect Disord 8:113–121, 1985

Serpell MG: Gabapentin in neuropathic pain syndromes: a randomised, double-blind, placebo-controlled trial. Pain 99:557–566, 2002

Shopsin B, Gershon S, Thompson H, et al. Psychoactive drugs in mania: a controlled comparison of lithium carbonate, chlorpromazine, and haloperidol. Arch Gen Psychiatry 32:34–42, 1975

Silberstein SD, Lipton RB, Dodick DW, et al: Efficacy and safety of topiramate for the treatment of chronic migraine: a randomized, double-blind, placebo-controlled trial. Headache 47:170–180, 2007

Small JG, Milstein V: Lithium interactions: lithium and electroconvulsive therapy. J Clin Psychopharmacol 10:346–350, 1990

Small JG, Klapper MH, Marhenke JD, et al: Lithium combined with carbamazepine or haloperidol in the treatment of mania. Psychopharmacol Bull 31:265–272, 1995

Smulevich AB, Khanna S, Eerdekens M, et al: Acute and continuation risperidone monotherapy in bipolar mania: a 3-week placebo-controlled trial followed by a 9-week double-blind trial of risperidone and haloperidol. Eur Neuropsychopharmacol 15:75–84, 2005

Spira PJ, Beran RG: Gabapentin in the prophylaxis of chronic daily headache: a randomized, placebo-controlled study. Neurology 61:1753–1759, 2003

Spring G, Schweid D, Gray C, et al: A double-blind comparison of lithium and chlorpromazine in the treatment of manic states. Am J Psychiatry 126:1306–1310, 1970

Stahl SM, Lombardo I, Loebel A, et al: Efficacy of ziprasidone in dysphoric mania: pooled analysis of 2 double-blind studies (abstract). Neuropsychopharmacology 30 (suppl 1):S239–S240, 2005

Stenlof K, Rossner S, Vercruysse F, et al: Topiramate in the treatment of obese subjects with drug-naive type 2 diabetes. Diabetes Obes Metab 9:360–368, 2007

Stokes PE, Shamoian CA, Stoll PM, et al: Efficacy of lithium as acute treatment of manic-depressive illness. Lancet 1:1319–1325, 1971

Suppes T, Webb A, Paul B, et al: Clinical outcome in a randomized 1-year trial of clozapine versus treatment as usual for patients with treatment-resistant illness and a history of mania. Am J Psychiatry 156:1164–1169, 1999

Suppes T, Chisholm KA, Dhavale D, et al: Tiagabine in treatment refractory bipolar disorder: a clinical case series. Bipolar Disord 4:283–289, 2002

Suppes T, Dennehy EB, Hirschfeld RM, et al: The Texas Implementation of Medication Algorithms: update to the algorithms for treatment of bipolar I disorder. J Clin Psychiatry 66:870–886, 2005

Suppes T, Eudicone J, McQuade R, et al: Efficacy and safety of aripiprazole in subpopulations with acute manic or mixed episodes of bipolar I disorder. J Affect Disord 107:145–154, 2008

Suppes T, Vieta E, Liu S, et al: Maintenance treatment for patients with bipolar I disorder: results from a North American study of quetiapine in combination with lithium or divalproex (trial 127). Am J Psychiatry 166:476–488, 2009

Swann AC, Bowden CL, Morris D, et al: Depression during mania: treatment response to lithium or divalproex. Arch Gen Psychiatry 54:37–42, 1997

Swann AC, Bowden CL, Calabrese JR, et al: Mania: differential effects of previous depressive and manic episodes on response to treatment. Acta Psychiatr Scand 101:444–451, 2000

Swann AC, Bowden CL, Calabrese JR, et al: Pattern of response to divalproex, lithium, or placebo in four naturalistic subtypes of mania. Neuropsychopharmacology 26:530–536, 2002

Swartz HA, Frank E: Psychotherapy for bipolar depression: a phase-specific treatment strategy? Bipolar Disord 3:11–22, 2001

Takahashi R, Sakuma A, Itoh K, et al: Comparison of efficacy of lithium carbonate and chlorpromazine in mania: report of collaborative study group on treatment of mania in Japan. Arch Gen Psychiatry 32:1310–1318, 1975

Thase ME, Macfadden W, Weisler RH, et al: Efficacy of quetiapine monotherapy in bipolar I and II depression: a double-blind, placebo-controlled study (the BOLDER II study). J Clin Psychopharmacol 26:600–609, 2006

Tohen M, Sanger TM, McElroy SL, et al: Olanzapine versus placebo in the treatment of acute mania. Olanzapine HGEH Study Group. Am J Psychiatry 156:702–709, 1999

Tohen M, Jacobs TG, Grundy SL, et al: Efficacy of olanzapine in acute bipolar mania: a double-blind, placebo-controlled study. The Olanzapine HGGW Study Group. Arch Gen Psychiatry 57:841–849, 2000

Tohen M, Baker RW, Altshuler LL, et al: Olanzapine versus divalproex in the treatment of acute mania. Am J Psychiatry 159:1011–1017, 2002a

Tohen M, Chengappa KN, Suppes T, et al: Efficacy of olanzapine in combination with valproate or lithium in the treatment of mania in patients partially nonresponsive to valproate or lithium monotherapy. Arch Gen Psychiatry 59:62–69, 2002b

Tohen M, Goldberg JF, Gonzalez-Pinto Arrillaga AM, et al: A 12-week, double-blind comparison of olanzapine vs haloperidol in the treatment of acute mania. Arch Gen Psychiatry 60:1218–1226, 2003

Tohen M, Kryzhanovskaya L, Carlson G, et al: Olanzapine versus placebo in the treatment of adolescents with bipolar mania. Am J Psychiatry 164:1547–1556, 2007

Tohen M, Bowden CL, Smulevich AB, et al: Olanzapine plus carbamazepine v. carbamazepine alone in treating manic episodes. Br J Psychiatry 192:135–143, 2008

Toplak H, Hamann A, Moore R, et al: Efficacy and safety of topiramate in combination with metformin in the treatment of obese subjects with type 2 diabetes: a randomized, double-blind, placebo-controlled study. Int J Obes (Lond) 31:138–146, 2007

Tremblay A, Chaput JP, Berube-Parent S, et al: The effect of topiramate on energy balance in obese men: a 6-month double-blind randomized placebo-controlled study with a 6-month open-label extension. Eur J Clin Pharmacol 63:123–134, 2007

Vajda F, Lander C, O'Brien T, et al: Australian pregnancy registry of women taking antiepileptic drugs (letter). Epilepsia 45:1466, 2004

Valenti M, Benabarre A, Garcia-Amador M, et al: Electroconvulsive therapy in the treatment of mixed states in bipolar disorder. Eur Psychiatry 23:53–56, 2008

Vieta E, Bourin M, Sanchez R, et al: Effectiveness of aripiprazole v. haloperidol in acute bipolar mania: double-blind, randomised, comparative 12-week trial. Br J Psychiatry 187:235–242, 2005

Vieta E, T'joen C, McQuade RD, et al: Efficacy of adjunctive aripiprazole to either valproate or lithium in bipolar mania patients partially nonresponsive to valproate/lithium monotherapy: a placebo-controlled study. Am J Psychiatry 165:1316–1325, 2008a

Vieta E, Suppes T, Eggens I, et al: Efficacy and safety of quetiapine in combination with lithium or divalproex for maintenance of patients with bipolar I disorder (international trial 126). J Affect Disord 109:251–263, 2008b

Wagner KD, Kowatch RA, Emslie GJ, et al: A double-blind, randomized, placebo-controlled trial of oxcarbazepine in the treatment of bipolar disorder in children and adolescents. Am J Psychiatry 163:1179–1186, 2006

Wang PS, Schneeweiss S, Avorn J, et al: Risk of death in elderly users of conventional vs. atypical antipsychotic medications. N Engl J Med 353:2335–2341, 2005

Wang PW, Yang YS, Chandler RA, et al: Adjunctive zonisamide for weight loss in euthymic bipolar disorder patients: a pilot study. J Psychiatr Res 42:451–457, 2008

Warrington L, Lombardo I, Loebel A, et al: Ziprasidone for the treatment of acute manic or mixed episodes associated with bipolar disorder. CNS Drugs 21:835–849, 2007

Weisler RH, Kalali AH, Ketter TA: A multicenter, randomized, double-blind, placebo-controlled trial of extended-release carbamazepine capsules as monotherapy for bipolar disorder patients with manic or mixed episodes. J Clin Psychiatry 65:478–484, 2004a

Weisler RH, Warrington L, Dunn J, et al: Adjunctive ziprasidone in bipolar mania: short-term and long-term data (NR358), in 2004 New Research Program and Abstracts, American Psychiatric Association 157th Annual Meeting, New York, NY, May 1–6, 2004. Washington, DC, American Psychiatric Association, 2004b, pp 132–133

Weisler RH, Keck PE Jr, Swann AC, et al: Extended-release carbamazepine capsules as monotherapy for acute mania in bipolar disorder: a multicenter, randomized, double-blind, placebo-controlled trial. J Clin Psychiatry 66:323–330, 2005

Yatham LN, Grossman F, Augustyns I, et al: Mood stabilisers plus risperidone or placebo in the treatment of acute mania: international, double-blind, randomised controlled trial. Br J Psychiatry 182:141–147, 2003

Yatham LN, Paulsson B, Mullen J, et al: Quetiapine versus placebo in combination with lithium or divalproex for the treatment of bipolar mania. J Clin Psychopharmacol 24:599–606, 2004

Yatham LN, Kennedy SH, O'Donovan C, et al: Canadian Network for Mood and Anxiety Treatments (CANMAT) guidelines for the management of patients with bipolar disorder: update 2007. Bipolar Disord 8:721–739, 2006

Zajecka JM, Weisler R, Sachs G, et al: A comparison of the efficacy, safety, and tolerability of divalproex sodium and olanzapine in the treatment of bipolar disorder. J Clin Psychiatry 63:1148–1155, 2002

Zarate CA Jr, Tohen M, Baldessarini RJ: Clozapine in severe mood disorders. J Clin Psychiatry 56:411–417, 1995

Zimbroff DL, Marcus RN, Manos G, et al: Management of acute agitation in patients with bipolar disorder: efficacy and safety of intramuscular aripiprazole. J Clin Psychopharmacol 27:171–176, 2007

CHAPTER 7

Management of Acute Major Depressive Episodes in Bipolar Disorders

Po W. Wang, M.D.

Terence A. Ketter, M.D.

Bipolar disorder is a group of disorders that share features of mood elevation and depressive episodes. However, bipolar disorder also may be thought of as having a core phenomenon of mood instability. For all practical purposes, however, nearly all contemporary studies of bipolar disorder use the classification currently set out by DSM-IV-TR (American Psychiatric Association 2000). As described in Chapter 2 of this volume, "DSM-IV-TR Diagnosis of Bipolar Disorders," this system classifies bipolar disorder into four major entities: bipolar I disorder, bipolar II disorder, cyclothymic disorder, and bipolar disorder not otherwise specified (NOS). Because of the limited data available for bipolar disorder NOS and cyclothymic disorder, the major focus of this chapter is on depression in the context of bipolar I disorder and bipolar II disorder.

Depression is commonly the predominant mood disturbance during the course of bipolar illness. Diagnosing and treating bipolar depression, by consequence, constitute one of the most common clinical challenges for clinicians and patients. In this chapter we review the treatment of acute major depressive episodes in patients with bipolar disorders, with special emphasis on evidence-based, practical, clinical information.

Treatment of Acute Bipolar Depression: A Shifting Paradigm

Because of a limited evidence base, substantial variations in response to therapeutic interventions across individuals, and the common phenomenon of treatment resistance, the optimal approach to acute bipolar depression is a topic of spirited debate.

Until recently, traditional approaches to bipolar depression such as lithium monotherapy or lithium (or other mood stabilizers) combined with antidepressants prevailed. The first of these approaches was based on the premise that lithium was a foundational treatment for all phases of bipolar disorder, in spite of limitations of data supporting its utility in acute bipolar depression. The second approach was based on the premise that bipolar depression was an analog of unipolar depression, combined with the abundance of robust data supporting the efficacy of antidepressants in unipolar depression, to yield the notion that antidepressants (counterbalanced by mood stabilizers) ought to be effective in bipolar depression, in spite of the limited evidence to support this view.

Increasingly, it is becoming clear that the evidence base to support traditional approaches to bipolar depression is inadequate. As discussed later in this chapter, this is becoming even more problematic with the emergence of other treatment options with more substantive evidence to support their use in acute bipolar depression. In this chapter we describe an evidence-based approach to the treatment of acute bipolar depression, starting with interventions with the most evidence to support their use.

Treatment of Acute Bipolar Depression: Balancing Benefits and Risks

Unfortunately, there are only limited systematic data and even sparser approved treatment options for acute bipolar depression, despite subsyndromal and syndromal depressive symptoms constituting the most pervasive aspects of mood disturbance in bipolar disorder. Thus, there are only two approved treatments for bipolar depression, the olanzapine plus fluoxetine combination (OFC) and quetiapine monotherapy (Figure 7–1, left, second from left), compared with nine approved treatments for mania and five approved treatments for longer-term treatment.

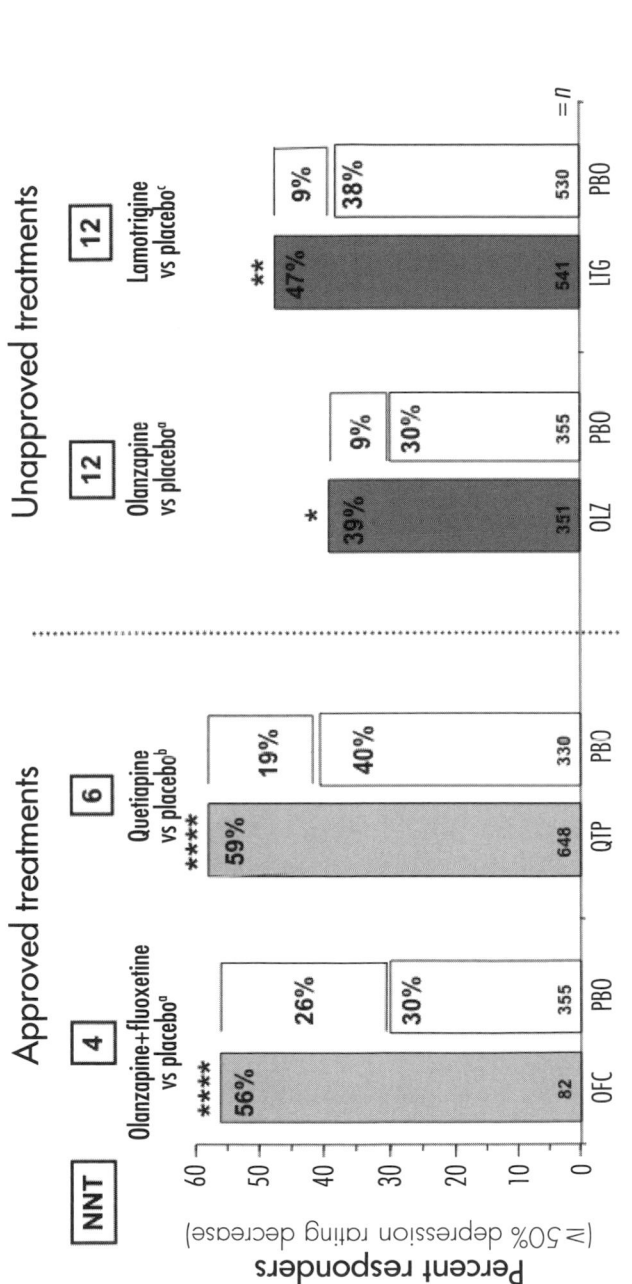

FIGURE 7–1. Overview of contemporary acute bipolar depression studies: treatment response.

Numbers needed to treat (NNT) for response, rates. The approved treatments have single-digit NNT for response. LTG=lamotrigine; PBO=placebo; OFC=olanzapine plus fluoxetine combination; OLZ=olanzapine; QTP=quetiapine. *$P<0.05$; **$P<0.01$; ****$P<0.0001$ versus placebo.

[a]Data from Tohen et al. 2003.

[b]Data from Calabrese et al. 2005; Thase et al. 2006.

[c]Data from Geddes et al. 2009.

The approved treatments for bipolar depression, as with approved treatments for other aspects of bipolar disorder, have single-digit numbers needed to treat (NNT) (Figure 7–1, top), indicating that treating fewer than 10 patients with an approved agent compared with placebo can be expected to yield one more responder. Thus, if efficacy were the sole consideration, the approved options would carry higher priorities than an unapproved treatment such as lamotrigine, which is associated with an NNT in the low teens (Figure 7–1, right).

However, the practice of evidence-based medicine entails considering not only efficacy data (i.e., giving higher priorities to treatments with lower NNTs), but also taking into account safety/tolerability data (i.e., giving higher priorities to treatments with higher numbers needed to harm [NNH]). In making treatment decisions, it is crucial to determine which choice optimizes for the individual patient the benefit-to-risk ratio, which may be characterized as the likelihood to be helped or harmed (LHH=NNH/NNT). In some instances, a higher NNT (e.g., as with lamotrigine) may be considered acceptable if it is accompanied by an even higher NNH. This is the evidence-based equivalent of the Hippocratic maxim "First, do no harm."

Balancing benefit and risk is arguably even more crucial when treating acute bipolar depression than when treating acute mania, because depressive symptoms are more chronic than mood elevation symptoms and entail greater sensitivity to side effects of interventions. Thus, clinicians need to integrate the efficacy data in Figure 7–1 with safety and tolerability data, as depicted in Figure 7–2. Although the approved treatments for bipolar depression have the benefit of efficacy, they are associated with comparable risks with respect to safety and tolerability.

Hence, as described in greater detail later in this chapter, for the olanzapine plus fluoxetine combination the NNT for response is 4 but the NNH for clinically significant (≥7%) weight gain is 6 (Figure 7–2, left), yielding an LHH of 1.5 (6/4). Put another way, patients with bipolar depression taking the olanzapine plus fluoxetine combination compared with placebo are only slightly (by a factor of 1.5) more likely to respond than they are likely to experience clinically significant weight gain. Similarly, for quetiapine monotherapy, the NNT for response is 6 but the NNH for sedation is 5 (Figure 7–2, second from left), yielding an LHH of 1.2 (6/5). In other words, patients with bipolar depression taking quetiapine monotherapy compared with placebo are slightly more likely to experience sedation than they are likely to respond.

The unapproved treatment lamotrigine monotherapy, aside from the risk of rare serious rash (seen in approximately 0.1% of patients), has the advantage of

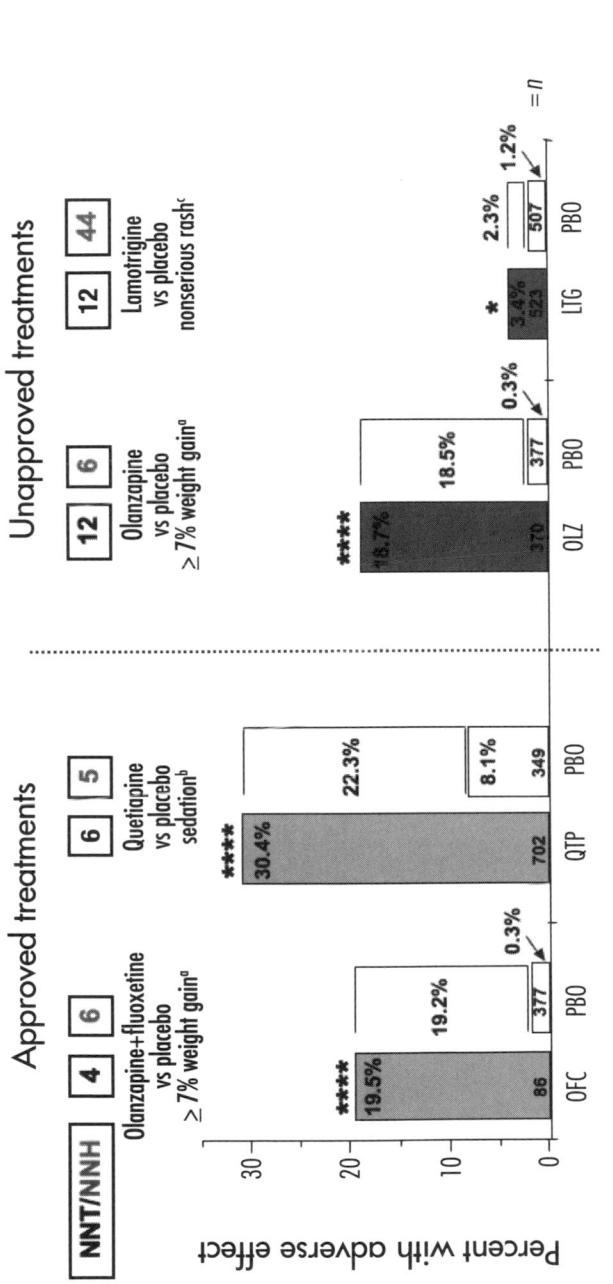

FIGURE 7–2. Overview of contemporary acute bipolar depression studies: adverse effects.

Numbers needed to treat (NNT) and numbers needed to harm (NNH), adverse effect rates. The approved treatments are associated with weight gain and sedation, which can limit their clinical utility. Benefit-risk analysis for the approved treatments (OFC, QTP) involves assessing whether the good efficacy merits the adverse effects (weight gain, sedation) risks. Benefit-risk analysis for the unapproved treatment LTG involves assessing whether the low risks of adverse effects merit the risk of inefficacy. Response rates accounting for NNT are depicted in Figure 7–1. LTG=lamotrigine; OFC=olanzapine plus fluoxetine combination; OLZ=olanzapine; PBO=placebo; QTP=quetiapine. *$P<0.05$; ****$P<0.0001$ versus placebo.
[a]Data from Tohen et al. 2003. [b]Data from Calabrese et al. 2005; Thase et al. 2006. [c]Data from Calabrese et al. 2008; Geddes et al. 2009.

having an uncommonly favorable safety/tolerability profile, as described in greater detail later. Specifically, lamotrigine compared with placebo carries negligible risks of clinically significant weight gain or sedation. Indeed, in many instances, nonserious rash (seen in 3.4% of bipolar depression patients across five controlled studies) may be the most common side effect leading to lamotrigine discontinuation. Thus, lamotrigine monotherapy of bipolar depression entails suboptimal efficacy (NNT for response of 12) potentially offset by advantageous safety/tolerability (NNH for benign rash of 44), yielding an LHH of 3.7 (44/12). Put another way, patients with bipolar depression taking lamotrigine monotherapy compared with placebo are considerably (by a factor of 3.7) more likely to respond than they are likely to experience benign rash. In addition, lamotrigine is approved for longer-term treatment to delay mood episodes in patients with bipolar disorder, particularly depressive episodes. Thus, some clinicians and patients may view lamotrigine monotherapy as a reasonable unapproved alternative to the two approved treatments for acute bipolar depression.

In contrast, another unapproved treatment, namely olanzapine monotherapy, appears substantially less attractive (Figure 7–2, second from right), because it has an NNT for response of 12 accompanied by an NNH for clinically significant weight gain of 6, yielding an LHH of 0.5 (6/12). In other words, patients taking olanzapine monotherapy compared with placebo are substantially (by a factor of 0.5) *less* likely to respond than they are likely to experience weight gain. Thus, it appears unlikely that clinicians and patients would view olanzapine monotherapy as an attractive unapproved alternative to the two approved treatments or to lamotrigine monotherapy.

Thus, optimal management of bipolar depression entails finding the agent(s) with the best combination of efficacy and safety/tolerability for the individual patient. For example, for the patient with very acute, severe bipolar depression, characterized by marked weight loss, insomnia, and psychomotor agitation, the approved treatments may be very attractive in view of their superior efficacy and the fact that the risks of weight gain and sedation may not be particularly problematic, at least in the short term. In contrast, for the patient with chronic, mild bipolar depression, characterized by weight gain, hypersomnia, and psychomotor retardation, the unapproved treatment lamotrigine may be attractive, in spite of its inferior efficacy, because it carries minimal risks of weight gain and sedation and in the longer term may help delay the return of depression. In yet another patient with a history of a serious rash, even the low risk of such a rash with lamotrigine may render this agent unacceptable.

Treatments for acute bipolar depression are reviewed later, using the four-tier system in presented in Table 7–1. This system is a hybrid approach, combining evidence-based medical information on efficacy and tolerability, with more empirical constructs such as familiarity and patient acceptability, to prioritize treatments in a fashion broadly consistent with North American clinical practice and treatment guidelines.

Tier I treatment options have U.S. Food and Drug Administration (FDA) approval for the treatment of acute bipolar depression and are supported by the most compelling evidence of efficacy. However, tolerability limitations of Tier I treatments may lead clinicians and patients, after comparing the risks and ben-

TABLE 7–1.　A four-tier approach to the management of acute bipolar depression

Tier	Priority	Status	Treatment options
I	High	Approved	Second-generation antipsychotics: olanzapine plus fluoxetine, quetiapine
II	High	High-priority unapproved	Mood stabilizers: lithium, lamotrigine
III	Intermediate	Other	Other mood stabilizers: divalproex, carbamazepine Other second-generation antipsychotics: olanzapine monotherapy, aripiprazole,[a] risperidone, ziprasidone, clozapine Adjunctive antidepressants Electroconvulsive therapy Adjunctive psychotherapy: psychoeducation, cognitive-behavioral therapy, family-focused therapy, interpersonal and social rhythm therapy
IV	Low	Novel adjuncts	Thyroid hormones Pramipexole Modafinil Topiramate Stimulants Sleep deprivation Light therapy Nutraceuticals Vagus nerve stimulation Transcranial magnetic stimulation

[a]Ineffective in controlled acute bipolar depression trials as of early 2009.

efits, to consider treatments in other tiers, particularly Tier II. Indeed, in clinical practice and in some treatment guidelines, Tier I treatments have been considered to have equal priority to or even lower priority than Tier II options.

Tier II treatment options lack FDA approval for the treatment of acute bipolar depression and have less compelling evidence of efficacy than Tier I options but arguably have mitigating advantages such as maintenance indications, tolerability, or familiarity that might make them attractive for a substantial number of patients. In clinical practice and in some treatment guidelines, these medications have been considered first-line interventions in spite of the absence of FDA indications for acute bipolar depression.

Tier III treatment options generally lack FDA approval for the treatment of acute bipolar depression and have even less compelling evidence of efficacy than Tier I or II options. In general, treatment guidelines do not consider these modalities to be first-line interventions but cite them as intermediate-priority options. However, some Tier III options have mitigating advantages such as maintenance indications, tolerability, or familiarity that might make them attractive for selected patients, and in certain circumstances some of these interventions may be considered early on (e.g., psychotherapy or electroconvulsive therapy in pregnant women with acute bipolar depression). For some of these treatments (e.g., adjunctive psychotherapy), advances in research, familiarity, and/or availability ultimately may be sufficient to merit their consideration for placement in higher tiers.

Tier IV treatment options generally lack FDA approval for the treatment of acute bipolar depression and have even more limited evidence of efficacy than Tier I, II, or III options. In general, treatment guidelines consider these modalities to be low-priority interventions. Nevertheless, some Tier IV options could prove attractive for carefully selected patients after consideration of Tier I–III treatments (e.g., patients treatment resistant or intolerant to Tier I–III treatments). For some of these treatments, advances in research may ultimately provide sufficient evidence to merit their consideration for placement in higher tiers.

Tier I: Approved Treatment Options for Acute Bipolar Depression

The approved treatments for acute bipolar depression are the olanzapine plus fluoxetine combination and quetiapine monotherapy. As noted previously and described in greater detail later in this chapter, both of these options have favorable efficacy (NNTs of 4 and 6, respectively; Figure 7–1, left side) but also have safety/tolerability challenges (NNHs of 6 and 5, respectively; Figure 7–2, left side). Thus, as noted earlier, tolerability limitations of Tier I treatments may lead clinicians and patients, after comparing the risks and benefits, to consider treatments in other tiers, particularly Tier II. Indeed, in clinical practice and in some treatment guidelines, Tier I treatments have commonly been considered to have equal or even lower priority than Tier II options. Also, because Tier I treatments were relatively recently approved, they are only noted as first- or second-line options in more recent North American guidelines (Suppes et al. 2005; Yatham et al. 2006).

Second-Generation Antipsychotics

Second-generation antipsychotics increasingly have been used in the management of bipolar disorders, initially in the treatment of acute mania and more recently in acute bipolar depression as well as longer-term treatment. These changes represent a substantial challenge to the older view that antipsychotics are mere adjuncts for acute mania that need to be minimized at other times in the management of bipolar disorders. Emerging data indicate that second-generation antipsychotics, although they share similar efficacy profiles for acute mania, may have differential efficacy profiles in bipolar depression.

Olanzapine Plus Fluoxetine Combination

In 2003, the combination of olanzapine plus fluoxetine, or OFC, became the first treatment approved for acute bipolar depression, based on the largest placebo-controlled trial ($N=833$) published to date on the treatment of acute bipolar depression (Tohen et al. 2003).

Olanzapine (mean final dosage 10 mg/day) monotherapy ($n=370$) and OFC (mean final dosages = olanzapine 7.5 mg/day, fluoxetine 40 mg/day) ($n=86$) were superior to placebo ($n=377$) during an 8-week, multicenter, randomized, double-blind, placebo-controlled trial in bipolar I disorder depression. The Montgomery-Åsberg Depression Rating Scale (MADRS) response ($\geq$50% MADRS decrease) rate with OFC (56.1%) was robustly superior to that with not only placebo (30.4%, $P<0.001$, NNT=4; Figure 7–1, left) but also that with olanzapine (39.0%, $P=0.006$), whereas olanzapine was modestly superior to placebo ($P=0.02$, NNT=12; Figure 7–1, second from right). Importantly, efficacy was evident as early as the end of the first week of treatment for both OFC and olanzapine monotherapy, and OFC was superior to olanzapine monotherapy by the end of week 4.

Somnolence, weight gain, increased appetite, and dry mouth were observed similarly in subjects treated with OFC therapy and olanzapine monotherapy, but nausea and diarrhea were reported at significantly higher rates in the OFC group. Rates of clinically significant (≥7%) weight gain were greater with OFC (19.5%) compared with placebo (0.3%, NNH=6; Figure 7–2, left), and with olanzapine (18.7%) compared with placebo (NNH=6; Figure 7–2, second from right). Rates of sedation also tended to be greater with OFC (20.9%) compared with placebo (12.5%, NNH=12), and with olanzapine (28.1%) compared with placebo (NNH=7). The incidence of treatment-emergent affective switch (mania induction) was low and did not differ between groups. Thus, OFC and to a more limited extent olanzapine appeared effective in depressed patients with bipolar I disorder, with sedation and weight gain being the most common adverse effects.

As discussed in the section on lamotrigine later in this chapter, a subsequent controlled trial found that OFC compared with lamotrigine in depressed patients with bipolar I disorder was slightly more effective but more poorly tolerated because of sedation and weight gain (Brown et al. 2006). As noted previously, the potential efficacy benefit of OFC needs to be considered in tandem with the risks of adverse effects, particularly weight gain, metabolic problems, and sedation (Figure 7–2, left) when embarking on this treatment modality.

Dosing guidelines in this chapter are provided for outpatients, the most common status of individuals presenting with bipolar depression. OFC is marketed in the United States in a single-capsule formulation. The U.S. prescribing information recommends starting OFC at olanzapine 6 mg/day plus fluoxetine 25 mg/day (6/25) and adjusting the dosage as necessary and tolerated to as high as olanzapine 12 mg/day plus fluoxetine 50 mg/day (12/50). There are five available capsule strengths: 3/25, 6/25, 6/50, 12/25, and 12/50. Starting with the 3/25 capsule is recommended in order to limit adverse effects in vulnerable patients, such as those with a predisposition to hypotensive reactions, hepatic impairment, combinations of slow olanzapine metabolism risk factors (elderly, female, non-smoker), or pharmacodynamic medication sensitivity. Because the rate of sedation with OFC was 20.9% in the pivotal trial (which started OFC at 6/25), clinicians may wish to initiate OFC at 3/25, even in patients lacking the previously mentioned vulnerability risk factors. The prescribing information also notes that the safety of OFC doses above 18/75 has not been evaluated in clinical studies, and OFC has not been systematically studied in patients younger than age 18 years or older than age 65 years.

Clinicians may prefer to administer the olanzapine and fluoxetine components separately to have greater control over titration and the ratio of olanzapine to fluoxetine. However, it should be noted that the OFC single-capsule formulation has the advantage of making it not possible for patients to take the fluoxetine component in the absence of olanzapine, thus decreasing the potential risk of treatment-emergent affective switch related to taking unopposed fluoxetine.

For clinicians who wish to administer the olanzapine and fluoxetine components separately, starting olanzapine at 2.5 mg/day at bedtime and increasing every 4–7 days as necessary and tolerated by 2.5 mg/day, initially targeting a dosage of 7.5 mg/day at bedtime, may enhance tolerability. Concurrently, fluoxetine may be started at 10 mg/day at bedtime, and increasing every 4–7 days as necessary and tolerated by 10 mg/day, initially targeting a dosage of 40 mg/day at bedtime, may enhance tolerability. Thus, with this approach the initial target dosages are olanzapine 7.5 mg/day plus fluoxetine 40 mg/day, which reflect the mean dosages in the registration study. In patients who tolerate but fail to respond to olanzapine 7.5 mg/day plus fluoxetine 40 mg/day, further increasing olanzapine by 2.5 mg/day and fluoxetine by 10 mg/day every 4–7 days as necessary and tolerated, to as high as olanzapine 12.5 mg/day plus fluoxetine 50 mg/day, yields dosages similar to the 12/50 maximum recommended in the U.S. prescribing information. Administering olanzapine and fluoxetine separately may permit fewer adverse effects, particularly in relationship to limiting exposure to olanzapine, which can cause sedation, weight gain, and metabolic problems. However, it must be kept in mind that dosages of olanzapine below 6 mg/day might provide inadequate antimanic coverage to counterbalance the risk of fluoxetine-induced treatment-emergent affective switch. Additional information regarding olanzapine and fluoxetine is provided in Chapter 13, "Mood Stabilizers and Antipsychotics," and Chapter 14, "Antidepressants, Anxiolytics/Hypnotics, and Other Medications."

In summary, OFC appears effective in acute bipolar depression, but safety and tolerability challenges may limit its utility, particularly in longer-term therapy. Controlled studies are needed to inform clinicians regarding the potential benefits and risks of continuing this treatment in patients who have experienced relief of acute bipolar depression.

Quetiapine

In 2006, quetiapine was the first monotherapy medication approved by the FDA for the treatment of acute bipolar depression, based on two 8-week, multicenter, randomized, double-blind, placebo-controlled trials (Calabrese et al. 2005; Thase et al. 2006). Perhaps equally as important was the inclusion of patients with bipolar II disorder as well as patients with bipolar I disorder, thus resulting in the first approval of an agent for the treatment of patients with bipolar II disorder. In 2008, extended-release quetiapine (quetiapine XR) received a similar indication for the treatment of acute bipolar depression.

In pooled analyses of the two quetiapine immediate-release formulation pivotal trials, quetiapine (300 mg/day and 600 mg/day) had antidepressant effects in patients with bipolar I disorder and patients with bipolar II disorder and in patients with or without rapid-cycling course of illness. Also, analysis of pooled data for both dosages of quetiapine for both trials revealed MADRS response rates of 59% for quetiapine and 40% for placebo, yielding for quetiapine versus placebo an NNT for MADRS response of 6 (Figure 7–1, second from left). However, a similar pooled analysis of safety/tolerability data yielded sedation rates of 30.4% for quetiapine and 8.1% for placebo, yielding for quetiapine versus placebo an NNH for sedation of 5 (Figure 7–2, second from left). Thus, as noted previously, the potential efficacy benefit of quetiapine needs to be considered along with the risks of adverse effects, particularly sedation, and to a lesser extent weight gain and metabolic problems, when embarking on this treatment modality.

In two recent additional 8-week, multicenter, randomized, double-blind, placebo-controlled studies, quetiapine 300 mg/day and quetiapine 600 mg/day were found to be superior to placebo (Olausson et al. 2008; Young et al. 2008). These two studies were of particular interest because they included lithium and paroxetine, respectively, as active comparators that failed to separate from placebo.

These controlled studies of quetiapine in bipolar depression were conducted in outpatient samples. Quetiapine immediate-release formulation was started at 50 mg the first evening, increased to 100 mg by the second night, to 200 mg by the third night, and to 300 mg/day by the fourth night. In patients randomly assigned to the higher dosage, quetiapine was further increased to 400 mg/day by the fifth night and to 600 mg/day by the eighth night. This relatively rapid titration yielded rapid improvement. However, as noted previously, in the two pivotal bipolar depression studies 30.4% of patients taking quetiapine experienced sedation, compared with 8.1% of those taking placebo (Figure 7–2, second from left).

This previously mentioned quetiapine initial dosing is described in the U.S. prescribing information, with the acknowledgment that both quetiapine 300 mg/day and quetiapine 600 mg/day were effective for bipolar depression but with the caveat that there was no additional benefit in the 600-mg/day group. Thus, in efforts to limit adverse effects such as sedation, clinicians may choose to make 300 mg/day the initial target dosage, and after 2–3 weeks, in patients who tolerate but fail to respond to 300 mg/day, further increase weekly by 100-mg increments as necessary and tolerated, to as high as 600 mg/day.

In some patients, the recommended titration may not be tolerated (most often because of sedation), so that more gradual increases (e.g., starting with 25 mg at bedtime and increasing daily by 25 mg) will be necessary. Smaller, less frequent dosage increases that are judiciously timed (e.g., on Friday and Saturday evenings to avoid affecting work or school performance) may yield fewer adverse effects with less functional impairment. Adjusting the timing of doses may yield benefit as well, with some patients splitting the dose between dinner and bedtime, or even taking the entire dose at dinner, noting less sedation the following morning. The minimum effective quetiapine dosage in bipolar depression has not been established, so that even if tolerability limits the final quetiapine dosage to less than the 300-mg/day initial target, this could be sufficient to yield benefit. Additional information regarding quetiapine is provided in Chapter 13 of this volume.

In summary, quetiapine appears effective in acute bipolar depression, but safety and tolerability challenges may limit its utility, particularly in longer-term therapy. As recent controlled studies suggest that adjunctive quetiapine (added to lithium or valproate) is effective in longer-term treatment in bipolar disorder, patients experiencing relief of acute bipolar depression may also be candidates for maintenance therapy, provided tolerability is adequate.

Tier II: High-Priority Unapproved Treatment Options for Acute Bipolar Depression

As noted previously, safety and tolerability limitations of the two Tier I approved treatments for bipolar depression may lead clinicians and patients to consider other options. When assessing such treatments, one approach is to first consider medications that are approved for bipolar maintenance. Such agents include lithium, lamotrigine, olanzapine, and aripiprazole. Among these agents, lithium and lamotrigine have the advantageous combination of generally acceptable (lithium) to excellent (lamotrigine) tolerability accompanied by at least some systematic data supporting their utility in the acute and/or prophylactic management of bipolar depression. These qualities have contributed to use of lithium and/or lamotrigine alone or in combination, with antidepressants being considered high-priority options for acute bipolar depression in multiple treatment guidelines (American Psychiatric Association 2002; Goodwin

2003; Grunze et al. 2002; Keck et al. 2004; Suppes et al. 2005; Yatham et al. 2006).
In contrast, the other approved maintenance therapies have tolerability (olanzapine) and/or efficacy (aripiprazole) limitations that make them lower-priority
options, as discussed in the section on Tier III treatment options for acute bipolar depression.

Mood Stabilizers

Mood stabilizers are considered foundational treatments for bipolar disorders.
Lithium and lamotrigine compared with divalproex and carbamazepine have
more evidence supporting their efficacy in acute bipolar depression.

Lithium

Lithium has been considered the gold-standard treatment for bipolar disorder
since its approval by the FDA for use in acute mania in 1970 and maintenance
treatment in 1974. Thus, lithium (monotherapy or in combination with an antidepressant) has been considered a first-line treatment for acute bipolar depression in multiple practice guidelines, including the 2002 revision of the
American Psychiatric Association's "Practice Guideline for the Treatment of
Patients With Bipolar Disorder" (American Psychiatric Association 2002), the
2003 British Association for Psychopharmacology bipolar disorder guideline
(Goodwin 2003), the 2004 expert consensus guideline for treatment of bipolar
disorder (Keck et al. 2004), the 2007 "Canadian Network for Mood and Anxiety
Treatments (CANMAT) Guidelines for the Management of Patients With Bipolar Disorder" (Yatham et al. 2006), the 2005 Texas Implementation of Medication Algorithms (Suppes et al. 2005), and the 2002 "World Federation of
Societies of Biological Psychiatry (WFSBP) Guidelines for Biological Treatment
of Bipolar Disorders" (Grunze et al. 2002).

In spite of its broad acceptance, the evidence base supporting the use of
lithium in acute bipolar depression is limited compared with the approved
treatments. Specifically, results pertaining to lithium efficacy in acute bipolar
depression in early studies were clouded by such studies using older, less established clinical trials methodology (e.g., crossover rather than randomized parallel
paradigms) and including mixed samples of patients with unipolar and bipolar
depression.

As reviewed by Zornberg and Pope (1993), eight controlled studies from
the 1960s and 1970s involving 145 patients found lithium superior to placebo in
bipolar depression (Baron et al. 1975; Donnelly et al. 1978; Fieve et al. 1968;
Goodwin et al. 1969, 1972; Greenspan et al. 1970; Mendels 1976; Noyes et al.

1974), whereas only one study (involving 18 patients who took lithium for only 7–10 days) found lithium to be no better than placebo (Stokes et al. 1971). Methodological limitations of these studies made interpretation challenging, but in a subset of five studies involving 80 patients with sufficient data (Baron et al. 1975; Goodwin et al. 1969, 1972; Mendels 1976; Noyes et al. 1974), only 36% of patients were deemed "unequivocal" lithium responders by Zornberg and Pope (1993).

In recent decades, the efficacy of lithium in bipolar depression increasingly has been challenged, perhaps related to a more heterogeneous patient population that includes patients with treatment-resistant forms of bipolar disorder. Thus, in a 10-week, multicenter trial, in 43 depressed patients with bipolar I disorder taking open lithium (mean final serum concentration 0.78 mEq/L) plus placebo, the response rate was only 34.9% (Nemeroff et al. 2001). It should be noted that response in this trial entailed having a final Hamilton Rating Scale for Depression (Ham-D) score of 7 or less, which is a degree of absolute improvement that is more commonly termed *remission*. Nevertheless, having less than 35% of patients meet this standard with open lithium treatment could be considered discouraging. Response rates in patients with lower (≤0.08 mEq/L) and higher (>0.08 mEq/L) final serum lithium concentrations were only 31.8% and 38.1%, respectively.

Moreover, as noted previously, in a recent multicenter, randomized, double-blind, placebo-controlled trial in depressed patients with bipolar I disorder or bipolar II disorder, 136 patients taking lithium 600 mg/day compared with 129 patients taking placebo had statistically similar MADRS response (≥50% decrease) rates (62.5% vs. 55.8%, NNT=15) (Young et al. 2008). The treatment-emergent affective switch rate was low with lithium but still higher than with placebo (2.2% and 0.8%, respectively). The relatively low dosage of lithium was one limitation of this study.

Lithium appears to have antidepressant effects that are less robust than its antimanic activity, both for acute and preventive treatment.

Thus, as noted in Chapter 6 of this volume, "Management of Acute Manic and Mixed Episodes in Bipolar Disorders," in pooled contemporary acute mania studies, lithium was superior to placebo, with the response rate for lithium being just over 50%, yielding an NNT for response compared with placebo of 4. However, as noted previously, in some controlled trials in acute bipolar depression, lithium response rates were considerably lower than 50% (Nemeroff et al. 2001; Zornberg and Pope 1993), and in one recent multicenter, randomized, double-blind, placebo-controlled study, lithium was no better than placebo, yielding an NNT for response compared with placebo of 15 (Young et al. 2008). In a pooled analysis of 10 maintenance studies from the 1970s, lithium yielded a lower rate of depressive relapse than placebo (21% vs. 37%, $P<0.0001$), with an NNT of 7 for depressive episode prevention for lithium compared with placebo (Goodwin et al. 2004). However, the antimanic effect was more robust, with lithium yielding a lower rate of manic relapse than with placebo (23% vs. 56%, $P<0.0001$), yielding an NNT for manic episode prevention for lithium compared with placebo of 3. Pooled data from the contemporary lamotrigine registration studies suggested lithium was generally less effective compared with the findings of studies from the 1970s but still showed an NNT for lithium compared with placebo for depression prevention that was substantially higher than that for mania prevention (49 vs. 8) (Goodwin et al. 2004). Taken together, these data suggest that lithium's antidepressant effects are less robust than its antimanic activity, for both acute and preventive treatment.

There are only limited data in homogeneous samples of patients with bipolar depression regarding direct comparisons of lithium antidepressant efficacy against other medications. In two older controlled studies, lithium was inferior (Fieve et al. 1968) and equivalent (Watanabe et al. 1975) to imipramine in acute bipolar depression. As noted previously, in a recent multicenter, randomized, double-blind, placebo-controlled study in depressed bipolar I disorder and bipolar II disorder patients, 255 patients taking quetiapine 300 mg/day and 263 taking quetiapine 600 mg/day (but not 136 taking lithium 600 mg/day) compared with 129 taking placebo had higher MADRS response rates, with the response rates for quetiapine compared with lithium being numerically but not statistically greater (Young et al. 2008). The relatively low dosage of lithium was one limitation of this study.

Lithium augmentation of antidepressants in treatment-resistant unipolar depression has been extensively studied. In a meta-analysis of 9 randomized, double-blind, placebo-controlled trials including a total of 234 patients, lithium augmentation compared with placebo augmentation yielded a higher mean response rate (45% vs. 18%), indicating an NNT of 4 for response with lithium compared with placebo augmentation (Bauer and Dopfmer 1999).

Antidepressants are commonly added to lithium in patients with acute bipolar depression. However, as described later in the section on adjunctive antidepressants, there are few systematic data supporting this practice. There are also limited data supporting increased efficacy with starting lithium along with antidepressants compared with antidepressants alone in bipolar depression, although there is one positive controlled study.

In a 5-week, randomized, double-blind, placebo-controlled trial in inpatients with melancholic bipolar depression, 20 patients taking lithium (900 mg/day, mean serum concentration 0.65 mEq/L) plus amitriptyline (225 mg/day) compared with 20 patients taking placebo plus amitriptyline (225 mg/day) yielded greater Ham-D decreases at week 5 but not at week 1 or 2 (Ebert et al. 1995).

Longer-term use of lithium may affect the more complex phenomenon of suicidality (suicide attempts and completed suicides). Tondo and colleagues found that longer-term (mean duration 6.4 years) lithium use was associated with a significantly lower incidence of suicidality in bipolar I disorder and bipolar II disorder patients followed for a total of 5,233 patient years (Tondo et al. 1998). Importantly, when lithium was discontinued naturalistically, there was a rebound increase in suicidality during the first year following discontinuation, which was greater than either the period prior to initiation of lithium treatment or the subsequent period after the first year following discontinuation. In addition, Goodwin and colleagues found that the risk of suicide was lower in 20,638 patients with bipolar disorder who were taking lithium, compared with divalproex (Goodwin et al. 2003).

Lithium lacks FDA approval for acute bipolar depression, so the U.S. prescribing information does not provide dosing recommendations for this application. In outpatients with acute bipolar depression, lithium is commonly started at 300 mg/day taken at bedtime. Because lithium has a half-life of approximately 1 day, the dosage may be increased every 3–5 days in increments of 300 mg/day, as necessary and tolerated, with final dosages commonly ranging between 900 mg/day and 1,200 mg/day, similar to the longer-term dosage recommended in the U.S. prescribing information, which suggests lithium be administered in two divided doses. However, clinicians and patients commonly endeavor to have most of or, if possible, the entire lithium dose taken at bedtime to enhance convenience and to have peak lithium serum concentrations and hence the major burden of adverse effects occur during sleep. Twelve-hour trough serum lithium concentrations may be checked upon reaching 900 mg/day for 5 days, targeting 0.8 mEq/L, which is toward the lower end of the 0.6–1.2 mEq/L maintenance therapy range recommended in the prescribing information. However, in patients who fail to tolerate 0.8 mEq/L, lithium serum concentrations as low as 0.5–0.6 mEq/L may still yield benefit, particularly if lithium is combined with other medications. Additional information regarding lithium is provided in Chapter 13 in this volume.

In summary, lithium may yield benefits in acute bipolar depression, but tolerability challenges may limit its utility. As lithium also yields benefits in longer-term treatment in bipolar disorder, patients experiencing relief of acute bipolar depression may also be candidates for lithium maintenance therapy.

Lamotrigine

Lamotrigine received approval from the FDA for maintenance treatment of bipolar I disorder in 2003. Although lamotrigine was effective for delaying overall (depressive, manic, hypomanic, and mixed episode) relapses and recurrences, lamotrigine was most effective in delaying depressive episodes (Goodwin et al. 2004). However, lamotrigine has not been approved for acute bipolar depression, despite early hopes for this agent based on an encouraging large, controlled study suggesting acute antidepressant efficacy of lamotrigine in bipolar depression (Calabrese et al. 1999). These encouraging early data contributed to lamotrigine being considered a high-priority option for acute bipolar depression in multiple treatment guidelines (American Psychiatric Association 2002; Goodwin 2003; Grunze et al. 2002; Keck et al. 2004; Suppes et al. 2005; Yatham et al. 2006). However, four subsequent multicenter, randomized, double-blind, placebo-controlled studies of lamotrigine in patients with bipolar I disorder or bipolar II disorder with acute depression were negative (Calabrese et al. 2008).

Thus, in five studies considered individually, lamotrigine did not differ significantly from placebo on primary efficacy outcome measures. However, lamotrigine was numerically (but not significantly) superior to placebo in all five studies considered individually, and in a meta-analysis involving all 1,030 patients with bipolar I disorder and bipolar II disorder, lamotrigine compared with placebo had significantly higher MADRS and Ham-D response ($>50\%$ improvement) rates and a significantly higher MADRS (final total<12) but not Ham-D (final total<8) remission rate (Geddes et al. 2009). Thus, the pooled MADRS response rate for lamotrigine (47%) was significantly greater than for placebo (38%, $P<0.01$), yielding an NNT for MADRS response for lamotrigine versus placebo of 12 (Figure 7–1, right). Lamotrigine was generally well tolerated, with negligible rates of sedation and weight gain, no patient experiencing serious rash, and nonserious rash incidence being 1.2% with placebo and 3.4% with lamotrigine ($P<0.05$), yielding an NNH for benign rash with lamotrigine compared with placebo of 44 (Figure 7–2, right). The incidence of treatment-emergent affective switch was similarly low for the lamotrigine and placebo groups (3.8% and 3.3%, respectively).

When considering the option of lamotrigine for acute bipolar depression, it is important to be aware that this modality may not be the most efficacious because it has a low-teen NNT for response that is less attractive than the approved treatments, which have single-digit NNTs. However, it is equally important to keep in mind that lamotrigine in most patients is exceedingly well tolerated, with negligible risks of sedation and weight gain, adverse effects that are substantial limitations of the approved treatments, and a high NNH for benign rash.

One challenge to such an approach comparing lamotrigine and the approved acute bipolar depression treatments is the fact that in the trials aimed at securing registration, these agents were compared with placebo rather than with one another. An evidence-based approach to this issue requires large multicenter, randomized, double-blind, head-to-head comparisons of these agents, ideally along with a placebo arm to aid in interpretation. Unfortunately, because of economic concerns, such trials are relatively uncommon. However, a recent multicenter, randomized, double-blind, head-to-head comparison of lamotrigine and OFC, in spite of lacking a placebo arm, may help inform clinicians and patients wishing to assess the benefit-to-risk ratio of lamotrigine compared with OFC.

For a study funded by the manufacturer of OFC, Brown and colleagues reported the results of a 7-week, multicenter, randomized, double-blind trial directly comparing the efficacy and safety of OFC (*n*=205) and lamotrigine monotherapy (*n*=205) for bipolar I disorder depression (Brown et al. 2006). OFC (mean modal dosage olanzapine 11 mg/day, fluoxetine 38 mg/day) compared with lamotrigine (mean modal dosage 106 mg/day) yielded significantly but modestly greater decreases from baseline to end point in MADRS total scores and Young Mania Rating Scale (YMRS) scores. OFC compared with lamotrigine tended to yield a higher MADRS response rate (68.8% vs. 59.7%, *P*=0.073). Thus, the NNT for response with OFC versus lamotrigine was 12 (Figure 7–3, left). Both treatments had similarly low rates of treatment-emergent affective switch.

In contrast, lamotrigine therapy was better tolerated, with fewer problems with metabolic adverse events (increases in weight, total cholesterol, and triglyceride levels), increased appetite, dry mouth, sedation, somnolence, and tremor, compared with OFC therapy. For example, the rates of clinically significant (≥7%) weight gain with OFC and lamotrigine were 23% and 0% (*P*< 0.001), respectively. Hence, the NNH for clinically significant weight gain with OFC versus lamotrigine was 5 (Figure 7–3, right). Thus, the LHH (NNH/NNT) for OFC versus lamotrigine was 0.4 (5/12). Put another way, patients with bipolar depression taking OFC compared with lamotrigine were *less* likely (by a factor of 0.4) to respond than they were likely to experience clinically significant weight gain.

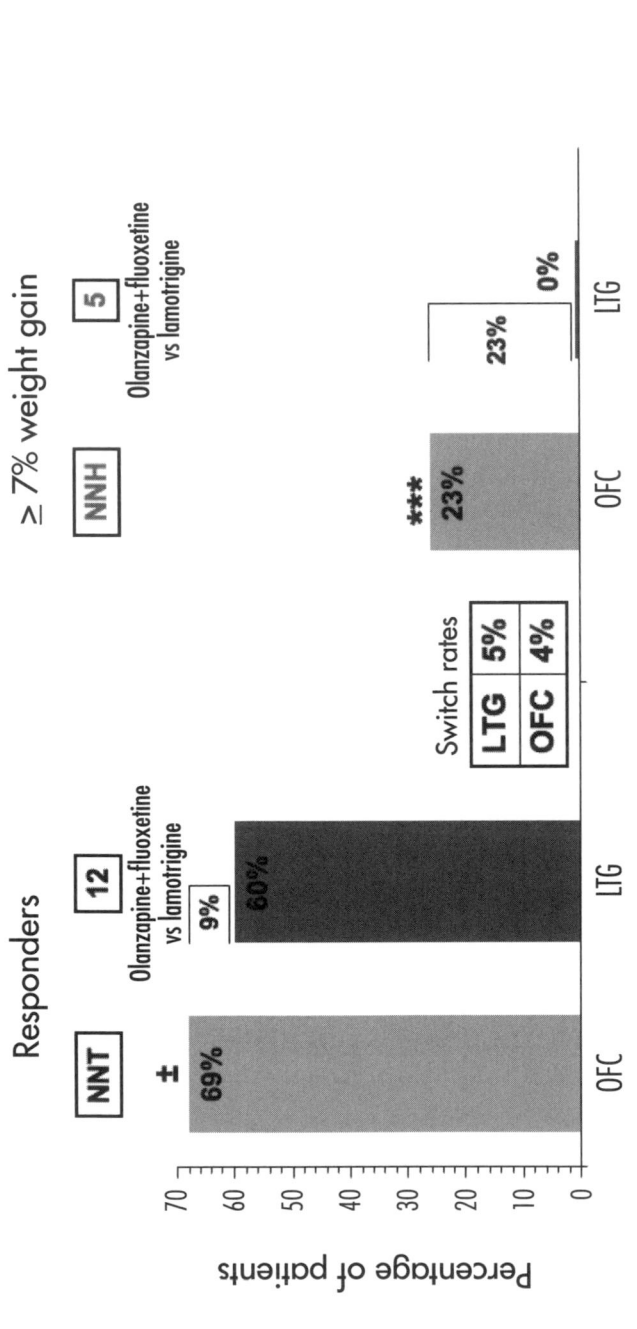

FIGURE 7–3.   Seven-week, randomized, double-blind study of lamotrigine (LTG) versus olanzapine plus fluoxe-tine combination (OFC) in acute bipolar I depression.

Number needed to treat (NNT) for response and number needed to harm (NNH) for clinically significant weight gain, response, and adverse effect rates. OFC compared with LTG yielded a modest increase in Montgomery-Åsberg Depression Rating Scale response rate but substantially more clini-cally significant (≥7%) weight gain. Rates of treatment-emergent affective switch were similar. Benefit-risk analysis involves assessing whether a 9% in-crease in response rate merits a 23% increase in rate of clinically significant weight gain. ±*P*<0.08; *** <0.001 OFC versus LTG.

Source.   Data adapted from Brown et al. 2006.

Taken together, the previous data support the view that for some patients with bipolar depression, when considering lamotrigine compared with OFC, lamotrigine's superior tolerability may mitigate its inferior efficacy, making it a reasonable unapproved alternative. Table 7–2 outlines the comparative benefits and risks with these two approaches.

In addition to the controlled efficacy data reviewed above, controlled and uncontrolled effectiveness studies suggest that lamotrigine may have a role in the treatment of acute bipolar depression. In a recent study, a heterogeneous cohort of 1,175 outpatients with bipolar I disorder received 12 weeks of adding open-label lamotrigine to concomitant medications (Ketter et al. 2006a). Thus, patients with comorbid medical and psychiatric disorders were not excluded unless in the opinion of the investigators these problems precluded participation. The most frequent abnormal baseline mood state was depression. Lamotrigine was well tolerated, with 74% of patients completing the study, no serious rash, and low incidences of nonserious rash and discontinuation due to rash, and Clinical Global Impression (CGI) for Bipolar Disorder severity and improvement scores indicated mood improvement. In additional analyses, there was no significant change in mean weight after lamotrigine monotherapy or adjunctive therapy, whereas quality-of-life scores improved significantly more in patients not receiving compared with those receiving concomitant antipsychotics (Zarzar et al. 2007).

Another recent controlled effectiveness study assessed 66 outpatients with bipolar I or II disorder enrolled in the Systematic Treatment Enhancement Program for Bipolar Disorder (STEP-BD) who had a current major depressive episode that was nonresponsive to a combination of adequate doses of established mood stabilizers plus at least one antidepressant (Nierenberg et al. 2006b). Again, patients with comorbid medical and psychiatric disorders were not excluded. Patients were randomized to receive open adjunctive lamotrigine, inositol, or risperidone for up to 16 weeks. There were no significant differences comparing any pair of treatments on the primary outcome measure, perhaps because of limited statistical power related to the small sample size. However, the recovery (attaining and maintaining euthymia for 8 weeks) rate with lamotrigine was 24%, whereas the recovery rate with inositol was 17% and with risperidone was 5%, and lamotrigine exhibited lower exit depression and CGI severity scores as well as greater Global Assessment of Function scores compared with inositol and risperidone.

In a recent uncontrolled effectiveness study, in 145 bipolar disorder patients, starting open lamotrigine (mean final dosage 236 mg/day), combined with a

TABLE 7–2. Comparison of benefits and risks of lamotrigine versus the olanzapine plus fluoxetine combination for acute bipolar depression

	Lamotrigine	Olanzapine plus fluoxetine
Benefits	Superior tolerability	Superior efficacy
	Less sedation (benefit if no insomnia)	More rapid onset of action
	Less weight gain (benefit if at normal or high weight)	More nocturnal sedation (benefit if insomnia)
	Less metabolic risk	More weight gain (benefit if at low weight)
Risks	Inferior efficacy	Inferior tolerability
	Slower onset of action (more titration)	More daytime sedation
	Less sedation (risk if insomnia)	More weight gain (risk if at normal or high weight)
	Less weight gain (risk if at low weight)	More metabolic risk
	More benign rash	
	More severe rash (rare)	
Ideal patients	Nonurgent efficacy need	Urgent efficacy need
	Hypersomnia	Insomnia
	Psychomotor retardation	Psychomotor agitation
	Overweight or obese	Underweight
	Not anxious	Anxious

mean of 2.1 other psychotropics, yielded several sustained (mean duration 394 days) significant benefits, including decreasing the percentage of patients with syndromal depression, increasing the percentage with euthymia, and improving mean ratings of overall illness (Ketter et al. 2008). Lamotrigine was not associated with sedation or weight gain, there was no serious rash, and only 3.5% discontinued lamotrigine because of benign rash.

Unlike most other mood stabilizers and second-generation antipsychotics, lamotrigine appears to have antidepressant effects that are *more* robust compared with its antimanic activity, for both acute and preventive treatment.

Thus, as noted in Chapter 6 of this book, in two multicenter, randomized, double-blind, placebo-controlled studies, lamotrigine was no more effective than placebo in acute mania (Bowden et al. 2000a; Goldsmith et al. 2003), with a pooled analysis yielding an NNT for response in acute mania for lamotrigine compared with placebo of 38. In contrast, as noted previously, a pooled analysis of five multicenter, randomized, double-blind, placebo-controlled studies yielded an NNT for response in acute bipolar depression for lamotrigine compared with placebo of 13. Pooled data from the lamotrigine registration studies yielded an NNT for lamotrigine compared with placebo for depression prevention that was substantially lower than that for mania prevention (15 vs. 49) (Goodwin et al. 2004). Taken together, these data suggest that lamotrigines antidepressant effects are *more* robust than its antimanic activity, for both acute and preventive treatment.

Lamotrigine lacks FDA approval for acute bipolar depression; therefore, the U.S. prescribing information does not provide dosing recommendations for this application. Thus, the prescribing information for the maintenance indication is described. Regardless of what mood state the patient is experiencing, it is crucial to gradually introduce lamotrigine in order to minimize the risk of treatment-emergent rash. Thus, the recommended initiation of lamotrigine includes starting at 25 mg/day and maintaining that dosage for the first 2 weeks. The dosage is then increased to 50 mg/day for the third and fourth weeks. Dosages may then be increased to 100 mg/day for the fifth week and to the target dosage of 200 mg/day by the sixth week. The U.S. prescribing information does not recommend dosages over 200 mg/day for bipolar maintenance treatment because in the registration studies 400 mg/day did not offer additional benefit. However, in patients who tolerate but fail to respond to 200 mg/day, increasing weekly by 25 mg/day as necessary and tolerated to as high as 400 mg/day is generally well tolerated and may yield benefit in some individuals.

Because divalproex inhibits metabolism of lamotrigine by approximately 50%, the dose of lamotrigine taken concurrently with divalproex needs to be halved. Thus, with concurrent divalproex, the recommended starting lamotrigine dosage is 25 mg every other day. However, taking 12.5 mg/day, though requiring splitting pills, may be preferable because this approach yields less fluctuation in blood levels and facilitates adherence. Lamotrigine is maintained at that dosage for the first 2 weeks, increased to 25 mg/day for the third and fourth weeks, increased to 50 mg/day for the fifth week, and to the target dosage of 100 mg/day by the sixth week.

Carbamazepine approximately doubles lamotrigine metabolism, so that the dosage of lamotrigine taken concurrently with carbamazepine needs to be doubled. Thus, when taken with carbamazepine, lamotrigine is started at 50 mg/day and maintained at that dosage for the first 2 weeks, increased to 100 mg/day for the third and fourth weeks, increased to 200 mg/day for the fifth week, and to the target dosage of 400 mg/day by the sixth week.

Although the titration regimen may seem complex, understanding the need to decrease the risk of serious rash and the drug-drug interactions between lamotrigine and divalproex or carbamazepine makes the schedule more comprehensible. The three available dosage titration packages (for lamotrigine without divalproex or carbamazepine, lamotrigine plus divalproex, or lamotrigine plus carbamazepine) can simplify the process further for clinicians and patients. Additional information regarding lamotrigine is provided in Chapter 13 of this volume.

In summary, lamotrigine may yield benefits in acute bipolar depression and provides uncommonly good tolerability. As lamotrigine also yields benefits in longer-term treatment in bipolar disorder, particularly in delaying return of depressive symptoms, patients experiencing relief of acute bipolar depression may also be candidates for lamotrigine maintenance therapy.

Tier III: Other Treatment Options for Acute Bipolar Depression

The management of bipolar depression is sufficiently challenging that clinical need commonly outstrips the previously mentioned evidence-based treatment options. In this section we consider other treatment options with even more limited evidence of efficacy than the previously mentioned Tier I and Tier II treatments. These alternatives include other mood stabilizers (divalproex and carbamazepine), other second-generation antipsychotics (olanzapine monotherapy, aripiprazole, risperidone, ziprasidone, and clozapine), electroconvulsive therapy (ECT), and adjunctive psychotherapy. In general, treatment guidelines do not consider these modalities to be first-line interventions but cite them as intermediate-priority options (American Psychiatric Association 2002; Goodwin 2003; Grunze et al. 2002; Keck et al. 2004; Suppes et al. 2005; Yatham et al. 2006).

Another important approach is to combine antimanic agents with standard antidepressants that are approved for unipolar major depressive disorder. This strategy has been considered first-line in European and Canadian guidelines (Goodwin 2003; Grunze et al. 2002; Yatham et al. 2006) but has been given lower priority in U.S. guidelines (American Psychiatric Association 2002; Keck et al. 2004; Suppes et al. 2005). The data supporting the efficacy of such practice is limited, and increasingly results of randomized controlled trials are challenging perceptions that this strategy ought to be a high priority. Thus, in the current hierarchy adjunctive antidepressants have been assigned to Tier III.

Some Tier III options have mitigating advantages such as maintenance indications, tolerability, or familiarity that might make them attractive for selected patients, and in certain circumstances some of these interventions may be considered early on (e.g., psychotherapy or ECT in pregnant women with acute bipolar depression). For some of these treatments (e.g., adjunctive psychotherapy), advances in research, familiarity, and/or availability ultimately may be sufficient to merit their consideration for placement in higher tiers.

Other Mood Stabilizers

The other mood stabilizers divalproex and carbamazepine, unlike lithium and lamotrigine, have less of an evidence base supporting their use in acute bipolar depression and lack indications for maintenance treatment in bipolar disorders. Nevertheless, limited systematic data support their consideration as alternative treatments in acute bipolar depression.

Anticonvulsant medications are commonly used in bipolar disorder. With diverse mechanisms of action, including sodium channel–blocking activity, enhancement of γ-aminobutyric acid (GABA), and inhibition of glutamate neurotransmission, in addition to lamotrigine, some, but not all, medications in this broad class, such as divalproex and carbamazepine, may have utility in the treatment of bipolar depression.

Divalproex

Divalproex was approved by the FDA for the treatment of acute mania in 1994. Three small controlled studies suggested that divalproex may have efficacy in bipolar depression (Davis et al. 2005; Ghaemi et al. 2007; Muzina 2008), and one study was less encouraging (Sachs et al. 2001). Limited statistical power and, in some instances, overly conservative dosing may have contributed to the modest statistical outcome of these controlled studies.

Pooling the data from the four small controlled acute bipolar depression studies yields divalproex and placebo remission (Davis et al. 2005) or response (Ghaemi et al. 2007; Muzina 2008; Sachs et al. 2001) rates of 40.6% (28/69) and 18.8% (13/69; $P=0.009$) and an NNT for remission/response of 5. Taken together, these data suggest that a large controlled trial of divalproex in bipolar depression is warranted.

Although a 52-week, multicenter, randomized, double-blind, parallel-group trial of divalproex, lithium, and placebo maintenance monotherapy failed to demonstrate a significant finding on the primary outcome measure (time to a manic episode) in patients with bipolar I disorder (Bowden et al. 2000b), divalproex antidepressant efficacy was suggested in post hoc analyses (Gyulai et al. 2003). Divalproex-treated patients had greater prevention of depressive symptom relapse compared with lithium-treated patients and had fewer study discontinuations caused by a depressive episode. Furthermore, in this study, patients developing depressive symptoms while taking divalproex, lithium, or placebo could be treated with selective serotonin reuptake inhibitors (SSRIs). Fewer patients taking divalproex and an SSRI, compared with placebo and an SSRI, discontinued early because of a depressive episode (Gyulai et al. 2003). Overall, divalproex-treated patients exhibited less worsening of depressive symptoms during maintenance compared with patients receiving lithium.

Although clinical perceptions tend to view divalproex as having more potent antimanic compared with antidepressant activity, the data from controlled trials thus far have failed to confirm this speculation.

Thus, as noted in Chapter 6 of this book, in pooled contemporary acute mania studies, divalproex was superior to placebo, with the response rate for divalproex being just under 50%, yielding an NNT for response compared with placebo of 7. However, as noted previously, in pooled analyses of data from the four small controlled acute bipolar depression studies, the NNT for remission/response for divalproex compared with placebo was 5. Moreover, in a multicenter, randomized, double-blind, placebo-controlled maintenance study, for divalproex compared with placebo, the NNTs for depression prevention and mania prevention were 11 and 22, respectively (Bowden et al. 2000b). More studies are necessary to assess the differential antimanic and antidepressant effects of divalproex in bipolar disorder.

Although data remain limited to date and more randomized, double-blind, placebo-controlled studies are needed, current literature suggests divalproex might have utility in the depressive phase of bipolar disorder but dosing may be particularly important.

Divalproex lacks FDA approval for acute bipolar depression, so the U.S. prescribing information does not provide dosing recommendations for this application. In outpatients with acute bipolar depression, divalproex may be started at 250 mg/day, dosing at bedtime. Dosages may be increased, as necessary and tolerated, every 4–7 days, initially targeting a dosage of 750 mg/day, before checking blood levels. This titration is considerably slower than that seen in acute mania and strives to decrease the risk of adverse effects, which are more common in depressed as compared with manic patients. Based on the available literature, blood levels of at least 80 μg/mL may have better efficacy than lower blood levels. Additional information regarding divalproex is provided in the Chapter 13 of this volume.

In summary, limited controlled data suggest that divalproex may yield benefits in acute bipolar depression, but this needs to be established in large controlled studies. As divalproex also appears to yield benefits in longer-term treatment in bipolar disorder, patients experiencing relief of acute bipolar depression may also be candidates for divalproex maintenance therapy.

Carbamazepine

Carbamazepine was approved by the FDA for the treatment of acute mania in 2004. The approved formulation was a proprietary beaded, extended-release capsule form of carbamazepine (ERC carbamazepine). There are limited controlled data regarding the acute antidepressant effects of carbamazepine. Although carbamazepine appears to have weaker antidepressant than antimanic properties, limited data suggest that it may provide benefit in acute bipolar depression.

In a 12-week, randomized, double-blind, placebo-controlled study, 47 patients taking carbamazepine (mean dosage 452 mg/day) compared with 23 taking placebo had a significantly higher Ham-D response rate (64% vs. 35%, NNT=4) (Zhang et al. 2007). The most common adverse effects with carbamazepine included dizziness, laboratory test abnormality, rash, fatigue, and headache.

In other controlled studies with active comparator and adjunctive and placebo on-off-on designs in treatment-resistant patients, carbamazepine yielded response rates of approximately one-third (Neumann et al. 1984; Post et al. 1986;

Small 1990). Unfortunately, most of these studies were limited by the use of small samples of heterogeneous (both bipolar and unipolar) highly treatment-resistant patients. The largest of these studies was a double-blind, placebo-controlled, off-on-off-on design in 24 bipolar and 11 unipolar depressed patients given carbamazepine (mean dosage 971 mg/day, mean serum concentration 9.3 ± 1.9 µg/mL) for a mean of 45 days, which found that approximately one-third of carbamazepine-treated patients met response criteria (Post et al. 1986).

In addition, a pooled analysis suggested that in patients with mixed episodes, ERC carbamazepine substantially decreased Ham-D total scores, which is consistent with the notion that this agent may have efficacy for the depressive component of bipolar disorder (Weisler et al. 2006).

Studies have suggested some positive response predictors of carbamazepine, including greater severity of depression, more discrete depressive episodes, less chronicity, and greater decreases in serum thyroxine concentrations with carbamazepine treatment (Post et al. 1986, 1991). Nevertheless, the available evidence suggests that carbamazepine appears to have weaker antidepressant than antimanic properties, and larger controlled studies are needed to definitively demonstrate the efficacy of carbamazepine in acute bipolar depression.

Optimal use of carbamazepine requires a thorough knowledge of its potential adverse effects (aplastic anemia, rash, hepatotoxicity, and teratogenicity) and significant pharmacokinetic interactions. In particular, the risk of drug-drug interactions is high, given the cytochrome P450 enzyme induction by carbamazepine and the high degree of polypharmacy common in bipolar disorder treatment. For a review of the pharmacokinetics and drug-drug interactions with carbamazepine, readers are referred to Chapter 13 of this volume.

Carbamazepine lacks FDA approval for acute bipolar depression, so the U.S. prescribing information does not provide dosing recommendations for this application. In outpatients with acute bipolar depression, carbamazepine is generally started at 200 mg/day, given at bedtime, and increased every 3–7 days by 200 mg/day. This titration is considerably slower than that seen in acute mania and strives to decrease the risk of adverse effects, which are more common in depressed as compared with manic patients. Even more gradual titration may be achieved by starting with 100 mg/day and increasing every 3–7 days by 100 mg/day. The target dosage is generally 600–1,200 mg/day, with blood levels commonly in the range of 4–12 µg/mL.

In summary, limited controlled data suggest the possibility that carbamazepine may have utility in acute bipolar depression as well as in longer-term treatment in bipolar disorder. Thus, large controlled clinical trials are needed to inform clinicians of the risks and benefits not only of carbamazepine in acute depression but also of continuing carbamazepine in patients who experience relief of acute bipolar depression. The lack of compelling evidence of efficacy along with complexity of administration related to drug interactions and tolerability challenges substantially limit the utility of this intervention.

Other Second-Generation Antipsychotics

Second-generation antipsychotics as a class have emerged to have efficacy in bipolar disorder, with olanzapine, risperidone, quetiapine, ziprasidone, and aripiprazole having FDA acute mania indications; olanzapine and aripiprazole monotherapy and adjunctive quetiapine having longer-term treatment indications; and OFC and quetiapine monotherapy having acute bipolar depression indications. Although clozapine lacks an FDA indication for the treatment of bipolar disorder, limited data suggest it may have utility, perhaps more to counter mood elevation compared with depressive symptoms. In addition, emerging evidence suggests second-generation antipsychotics may be useful adjuncts to antidepressants in unipolar major depressive disorder. Randomized, placebo-controlled studies of second-generation antipsychotics suggest heterogeneity within this class with respect to efficacy for acute bipolar depression, with quetiapine monotherapy having moderate efficacy (NNT=6), olanzapine monotherapy having modest efficacy (NNT=12), and aripiprazole monotherapy (NNT=44) and ziprasidone monotherapy lacking efficacy. The data are much more limited regarding the utility of risperidone and clozapine in treating acute bipolar depression.

Olanzapine

Olanzapine appears to have modest acute antidepressant effects, which are less robust compared with its acute antimanic activity or compared with the antidepressant effects of OFC.

Thus, as noted previously, olanzapine monotherapy appeared to have modest efficacy in acute bipolar depression, with a MADRS response rate (39%) significantly exceeding that of placebo (30%), yielding an NNT for response for olanzapine compared with placebo of 12 (Figure 7–1, second from right) (Tohen et al. 2003). In contrast, as noted in Chapter 6 of this book, for acute manic/mixed episodes olanzapine had a more robust effect, with an NNT for response for olanzapine compared with placebo of 5. Also, OFC appears to have more robust efficacy than olanzapine in acute bipolar depression, with a MADRS response rate (56%) significantly exceeding that of placebo (30%) and an NNT for response for OFC compared with placebo of 4 (Figure 7–1, left). Indeed, OFC yielded a MADRS response rate significantly exceeding that of olanzapine, with an NNT for response for OFC compared with olanzapine of 6.

Similarly, maintenance data indicate olanzapine may have modest preventive antidepressant effects, which are less robust compared with its preventive antimanic activity. Thus, in the pivotal maintenance study, olanzapine compared with placebo yielded a significantly longer time to depressive relapse and a nonsignificantly lower rate of depressive relapse (30.2% vs. 39.0%, $P=0.11$) and an NNT for depressive episode prevention for olanzapine compared with placebo of 12 (Tohen et al. 2006). In contrast, olanzapine compared with placebo yielded not only a significantly longer time to manic/mixed relapse but also a significantly lower rate of manic/mixed relapse (16.4% vs. 41.2%, $P<0.001$), yielding an NNT for manic/mixed episode prevention for olanzapine compared with placebo of 5. Thus, for both response in acute bipolar depression and prevention of depressive episodes, olanzapine compared with placebo had an NNT of 12, whereas for both response in acute manic/mixed episodes and prevention of manic/mixed episodes, olanzapine compared with placebo had an NNT of 5.

In contrast to lamotrigine, which has an extremely favorable tolerability profile that may mitigate a double-digit NNT for acute bipolar depression, olanzapine has a tolerability profile similar to that of OFC. Thus, both OFC and olanzapine compared with placebo had an NNH for clinically significant weight gain of 6 (Figure 7–2, left and second from right). Taken together, these data suggest that olanzapine monotherapy is not a high-priority option for acute bipolar depression, a fact evident in multiple treatment guidelines (Grunze et al. 2002; Keck et al. 2004; Suppes et al. 2005; Yatham et al. 2006).

Because olanzapine monotherapy lacks FDA approval for acute bipolar depression, the U.S. prescribing information does not provide dosing recommendations for this application. In a large controlled acute bipolar depression study, olanzapine monotherapy was started at 5 mg/day and could be increased daily by 5 mg/day to as high as 20 mg/day, with a mean final dosage of 10 mg/day (Tohen et al. 2003). Because that approach yielded sedation in 28.1% of patients, clinicians may prefer to titrate more conservatively in order to limit adverse effects, starting olanzapine at 2.5 mg/day at bedtime and increasing every 4–7 days as necessary and tolerated by 2.5 mg/day, initially targeting a dosage of 10 mg/day at bedtime. Occasionally patients who tolerate but fail to respond to 10 mg/day may benefit from continuing to gradually increase olanzapine every 4–7 days as necessary and tolerated by 2.5 mg/day to as high as 20 mg/day.

In summary, controlled data indicate that olanzapine has modest utility in acute bipolar depression; however, OFC is a more attractive option in view of its having more robust efficacy and comparable tolerability. Although olanzapine has a bipolar disorder longer-term treatment indication, its effects appear less robust in preventing depression compared with mania, and safety and tolerability concerns limit its utility.

Aripiprazole

Aripiprazole was approved by the FDA for the treatment of acute manic and mixed episodes in 2004, for longer-term treatment of bipolar I disorder in 2005, as adjunctive (added to antidepressants) treatment of acute major depressive disorder in 2007, and as adjunctive (added to lithium or valproate) treatment of acute manic and mixed episodes in 2008. It appears that aripiprazole monotherapy is not effective in acute bipolar depression or prevention of bipolar depression but is effective in acute manic/mixed episodes and prevention of manic/mixed episodes.

Thus, two recently completed, 8-week, randomized, parallel-group, placebo-controlled studies for treatment of acute bipolar I disorder depression did not find aripiprazole (initiated at 10 mg/day, flexibly dosed between 5–30 mg/day, with a pooled mean dosage of 16.5 mg/day) superior to placebo (Thase et al. 2008). An analysis using pooled data for the two studies showed that the response rate in 337 patients taking aripiprazole (mean dosage 16.5 mg/day) was similar to that in 353 patients taking placebo (44% vs. 42%), yielding an NNT for response for aripiprazole compared with placebo of 44. Adverse effects (akathisia, insomnia, nausea, fatigue, and restlessness) and rates of early discontinuation due to adverse events were higher with aripiprazole compared with placebo. Citing high discontinuation rates, the authors speculated that the dosing may have been too aggressive for acute bipolar depression. Interestingly, in both studies aripiprazole did have superior antidepressant effects compared with placebo at several time points up to weeks 5–6, but the aripiprazole benefit attenuated at weeks 7–8, resulting in loss of statistical significance, suggesting some potential attenuation of aripiprazole's potential antidepressant effects over time. In contrast, as noted in Chapter 6 of this book, aripiprazole was effective for acute manic/mixed episodes, with an NNT for response for aripiprazole compared with placebo of 5.

Similarly, maintenance data indicate aripiprazole may lack preventive antidepressant effects but has preventive antimanic effects. Thus, in the pivotal maintenance study, aripiprazole compared with placebo yielded similar times to depressive relapse and similar rates of depressive relapse (13% vs. 12%) and an NNT for depressive episode prevention for aripiprazole compared with placebo of 64 (Keck et al. 2006a). In contrast, aripiprazole compared with placebo yielded not only a significantly longer time to manic/mixed relapse but also a significantly lower rate of manic/mixed relapse (13.0% vs. 30.1%, $P<0.05$) and an NNT for manic/mixed episode prevention for aripiprazole compared with placebo of 5. Thus, for response in acute bipolar depression and for prevention of depressive episodes, aripiprazole compared with placebo had NNTs of 44 and 64, respectively, whereas both for response in acute manic/mixed episodes and for prevention of manic/mixed episodes, aripiprazole compared with placebo had an NNT of 5.

Although controlled data indicate aripiprazole monotherapy lacks efficacy in acute bipolar depression, it remains to be established whether aripiprazole combined with antidepressants yields benefits in acute bipolar depression. This question is of considerable interest in view of the more robust efficacy of OFC compared with olanzapine in bipolar depression and data suggesting that second-generation antipsychotics combined with antidepressants offer benefit in acute unipolar depression. Indeed, in late 2007, aripiprazole received the first FDA approval for adjunctive (added to antidepressants) treatment of acute unipolar depression, based on two 6-week, multicenter, randomized, double-blind, placebo-controlled trials (Berman et al. 2007; Marcus et al. 2008). However, the brief (6-week) duration of these adjunctive aripiprazole in unipolar depression studies may be a limitation because the potential benefit of aripiprazole monotherapy in acute bipolar depression appeared to attenuate after 6 weeks. Taken together, the controlled data reviewed previously as well as case series data suggesting utility of adjunctive aripiprazole in acute bipolar depression (Kemp et al. 2007; Ketter et al. 2006b; McElroy et al. 2007; Sokolski 2007) suggest that a large controlled study of adjunctive aripiprazole in acute bipolar depression is warranted.

As aripiprazole monotherapy lacks FDA approval for acute bipolar depression, the U.S. prescribing information does not provide dosing recommendations for this application. In the controlled acute bipolar depression trials, aripiprazole was started at 10 mg/day (5 mg twice daily), and dosages could be adjusted weekly by 5 mg/day, with final dosages ranging from 5 mg/day to 30 mg/day and a pooled mean dosage of 16.5 mg/day. However, this approach yielded adverse effects such as akathisia, insomnia, and nausea, with rates ranging between approximately 14% and 28% of patients. Thus, clinicians may wish to initiate aripiprazole more gradually in order to limit adverse effects, using the approach suggested in the U.S. prescribing information for the adjunctive (added to antidepressants) treatment of unipolar major depressive disorder, starting at 2–5 mg/day and titrating to a recommended dosage of 5–10 mg/day. Akathisia may attenuate with dosage reduction or addition of a benzodiazepine such as lorazepam. Occasionally patients may find aripiprazole sedating, requiring shifting the medication to bedtime. In view of the findings of the controlled acute bipolar depression studies, clinicians should monitor carefully for attenuation of benefit between the fifth and eighth week of therapy.

In summary, controlled data indicate that aripiprazole monotherapy lacks efficacy in acute bipolar depression. Although aripiprazole has a bipolar disorder longer-term treatment indication, its effects appear less robust in preventing depression compared with mania. Controlled trials are needed to assess whether adjunctive aripiprazole has utility in acute bipolar depression.

Risperidone

Risperidone received FDA approval for the treatment of acute mania in 2003 but lacks acute bipolar depression and bipolar maintenance indications. As with other second-generation antipsychotics, adjunctive risperidone appears to yield benefit in treatment-resistant unipolar depression (Mahmoud et al. 2007).

Open studies suggested that adjunctive risperidone had some utility in acute bipolar depression (McIntyre et al. 2004; Vieta et al. 2001). However, there have been no placebo-controlled trials investigating risperidone in acute bipolar depression. Two randomized, active-controlled, adjunctive risperidone trials in acute bipolar depression were not particularly encouraging, but limited statistical power and lack of placebo control groups make interpretation of these studies challenging.

In a 12-week, randomized, double-blind study, adjunctive risperidone (mean maximum dosage 2.15 mg/day) plus placebo, paroxetine (mean maximum dosage 35.0 mg/day) plus placebo, and combined risperidone (mean maximum dosage 1.16 mg/day) plus paroxetine (mean maximum dosage 22.0 mg/day) were added to mood stabilizers in 21 bipolar I disorder and 9 bipolar II disorder patients with acute depression (Shelton and Stahl 2004). Risperidone was started at 1 mg/day and increased weekly by 1 mg/day to as high as 4 mg/day. Paroxetine was started at 20 mg/day and increased weekly by 10 mg/day to as high as 40 mg/day. All three groups experienced similar modest Ham-D response rates: 30% (3/10), 20% (2/10), and 30% (3/10) for adjunctive risperidone plus placebo, paroxetine plus placebo, and risperidone plus paroxetine, respectively. Somnolence, appetite increase, weight gain, diarrhea, and sexual dysfunction were the most common adverse effects. There was minimal treatment-emergent affective switch because only 1 patient (taking paroxetine plus placebo) developed mild hypomania. Thus, this study did not demonstrate efficacy differences between adding risperidone or paroxetine to mood stabilizer therapy for bipolar depression, nor did it suggest an added effect of the combination of risperidone and paroxetine. Interpretation of the absence of differences between treatments in this underpowered study is challenging.

In a STEP-BD 16-week, multicenter, randomized, open effectiveness study, 66 patients with bipolar I disorder or bipolar II disorder with depression resistant to mood stabilizer plus antidepressant combination therapy received adjunctive risperidone (mean dosage 1.5 mg/day), lamotrigine (mean dosage 138 mg/day), or inositol (mean dosage 9,429 mg/day) (Nierenberg et al. 2006b). Risperidone was started at 0.5–1 mg/day and titrated as high as 6 mg/day. The rate of durable recovery (euthymia for 8 weeks) was numerically lower with adjunctive risperidone (4.6%) compared with adjunctive lamotrigine (23.8%) and adjunctive inositol (17.4%), but perhaps because of limited statistical power these differences did not reach statistical significance. Thus, adding risperidone yielded very little improvement. Treatment-emergent affective switch was seen in 13% with risperidone, 19% with lamotrigine, and 13% with inositol.

Risperidone monotherapy lacks FDA approval for acute bipolar depression, so the U.S. prescribing information does not provide dosing recommendations for this application. In order to limit adverse effects, risperidone in acute bipolar depression may be started at 0.25–0.5 mg/day and increased as necessary and tolerated every 4–7 days by 0.25–0.5 mg/day, with an initial target dosage of 1–2 mg/day.

In summary, the previous data regarding the efficacy of risperidone in acute bipolar depression are not particularly encouraging, but large, randomized, double-blind, placebo-controlled trials are needed to systematically investigate this issue.

Ziprasidone

Ziprasidone received FDA approval for the treatment of acute mania in 2004 but lacks acute bipolar depression and bipolar maintenance indications. In view of its 5-HT$_{1A}$ receptor agonist and serotonin and norepinephrine reuptake inhibitor effects, ziprasidone might be expected to have antidepressant effects. However, two recent controlled clinical trials of ziprasidone monotherapy in acute bipolar depression were negative (Sachs et al. 2009), in contrast with some encouraging limited case report (Mech 2008) and case series (Wang et al. 2008) data.

As with other second-generation antipsychotics, adjunctive ziprasidone ultimately may prove to yield benefit in treatment-resistant unipolar depression (Dunner et al. 2007).

As lower (e.g., less than 80 mg/day) compared with higher (e.g., at least 80 mg/day) ziprasidone dosages may increase the risk of akathisia (Oral et al. 2006), optimal titration of this agent may involve avoiding lower dosages to prevent akathisia or abruptly increasing to higher dosages if akathisia develops at lower dosages. Adjunctive lorazepam used in clinical acute mania trials may have decreased problems with akathisia.

Ziprasidone monotherapy lacks FDA approval for acute bipolar depression, so the U.S. prescribing information does not provide dosing recommendations for this application. In order to limit adverse effects (particularly akathisia at low dosages), ziprasidone in acute bipolar depression may be started at 80 mg/day at dinnertime or at bedtime with a snack and increased as necessary and tolerated daily by 20 mg/day, with an initial target dosage of 160 mg/day, which is the recommended maximum dosage in the U.S. prescribing information. In patients who tolerate but fail to respond to 160 mg/day, continuing to increase ziprasidone as necessary and tolerated daily by 20 mg/day to as high as 240–320 mg/day may yield additional benefit. Higher dosages tend to yield sedation and appetite suppression. If akathisia develops with the first-day dose (80 mg/day), abruptly increasing to 160 mg/day and, if appropriate, adding or increasing benzodiazepine may offer benefit. If sedation develops with the first-day dose (80 mg/day), decreasing daily by 20 mg/day (monitoring carefully for akathisia) may yield benefit. Attaining a ziprasidone dosage of at least 160 mg/day before beginning to taper other agents may help avoid akathisia when crossing over from another second-generation antipsychotic to ziprasidone. It is important that ziprasidone be ingested with food, which doubles ziprasidone absorption.

In summary, two large, randomized, double-blind, placebo-controlled trials failed to demonstrate efficacy of ziprasidone monotherapy in acute bipolar depression, making it a low-priority intervention for this application. As with aripiprazole, controlled trials are needed to assess whether adjunctive ziprasidone has utility in acute bipolar depression.

Clozapine

Clozapine received FDA approval for the treatment of schizophrenia in 1990 but lacks any indication for bipolar disorder. However, the antidepressant properties are of potential interest because clozapine is the only agent approved for decreasing suicidal behavior in patients with schizophrenia (Meltzer et al. 2003).

There are no controlled trials of clozapine in acute bipolar depression. Case reports and case series suggest clozapine may help occasional patients with treatment-refractory bipolar or unipolar depression, particularly with psychotic features (Banov et al. 1994; Dassa et al. 1993; Hrdlicka 2002; Jeyapaul and Vieweg 2006; Náhunek et al. 1973; Parsa et al. 1991; Privitera et al. 1993; Ranjan and Meltzer 1996; Vangala et al. 1999). The mean maximum clozapine dosage in 13 patients with unipolar or bipolar depression from 7 of these reports was 286 mg/day (range 125–650 mg/day) (Banov et al. 1994; Dassa et al. 1993; Jeyapaul and Vieweg 2006; Parsa et al. 1991; Privitera et al. 1993; Ranjan and Meltzer 1996; Vangala et al. 1999). However, it appears that in aggregate, clozapine may have less therapeutic potential in depressive as compared with manic/mixed states.

As compiled by Zarate et al. (1995) across five observational studies of clozapine (Banov et al. 1994; Battegay et al. 1977; Leppig et al. 1989; McElroy et al. 1991; Suppes et al. 1992), the response rate with clozapine in manic or mixed psychotic states (57/79, 77%) was significantly higher than in major depressive syndromes (30/58, 52%).

Clozapine monotherapy lacks FDA approval for acute bipolar depression, so the U.S. prescribing information does not provide dosing recommendations for this application. Clozapine dosages in patients with mood disorders tend to be considerably lower than in patients with schizophrenia. In order to limit adverse effects (particularly sedation), clozapine in acute bipolar depression may be started at 12.5 mg/day at bedtime and increased as necessary and tolerated every 4–7 days by 12.5 mg/day, with an initial target dosage of 100 mg/day. In patients who tolerate but fail to respond to 100 mg/day, continuing to increase as necessary and tolerated by 12.5 mg/day every 4–7 days to as high as 300 mg/day, which is one-third of the recommended maximum dosage for patients with schizophrenia in the U.S. prescribing information, may yield additional benefit. Occasional patients with bipolar depression may need and tolerate dosages higher than 300 mg/day.

In summary, in view of the challenging adverse effect profile of this agent, clozapine is usually held in reserve for patients with treatment-resistant illness. Controlled trials of clozapine in acute bipolar depression are needed to inform clinical practice.

Adjunctive Antidepressants

The role of antidepressants in the management of bipolar disorder is controversial. European experts are more enthusiastic than their North American counterparts regarding the utility of these agents in bipolar disorder, believing antidepressants are effective in acute bipolar depression and do not entail an excessive risk of treatment-emergent affective switch (Gijsman et al. 2004; Goodwin 2003). However, North American experts are less sanguine about these agents, raising concerns regarding efficacy as well as the risks of mood switches in the short term and cycle acceleration in the longer term (Ghaemi et al. 2003; Suppes et al. 2005). However, on both sides of the Atlantic Ocean there is general consensus that antidepressants in patients with bipolar disorder need to be administered with concurrent mood stabilizers or antimanic agents (Goodwin 2003; Suppes et al. 2005), although on occasion the contrary view has been argued for patients with bipolar II disorder (Amsterdam and Shults 2008).

Important contributors to this controversy are the paucity of controlled data supporting antidepressants in acute bipolar depression and the emergence of substantial controlled data supporting other agents. Nevertheless, in the mid-2000s, even in North America, antidepressants were still the most commonly used initial treatments for patients with bipolar disorder (Baldessarini et al. 2007).

Thus, it is becoming increasingly clear that the role of antidepressants in bipolar disorder is being reevaluated. Hence, whereas older treatment guidelines and even some newer treatment guidelines considered antidepressants first- or second-line interventions for acute bipolar depression (American Psychiatric Association 2002; Goodwin 2003; Grunze et al. 2002; Keck et al. 2004; Yatham et al. 2006), in some instances more recent expert opinion in North America has given these agents considerably lower priority (Suppes et al. 2005).

An increasing evidence base suggests that antidepressants may have substantial efficacy and tolerability limitations in the management of acute bipolar depression. Thus, there is broad consensus that antidepressant monotherapy is not recommended in acutely depressed patients with bipolar I disorder, in view of the risk of treatment-emergent affective switch (Goodwin 2003; Suppes et al. 2005). However, there is some controversy regarding the use of an antidepressant monotherapy in acutely depressed patients with bipolar II disorder (Amsterdam and Shults 2008).

In this section we begin with a review of the evidence from large placebo-controlled studies that, taken together, challenges the notion that antidepressants combined with antimanic agents ought to be considered high-priority options in the management of acute bipolar depression. This is followed by a review of the data regarding individual antidepressants in the management of acute bipolar depression.

Paradigm Challenging Multicenter, Randomized, Double-Blind, Placebo-Controlled Trials

The largest randomized controlled study to date to assess the utility of combining antidepressants with mood stabilizers in acute bipolar depression was not encouraging. Sachs and colleagues reported on a multicenter, randomized, double-blind, placebo-controlled effectiveness study from the STEP-BD, in which 366 subjects with bipolar depression (68% bipolar I disorder, 32% bipolar II disorder) were assigned to receive up to 26 weeks of treatment with a mood stabilizer plus adjunctive antidepressant therapy (bupropion, median dosage 300 mg/day, n=86; or paroxetine, median dosage 30 mg/day, n=93) or a mood stabilizer plus a matching placebo (n=187) (Sachs et al. 2007). The primary outcome was the percentage of subjects in each treatment group achieving "durable recovery" (8 consecutive weeks of euthymic mood). Among the subjects receiving de facto mood stabilizer without antidepressant (i.e., mood stabilizer plus a matching placebo), 27.3% (51/187) had durable recovery, which was numerically but not statistically greater than the 23.5% (42/179) receiving a mood stabilizer plus adjunctive antidepressant combined therapy who had durable recovery (P=0.40) (Figure 7–4, left). Thus, adding bupropion or paroxetine to mood stabilizers did not appear to add incremental benefit compared with mood stabilizers alone. The small deleterious effect of adding bupropion or paroxetine (a recovery rate that was 3.8% lower) translated into an NNH for not achieving recovery of 26 for bupropion or paroxetine plus mood stabilizers compared with mood stabilizers without bupropion or paroxetine. Put another way, 26 patients would need to be treated with bupropion or paroxetine plus mood stabilizers to yield one fewer recovery compared with treating with mood stabilizers without bupropion or paroxetine. However, addition of bupropion or paroxetine also did not appear to be associated with higher rates of treatment-emergent affective switch because these rates were statistically similar in the two groups. Thus, 10.1% (18/179) of patients taking bupropion or paroxetine plus mood stabilizer and 10.7% (20/187) patients taking mood stabilizer without bupropion or paroxetine had treatment-emergent affective switch.

The largest randomized controlled study to date to assess the utility of adding antidepressants to lithium in acute bipolar I depression was also not encouraging. In the study, 43 patients taking lithium plus placebo, 33 taking lithium

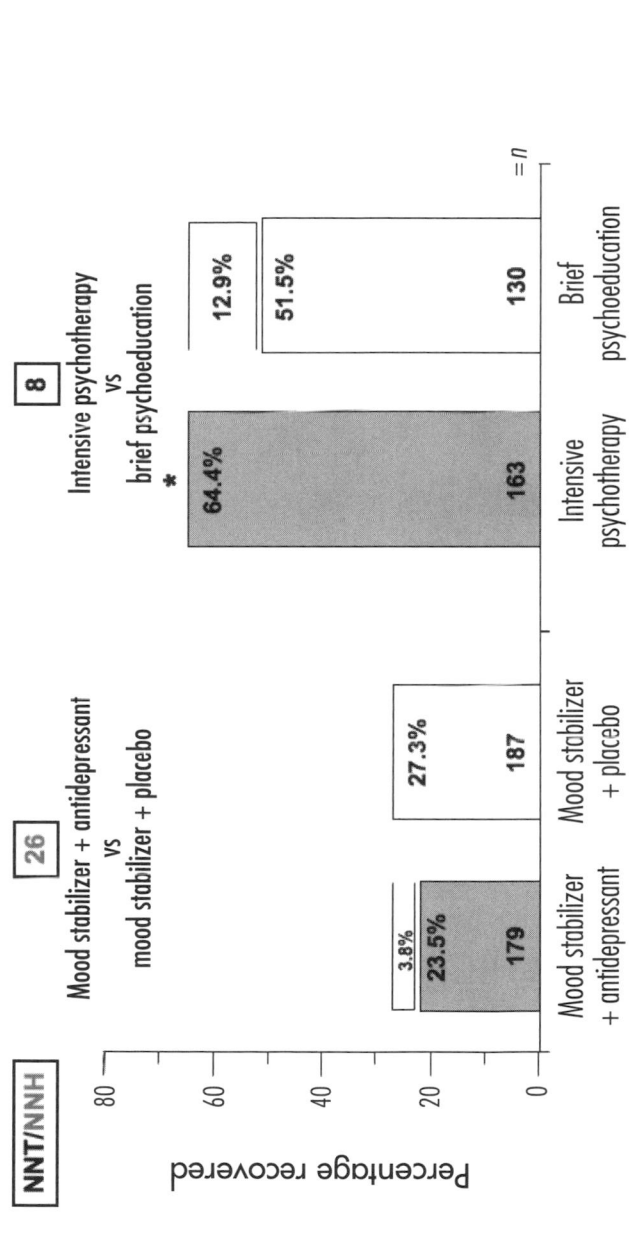

FIGURE 7–4. **Systematic Treatment Enhancement Program for Bipolar Disorder randomized acute bipolar depression effectiveness studies.**

Number needed to treat (NNT) and number needed to harm (NNH) for recovery, recovery rates. Adjunctive antidepressants (added to mood stabilizers) and adjunctive placebo yielded statistically similar, modest recovery rates (23.5% vs. 27.3%, *left*) (Sachs et al. 2007), highlighting the need for additional treatment options such as adjunctive intensive psychotherapy; which, compared with adjunctive brief psychoeducation, yielded a significantly higher recovery rate (64.4% vs. 51.5%, NNT=8, *right*) (Miklowitz et al. 2007). The NNT of 8 for intensive adjunctive psychotherapy was comparable to the single-digit NNT seen with FDA-approved pharmacotherapies across phases of bipolar disorders. *$P<0.05$ versus adjunctive brief psychoeducation.

plus paroxetine (paroxetine mean dosage 33 mg/day), and 36 taking lithium plus imipramine (imipramine mean dosage 167 mg/day) had statistically similar response (final Ham-D score ≤7) rates (34.9%, 45.5%, and 38.9%, respectively), and all three groups had statistically similar decreases in Ham-D total scores (Nemeroff et al. 2001). Thus, in the entire sample the NNTs for Ham-D response compared with adjunctive placebo were 10 for adjunctive paroxetine and 25 for adjunctive imipramine. It should be noted that response in this trial entailed having a Ham-D score of 7 or less, which is considered to be remission. Rates of incidence of treatment-emergent affective switch for lithium plus placebo, lithium plus paroxetine, and lithium plus imipramine were 2.3%, 0%, and 7.7%, respectively. The mean final serum lithium concentration for the entire sample was 0.78 mEq/L. In the subgroup of patients with serum lithium concentrations of 0.8 mEq/L or less, response rates were 31.8%, 52.6%, and 36.8%, and both adjunctive antidepressants compared with adjunctive placebo yielded larger decreases in Ham-D total scores. Thus, in this subgroup the NNTs for Ham-D response compared with adjunctive placebo were 5 for adjunctive paroxetine and 20 for adjunctive imipramine. In contrast, in the subgroup of patients with serum lithium concentrations of greater than 0.8 mEq/L, Ham-D response rates were 38.1%, 35.7%, and 41.2%, and all three groups had statistically similar decreases in depression scores. Thus, it may be that aiming for lithium serum concentrations greater than 0.8 mEq/L is preferable to combination therapy with an antidepressant unless lithium cannot be tolerated at such serum concentrations.

Paroxetine

Paroxetine is an SSRI antidepressant that aside from sedation, weight gain, and sexual dysfunction is generally well tolerated. However, as noted previously, in the two largest randomized, double-blind, placebo-controlled studies to date of adjunctive (added to mood stabilizers and/or antimanic agents) antidepressants in bipolar depression, adjunctive paroxetine was no better than adjunctive placebo (Nemeroff et al. 2001; Sachs et al. 2007). Moreover, as noted previously, in a recent 8-week, multicenter, randomized, double-blind, placebo-controlled trial in depressed patients with bipolar I disorder or bipolar II disorder, 118 patients taking paroxetine monotherapy 20 mg/day did no better than 121 patients taking placebo, in that these groups had statistically similar MADRS response (≥50% decrease) rates (55.1% vs. 52.9%, NNT=46) (Olausson et al. 2008). Treatment-emergent affective switch rates with paroxetine and placebo were similar (10.7% and 8.9%, respectively). In contrast, quetiapine at 300 mg/day and quetiapine at 600 mg/day compared with placebo and paroxetine had higher

MADRS response rates (66.8% and 67.2%, respectively) as well as lower treatment-emergent affective switch rates (2.1% and 4.1%, respectively).

Adjunctive paroxetine may entail a lower risk of treatment-emergent affective switch compared with some other adjunctive antidepressants. Thus, in two large controlled studies, the rate of treatment-emergent affective switch with adjunctive paroxetine was no different from that with adjunctive placebo (Nemeroff et al. 2001; Sachs et al. 2007). In one of these trials the incidence of treatment-emergent affective switch for lithium plus paroxetine was 0%, compared with 2.3% with lithium plus placebo and 7.7% with lithium plus imipramine (Nemeroff et al. 2001).

Paroxetine adjunctive therapy in acute bipolar depression was evaluated in two additional double-blind, active-controlled studies. In one study adjunctive paroxetine had a lower rate of treatment-emergent affective switch compared with adjunctive venlafaxine (Vieta et al. 2002), and in the other adjunctive paroxetine was better tolerated than adding a second mood stabilizer (Young et al. 2000).

Taken together, this evidence is considered by European (Goodwin 2003; Grunze et al. 2002) and Canadian (Yatham et al. 2006) experts, but not by some American experts (Suppes et al. 2005), to be sufficient for adjunctive use of SSRIs such as paroxetine to be considered a high-priority option in the management of acute bipolar depression.

Bupropion

Bupropion is an atypical antidepressant that, compared with other antidepressants, is generally well tolerated (not associated with sedation, weight gain, or sexual dysfunction) and when used adjunctively may entail a lower risk of treatment-emergent affective switch. Thus, in the largest randomized, double-blind, placebo-controlled study to date of adjunctive antidepressants (added to mood stabilizers and/or antimanic agents) in bipolar depression, the rate of treatment-emergent affective switch with adjunctive bupropion was no different from that with adjunctive placebo (Sachs et al. 2007). However, in this study adjunctive bupropion (as well as adjunctive paroxetine) was no more effective than adjunctive placebo. Some older placebo-controlled studies demonstrating bupropion monotherapy efficacy in hospitalized depressed subjects included more bipolar than unipolar patients (Fabre et al. 1983; Merideth and Feighner 1983).

In additional double-blind, active-controlled studies, adjunctive bupropion had lower rates of treatment-emergent affective switch compared with adjunctive venlafaxine (Post et al. 2006) and adjunctive desipramine (Sachs et al. 1994).

Also, in an 8-week, randomized, single-blind rater study, adjunctive bupropion (mean dose 250 mg) compared with adjunctive topiramate (mean dose 176 mg) yielded a similar Ham-D response (≥50% decrease) rate (59% vs. 56%), a nonsignificantly lower adverse effect discontinuation rate (22% vs. 33%), and significantly less weight loss (1.2 kg vs. 5.8 kg), suggesting adjunctive topiramate yields weight loss in bipolar depression (McIntyre et al. 2002). The small sample size limits the interpretation of this study.

Taken together, this evidence is considered by European (Goodwin 2003; Grunze et al. 2002) and Canadian (Yatham et al. 2006) experts but not by some American experts (Suppes et al. 2005) to be sufficient for adjunctive use of bupropion to be considered a high-priority option in the management of acute bipolar depression.

Fluoxetine

Fluoxetine is an SSRI antidepressant that, aside from gastrointestinal adverse effects and sexual dysfunction, is generally well tolerated. As noted previously, fluoxetine combined with olanzapine was the first treatment approved for acute bipolar depression (Tohen et al. 2003). Fluoxetine has been studied in bipolar depression in four additional controlled studies. However, methodological limitations make the interpretation of these findings challenging (Amsterdam and Shults 2005; Amsterdam et al. 1998, 2004; Cohn et al. 1989).

Taken together, this evidence is considered by European (Goodwin 2003; Grunze et al. 2002) and Canadian (Yatham et al. 2006) experts, but not by some American experts (Suppes et al. 2005), to be sufficient for adjunctive use of SSRIs such as fluoxetine to be considered a high-priority option in the management of acute bipolar depression.

Venlafaxine

Venlafaxine is a serotonin-norepinephrine reuptake inhibitor antidepressant that aside from gastrointestinal adverse effects, sexual dysfunction, and blood pressure increases may be generally well tolerated. However, as noted previously, controlled studies suggest the rate of treatment-emergent affective switch with adjunctive venlafaxine in bipolar depression is higher than with adjunctive bupropion or adjunctive sertraline (Post et al. 2006) or than with adjunctive paroxetine (Vieta et al. 2002). Although these controlled studies also suggested adjunctive venlafaxine had similar antidepressant efficacy in bipolar depression compared with adjunctive bupropion and adjunctive sertraline (Post et al. 2006) and adjunctive paroxetine (Vieta et al. 2002), the absence of placebo control groups, and in one trial limited statistical power, makes interpretation of these findings challenging. Two additional studies assessed venlafaxine in patients with bipolar II disorder depression, but methodological limitations make interpretation of these studies challenging (Amsterdam and Shults 2008; Amsterdam et al. 1998).

Taken together, this evidence suggests that the increased risk of treatment-emergent affective switch with venlafaxine compared with SSRIs or bupropion is sufficient to warrant extra caution when using venlafaxine, holding it in reserve for patients with inadequate efficacy or tolerability with SSRIs or bupropion. Indeed, several treatment guidelines to different degrees reflect such a lower priority for venlafaxine (American Psychiatric Association 2002; Grunze et al. 2002; Keck et al. 2004; Yatham et al. 2006).

Tricyclic Antidepressants

Tricyclic antidepressants (TCAs), because of a more problematic adverse effect profile, including a greater risk of treatment-emergent affective switch, have been superceded by newer agents in the treatment of acute bipolar depression. In aggregate, placebo-controlled studies of TCAs in acute bipolar depression have not been particularly encouraging with respect to not only tolerability but also efficacy.

As noted previously, in the largest randomized controlled study to date assessing the utility of adding antidepressants to lithium in patients with acute bipolar I depression, lithium plus imipramine (imipramine mean dosage 167 mg/day), lithium plus paroxetine (paroxetine mean dosage 33 mg/day), and lithium plus placebo yielded statistically similar response (final Ham-D score≤7) rates of 38.9%, 45.5%, and 34.9%, respectively (Nemeroff et al. 2001). Rates of incidence of treatment-emergent affective switch for lithium plus imipramine, lithium plus paroxetine, and lithium plus placebo were 7.7%, 0%, and 2.3%, respectively.

In another randomized, controlled bipolar I depression study, fluoxetine (mean dosage approximately 60 mg/day), imipramine (mean dosage approximately 170 mg/day), and placebo yielded treatment-emergent affective switch rates of 0%, 6.7%, and 3.4%, respectively, and for patients who remained in the study for at least 3 weeks, Ham-D response rates were significantly greater with fluoxetine compared with imipramine and placebo (86%, 57%, and 38%) (Cohn et al. 1989).

In another randomized, controlled study in depressed patients with bipolar I disorder resistant to mood stabilizers, adjunctive bupropion (mean dosage 358 mg/day) and adjunctive desipramine (mean dosage 140 mg/day) yielded similar Ham-D response (≥50% decrease) rates (63% vs. 71%) (Sachs et al. 1994).

Four nonresponders crossed over to the other adjunctive antidepressant again failed to respond, lowering the aggregate response rates (55% and 50%). However, bupropion compared with desipramine had a lower aggregate treatment-emergent affective switch rate (11% vs. 30%).

As reviewed by Zornberg and Pope (1993), in one older controlled study in 29 depressed patients with bipolar I disorder, imipramine was superior to not only placebo but also lithium (Fieve et al. 1968), but in other older acute bipolar depression studies, imipramine was equivalent to lithium ($n=5$) (Watanabe et al. 1975), equivalent to moclobemide ($n=33$) (Baumhackl et al. 1989), and inferior to tranylcypromine ($n=56$) (Himmelhoch et al. 1991).

A meta-analysis of six controlled trials (Cohn et al. 1989; De Wilde and Doogan 1982; Himmelhoch et al. 1991; Nemeroff et al. 2001; Sachs et al. 1994; Silverstone 2001) found that the incidence of treatment-emergent affective switch was significantly higher in patients taking TCAs (10.3%, 19/184) compared with patients taking other antidepressants (SSRIs, monoamine oxidase inhibitors [MAOIs], or bupropion, 3.2%, 6/186) (Gijsman et al. 2004).

Female gender was a risk factor for antidepressant treatment-emergent affective switch in a 3-year, randomized, double-blind, placebo-controlled trial of imipramine plus lithium compared with lithium monotherapy in 75 patients with bipolar I disorder (Quitkin et al. 1981) but not in a later uncontrolled retrospective study of 53 patients with bipolar disorder (Goldberg and Whiteside 2002).

Taken together, the previous evidence suggests that the increased risk of somatic adverse effects and treatment-emergent affective switch with TCAs compared with SSRIs or bupropion is sufficient to warrant extra caution when using TCAs, holding them in reserve for patients with inadequate efficacy or tolerability with SSRIs or bupropion. Indeed, treatment guidelines uniformly reflect such a lower priority for TCAs (American Psychiatric Association 2002; Grunze et al. 2002; Keck et al. 2004; Suppes et al. 2005; Yatham et al. 2006).

Monoamine Oxidase Inhibitors

MAOIs increase monoamine neurotransmission by attenuating degradation rather than blocking reuptake. Older agents such as tranylcypromine irreversibly inhibit both monoamine oxidase A and monoamine oxidase B and entail substantial risks of adverse effects and drug interactions and require dietary restrictions. However, a controlled trial suggested tranylcypromine had superior efficacy compared with imipramine in bipolar depression.

In a 6-week, randomized, double-blind trial in anergic bipolar (43% Type I, 57% Type II) depression among patients who completed at least 4 weeks, tranylcypromine (30–60 mg/day) monotherapy compared with imipramine (150–300 mg/day) monotherapy yielded a higher Ham-D ($\geq$50% decrease) response rate (81% vs. 48%) and a similar rate of treatment-emergent affective switch (21% vs. 25%) (Himmelhoch et al. 1991). Across both treatments the switch rate was higher in patients with bipolar I disorder compared with patients with bipolar II disorder (38% vs. 13%).

Newer agents such as the reversible inhibitor of monoamine oxidase A moclobemide and transdermal selegiline address some of the safety and tolerability limitations of tranylcypromine but have less evidence of efficacy. Controlled data are lacking for transdermal selegiline in bipolar disorder but there are some controlled active comparator data for moclobemide in acute bipolar depression.

A pooled analysis of early randomized, double-blind, acute depression trials found that in the subset of patients with bipolar I disorder, moclobemide compared with comparator antidepressants yielded a nonsignificantly higher CGI improvement response (good/very good) rate (59.8% vs. 48.7%) (Angst and Stabl 1992).

In an 8-week, multicenter, randomized, double-blind trial in patients with acute bipolar I depression, approximately half of whom were taking mood stabilizers (primarily lithium), moclobemide (450–750 mg/day) compared with imipramine (150–250 mg/day) yielded a nonsignificantly lower Ham-D response ($\geq$50% decrease) rate (46% vs. 53%) but significantly less dry mouth, constipation, diaphoresis, palpitations, and tremor, and nonsignificantly less weight gain and withdrawal caused by treatment-emergent affective switch (2.5% vs. 8.0%) (Silverstone 2001).

Taken together, the previous evidence suggests that the increased risk of somatic adverse effects and drug interactions with irreversible monoamine oxidase A and monoamine oxidase B inhibitors such as tranylcypromine is sufficient to warrant extra caution when using such agents, holding them in reserve for patients with inadequate efficacy or tolerability with SSRIs or bupropion. Indeed, treatment guidelines uniformly reflect such a lower priority (American Psychiatric Association 2002; Grunze et al. 2002; Keck et al. 2004; Suppes et al. 2005; Yatham et al. 2006). Although better tolerated, moclobemide and transdermal selegiline have sufficiently limited efficacy data that generally they are also considered to have lower priority than SSRIs or bupropion.

Efficacy Limitations of Adjunctive Antidepressants

European psychiatrists have a more positive opinion than their North American counterparts of the efficacy and tolerability of antidepressants in acute bipolar depression. Recent European meta-analyses concluded that five randomized, controlled bipolar depression trials involving a total of 779 patients indicated that antidepressants compared with placebo had superior efficacy and a similar rate of treatment-emergent affective switch (Gijsman et al. 2004). However, these analyses had substantial limitations: 1) two trials were adjunctive (Nemeroff et al. 2001; Tohen et al. 2003), one involved partial adjunctive use (Cohn et al. 1989), and two involved monotherapy (Himmelhoch et al. 1982; Mendlewicz and Youdim 1980); 2) two trials included both unipolar and bipolar patients (Himmelhoch et al. 1982; Mendlewicz and Youdim 1980); and 3) almost 59% of the patients came from one trial (Tohen et al. 2003).

In a naturalistic STEP-BD study, Sachs and colleagues reported preliminary outcomes for the first 1,000 subjects enrolled in the STEP-BD, assessing treatment outcomes of the first episode of depression to occur during the first year of participation in the study (Sachs 2003). Thus, 181 subjects experienced a new onset major depressive episode. Surprisingly, adding compared with not adding a antidepressant or lamotrigine tended to yield a *longer* time to durable recovery (8 consecutive weeks of euthymic mood) and a *lower* rate of treatment-emergent affective switch (adding antidepressant—8.6%, adding lamotrigine—8.8%, adding neither—14.6%). These results are broadly consistent with the STEP-BD randomized controlled trial described previously (Figure 7–1, left), in which adjunctive antidepressants compared with adjunctive placebo yielded nonsignificantly lower recovery and switch rates (Sachs et al. 2007). Taken together, these studies suggest that the risk of inefficacy rather than the risk of switching may be the more substantive limitation of adjunctive antidepressants in acute bipolar depression.

In another naturalistic effectiveness study, only 34% (189/549) of Stanley Foundation Bipolar Network patients receiving adjunctive antidepressants for new-onset major depressive episodes continued these agents for at least 60 days (Altshuler et al. 2003).

Tolerability Limitations of Adjunctive Antidepressants

Antidepressant medications may induce treatment-emergent affective switch (mood elevation episodes) or accelerate episode frequency (cycle acceleration). In a small retrospective study, antidepressant therapy was less effective in 41 bipolar patients with depression compared with 37 unipolar patients with depression, with the former having a lower short-term response rate (48.7% vs. 68.4%) and, among responders, a 3.4 times higher relapse rate (53.8% vs. 15.8%) (Ghaemi et al. 2004). Approximately one-quarter (25.6%) of patients with bipolar disorder developed cycle acceleration, whereas approximately one-half (48.8%) experienced treatment-emergent affective switch. Patients with bipolar disorder taking concurrent antimanic medications compared with those not taking concurrent antimanic medications had a lower treatment-emergent affective switch rate (31.6% vs. 84.2%).

These tolerability limitations have attracted the attention of researchers for over two decades. Thus, in the late 1980s Wehr and associates reported a case series of six patients with bipolar disorder, in whom cycle length shortened during TCA treatment (Wehr et al. 1988). Several other case series found similar results of rapid-cycling course of illness associated with antidepressant treatment (Wehr and Goodwin 1979; Wehr et al. 1988). Using life-charting methodology (Denicoff et al. 1997), Altshuler and colleagues evaluated the course of illness of 51 patients with treatment-refractory bipolar disorder to examine the potential effect of heterocyclic antidepressants on the emergence of manic episodes and cycle acceleration (Altshuler et al. 1995). During antidepressant treatment, 35% of mood switches from depression to mania and 26% of cycle accelerations were deemed likely to be antidepressant induced. Interestingly, most of these patients were not taking mood stabilizers, which is a common treatment inadequacy encountered in clinical practice. The rates of treatment-emergent affective switch (occurring within the first 3 months of antidepressant therapy) ranged from 8% to 15% in the SFBN and STEP-BD samples of patients with bipolar depression.

In spite of these case series, naturalistic studies, and uncontrolled trials suggesting that use of antidepressant medications in patients with bipolar disorder carries a liability of treatment-emergent affective switch, it is important to note that no large randomized, placebo-controlled, parallel-group trial has validated this adverse effect. In part, this may be because of such highly structured studies excluding patients with more severe illness such as rapid cycling or with psychiatric or medical comorbidities such as substance abuse disorders (Visser and Van Der Mast 2005) and hypothyroidism (Bottlender et al. 2000), which may be associated with a greater risk of treatment-emergent affective switch. In addition, subjects in controlled trials compared with routine clinical care may be monitored more carefully for concurrent use of mood-stabilizing medications (Goldberg et al. 2001).

As noted previously, the risk of treatment-emergent affective switch appears to vary across antidepressants, with TCAs appearing to entail particularly high risk (Boerlin et al. 1998; Bottlender et al. 1998, 2000), possibly as much as three times that of other classes of antidepressant medications, based on meta-analysis (Gijsman et al. 2004). Arguably, the serotonin-norepinephrine reuptake inhibitor venlafaxine has more similarity (e.g., shared noradrenergic effects) to TCAs than other contemporary antidepressants, perhaps contributing to clinical observations of venlafaxine yielding higher rates of treatment-emergent affective switch than bupropion and sertraline (Post et al. 2006), as well as paroxetine (Vieta et al. 2002).

Summary of Adjunctive Antidepressants in Acute Bipolar Depression

Emerging data on substantive efficacy limitations, and perhaps to a lesser degree tolerability limitations (e.g., risk of treatment-emergent affective switch), suggest that the role of adjunctive antidepressants in acute bipolar depression needs to be reconsidered. Thus, the historically important approach of administering antidepressants along with mood stabilizers ultimately may be superceded by other strategies. Currently, this is a topic of at times spirited controversy. It may be that certain antimanic agents combined with specific antidepressants (e.g., OFC) prove effective without increased switch risk, whereas other combinations (e.g., lithium plus TCAs) prove ineffective with excessive switch risk. Additional controlled trials are needed to help clarify this issue. Variability across patients is substantial, and there may be a minority (perhaps 15%) of patients with acute bipolar depression in whom adding an antidepressant to an antimanic agent is effective not only acutely but also during longer-term therapy. Hopefully, research will ultimately aid clinicians in identifying bipolar disorder patients with the potential for such excellent responses to adjunctive antidepressants. Until that time, clinicians and patients will have to rely on carefully individualized benefit-risk analyses using the limited information available.

Electroconvulsive Therapy

ECT is a well-established treatment option for acute depression supported by multiple randomized controlled trials, commonly in heterogeneous samples of bipolar and unipolar patients with depression. Thus, meta-analyses of randomized controlled trials in mixed-age samples of depressed unipolar and bipolar disorder patients revealed superior efficacy for 1) real compared with simulated ECT; 2) ECT compared with pharmacotherapy (including TCAs, MAOIs, paroxetine, and lithium); 3) bilateral compared with unilateral ECT; and 4) high compared with low electrical stimulus ECT (UK ECT Review Group 2003).

ECT may be particularly effective for psychotic depression, in older patients with depression, and in patients with atypical depression, and has a rapid onset of antidepressant effect.

A meta-analysis of 44 acute psychotic depression studies revealed superior efficacy with ECT compared with 1) antidepressant (tricyclic or MAOI) monotherapy, 2) antipsychotic (first-generation) monotherapy, and 3) antidepressant plus antipsychotic combination therapy, although the latter fell short of statistical significance (Parker et al. 1992).

In one study, the Ham-D remission rate was higher in psychotic (83%, 64/77) compared with nonpsychotic (71%, 125/176) patients with unipolar depression. In another report, ECT response increased with age (O'Connor et al. 2001). In yet another study, the Ham-D remission rate was higher in patients with atypical depression (81%, 29/36) compared with those with typical depression (67%, 304/453) (Husain et al. 2008), with over half of patients experiencing initial first response by the end of the first week (Husain et al. 2004).

There are fewer data addressing ECT efficacy in exclusively bipolar samples, or in bipolar depression compared with unipolar depression. A review by Zornberg and Pope (1993) found that ECT efficacy in acute bipolar depression was 1) superior to TCAs or MAOIs in five studies, 2) similar to TCAs in two studies, and 3) similar in patients with bipolar or unipolar depression in five studies; although in one study, ECT was inferior in patients with bipolar depression compared with those with unipolar depression (Homan et al. 1982).

Three more recent studies also supported similar ECT efficacy in bipolar compared with unipolar depression (Daly et al. 2001; Grunhaus et al. 2002; Sackeim and Prudic 2005). Of interest, two of these studies found that bipolar compared with unipolar patients required significantly fewer ECT treatments, a finding previously reported in a retrospective case series by another group (Perris and d'Elia 1966).

Treatment-emergent affective switch with ECT has been reported with variable incidence. A retrospective study cited a switch rate in patients with bipolar depression of 38% (15/40) with ECT, but this was statistically similar to the rate without treatment (29%, 6/21) (Angst et al. 1992). In contrast, a prospective analysis found a switch rate of only 3% (2/66) with ECT in patients with bipolar depression (Daly et al. 2001).

Concerns based on case reports regarding the risks of delirium, seizures, and prolonged apnea resulted in recommendations that lithium not be combined with ECT (Small and Milstein 1990).

In summary, in patients with severe, psychotic, catatonic, or acutely suicidal depression and depression during pregnancy, ECT should be considered and offered as an early option. However, as advocated in many treatment guidelines (American Psychiatric Association 2002; Goodwin 2003; Suppes et al.

2005; Yatham et al. 2006), in less challenging circumstances ECT generally should be held in reserve for patients intolerant of or refractory to pharmacotherapy because of stigma, consent challenges, or logistical concerns such as coordination of care and aftercare, as well as the risk of interruption of function related to cognitive adverse effects.

Adjunctive Psychotherapy

Emerging data from controlled trials indicate the increasing importance of adjunctive psychosocial interventions in the management of bipolar disorders, as discussed in detail in Chapter 15 of this volume, "Adjunctive Psychosocial Interventions in the Management of Bipolar Disorders."

The most studied psychosocial interventions in patients with bipolar disorders have been psychoeducation (Colom et al. 2003), cognitive-behavioral therapy (CBT) (Lam et al. 2003), family-focused therapy (FFT) (Miklowitz et al. 2003), and interpersonal and social rhythm therapy (IPSRT) (Frank et al. 2005). These treatments may have illness phase–specific features, with optimal time of administration being during depression or euthymia as opposed to during mania and with acute and preventive effects being greater against depressive as compared with the mood elevation aspects of the illness (Swartz and Frank 2001). Indeed, some data suggest that psychoeducation (Colom et al. 2003), FFT (Miklowitz et al. 2003), and IPSRT (Frank et al. 2005) may have greater ability to counter depressive as compared with mood elevation symptoms. However, other data suggest psychoeducation (Perry et al. 1999) and CBT (Lam et al. 2003) may have greater ability to counter mood elevation as compared with depressive symptoms.

Studies have emphasized the use of psychosocial interventions in relapse/ recurrence prevention in patients with bipolar disorder during euthymia or heterogeneous mood states (Colom et al. 2003; Frank et al. 2005; Lam et al. 2003; Miklowitz et al. 2003; Perry et al. 1999; Scott et al. 2001) more than in acute bipolar depression (Miklowitz et al. 2007; Zaretsky et al. 1999). However, in a pilot study by Zaretsky et al. (1999), 20 weekly CBT sessions yielded similar Ham-D decreases in 11 patients with bipolar disorder with depression and 11 matched patients with unipolar depression.

The largest psychosocial intervention study to date in acute bipolar depression was a STEP-BD, 9-month, multicenter, randomized, controlled effectiveness trial, in which 163 patients who received adjunctive intensive (thirty 50-minute sessions over 9 months) CBT, FFT, or IPSRT, compared with 130 patients who received a much more limited brief (three 50-minute sessions) psychoeducational control intervention, recovered more quickly and had a higher recovery rate (64.4% vs. 51.5%, NNT=8; Figure 7–4, right) (Miklowitz et al. 2007). This NNT of 8 was comparable with the single-digit NNT seen with FDA-approved pharmacotherapies across phases of bipolar disorders. This and other psychotherapy studies are discussed in detail in Chapter 15 of this volume. In contrast, as noted previously, in another STEP-BD multicenter, randomized, controlled study in acute bipolar depression, the effectiveness of adjunctive antidepressants (added to mood stabilizers) was no better or worse than adjunctive placebo, with both interventions yielding only modest recovery rates (23.5% vs. 27.3%; Figure 7–4, left) (Sachs et al. 2007), highlighting the need for additional treatment options such as adjunctive psychosocial interventions for acute bipolar depression.

Taken together, these data indicate an increasingly important role for adjunctive psychosocial interventions in the management of acute bipolar depression, which has already been acknowledged in multiple treatment guidelines (American Psychiatric Association 2002; Goodwin 2003; Keck et al. 2004). Should additional controlled data confirm the STEP-BD acute bipolar depression studies suggesting limited efficacy of adjunctive antidepressants (Sachs et al. 2007) and more substantive efficacy of adjunctive intensive psychotherapy (Miklowitz et al. 2007), reevaluation of the relative priorities of these approaches will be necessary.

In summary, emerging data support the use of adjunctive psychosocial interventions in acute bipolar depression. With evidence from additional controlled trails, it is anticipated that these treatments will become increasingly important options.

Tier IV: Novel Adjunctive Treatments

Treatment resistance or intolerance is sufficiently common in patients with bipolar disorders, that even the previously mentioned armamentarium is insufficient to meet clinical needs. This section describes novel adjunctive treatments with even more limited evidence of efficacy than the previously mentioned treatments. These treatments include thyroid hormones, pramipexole, modafinil, topiramate, stimulants, sleep deprivation, light therapy, nutriceuticals, vagus nerve stimulation (VNS), and transcranial magnetic stimulation. In general, treatment guidelines consider these modalities to be low-priority interventions (American Psychiatric Association 2002; Goodwin 2003; Grunze et al. 2002; Keck et al. 2004; Suppes et al. 2005; Yatham et al. 2006). Nevertheless, some Tier IV options could prove attractive for carefully selected patients after consideration of Tier I–III treatments (e.g., patients treatment resistant or intolerant to Tier I–III treatments). For some of these treatments, advances in research may ultimately provide sufficient evidence to merit their consideration for placement in higher tiers.

Adjunctive Thyroid Hormones

An extensive literature links mood disorders to disturbances of the hypothalamic-pituitary-thyroid axis. L-thyroxine (T_4) and L-triiodothyronine (T_3, also referred to as liothyronine) are used not only in the treatment of hypothyroidism, which is common in patients with mood disorders, but also as adjuncts in the management of primary mood disorders.

Physiological Doses of T_3 in Mood Disorders

Adjunctive T_3 has been used in physiological doses, primarily combined with other agents (most often antidepressants), to accelerate treatment response in nonrefractory depression and to enhance treatment response in treatment-resistant depression. Thus, meta-analyses of controlled studies suggested that adjunctive T_3 added to TCAs accelerated TCA response in nonrefractory unipolar depression and less consistently enhanced treatment response in TCA-resistant and SSRI-resistant depression.

A meta-analysis of six controlled trials involving a total of 125 patients with nonrefractory unipolar depression indicated that adjunctive T_3 (20–62.5 μg/day) compared with adjunctive placebo accelerated response to TCAs (overall, and in 5 of 6 trials), with women compared with men being more likely to benefit (Altshuler et al. 2001).

A meta-analysis of eight controlled trials (four trials including both unipolar and bipolar disorder patients, four trials including only unipolar patients) involving a total of 292 patients with TCA-resistant depression indicated an NNT for response with adjunctive T_3 (20–50 μg/day) compared with control of 5 (Aronson et al. 1996). However, considering only the subset of four randomized, double-blind, controlled trials yielded an NNT for response with adjunctive T_3 compared with control of 13. Two controlled studies of combining T_3 with SSRIs have had varying results in unipolar depression (Appelhof et al. 2004; Cooper-Kazaz et al. 2007).

In a recent Sequenced Treatment Alternatives to Relieve Depression (STAR*D) 14-week, randomized, open-label effectiveness study of treatment-resistant or treatment-intolerant unipolar depression, 73 patients adding

T_3 (mean final dosage 45 μg/day) compared with 69 patients adding lithium (mean final dosage 860 μg/day, 0.6 mEq/L) had similar efficacy (remission rates of 24.7% vs. 15.9%, *P*=NS) but better tolerability (adverse effect discontinuation rates 23.2% vs. 9.6%) (Nierenberg et al. 2006a).

Conservative T_3 dosing may be prudent in mood disorder patients, who may be at increased risk for central nervous system adverse effects such as anxiety and tremor. In such patients, tolerability may be enhanced by starting T_3 at 5 μg/day taken in the morning, increasing weekly by 5 μg/day as indicated by clinical response and/or serum T_3 and thyrotropin concentrations, pausing for 2 weeks at 25 μg/day to assess efficacy and tolerability, and then increasing weekly by 5 μg/day as necessary and tolerated and as indicated by clinical response and/or serum T_3 and thyrotropin concentrations to as high as 50 μg/day. Mean dosages in mood disorder studies have commonly ranged from approximately 25 to 50 μg/day.

Supraphysiological Doses of T₄ in Mood Disorders

Supraphysiological doses of T_4 have been less extensively studied and used than physiological doses of T_3 in patients with mood disorders. It may be that at physiological doses, adjunctive T_4 compared with adjunctive T_3 has less potency in treatment-resistant depression (Joffe and Singer 1990).

Limited uncontrolled studies suggest that supraphysiological doses of T_4 (up to 500 μg/day) may offer benefit in treatment-resistant acute bipolar depression (Bauer et al. 1998) and in treatment-resistant rapid-cycling bipolar disorder (Bauer and Whybrow 1990), as discussed in Chapter 9 of this volume, "Management of Rapid-Cycling Bipolar Disorders." In general, long-term administration of supraphysiological doses of T_4 does not appear to alter bone mineral density in women with mood disorders (Bauer et al. 2004; Gyulai et al. 2001), although this may occur in sporadic individuals (Bauer et al. 2004).

Supraphysiological T_4 in mood disorder studies has been started at 50 μg/day and increased as necessary and tolerated every 3–7 days by 50 μg/day to as high as 500 μg/day (approximately twice the U.S. prescribing information recommended dosage), aiming to suppress thyrotropin and increase free T_4 by at least 50% compared with baseline (Bauer et al. 2002). Mean dosages in such studies have commonly ranged from approximately 300 to 500 μg/day. Supraphysiological doses of T_4 compared with physiological doses of T_3 have not been used as extensively in mood disorder patients, and considerable caution is warranted regarding careful selection of medically appropriate (particularly with respect to cardiac and bone health) patients.

Physiological Doses of T₃ Combined With T₄

On occasion, T_3 may be combined with T_4 in patients with hypothyroidism, but this has not been systematically assessed in patients with bipolar disorders. Although there have been controlled studies of the T_3 (dosages ranging between 7.5 and 25 μg/day) plus T_4 combination in patients with hypothyroidism, findings regarding the mood, cognitive, and somatic effects and patient preference benefits have been variable.

Although an early controlled study was encouraging (Bunevicius et al. 1999), subsequent studies were generally discouraging, and in a meta-analysis of nine controlled studies, the T_3 plus T_4 combination was no better than T_4 monotherapy with respect to measures of mood and well-being, although there was a tendency toward patients preferring the T_3 plus T_4 combination over T_4 monotherapy (Joffe et al. 2007).

Additional information regarding thyroid hormones is provided in Chapter 14 of this volume.

Adjunctive Pramipexole

Dopamine neurotransmission plays an important role in reward and motivation neural circuits. Thus, dopamine agonists may have a role in the treatment of bipolar depression. Two small, 6-week, randomized, double-blind, placebo-controlled studies suggested the utility of adjunctive use of the dopamine agonist pramipexole in bipolar depression.

In one study of nonpsychotic bipolar I disorder and bipolar II disorder outpatients with depression resistant to lithium, divalproex, carbamazepine, lamotrigine, and/or gabapentin, 12 patients receiving adjunctive pramipexole (mean final dosage 1.7 mg/day) compared with 12 patients receiving adjunctive placebo had a higher Ham-D response (≥50% reduction) rate (67% vs. 20%) (Goldberg et al. 2004). Pramipexole was started at 0.125 mg twice daily and increased by 0.25 mg/day every 3–5 days to a target range of 1.0–2.5 mg/day. Subjects who remained nonresponders at the target dosage could increase the pramipexole dosage up to 5 mg/day. One patient taking pramipexole dropped out because of psychotic mania.

In another study of bipolar II disorder patients with depression resistant to mood stabilizers, 11 patients receiving adjunctive pramipexole (mean final dosage 1.7 mg/day) compared with 11 patients receiving adjunctive placebo had a higher MADRS response (>50% decrease) rate (60% vs. 9%) (Zarate et al. 2004). Pramipexole was initiated at 0.125 mg three times a day and increased every 5–7 days by 0.125 mg three times a day to achieve the target range of 1–3 mg/

day. The maximum dosage allowable was 4.5 mg/day. Three subjects (one on pramipexole and two on placebo) developed hypomanic symptoms.

Together these two small controlled studies suggest that adjunctive pramipexole may have utility in bipolar depression. However, both had remarkably low placebo response rates, and the small sample sizes make these positive findings tentative. For example, for each study, reassigning a single adjunctive pramipexole subject from responder to nonresponder status, or a single adjunctive placebo subject from nonresponder to responder status, would have made the results nonsignificant. Larger controlled studies are needed to confirm these encouraging data regarding the utility of adjunctive pramipexole in bipolar depression.

Using more gradual initiation than that in the controlled studies may enhance tolerability. Therefore, it may be prudent to start pramipexole at 0.125 mg/day and increase as necessary and tolerated on a daily basis by 0.125 mg/day to an initial target range of 1–2 mg/day. In patients who tolerate but fail to respond to 2 mg/day, continuing to increase as necessary and tolerated on a daily basis by 0.125 mg/day to as high as 4.5 mg/day may yield benefit. As pramipexole may be sedating, a single daily dose at bedtime may be preferred, providing it does not yield nausea or other adverse effects. Additional information regarding pramipexole is provided in Chapter 14 of this volume.

Adjunctive Modafinil

Modafinil is approved for improving wakefulness in patients with excessive sleepiness associated with narcolepsy, obstructive sleep apnea, and shift-work sleep disorder, and may improve mood ratings in healthy volunteers (Taneja et al. 2007) and used adjunctively may relieve residual fatigue and sleepiness in unipolar major depressive disorder patients with partial responses to antidepressants (Fava et al. 2005). A recent controlled trial suggested adjunctive modafinil may have utility in acute bipolar depression.

In a 6-week, multicenter, randomized, double-blind, placebo-controlled study in patients with bipolar depression inadequately responsive to a mood stabilizer with or without concomitant antidepressant therapy, 41 patients taking adjunctive modafinil (mean dosage 177 mg/day) compared with 44 patients taking adjunctive placebo had a higher response rate (44% vs. 23%) and remission rate (39% vs. 18%) and a similar treatment-emergent affective switch rate (4.9% vs. 11.4%) (Frye et al. 2007). Headache was the most common other side effect with modafinil. Larger controlled studies are needed to confirm these encouraging data regarding the utility of adjunctive modafinil in bipolar depression.

In the previously mentioned controlled study of patients with acute bipolar depression, adjunctive modafinil was started at 100 mg each morning and after 1 week was increased to 100 mg twice daily (morning and noon so as to not interfere with sleep), with the mean final dosage being 177 mg/day. Occasional patients may tolerate and benefit from further increasing modafinil as necessary and tolerated by 100 mg on a weekly basis to as high as 400 mg/day. Some patients may prefer a single daily dose in the morning. Additional information regarding modafinil is provided in Chapter 14 of this volume.

Adjunctive Topiramate

Topiramate is a fructopyranose sulfamate that blocks sodium channels, inhibits carbonic anhydrase, and positively modulates $GABA_A$ receptors. Topiramate also blocks AMPA/kainate gated ion channels, and therefore it may have antiglutamatergic properties, somewhat similar to lamotrigine. Early case reports and open case series in patients with bipolar disorders were encouraging, as reviewed by Suppes (2002). However, interpretation of results of such nonrandomized open label trials is challenging.

Indeed, four multicenter, randomized, double-blind, placebo-controlled, and lithium-controlled trials involving a total of over 1,300 patients with acute mania demonstrated lithium efficacy and topiramate inefficacy, although topiramate compared with both placebo and lithium yielded weight loss, with the weight change for these groups being −1.60 kg, −0.40 kg, and −0.16 kg, respectively (Kushner et al. 2006).

In an 8-week, randomized, single-blind rater study in 36 bipolar (19 bipolar I disorder, 17 bipolar II disorder) outpatients with mood stabilizer (lithium or divalproex)–resistant depression, 18 patients taking adjunctive topiramate (mean dose 176 mg) compared with 18 patients taking adjunctive bupropion (mean dose 250 mg) had a similar Ham-D response (≥50% decrease) rate (56% vs. 59%), a nonsignificantly higher adverse effect discontinuation rate (33% vs. 22%), and significantly more weight loss (5.8 kg vs. 1.2 kg), suggesting adjunctive topiramate yields weight loss in bipolar depression (McIntyre et al. 2002). The lack of a placebo control group and inadequate statistical power make the absence of a difference in antidepressant effects of topiramate and bupropion sustained release challenging to interpret. Additional information regarding topiramate is provided in Chapter 14 of this volume.

Adjunctive Stimulants

Similar to the rationale for using adjunctive pramipexole for treatment-resistant depression, psychostimulant medications have robust dopaminergic activity that may modulate cerebral reward and motivation systems. Stimulants have been suggested to have utility in bipolar depression, supported by case series (Carlson et al. 2004; Lydon and El-Mallakh 2006) and open studies (El-Mallakh 2000) but no randomized controlled trials. However, such effects could be in part because of mood destabilization because they may be short-lived (Shopsin and Gershon 1978) and have been associated with subsyndromal mood elevation symptoms (e.g., irritability) and syndromal hypomania and mania with psychosis (El-Mallakh 2000; Murphy et al. 1973; Shopsin and Gershon 1978). Moreover, these medicines have abuse potential. Therefore, use of adjunctive psychostimulants in acute bipolar depression should only be embarked upon with considerable caution.

Adjunctive Sleep Deprivation

Circadian rhythm disturbances appear to be significant contributors to the pathophysiology of bipolar disorders, so that the effects of adjunctive chronobiological interventions such as sleep deprivation and light therapy have been assessed in patients with bipolar disorders.

Depriving of an entire night (and in some instances even only the second half of the night) of sleep may have both beneficial and adverse effects in patients with mood disorders. Pooled analysis of 61 studies involving over 1,700 patients with bipolar or unipolar depression found an overall acute response (marked improvement) rate with sleep deprivation of approximately 60% (Wu and Bunney 1990). Higher response rates (as high as 80%) may be seen in patients with bipolar compared with unipolar depression (Barbini et al. 1998; Szuba et al. 1994). In contrast to depression, anxiety appears to worsen with sleep deprivation (Roy-Byrne et al. 1986).

The time course of improvement in depression with sleep deprivation was assessed in a pooled analysis of eight studies, which indicated in responders that depression attenuated throughout the day prior to and the night of sleep deprivation as well as the following day, plateauing between 1 P.M. and 5 P.M. and relapsing the next morning after recovery sleep (Wu and Bunney 1990). In nonresponders, depression appeared essentially unchanged throughout this entire period. Diurnal mood variation with attenuation of depression throughout the day may be a marker for sleep deprivation response (Wehr et al. 1985).

Although sleep deprivation may yield abrupt (overnight) antidepressant response, the improvement is transient (lasting 1–2 days) and mood may destabilize (Riemann et al. 2002; Wright 1993); therefore, sleep deprivation has not had major clinical application and is most often reserved for treatment-resistant patients.

Attempts to sustain the benefits of sleep deprivation with lithium, transcranial magnetic stimulation (TMS), light therapy, sleep-phase advance, and antidepressant medication have had inconsistent results (Benedetti et al. 2001a, 2001b, 2003). However, limited controlled evidence suggests that adjunctive sleep deprivation may accelerate antidepressant response to lithium (Baxter et al. 1986; Szuba et al. 1994).

Adjunctive Light Therapy

The antidepressant effects of light therapy have been studied for over two decades, originally for the treatment of seasonal affective disorder (SAD) (Rosenthal et al. 1984) and more recently for the treatment of nonseasonal depression (Kripke 1998). Light therapy commonly involves exposure to bright light upon awakening in the morning (Lam et al. 2006), although dawn simulation presented toward the end of sleep has also been assessed (Terman and Terman 2006).

SAD may account for at least 10% of all mood disorders and is a risk factor for bipolarity because in some samples, close to 50% of SAD patients may have bipolar disorders (30% bipolar I disorder, 20% bipolar II disorder) (Faedda et al. 1993). The most common form of SAD, winter SAD, involves hyperphagic, hypersomnic, anergic depression in the fall and winter, with remission or a switch to mood elevation (particularly hypomania) in the spring and summer (Rosenthal et al. 1984). However, other patients may have summer SAD—that is, summer depression and winter mood elevation (Wehr et al. 1987).

Light therapy and SAD do not appear to have specificity for one another because both light therapy and antidepressant medications appear effective in both SAD and nonseasonal depression.

A meta-analysis of randomized, controlled light therapy studies demonstrated significant antidepressant effects for 1) bright light treatment for SAD, 2) dawn simulation for SAD, and 3) bright light treatment for nonseasonal depression but not adjunctive bright light treatment (added to medications) for nonseasonal depression (Golden et al. 2005). Similarly, in a meta-analysis of 20 studies of light therapy in treating nonseasonal depression, adjunctive light therapy compared with control interventions appeared to be effective when using morning light treatment and in sleep deprivation responders (Tuunainen et al. 2004). Although early light therapy trials had methodological limitations, studies have increasingly incorporated refinements seen in pharmacotherapy trials.

For example, in a recent 8-week, multicenter, randomized, double-blind, active-control study in subjects with winter SAD (94.9% unipolar, 5.1% bipolar II disorder), 48 patients receiving light therapy (white fluorescent light with ultraviolet filter, rated at 10,000 lux 14 inches from screen to cornea) for 30 minutes each morning compared with 48 patients taking fluoxetine 20 mg/day had similar final Ham-D response ($\geq$50% decrease) rates (67% for both groups), but in a post hoc analysis light therapy yielded a significantly greater Ham-D decrease at week one but not thereafter (Lam et al. 2006). In this study, no patient experienced treatment-emergent affective switch.

Light therapy appears to have a rapid onset of antidepressant effect (commonly within 1 week) (Martiny et al. 2004) and is generally well tolerated, with the most common adverse effects including jumpiness/jitteriness, headache, and nausea (Terman and Terman 1999). Overactivity/excitation/elation may have greater emergence with morning light and greater remission with evening light (Terman and Terman 1999). Thus, individual adjustments of dosing and treatment time of day may be necessary for optimal outcomes.

Treatment-emergent affective switch with light therapy has been observed in patients with SAD as well as with nonseasonal depression. Considered collectively, 10 studies that reported switches suggested risks of 30% of 29 patients with bipolar depression and 25% of 84 patients with unspecified depression (Wu and Bunney 1990). Rapid cyclers may be at increased risk for such reactions. Thus, a subsequent study of 206 patients with bipolar depression who were not rapid cyclers treated with three cycles of adjunctive sleep deprivation found a lower switch rate, observing hypomania in 5.8% and mania in 4.9% of patients (Colombo et al. 1999). In a meta-analysis of 20 studies of light therapy in treating nonseasonal depression, hypomania was more common with bright light therapy compared with control interventions (NNH=8) (Tuunainen et al. 2004).

As noted previously, morning compared with evening light therapy may be more likely to destabilize mood (Kripke 1991). In rapid-cycling bipolar disorder, midday compared with early-morning light therapy may be more likely to relieve depression without destabilizing mood (Leibenluft et al. 1995).

Taken together, the previous findings suggest that with suitable precautions adjunctive light therapy may prove to be useful in patients with bipolar disorders. However, the impact of this intervention on the clinical management of patients with bipolar disorders has been limited. Indeed, it has been argued that light therapy is generally underappreciated and underutilized because insurers commonly deny reimbursement, and psychiatry residency programs do not typically provide clinical training in this modality (Golden et al. 2005).

Adjunctive Nutriceuticals

Patients may be actively involved in their own treatment whether or not it is evident during scheduled appointments. Patients frequently investigate a wide range of treatment options, some well studied and others only anecdotal. Acupuncture, homeopathy, or dietary supplements (nutriceuticals) with no known contraindications may be allowed, to encourage patient empowerment in his or her treatment. However, it remains important to remind patients that such interventions may have significant interactions and adverse effects, such as treatment-emergent affective switch or drug-drug interactions (e.g., with St. John's wort). Similar to other treatments, complementary and alternative medicine interventions should be recorded in the clinical chart along with associated clinical changes.

This section focuses on the use of various adjunctive dietary supplements, which have been assessed in uncontrolled and controlled studies in patients with mood disorders. Across interventions and across studies, efficacy has been variable. Although tolerability has generally been good, there have been sporadic reports of treatment-emergent affective switch.

The omega-3 polyunsaturated fatty acids eicosapentaenoic acid (EPA) and docosahexaenoic acid (DHA) are naturally occurring substances that like lithium and valproate have effects on intracellular signaling that include inhibiting protein kinase C and hence may have utility in bipolar disorders. Controlled studies of adjunctive EPA and DHA in bipolar depression and unipolar depression have had variable results.

In randomized controlled trials in treatment-resistant bipolar depression and rapid cycling, adjunctive omega-3 fatty acid therapy yielded benefit in two studies (Frangou et al. 2006; Stoll et al. 1999) but was no better than placebo in one study (Keck et al. 2006b). Omega-3 fatty acid dosages varied across studies: EPA 6.2 g/day plus DHA 3.4 g/day (Stoll et al. 1999), EPA 6 g/day (Keck et al. 2006b), and EPA 1 or 2 g/day (Frangou et al. 2006). Also, a 10-patient pilot monotherapy preventive study of DHA 2 g/day in pregnant women with bipolar disorder was negative (Marangell et al. 2006). Omega-3 fatty acids were generally well tolerated.

Inositol is a naturally occurring substance that is important in intracellular signaling, and inositol depletion has been proposed as a mechanism of action of lithium, so that it could have utility in bipolar disorders. Controlled studies of adjunctive inositol in bipolar depression and unipolar depression have also had variable results.

In randomized, controlled studies in treatment-resistant bipolar depression, adjunctive inositol was no better than placebo in two trials (Chengappa et al. 2000; Eden Evins et al. 2006) and no better or worse than adjunctive lamotrigine or adjunctive risperidone in one study (Nierenberg et al. 2006b). In these studies, inositol was started at 2.5–6 g/day, increased every 2–7 days by 4–6 g/day to as high as 6–25 g/day, with mean final dosages ranging between approximately 9.5 and 14 g/day administered in three divided doses. Also, meta-analysis of four controlled trials involving a total of 144 patients with bipolar or unipolar depression failed to reveal benefit with inositol (Taylor et al. 2004b). Inositol was generally well tolerated, but there have been case reports of treatment-emergent affective switch (Levine et al. 1996).

The vitamin folate is a methyl donor for multiple reactions that influence, among other things, amino acid metabolism and methylation of homocysteine to form S-adenosyl-l-methionine (SAMe, discussed later in this chapter). Moreover, low plasma and red blood folate concentrations have been observed in unipolar major depressive disorder; therefore, folate administration might have antidepressant effects. Controlled studies of folate in bipolar depression are lacking and in unipolar depression have had variable results.

Thus, meta-analysis of three 8-week, controlled trials involving a total of 247 patients with unipolar depression suggested possible benefit with folate as an adjunct but not as an alternative to antidepressants (Taylor et al. 2004a). These studies used folate 500 μg/day, and 5-methyltetrahydrofolate at dosages of 15 mg/day and 50 mg/day. Folate was generally well tolerated.

St. John's wort (extracts of *Hypericum perforatum*) is a naturally occurring substance with affinity for several neuroreceptors; therefore, its effects upon serotonin reuptake and monoamine oxidase inhibition could yield antidepressant effects. Controlled studies of St. John's wort in bipolar depression are lacking and in unipolar depression have had variable results.

Meta-analysis of 36 randomized, double-blind, placebo-controlled trials involving 3,320 patients indicated that St. John's wort efficacy compared with placebo was similar in patients with syndromal unipolar depression but superior in heterogeneous samples of patients with syndromal and subsyndromal unipolar depression (Linde et al. 2005). Also, meta-analysis of 14 randomized, double-blind, controlled trials involving 2,283 patients indicated that St. John's wort compared with antidepressants had similar efficacy in patients with unipolar depression (syndromal in 13/14 studies, subsyndromal in 1/14 studies) (Linde et al. 2005). Thus, St. John's wort may offer benefit in patients with mild to moderate unipolar depression. Dosages in these studies ranged between 350 and 1,500 mg/day, with 900 mg/day being the most common dosage. St. John's wort was generally well tolerated, but drug interactions, presumably related to induction of cytochrome P450 3A4 and possibly 2C19 (Markowitz et al. 2003; Wang et al. 2004), and treatment-emergent affective switch have been reported (Moses and Mallinger 2000; Nierenberg et al. 1999; O'Breasail and Argouarch 1998; Schneck 1998).

SAMe is a naturally occurring methyl donor involved in cerebral transmethylation reactions that affect, among other things, monoamine neurotransmission and thus could have activity in mood disorders. SAMe has been prescribed for depression in Europe for over 30 years and has been available as an over-the-counter dietary supplement in the United States since the late 1990s. Dosages for depression commonly range from 400 to 1,600 mg/day.

In meta-analyses of controlled depression studies, SAMe efficacy was superior to placebo and similar to TCAs (Bressa 1994). Although SAMe is generally well tolerated, treatment-emergent affective switch has been reported with SAMe in patients with bipolar depression. Thus, SAMe yielded switches in 9/11 bipolar and 0/11 unipolar patients in one report (Carney et al. 1989) and 2/6 bipolar and 0/3 unipolar patients in another (Lipinski et al. 1984). Hence, it appears prudent to avoid SAMe in patients with bipolar disorders, particularly in the absence of an antimanic agent.

Adjunctive Vagus Nerve Stimulation

VNS involves surgical implantation of an electronic device similar to a pacemaker with an electrode connecting it to the left vagus nerve and delivering low-frequency, chronic intermittent-pulsed electrical signals to the left vagus nerve, yielding deep brain and limbic cortical stimulation. VNS was approved for the adjunctive treatment of medically refractory partial-onset seizures in adults and adolescents over 12 years of age in 1997 and in 2005 was approved by the FDA for the adjunctive long-term treatment of chronic or recurrent depression resistant to four or more antidepressants in adults but not for rapid-cycling bipolar disorder.

In a multicenter, randomized, controlled, masked trial, adjunctive VNS appeared to have modest efficacy (NNTs for response of 20 and 11 on the primary and a secondary outcome measure, respectively) in patients with treatment-resistant unipolar or bipolar depression (Rush et al. 2005a). A 12-month, multicenter, nonrandomized, controlled, naturalistic treatment as usual comparator study was more encouraging (NNT=8) (George et al. 2005). In these studies, patients with bipolar disorders accounted for approximately 10% of participants, but patients with a history of psychosis or rapid-cycling bipolar disorder were excluded. Adjunctive VNS was generally well tolerated, but treatment-emergent affective switch occurred sporadically.

In a 10-week, multicenter, randomized, controlled, masked trial in chronically ill, treatment-resistant, nonpsychotic, unipolar (n=210) and bipolar (n=25) depression, adjunctive VNS compared with adjunctive sham VNS yielded a nonsignificantly higher Ham-D response ($\geq$50% decrease, primary outcome) rate (15.2% vs. 10.0%, NNT=20) but a significantly higher Inventory of Depressive Symptomatology–Self-Report response ($\geq$50% decrease, secondary outcome) rate (17.0% vs. 7.3%, NNT=11) (Rush et al. 2005a). VNS was generally well tolerated, with voice alteration, increased cough, neck pain, dyspnea, and dysphagia being the most common adverse effects, and only 1.3% (3/235) leaving the study because of adverse events. Two of 235 patients (0.9%) had treatment-emergent affective switch (YMRS$\geq$15), which occurred at or within 8 weeks of VNS initiation and resolved spontaneously after 1–2 weeks without altering of VNS treatment. One of these patients had a prior diagnosis of bipolar I disorder.

In a 12-month, multicenter, open, uncontrolled, extension study in unipolar (n=185) and bipolar (n=20) patients, VNS plus treatment as usual yielded a final Ham-D response ($\geq$50% decrease) rate of 27% (Rush et al. 2005b). Voice alteration, dyspnea, and neck pain were the most frequent adverse events. Six of 205 patients (2.9%, including the three patients mentioned in the preceding paragraph) had treatment-emergent affective switch (YMRS$\geq$15), and in one of these patients VNS was turned off during a manic episode. Three of these patients had a prior diagnosis of bipolar disorder.

In a 12-month, multicenter, nonrandomized, controlled, naturalistic study in treatment-resistant, nonpsychotic, unipolar (n=178) and bipolar (n=22) depression, VNS plus treatment as usual compared with treatment as usual only was associated with a significantly higher final Ham-D response ($\geq$50% decrease) rate (27% vs. 13%, NNT=8) (George et al. 2005). Bipolar and unipolar disorder patients had similar response rates.

Encouraging uncontrolled open-label case (Bajbouj et al. 2006) and case series (Marangell et al. 2008) data suggest that controlled trials of adjunctive VNS in treatment-resistant rapid-cycling bipolar disorder are warranted.

The cost and invasiveness of VNS and the relatively modest efficacy raise cost-benefit concerns. Indeed, often patients find their insurance companies deny reimbursement for VNS.

Adjunctive Transcranial Magnetic Stimulation

TMS strives to relieve depression by administration of nonconvulsive stimulation (with high frequency) or inhibition (with low frequency) of cerebral activity. In late 2008, the NeuroStar TMS system was approved for the treatment of (unipolar) major depressive disorder in patients who fail to achieve satisfactory improvement from one prior antidepressant at or above the minimal effective dose and duration in the current episode.

The NeuroStar TMS registration trial was a multicenter, randomized, sham-controlled study in patients with unipolar major depressive disorder resistant to one to four antidepressant medications during the current or most recent episode (O'Reardon et al. 2007). The study excluded patients with histories of psychosis, bipolar disorder, obsessive-compulsive disorder, posttraumatic stress disorder, eating disorder, resistance to ECT, prior TMS or VNS treatment, pregnancy, seizure disorders or medical or medication risk factors for seizure disorders, or ferromagnetic material in or in close proximity to the head. After a 1-week lead-in phase without psychotropic treatment (other than limited anxiolytics/hypnotics), patients received active TMS or sham treatment 5 days per week for 6 weeks, followed by 3 weeks of tapering active TMS or sham treatment and starting antidepressant medication.

The left dorsolateral prefrontal cortex was the treatment location, 5 cm anterior to the motor threshold location. TMS was administered at 120% magnetic field intensity relative to the patient's observed motor threshold, at a repetition rate of 10 magnetic pulses per second, with a stimulus train duration (on time) of 4 seconds and an intertrain interval (off time) of 26 seconds, yielding a total of 80 magnetic pulses per minute of treatment. Treatment sessions lasted 37.5 minutes and thus involved 3,000 (37.5×80) magnetic pulses.

For the primary outcome measure (baseline to week 4 MADRS decrease), 155 patients receiving active TMS compared with 146 receiving sham TMS tended to show benefit ($P=0.057$). When four active and two sham TMS patients with baseline MADRS scores < 20 were excluded, the trend became statistically significant ($P=0.038$). At the week 6 secondary efficacy time point, active TMS also tended to be superior to sham TMS for the entire sample ($P=0.057$) and for the subset of patients with baseline MADRS > 20 ($P=0.052$). In contrast, MADRS response (≥50% decrease from baseline) rates were significantly higher for active TMS compared with sham TMS, not only at week 4 (18.1% compared with 11.0%, $P=0.045$, NNT$=15$), but also at week 6 (23.9% compared with 12.3%, $P=0.007$, NNT$=9$). Application site pain was more common with active TMS than with sham TMS (35.8% compared with 3.8%), and although this had the potential to compromise blinding, it was not related to the primary outcome measure. No seizure was reported in this study as well as in additional experience, involving a total of 10,000 outpatient TMS sessions (Janicak et al. 2008).

There are at least seven parameters involved in TMS: 1) number of trains per session, 2) duration of trains, 3) stimulation frequency, 4) stimulation intensity, 5) stimulation location, 6) number of sessions per week, and 7) total number of sessions. Results in prior smaller controlled studies were variable, perhaps understandably, given the number of parameters involved. For example, in randomized, controlled studies in patients with treatment-resistant bipolar depression, antidepressant effects with TMS as compared with sham TMS were superior in one trial (Dolberg et al. 2002) and similar in another trial (Nahas et al. 2003).

In an open uncontrolled case series, high-frequency right prefrontal TMS yielded decreases in Bech-Rafaelsen Mania Scale scores (Michael and Erfurth 2004). TMS is generally well tolerated, but adverse effects may include seizures (Tharayil et al. 2005) and treatment-emergent affective switch (Garcia-Toro 1999), although the risk of the latter may be no greater than with sham TMS (Xia et al. 2008).

TMS is contraindicated in patients with 1) conductive, ferromagnetic, or other magnetic-sensitive metals in the head or within 30 cm of the treatment coil; or 2) any (even more than 30 cm away from the treatment coil) implanted devices activated or controlled by physiological signals, such as pacemakers, implantable (and even wearable) cardioverter defibrillators, and vagus nerve stimilators. The United States NeuroStar TMS System user manual also includes warnings regarding the risks of seizures and worsening of depression or suicidality (an antidepressant class warning). Patients must wear earplugs or similar hearing protection devices with a rating of 30 db of noise reduction, and similar protection is also advised for the clinical operator. In controlled trials, the most common adverse events were headache and temporary mild discomfort at the site of stimulation during and/or shortly after treatment.

In summary, TMS is a generally well-tolerated, recently approved treatment for unipolar major depressive disorder, with a high single-digit NNT for response compared with sham TMS. Large randomized controlled trails are needed to assess the efficacy and safety of TMS in acute bipolar depression.

Special Subpopulations With Bipolar Depression

Optimal practice of evidence-based medicine involves applying findings of medical research in a fashion that yields the most favorable benefit-risk ratio for individual patients. This section describes several subpopulations with distinctive therapeutic implications for clinical decision making in the management of acute bipolar depression.

Patients With a Prior History of Antidepressant-Induced Affective Switch or Rapid Cycling

Patients with a prior history of antidepressant-induced treatment-emergent affective switch or rapid cycling are at particularly high risk for mood destabilization if treated with antidepressants (Truman et al. 2007; Wehr et al. 1979). In such patients, it appears prudent to emphasize mood stabilizers, second-generation antipsychotics, and nonantidepressant interventions (including psychotherapy and ECT) rather than antidepressants in efforts to attenuate the risk of switching. If antidepressants are used, it is prudent to avoid antidepressant(s) that have destabilized mood in the past and, if feasible, even classes of antidepressants that have destabilized mood in the past. It is crucial to have sufficient antimanic coverage. The optimal duration of antidepressant administration after achieving response or remission may range from as brief as a few days (i.e., not waiting for recovery from the acute episode) to as long as 2 months, depending on the degree of historical mood instability.

Patients With Depression-Mania-Interval Sequence

Patients with the sequence of first depression, then mania, then interval of euthymia (DMI sequence) may be at particularly high risk of treatment-emergent affective switch with antidepressants because mood elevation "naturally" follows depression (Kessing 1999). Also, patients with the DMI sequence appear to have poorer responses to lithium maintenance compared with the "classic" sequence of first mania, then depression, then interval of euthymia (MDI sequence) (Faedda et al. 1991; Grof et al. 1987; Haag et al. 1987; Kukopulos et al. 1980; Maj et al. 1989). However, the utility of these observations appears to be limited by the existence of a substantial number of patients who have irregular episode sequences. Nevertheless, in patients with a clear DMI sequence, it appears prudent to emphasize mood stabilizers, second-generation antipsychotics, and nonantidepressant interventions in efforts to attenuate the risk of switching and to limit the duration of adjunctive antidepressant exposure, in some instances to as little as a few days after achieving response or remission.

Patients With a Prior History of Psychotic Mania

Because of the severity of mania in patients with a history of psychotic mania (particularly with antidepressants), the consequences of a treatment-emergent affective switch may be sufficient to warrant minimizing administration of antidepressant medications. Thus, in such patients, it appears prudent to emphasize mood stabilizers, second-generation antipsychotics, and nonantidepressant interventions in efforts to attenuate the risk of switching. If antidepressants are necessary, combinations of mood stabilizers and second-generation antipsychotics may be necessary to provide sufficient protection against the risk of treatment-emergent affective switch.

Patients With Bipolar II Disorder

Bipolar II disorder is a condition with substantial interpatient variability. Thus, some patients with bipolar II disorder may have an illness more like major depressive disorder, with relatively infrequent recurrent pure (with minimal mixed features) depressive episodes, and rare hypomanias, and, with antidepressants, may experience relief of depression without treatment-emergent affective switch into hypomania or accelerating episodes. Antidepressants may be considered foundational treatments for such patients and may prove to be effective not only acutely but also in longer-term treatment. In academic centers with specialty clinics, such patients may more often be referred to major depressive disorder clinics, where clinicians may view antidepressants as treatments of choice for this type of patient with bipolar II disorder.

However, other patients with bipolar II disorder may have an illness more akin to bipolar I disorder, with relatively frequent recurrent depressive episodes that include mixed features (in some instances concurrently experiencing syndromal depression and hypomania [i.e., dysphoric hypomania]), common hypomanias, in some instances rapid cycling, and with antidepressants experience inadequate relief of depression and/or treatment-emergent affective switch or cycle acceleration. For such patients, mood stabilizers or atypical antipsychotics, instead of antidepressants, may be considered foundational treatments. In academic centers such patients may more often be referred to bipolar disorder clinics, where clinicians may view antidepressants as potentially problematic for this type of patient with bipolar II disorder.

Clinicians in the community, compared with providers in subspecialty major depressive disorder or bipolar disorder clinics, arguably face greater challenges related to encountering a full spectrum of clinical heterogeneity in patients with bipolar II disorder and need to administer carefully individually tailored treatments, balancing the relative risks and benefits of intervening with antidepressants.

Conclusion

The depressive phase of bipolar disorder is particularly challenging because of the chronicity of syndromal and subsyndromal symptoms, the significant morbidity and mortality, the common phenomenon of treatment resistance, and the limited evidence base to inform clinical practice. Thus, clinical need is profoundly underaddressed by the two FDA-approved medications for the treatment of acute bipolar depression (olanzapine plus fluoxetine combination and quetiapine monotherapy) when compared with the nine approved for treatment of acute mania and the five approved for bipolar prophylaxis.

The hierarchy of prioritized treatment options in Table 7–1 provides a schema for clinicians seeking to apply the limited but dynamic medical evidence base to the management of acute bipolar depression. The treatments in Tier I (OFC and quetiapine monotherapy) merit high priority because they have the most compelling evidence of efficacy in acute bipolar depression.

However, tolerability limitations of the Tier I treatments commonly result in clinicians preferring to use unapproved treatments such as the Tier II treatments (lithium and lamotrigine), which also receive high priority. Lithium and lamotrigine have less compelling evidence of efficacy compared with the approved treatments but have mitigating qualities such as tolerability and maintenance indications that may lead to their use instead of the approved treatments.

Adjunctive antidepressants (Tier III options) are also commonly used in spite of having even more limited evidence of efficacy compared with lithium or lamotrigine and concerns regarding the risk of treatment-emergent affective switch. Determining the appropriate priority for adjunctive antidepressants in bipolar disorder in general and for individual patients in particular constitutes one of the most controversial challenges faced by researchers and clinicians. Adjunctive antidepressants are still deemed to be high-priority options by some researchers, particularly in Europe, and many clinicians, even in North America. Additional research is needed to provide an adequate evidence base to address this important issue.

The other treatments in Tier III (other mood stabilizers, other second-generation antipsychotics, ECT, and adjunctive psychotherapy) merit intermediate priority because they also have limited evidence of efficacy in acute bipolar depression. However, Tier III options may be attractive for selected patients and in certain circumstances considered early on (e.g., psychotherapy or ECT in pregnant women with acute bipolar depression). For some of these treatments (e.g., aripiprazole monotherapy and ziprasidone monotherapy and ECT), the efficacy and/or tolerability limitations leading to their placement in Tier III are already clear. For other Tier III treatments (e.g., adjunctive psychotherapy), advances in research, familiarity, and/or availability ultimately may be sufficient to merit their consideration for placement in higher tiers.

The Tier IV treatment options (thyroid hormones, pramipexole, modafinil, topiramate, stimulants, sleep deprivation, light therapy, nutriceuticals, vagus nerve stimulation, and transcranial magnetic stimulation) have even more limited evidence of efficacy than Tier I, II, or III options and are considered low-priority interventions, and are most often reserved for patients who are treatment resistant or intolerant to Tier I–III treatments. However, for some of these treatments (e.g., pramipexole and modafinil) advances in research may ultimately provide sufficient evidence to merit their consideration for placement in higher tiers.

Data to support the evidence-based management of acute bipolar depression are beginning to emerge. Table 7–3 provides selected clinical decisions and evidence-based recommendations. Clearly, additional research is needed to better inform practice and enable clinicians and patients to address the substantial clinical challenges encountered in the management of bipolar depression.

Case Study: Management of Acute Bipolar Depression

Ms. Black is a 31-year-old, married, Caucasian attorney with a history of "mood swings" since her midteens. In her teenage years, she developed depressive episodes manifested by pervasive sadness, anhedonia, social isolation, hypersomnia (sleeping 11–12 hours per night), lethargy, guilty ruminations, increased appetite with weight gain, and passive thoughts of death. These episodes lasted about 2–4 weeks, followed by 2–4 weeks of her mood returning to a baseline level of poor self-esteem and sleeping 9–10 hours per night but with good occupational and social function. Her mood would continuously alternate between these two states of functionally disabling depression and intervals with adequate function but poor self-esteem.

At age 21, while in college, Ms. Black first sought psychiatric care and was diagnosed with "double depression" (major depressive disorder plus dysthymic disorder). Fluoxetine up to 20 mg/day for 2 months was ineffective, with dosage limited by intolerable nausea. Sertraline up to 100 mg/day for 2 months was also ineffective, with dosage this time limited by intolerable diarrhea. Venlafaxine extended-release formulation was started at 37.5 mg/day and yielded relief of

TABLE 7–3. Selected clinical decisions and evidence-based recommendations

Clinical decision	Evidence-based recommendations/references
Initial treatment of acute bipolar depression	
High-priority options	Olanzapine plus fluoxetine (Brown et al. 2006; Tohen et al. 2003)
	Quetiapine (Calabrese et al. 2005; Thase et al. 2006)
	Lithium (Zornberg et al. 1993)
	Lamotrigine (Brown et al. 2006; Calabrese et al. 2008)
Controversial option	Mood stabilizer plus antidepressant (Gijsman et al. 2004; Nemeroff et al. 2001; Sachs et al. 2007)
Bipolar depression breaking through mood stabilizer	Optimize mood stabilizer dosage (Nemeroff et al. 2001)
Bipolar depression despite optimized mood stabilizer	Add second mood stabilizer? (Young et al. 2000)
	Add antidepressant? (Gijsman et al. 2004; Nemeroff et al. 2001; Young et al. 2000)
Avoid venlafaxine and tricyclic antidepressants because of higher switch risk	Higher switch rate with venlafaxine (Post et al. 2006; Vieta et al. 2002)
	Higher switch rate with tricyclic antidepressants (Cohn et al. 1989; Gijsman et al. 2004; Himmel-hoch et al. 1991; Nemeroff et al. 2001; Sachs et al. 1994; Silverstone 2001)

depression within 1 week, and the patient reported feeling as if her whole life had been abnormally depressed until therapy with venlafaxine. She began to recognize multiple new opportunities in her life and experienced gradually increasing self-confidence, graduating with honors and deciding to apply to graduate school. One month after Ms. Black moved across the country to attend law school, she had a return of the depressive symptoms. The patient lost confidence in treatment and did not see a psychiatrist for another 2 years. However, as her depressive symptoms worsened to the point of interfering with her academic function, she returned to psychiatric care and started taking bupropion sustained-release formulation 100 mg/day, which was discontinued after 1 week because of intolerable irritability, agitation, and insomnia. As a result of the inefficacy of prior antidepressant medication trials, a psychopharmacology consultation was sought.

Upon careful questioning of both the patient and her fiancé, it was determined that over the last 2 years she had experienced frequent 2-week periods with improved function, during which she could catch up on her lost productivity and felt that she was more talented and energetic than the rest of her class because she could rapidly more than make up for times with decreased productivity. During these productive periods, she would be more gregarious but also on occasion irritable, particularly if others (including her fiancé) interfered with her work. She slept 7 hours, in contrast to requiring the usual 9–10 hours, and felt energetic rather than drowsy during the day. Her thoughts would come quickly, and her physical activity was increased to a level that at least some peers found excessive. She had increased libido, which both she and her fiancé agreed helped enhance intimacy in their relationship.

Ms. Black had no significant medical problems. She used marijuana in her late teens but had not used any other illicit drugs or abused alcohol. She denied any history of psychosis or psychiatric hospitalization. She reported a family history of depression in a brother and her maternal grandmother, and her mother was taking divalproex and paroxetine for bipolar depression.

Ms. Black was informed that her history indicated a diagnosis of bipolar II disorder. After a discussion of the potential benefits and risks of various treatments for bipolar depression, Ms. Black agreed to a trial of lamotrigine. Following the recommended gradual titration, a dosage of 200 mg/day of lamotrigine was reached after 6 weeks, at which point she began to report improvement in her mood and over the next month experienced remission of depressive symptoms. She reported tolerating lamotrigine well. She continued with euthymic mood for 4 years, until a month after the birth of her first child. Immediately prior to and during pregnancy she had tried to taper and discontinue lamotrigine but eventually plateaued the dosage at 100 mg/day in order to control symptoms of irritability and depression. One week after delivery, after deciding to forgo breastfeeding, she increased lamotrigine back to 200 mg/day. Three weeks later she developed a major depressive episode. Mood stabilized after lamotrigine was increased to 250 mg and remained stable for another 15 months until the birth of her second child. She suffered another major depressive episode, again within 1 month of delivery, this time despite uninterrupted treatment with lamotrigine 250 mg/day, but has since been stable for 3 years, after lamotrigine was increased to 300 mg/day.

In summary, this woman who struggled with depression had inadequate efficacy and/or tolerability to fluoxetine, sertraline, and bupropion, and a switch out of depression with venlafaxine. Careful assessment including information from a significant other revealed a diagnosis of bipolar II disorder. Based on generally very good tolerability, and the potential for preventing depression, and in spite of the limited efficacy in acute depression, the patient received a trial of lamotrigine. She was fortunate enough to have an acute antidepressant response with lamotrigine monotherapy—although she experienced postpartum breakthroughs that ultimately required increasing the dosage of lamotrigine to 300 mg/day, which was well tolerated—and has maintained stable mood for 3 years. One concern is that should she have another child, she may be at risk for yet another postpartum breakthrough depression.

References

Altshuler LL, Post RM, Leverich GS, et al: Antidepressant-induced mania and cycle acceleration: a controversy revisited. Am J Psychiatry 152:1130–1138, 1995

Altshuler LL, Bauer M, Frye MA, et al: Does thyroid supplementation accelerate tricyclic antidepressant response? A review and meta-analysis of the literature. Am J Psychiatry 158:1617–1622, 2001

Altshuler L, Suppes T, Black D, et al: Impact of antidepressant discontinuation after acute bipolar depression remission on rates of depressive relapse at 1-year follow-up. Am J Psychiatry 160:1252–1262, 2003

American Psychiatric Association: Diagnostic and Statistical Manual of Mental Disorders, 4th Edition, Text Revision. Washington, DC, American Psychiatric Association, 2000

American Psychiatric Association: Practice guideline for the treatment of patients with bipolar disorder (revision). Am J Psychiatry 159:1–50, 2002

Amsterdam JD, Shults J: Comparison of fluoxetine, olanzapine, and combined fluoxetine plus olanzapine initial therapy of bipolar type I and type II major depression—lack of manic induction. J Affect Disord 87:121–130, 2005

Amsterdam JD, Shults J: Comparison of short-term venlafaxine versus lithium monotherapy for bipolar II major depressive episode: a randomized open-label study. J Clin Psychopharmacol 28:171–181, 2008

Amsterdam JD, Garcia-Espana F, Fawcett J, et al: Efficacy and safety of fluoxetine in treating bipolar II major depressive episode. J Clin Psychopharmacol 18:435–440, 1998

Amsterdam JD, Shults J, Brunswick DJ, et al: Short-term fluoxetine monotherapy for bipolar type II or bipolar NOS major depression—low manic switch rate. Bipolar Disord 6:75–81, 2004

Angst J, Stabl M: Efficacy of moclobemide in different patient groups: a meta-analysis of studies. Psychopharmacology (Berl) 106(suppl):S109–S113, 1992

Angst J, Angst K, Baruffol I, et al: ECT-induced and drug-induced hypomania. Convuls Ther 8:179–185, 1992

Appelhof BC, Brouwer JP, van Dyck R, et al: Triiodothyronine addition to paroxetine in the treatment of major depressive disorder. J Clin Endocrinol Metab 89:6271–6276, 2004

Aronson R, Offman HJ, Joffe RT, et al: Triiodothyronine augmentation in the treatment of refractory depression: a meta-analysis. Arch Gen Psychiatry 53:842–848, 1996

Bajbouj M, Danker-Hopfe H, Heuser I, et al: Long-term outcome of vagus nerve stimulation in rapid-cycling bipolar disorder. J Clin Psychiatry 67:837–838, 2006

Baldessarini RJ, Leahy L, Arcona S, et al: Patterns of psychotropic drug prescription for U.S. patients with diagnoses of bipolar disorders. Psychiatr Serv 58:85–91, 2007

Banov MD, Zarate CA Jr, Tohen M, et al: Clozapine therapy in refractory affective disorders: polarity predicts response in long-term follow-up. J Clin Psychiatry 55:295–300, 1994

Barbini B, Colombo C, Benedetti F, et al: The unipolar-bipolar dichotomy and the response to sleep deprivation. Psychiatry Res 79:43–50, 1998

Baron M, Gershon ES, Rudy V, et al: Lithium carbonate response in depression: prediction by unipolar/bipolar illness, average-evoked response, catechol-O-methyl transferase, and family history. Arch Gen Psychiatry 32:1107–1111, 1975

Battegay R, Cotar B, Fleischhauer J, et al: Results and side effects of treatment with clozapine (Leponex R). Compr Psychiatry 18:423–428, 1977

Bauer MS, Whybrow PC: Rapid cycling bipolar affective disorder, II: treatment of refractory rapid cycling with high-dose levothyroxine: a preliminary study. Arch Gen Psychiatry 47:435–440, 1990

Bauer M, Hellweg R, Graf KJ, et al: Treatment of refractory depression with high-dose thyroxine. Neuropsychopharmacology 18:444–455, 1998

Bauer M, Dopfmer S: Lithium augmentation in treatment-resistant depression: meta-analysis of placebo-controlled studies. J Clin Psychopharmacol 19:427–434, 1999

Bauer M, Berghöfer A, Bschor T, et al: Supraphysiological doses of L-thyroxine in the maintenance treatment of prophylaxis-resistant affective disorders. Neuropsychopharmacology 27:620–628, 2002

Bauer M, Fairbanks L, Berghöfer A, et al: Bone mineral density during maintenance treatment with supraphysiological doses of levothyroxine in affective disorders: a longitudinal study. J Affect Disord 83:183–190, 2004

Baumhackl U, Bizière K, Fischbach R, et al: Efficacy and tolerability of moclobemide compared with imipramine in depressive disorder (DSM-III): an Austrian double-blind, multicentre study. Br J Psychiatry Suppl (6):78–83, 1989

Baxter LR Jr, Liston EH, Schwartz JM, et al: Prolongation of the antidepressant response to partial sleep deprivation by lithium. Psychiatry Res 19:17–23, 1986

Benedetti F, Barbini B, Campori E, et al: Sleep phase advance and lithium to sustain the antidepressant effect of total sleep deprivation in bipolar depression: new findings supporting the internal coincidence model? J Psychiatr Res 35:323–329, 2001a

Benedetti F, Campori E, Barbini B, et al: Dopaminergic augmentation of sleep deprivation effects in bipolar depression. Psychiatry Res 104:239–246, 2001b

Benedetti F, Colombo C, Serretti A, et al: Antidepressant effects of light therapy combined with sleep deprivation are influenced by a functional polymorphism within the promoter of the serotonin transporter gene. Biol Psychiatry 54:687–692, 2003

Berman RM, Marcus RN, Swanink R, et al: The efficacy and safety of aripiprazole as adjunctive therapy in major depressive disorder: a multicenter, randomized, double-blind, placebo-controlled study. J Clin Psychiatry 68:843–853, 2007

Boerlin HL, Gitlin MJ, Zoellner LA, et al: Bipolar depression and antidepressant-induced mania: a naturalistic study. J Clin Psychiatry 59:374–379, 1998

Bottlender R, Rudolf D, Strauss A, et al: Antidepressant-associated maniform states in acute treatment of patients with bipolar-I depression. Eur Arch Psychiatry Clin Neurosci 248:296–300, 1998

Bottlender R, Rudolf D, Strauss A, et al: Are low basal serum levels of the thyroid stimulating hormone (b-TSH) a risk factor for switches into states of expansive syndromes (known in Germany as "maniform syndromes") in bipolar I depression? Pharmacopsychiatry 33:75–77, 2000

Bowden C, Calabrese J, Ascher J, et al: Spectrum of efficacy of lamotrigine in bipolar disorder: overview of double-blind placebo-controlled studies (291). Abstract presented at the 39th Annual Meeting of the American College of Neuropsychopharmacology, San Juan, Puerto Rico, December 10–14, 2000a

Bowden CL, Calabrese JR, McElroy SL, et al: A randomized, placebo-controlled 12-month trial of divalproex and lithium in treatment of outpatients with bipolar I disorder. Divalproex Maintenance Study Group. Arch Gen Psychiatry 57:481–489, 2000b

Bressa GM: S-adenosyl-L-methionine (SAMe) as antidepressant: meta-analysis of clinical studies. Acta Neurol Scand Suppl 154:7–14, 1994

Brown EB, McElroy SL, Keck PE Jr, et al: A 7-week, randomized, double-blind trial of olanzapine/fluoxetine combination versus lamotrigine in the treatment of bipolar I depression. J Clin Psychiatry 67:1025–1033, 2006

Bunevicius R, Kazanavicius G, Zalinkevicius R, et al: Effects of thyroxine as compared with thyroxine plus triiodothyronine in patients with hypothyroidism. N Engl J Med 340:424–429, 1999

Calabrese JR, Bowden CL, Sachs GS, et al: A double-blind placebo-controlled study of lamotrigine monotherapy in outpatients with bipolar I depression. Lamictal 602 Study Group. J Clin Psychiatry 60:79–88, 1999

Calabrese JR, Keck PE Jr, Macfadden W, et al: A randomized, double-blind, placebo-controlled trial of quetiapine in the treatment of bipolar I or II depression. Am J Psychiatry 162:1351–1360, 2005

Calabrese JR, Huffman RF, White RL, et al: Lamotrigine in the acute treatment of bipolar depression: results of five double-blind, placebo-controlled clinical trials. Bipolar Disord 10:323–333, 2008

Carlson PJ, Merlock MC, Suppes T: Adjunctive stimulant use in patients with bipolar disorder: treatment of residual depression and sedation. Bipolar Disord 6:416–420, 2004

Carney MW, Chary TK, Bottiglieri T, et al: The switch mechanism and the bipolar/unipolar dichotomy. Br J Psychiatry 154:48–51, 1989

Chengappa KN, Levine J, Gershon S, et al: Inositol as an add-on treatment for bipolar depression. Bipolar Disord 2:47–55, 2000

Cohn JB, Collins G, Ashbrook E, et al: A comparison of fluoxetine, imipramine and placebo in patients with bipolar depressive disorder. Int Clin Psychopharmacol 4:313–322, 1989

Colom F, Vieta E, Martinez-Aran A, et al: A randomized trial on the efficacy of group psychoeducation in the prophylaxis of recurrences in bipolar patients whose disease is in remission. Arch Gen Psychiatry 60:402–407, 2003

Colombo C, Benedetti F, Barbini B, et al: Rate of switch from depression into mania after therapeutic sleep deprivation in bipolar depression. Psychiatry Res 86:267–270, 1999

Cooper-Kazaz R, Apter JT, Cohen R, et al: Combined treatment with sertraline and liothyronine in major depression: a randomized, double-blind, placebo-controlled trial. Arch Gen Psychiatry 64:679–688, 2007

Daly JJ, Prudic J, Devanand DP, et al: ECT in bipolar and unipolar depression: differences in speed of response. Bipolar Disord 3:95–104, 2001

Dassa D, Kaladjian A, Azorin JM, et al: Clozapine in the treatment of psychotic refractory depression. Br J Psychiatry 163:822–824, 1993

Davis LL, Bartolucci A, Petty F: Divalproex in the treatment of bipolar depression: a placebo-controlled study. J Affect Disord 85:259–266, 2005

De Wilde JE, Doogan DP: Fluvoxamine and chlorimipramine in endogenous depression. J Affect Disord 4:249–259, 1982

Denicoff KD, Smith-Jackson EE, Disney ER, et al: Preliminary evidence of the reliability and validity of the prospective life-chart methodology (LCM-p). J Psychiatr Res 31:593–603, 1997

Dolberg OT, Dannon PN, Schreiber S, et al: Transcranial magnetic stimulation in patients with bipolar depression: a double blind, controlled study. Bipolar Disord 4 (suppl 1):94–95, 2002

Donnelly EF, Goodwin FK, Waldman IN, et al: Prediction of antidepressant responses to lithium. Am J Psychiatry 135:552–556, 1978

Dunner DL, Amsterdam JD, Shelton RC, et al: Efficacy and tolerability of adjunctive ziprasidone in treatment-resistant depression: a randomized, open-label, pilot study. J Clin Psychiatry 68:1071–1077, 2007

Ebert D, Jaspert A, Murata H, et al: Initial lithium augmentation improves the antidepressant effects of standard TCA treatment in non-resistant depressed patients. Psychopharmacology (Berl) 118:223–225, 1995

Eden Evins A, Demopulos C, Yovel I, et al: Inositol augmentation of lithium or valproate for bipolar depression. Bipolar Disord 8:168–174, 2006

El-Mallakh RS: An open study of methylphenidate in bipolar depression. Bipolar Disord 2:56–59, 2000

Fabre LF, Brodie HK, Garver D, et al: A multicenter evaluation of bupropion versus placebo in hospitalized depressed patients. J Clin Psychiatry 44:88–94, 1983

Faedda GL, Baldessarini RJ, Tohen M, et al: Episode sequence in bipolar disorder and response to lithium treatment. Am J Psychiatry 148:1237–1239, 1991

Faedda GL, Tondo L, Teicher MH, et al: Seasonal mood disorders: patterns of seasonal recurrence in mania and depression (letter). Arch Gen Psychiatry 50:17–23, 1993

Fava M, Thase ME, DeBattista C: A multicenter, placebo-controlled study of modafinil augmentation in partial responders to selective serotonin reuptake inhibitors with persistent fatigue and sleepiness. J Clin Psychiatry 66:85–93, 2005

Fieve RR, Platman SR, Plutchik RR: The use of lithium in affective disorders, I: acute endogenous depression. Am J Psychiatry 125:487–491, 1968

Frangou S, Lewis M, McCrone P: Efficacy of ethyl-eicosapentaenoic acid in bipolar depression: randomised double-blind placebo-controlled study. Br J Psychiatry 188:46–50, 2006

Frank E, Kupfer DJ, Thase ME, et al: Two-year outcomes for interpersonal and social rhythm therapy in individuals with bipolar I disorder. Arch Gen Psychiatry 62:996–1004, 2005

Frye MA, Grunze H, Suppes T, et al: A placebo-controlled evaluation of adjunctive modafinil in the treatment of bipolar depression. Am J Psychiatry 164:1242–1249, 2007

Garcia-Toro M: Acute manic symptomatology during repetitive transcranial magnetic stimulation in a patient with bipolar depression. Br J Psychiatry 175:491, 1999

Geddes JR, Calabrese JR, Goodwin GM: Lamotrigine for treatment of bipolar depression: independent meta-analysis and meta-regression of individual patient data from five randomised trials. Br J Psychiatry 194:4–9, 2009

George MS, Rush AJ, Marangell LB, et al: A one-year comparison of vagus nerve stimulation with treatment as usual for treatment-resistant depression. Biol Psychiatry 58:364–373, 2005

Ghaemi SN, Hsu DJ, Soldani F, et al: Antidepressants in bipolar disorder: the case for caution. Bipolar Disord 5:421–433, 2003

Ghaemi SN, Rosenquist KJ, Ko JY, et al: Antidepressant treatment in bipolar versus unipolar depression. Am J Psychiatry 161:163–165, 2004

Ghaemi SN, Gilmer WS, Goldberg JF, et al: Divalproex in the treatment of acute bipolar depression: a preliminary double-blind, randomized, placebo-controlled pilot study. J Clin Psychiatry 68:1840–1844, 2007

Gijsman HJ, Geddes JR, Rendell JM, et al: Antidepressants for bipolar depression: a systematic review of randomized, controlled trials. Am J Psychiatry 161:1537–1547, 2004

Goldberg JF, Whiteside JE: The association between substance abuse and antidepressant-induced mania in bipolar disorder: a preliminary study. J Clin Psychiatry 63:791–795, 2002

Goldberg JF, Harrow M, Whiteside JE: Risk for bipolar illness in patients initially hospitalized for unipolar depression. Am J Psychiatry 158:1265–1270, 2001

Goldberg JF, Burdick KE, Endick CJ: Preliminary randomized, double-blind, placebo-controlled trial of pramipexole added to mood stabilizers for treatment-resistant bipolar depression. Am J Psychiatry 161:564–566, 2004

Golden RN, Gaynes BN, Ekstrom RD, et al: The efficacy of light therapy in the treatment of mood disorders: a review and meta-analysis of the evidence. Am J Psychiatry 162:656–662, 2005

Goldsmith DR, Wagstaff AJ, Ibbotson T, et al: Lamotrigine: a review of its use in bipolar disorder. Drugs 63:2029–2050, 2003

Goodwin FK, Murphy DL, Bunney WE Jr: Lithium-carbonate treatment in depression and mania: a longitudinal double-blind study. Arch Gen Psychiatry 21:486–496, 1969

Goodwin FK, Murphy DL, Dunner DL, et al: Lithium response in unipolar versus bipolar depression. Am J Psychiatry 129:44–47, 1972

Goodwin FK, Fireman B, Simon GE, et al: Suicide risk in bipolar disorder during treatment with lithium and divalproex. JAMA 290:1467–1473, 2003

Goodwin GM: Evidence-based guidelines for treating bipolar disorder: recommendations from the British Association for Psychopharmacology. J Psychopharmacol 17:149–173; discussion 147, 2003

Goodwin GM, Bowden CL, Calabrese JR, et al: A pooled analysis of 2 placebo-controlled 18-month trials of lamotrigine and lithium maintenance in bipolar I disorder. J Clin Psychiatry 65:432–441, 2004

Greenspan K, Schildkraut JJ, Gordon EK, et al: Catecholamine metabolism in affective disorders, 3: MHPG and other catecholamine metabolites in patients treated with lithium carbonate. J Psychiatr Res 7:171–183, 1970

Grof E, Haag M, Grof P, et al: Lithium response and the sequence of episode polarities: preliminary report on a Hamilton sample. Prog Neuropsychopharmacol Biol Psychiatry 11:199–203, 1987

Grunhaus L, Schreiber S, Dolberg OT, et al: Response to ECT in major depression: are there differences between unipolar and bipolar depression? Bipolar Disord 1 (suppl 4): 91–93, 2002

Grunze H, Kasper S, Goodwin G, et al: World Federation of Societies of Biological Psychiatry (WFSBP) guidelines for biological treatment of bipolar disorders. Part I: treatment of bipolar depression. World J Biol Psychiatry 3:115–124, 2002

Gyulai L, Bauer M, Garcia-Espana F, et al: Bone mineral density in pre-and post-menopausal women with affective disorder treated with long-term L-thyroxine augmentation. J Affect Disord 66:185–191, 2001

Gyulai L, Bowden CL, McElroy SL, et al: Maintenance efficacy of divalproex in the prevention of bipolar depression. Neuropsychopharmacology 28:1374–1382, 2003

Haag H, Heidorn A, Haag M, et al: Sequence of affective polarity and lithium response: preliminary report on Munich sample. Prog Neuropsychopharmacol Biol Psychiatry 11:205–208, 1987

Himmelhoch JM, Fuchs CZ, Symons BJ: A double-blind study of tranylcypromine treatment of major anergic depression. J Nerv Ment Dis 170:628–634, 1982

Himmelhoch JM, Thase ME, Mallinger AG, et al: Tranylcypromine versus imipramine in anergic bipolar depression. Am J Psychiatry 148:910–916, 1991

Homan S, Lachenbruch PA, Winokur G, et al: An efficacy study of electroconvulsive therapy and antidepressants in the treatment of primary depression. Psychol Med 12:615–624, 1982

Hrdlicka M: Combination of clozapine and maprotiline in refractory psychotic depression. Eur Psychiatry 17:484, 2002

Husain MM, Rush AJ, Fink M, et al: Speed of response and remission in major depressive disorder with acute electroconvulsive therapy (ECT): a Consortium for Research in ECT (CORE) report. J Clin Psychiatry 65:485–491, 2004

Husain MM, McClintock SM, Rush AJ, et al: The efficacy of acute electroconvulsive therapy in atypical depression. J Clin Psychiatry 69:406–411, 2008

Janicak PG, O'Reardon JP, Sampson SM, et al: Transcranial magnetic stimulation in the treatment of major depressive disorder: a comprehensive summary of safety experience from acute exposure, extended exposure, and during reintroduction treatment. J Clin Psychiatry 69:222–232, 2008

Jeyapaul P, Vieweg R: A case study evaluating the use of clozapine in depression with psychotic features. Ann Gen Psychiatry 5:20, 2006

Joffe RT, Singer W: A comparison of triiodothyronine and thyroxine in the potentiation of tricyclic antidepressants. Psychiatry Res 32:241–251, 1990

Joffe RT, Brimacombe M, Levitt AJ, et al: Treatment of clinical hypothyroidism with thyroxine and triiodothyronine: a literature review and metaanalysis. Psychosomatics 48:379–384, 2007

Keck PE Jr, Perlis RH, Otto MW, et al: The expert consensus guideline series: medication treatment of bipolar disorder 2004. Postgrad Med Special Report 1–120, 2004

Keck PE Jr, Calabrese JR, McQuade RD, et al: A randomized, double-blind, placebo-controlled 26-week trial of aripiprazole in recently manic patients with bipolar I disorder. J Clin Psychiatry 67:626–637, 2006a

Keck PE Jr, Mintz J, McElroy SL, et al: Double-blind, randomized, placebo-controlled trials of ethyl-eicosapentanoate in the treatment of bipolar depression and rapid cycling bipolar disorder. Biol Psychiatry 60:1020–1022, 2006b

Kemp DE, Gilmer WS, Fleck J, et al: Aripiprazole augmentation in treatment-resistant bipolar depression: early response and development of akathisia. Prog Neuropsychopharmacol Biol Psychiatry 31:574–577, 2007

Kessing LV: The effect of the first manic episode in affective disorder: a case register study of hospitalised episodes. J Affect Disord 53:233–239, 1999

Ketter TA, Greist JH, Graham JA, et al: The effect of dermatologic precautions on the incidence of rash with addition of lamotrigine in the treatment of bipolar I disorder: a randomized trial. J Clin Psychiatry 67:400–406, 2006a

Ketter TA, Wang PW, Chandler RA, et al: Adjunctive aripiprazole in treatment-resistant bipolar depression. Ann Clin Psychiatry 18:169–172, 2006b

Ketter TA, Brooks JO, Hoblyn JC, et al: Effectiveness of lamotrigine in bipolar disorder in a clinical setting. J Psychiatr Res 43:13–23, 2008

Kripke DF: Timing of phototherapy and occurrence of mania. Biol Psychiatry 29:1156–1157, 1991

Kripke DF: Light treatment for nonseasonal depression: speed, efficacy, and combined treatment. J Affect Disord 49:109–117, 1998

Kukopulos A, Reginaldi D, Laddomada P, et al: Course of the manic-depressive cycle and changes caused by treatment. Pharmakopsychiatr Neuropsychopharmakol 13:156–167, 1980

Kushner SF, Khan A, Lane R, et al: Topiramate monotherapy in the management of acute mania: results of four double-blind placebo-controlled trials. Bipolar Disord 8:15–27, 2006

Lam DH, Watkins ER, Hayward P, et al: A randomized controlled study of cognitive therapy for relapse prevention for bipolar affective disorder: outcome of the first year. Arch Gen Psychiatry 60:145–152, 2003

Lam RW, Levitt AJ, Levitan RD, et al: The Can-SAD study: a randomized controlled trial of the effectiveness of light therapy and fluoxetine in patients with winter seasonal affective disorder. Am J Psychiatry 163:805–812, 2006

Leibenluft E, Turner EH, Feldman-Naim S, et al: Light therapy in patients with rapid cycling bipolar disorder: preliminary results. Psychopharmacol Bull 31:705–710, 1995

Leppig M, Bosch B, Naber D, et al: Clozapine in the treatment of 121 out-patients. Psychopharmacology (Berl) 99(suppl): S77–S79, 1989

Levine J, Witztum E, Greenberg BD, et al: Inositol-induced mania? (letter) Am J Psychiatry 153:839, 1996

Linde K, Berner M, Egger M, et al: St John's wort for depression: meta-analysis of randomised controlled trials. Br J Psychiatry 186:99–107, 2005

Lipinski JF, Cohen BM, Frankenburg F, et al: Open trial of S-adenosylmethionine for treatment of depression. Am J Psychiatry 141:448–450, 1984

Lydon E, El-Mallakh RS: Naturalistic long-term use of methylphenidate in bipolar disorder. J Clin Psychopharmacol 26:516–518, 2006

Mahmoud RA, Pandina GJ, Turkoz I, et al: Risperidone for treatment-refractory major depressive disorder: a randomized trial. Ann Intern Med 147:593–602, 2007

Maj M, Pirozzi R, Starace F: Previous pattern of course of the illness as a predictor of response to lithium prophylaxis in bipolar patients. J Affect Disord 17:237–241, 1989

Marangell LB, Suppes T, Ketter TA, et al: Omega-3 fatty acids in bipolar disorder: clinical and research considerations. Prostaglandins Leukot Essent Fatty Acids 75:315–321, 2006

Marangell LB, Suppes T, Zboyan HA, et al: A 1-year pilot study of vagus nerve stimulation in treatment-resistant rapid-cycling bipolar disorder. J Clin Psychiatry 69:183–189, 2008

Marcus RN, McQuade RD, Carson WH, et al: The efficacy and safety of aripiprazole as adjunctive therapy in major depressive disorder: a second multicenter, randomized, double-blind, placebo-controlled study. J Clin Psychopharmacol 28:156–165, 2008

Markowitz JS, Donovan JL, DeVane CL, et al: Effect of St John's wort on drug metabolism by induction of cytochrome P450 3A4 enzyme. JAMA 290:1500–1504, 2003

Martiny K, Lunde M, Simonsen C, et al: Relapse prevention by citalopram in SAD patients responding to 1 week of light therapy. A placebo-controlled study. Acta Psychiatr Scand 109:230–234, 2004

McElroy SL, Dessain EC, Pope HG Jr, et al: Clozapine in the treatment of psychotic mood disorders, schizoaffective disorder, and schizophrenia. J Clin Psychiatry 52:411–414, 1991

McElroy SL, Suppes T, Frye MA, et al: Open-label aripiprazole in the treatment of acute bipolar depression: a prospective pilot trial. J Affect Disord 101:275–281, 2007

McIntyre RS, Mancini DA, McCann S, et al: Topiramate versus bupropion SR when added to mood stabilizer therapy for the depressive phase of bipolar disorder: a preliminary single-blind study. Bipolar Disord 4:207–213, 2002

McIntyre RS, Mancini DA, Srinivasan J, et al: The antidepressant effects of risperidone and olanzapine in bipolar disorder. Can J Clin Pharmacol 11:e218–e826, 2004

Mech AW: High-dose ziprasidone monotherapy in bipolar I disorder patients with depressed or mixed episodes. J Clin Psychopharmacol 28:240–241, 2008

Meltzer HY, Alphs L, Green AI, et al: Clozapine treatment for suicidality in schizophrenia: International Suicide Prevention Trial (InterSePT). Arch Gen Psychiatry 60:82–91, 2003

Mendels J: Lithium in the treatment of depression. Am J Psychiatry 133:373–378, 1976

Mendlewicz J, Youdim MB: Antidepressant potentiation of 5-hydroxytryptophan by L-deprenil in affective illness. J Affect Disord 2:137–146, 1980

Merideth CH, Feighner JP: The use of bupropion in hospitalized depressed patients. J Clin Psychiatry 44:85–87, 1983

Michael N, Erfurth A: Treatment of bipolar mania with right prefrontal rapid transcranial magnetic stimulation. J Affect Disord 78:253–257, 2004

Miklowitz DJ, George EL, Richards JA, et al: A randomized study of family focused psychoeducation and pharmacotherapy in the outpatient management of bipolar disorder. Arch Gen Psychiatry 60:904–912, 2003

Miklowitz DJ, Otto MW, Frank E, et al: Intensive psychosocial intervention enhances functioning in patients with bipolar depression: results from a 9-month randomized controlled trial. Am J Psychiatry 164:1340–1347, 2007

Moses EL, Mallinger AG: St. John's wort: three cases of possible mania induction. J Clin Psychopharmacol 20:115–117, 2000

Murphy DL, Goodwin FK, Brodie HK, et al: L-dopa, dopamine, and hypomania. Am J Psychiatry 130:79–82, 1973

Muzina DJ, Ganocy S, Khalife S, et al: A double-blind, placebo-controlled study of divalproex extended-release in newly diagnosed mood stabilizer naive patients with acute bipolar depression (NR3-028), in New Research Abstracts of the 161st Annual Meeting of the American Psychiatric Association, Washington, DC, May 3–8, 2008, p 101

Nahas Z, Kozel FA, Li X, et al: Left prefrontal transcranial magnetic stimulation (TMS) treatment of depression in bipolar affective disorder: a pilot study of acute safety and efficacy. Bipolar Disord 5:40–47, 2003

Náhunek K, Rodová A, Svestka J, et al: Clinical experience with clozapine in endogenous depression. Act Nerv Super (Praha) 15:111, 1973

Nemeroff CB, Evans DL, Gyulai L, et al: Double-blind, placebo-controlled comparison of imipramine and paroxetine in the treatment of bipolar depression. Am J Psychiatry 158:906–912, 2001

Neumann J, Seidel K, Wunderlich HP: Comparative studies of the effect of carbamazepine and trimipramine in depression, in Anticonvulsants in Affective Disorders. Edited by Emrich HM, Okuma T, Müller AA. Amsterdam, The Netherlands, Excerpta Medica, 1984, pp 160–166

Nierenberg AA, Burt T, Matthews J, et al: Mania associated with St. John's wort. Biol Psychiatry 46:1707–1708, 1999

Nierenberg AA, Fava M, Trivedi MH, et al: A comparison of lithium and T(3) augmentation following two failed medication treatments for depression: a STAR*D report. Am J Psychiatry 163:1519–1530; quiz 1665, 2006a

Nierenberg AA, Ostacher MJ, Calabrese JR, et al: Treatment-resistant bipolar depression: a STEP-BD equipoise randomized effectiveness trial of antidepressant augmentation with lamotrigine, inositol, or risperidone. Am J Psychiatry 163:210–216, 2006b

Noyes R Jr, Dempsey GM, Blum A, et al: Lithium treatment of depression. Compr Psychiatry 15:187–193, 1974

O'Breasail AM, Argouarch S: Hypomania and St John's wort. Can J Psychiatry 43:746–747, 1998

O'Connor MK, Knapp R, Husain M, et al: The influence of age on the response of major depression to electroconvulsive therapy: a C.O.R.E. report. Am J Geriatr Psychiatry 9:382–390, 2001

Olausson B, McElroy S, Chang W, et al: A double-blind, placebo-controlled study of quetiapine and paroxetine in adults with bipolar depression (EMBOLDEN II) (590), in 55th Annual Convention and Scientific Program of the Society of Biological Psychiatry, Washington, DC, May 1–3, 2008. Biol Psychiatry 63:188S, 2008

Oral ET, Altinbas K, Demirkiran S: Sudden akathisia after a ziprasidone dose reduction (letter). Am J Psychiatry 163:546, 2006

O'Reardon JP, Solvason HB, Janicak PG, et al: Efficacy and safety of transcranial magnetic stimulation in the acute treatment of major depression: a multisite randomized controlled trial. Biol Psychiatry 62:1208–1216, 2007

Parker G, Roy K, Hadzi-Pavlovic D, et al: Psychotic (delusional) depression: a meta-analysis of physical treatments. J Affect Disord 24:17–24, 1992

Parsa MA, Ramirez LF, Loula EC, et al: Effect of clozapine on psychotic depression and parkinsonism. J Clin Psychopharmacol 11:330–331, 1991

Perris C, d'Elia G: A study of bipolar (manic-depressive) and unipolar recurrent depressive psychoses, IX: therapy and prognosis. Acta Psychiatr Scand Suppl 194:153–171, 1966

Perry A, Tarrier N, Morriss R, et al: Randomised controlled trial of efficacy of teaching patients with bipolar disorder to identify early symptoms of relapse and obtain treatment. BMJ 318:149–153, 1999

Post RM, Uhde TW, Roy-Byrne PP, et al: Antidepressant effects of carbamazepine. Am J Psychiatry 143:29–34, 1986

Post RM, Altshuler LL, Ketter TA, et al: Antiepileptic drugs in affective illness. Clinical and theoretical implications. Adv Neurol 55:239–277, 1991

Post RM, Altshuler LL, Leverich GS, et al: Mood switch in bipolar depression: comparison of adjunctive venlafaxine, bupropion and sertraline. Br J Psychiatry 189:124–131, 2006

Privitera MR, Lamberti JS, Maharaj K: Clozapine in a bipolar depressed patient (letter). Am J Psychiatry 150:986, 1993

Quitkin FM, Kane J, Rifkin A, et al: Prophylactic lithium carbonate with and without imipramine for bipolar 1 patients. A double-blind study. Arch Gen Psychiatry 38:902–907, 1981

Ranjan R, Meltzer HY: Acute and long-term effectiveness of clozapine in treatment-resistant psychotic depression. Biol Psychiatry 40:253–258, 1996

Riemann D, Voderholzer U, Berger M: Sleep and sleep-wake manipulations in bipolar depression. Neuropsychobiology 45 (suppl 1):7–12, 2002

Rosenthal NE, Sack DA, Gillin JC, et al: Seasonal affective disorder. A description of the syndrome and preliminary findings with light therapy. Arch Gen Psychiatry 41:72–80, 1984

Roy-Byrne PP, Uhde TW, Post RM: Effects of one night's sleep deprivation on mood and behavior in panic disorder. Patients with panic disorder compared with depressed patients and normal controls. Arch Gen Psychiatry 43:895–899, 1986

Rush AJ, Marangell LB, Sackeim HA, et al: Vagus nerve stimulation for treatment-resistant depression: a randomized, controlled acute phase trial. Biol Psychiatry 58:347–354, 2005a

Rush AJ, Sackeim HA, Marangell LB, et al: Effects of 12 months of vagus nerve stimulation in treatment-resistant depression: a naturalistic study. Biol Psychiatry 58:355–363, 2005b

Sachs G: Mood stabilizers vs. standard antidepressants for treatment of bipolar depression. Paper presented at the 42nd annual meeting of the American College of Neuropsychopharmacology, San Juan, Puerto Rico, December 7–11, 2003

Sachs GS, Lafer B, Stoll AL, et al: A double-blind trial of bupropion versus desipramine for bipolar depression. J Clin Psychiatry 55:391–393, 1994

Sachs G, Altshuler L, Ketter T, et al: Divalproex versus placebo for the treatment of bipolar depression (232). Presentation at the 40th annual meeting of the American College of Neuropsychopharmacology, Waikoloa, HI, December 9–13, 2001

Sachs GS, Nierenberg AA, Calabrese JR, et al: Effectiveness of adjunctive antidepressant treatment for bipolar depression. N Engl J Med 356:1711–1722, 2007

Sachs G, Lombardo I, Yang R, et al: Learnings from the Ziprasidone Bipolar Depression Program, in Fifth Annual Scientific Meeting of the International Society for CNS Clinical Trials and Methodology, Washington, DC, March 3–5, 2009

Sackeim HA, Prudic J: Length of the ECT course in bipolar and unipolar depression. J ECT 21:195–197, 2005

Schneck C: St. John's wort and hypomania (letter). J Clin Psychiatry 59:689, 1998

Scott J, Garland A, Moorhead S: A pilot study of cognitive therapy in bipolar disorders. Psychol Med 31:459–467, 2001

Shelton RC, Stahl SM: Risperidone and paroxetine given singly and in combination for bipolar depression. J Clin Psychiatry 65:1715–1719, 2004

Shopsin B, Gershon S: Dopamine receptor stimulation in the treatment of depression: piribedil (ET-495). Neuropsychobiology 4:1–14, 1978

Silverstone T: Moclobemide vs. imipramine in bipolar depression: a multicentre double-blind clinical trial. Acta Psychiatr Scand 104:104–109, 2001

Small JG: Anticonvulsants in affective disorders. Psychopharmacol Bull 26:25–36, 1990

Small JG, Milstein V: Lithium interactions: lithium and electroconvulsive therapy. J Clin Psychopharmacol 10:346–350, 1990

Sokolski KN: Adjunctive aripiprazole in bipolar I depression. Ann Pharmacother 41:35–40, 2007

Stokes PE, Shamoian CA, Stoll PM, et al: Efficacy of lithium as acute treatment of manic-depressive illness. Lancet 1:1319–1325, 1971

Stoll AL, Severus WE, Freeman MP, et al: Omega 3 fatty acids in bipolar disorder: a preliminary double-blind, placebo-controlled trial. Arch Gen Psychiatry 56:407–412, 1999

Suppes T: Review of the use of topiramate for treatment of bipolar disorders. J Clin Psychopharmacol 22:599–609, 2002

Suppes T, McElroy SL, Gilbert J, et al: Clozapine in the treatment of dysphoric mania. Biol Psychiatry 32:270–280, 1992

Suppes T, Dennehy EB, Hirschfeld RM, et al: The Texas Implementation of Medication Algorithms: update to the algorithms for treatment of bipolar I disorder. J Clin Psychiatry 66:870–886, 2005

Swartz HA, Frank E: Psychotherapy for bipolar depression: a phase-specific treatment strategy? Bipolar Disord 3:11–22, 2001

Szuba MP, Baxter LR Jr, Altshuler LL, et al: Lithium sustains the acute antidepressant effects of sleep deprivation: preliminary findings from a controlled study. Psychiatry Res 51:283–295, 1994

Taneja I, Haman K, Shelton RC, et al: A randomized, double-blind, crossover trial of modafinil on mood. J Clin Psychopharmacol 27:76–79, 2007

Taylor MJ, Carney SM, Goodwin GM, et al: Folate for depressive disorders: systematic review and meta-analysis of randomized controlled trials. J Psychopharmacol 18:251–256, 2004a

Taylor MJ, Wilder H, Bhagwagar Z, et al: Inositol for depressive disorders. Cochrane Database Syst Rev CD004049, 2004b

Terman M, Terman JS: Bright light therapy: side effects and benefits across the symptom spectrum. J Clin Psychiatry 60:799–809, 1999

Terman M, Terman JS: Controlled trial of naturalistic dawn simulation and negative air ionization for seasonal affective disorder. Am J Psychiatry 163:2126–2133, 2006

Tharayil BS, Gangadhar BN, Thirthalli J, et al: Seizure with single-pulse transcranial magnetic stimulation in a 35-year-old otherwise-healthy patient with bipolar disorder. J ECT 21:188–189, 2005

Thase ME, Macfadden W, Weisler RH, et al: Efficacy of quetiapine monotherapy in bipolar I and II depression: a double-blind, placebo-controlled study (the BOLDER II study). J Clin Psychopharmacol 26:600–609, 2006

Thase ME, Jonas A, Khan A, et al: Aripiprazole monotherapy in nonpsychotic bipolar I depression: results of 2 randomized, placebo-controlled studies. J Clin Psychopharmacol 28:13–20, 2008

Tohen M, Vieta E, Calabrese J, et al: Efficacy of olanzapine and olanzapine-fluoxetine combination in the treatment of bipolar I depression. Arch Gen Psychiatry 60:1079–1088, 2003

Tohen M, Calabrese JR, Sachs GS, et al: Randomized, placebo-controlled trial of olanzapine as maintenance therapy in patients with bipolar I disorder responding to acute treatment with olanzapine. Am J Psychiatry 163:247–256, 2006

Tondo L, Baldessarini RJ, Hennen J, et al: Lithium treatment and risk of suicidal behavior in bipolar disorder patients. J Clin Psychiatry 59:405–414, 1998

Truman CJ, Goldberg JF, Ghaemi SN, et al: Self-reported history of manic/hypomanic switch associated with antidepressant use: data from the Systematic Treatment Enhancement Program for Bipolar Disorder (STEP-BD). J Clin Psychiatry 68:1472–1479, 2007

Tuunainen A, Kripke DF, Endo T: Light therapy for non-seasonal depression. Cochrane Database Syst Rev CD004050, 2004

UK ECT Review Group: Efficacy and safety of electroconvulsive therapy in depressive disorders: a systematic review and meta-analysis. Lancet 361:799–808, 2003

Vangala VR, Brown ES, Suppes T: Clozapine associated with decreased suicidality in bipolar disorder: a case report. Bipolar Disord 1:123–124, 1999

Vieta E, Goikolea JM, Corbella B, et al: Risperidone safety and efficacy in the treatment of bipolar and schizoaffective disorders: results from a 6-month, multicenter, open study. J Clin Psychiatry 62:818–825, 2001

Vieta E, Martinez-Aran A, Goikolea JM, et al: A randomized trial comparing paroxetine and venlafaxine in the treatment of bipolar depressed patients taking mood stabilizers. J Clin Psychiatry 63:508–512, 2002

Visser HM, Van Der Mast RC: Bipolar disorder, antidepressants and induction of hypomania or mania. A systematic review. World J Biol Psychiatry 6:231–241, 2005

Wang LS, Zhou G, Zhu B, et al: St John's wort induces both cytochrome P450 3A4-catalyzed sulfoxidation and 2C19-dependent hydroxylation of omeprazole. Clin Pharmacol Ther 75:191–197, 2004

Wang PW, Keller KL, Hill S, et al: Effectiveness of open adjunctive ziprasidone in obese and overweight bipolar disorder patients (606), in 55th Annual Convention and Scientific Program of the Society of Biological Psychiatry, Washington, DC, May 1–3, 2008. Biol Psychiatry 63 (suppl 7):193S–194S, 2008

Watanabe S, Ishino H, Otsuki S: Double-blind comparison of lithium carbonate and imipramine in treatment of depression. Arch Gen Psychiatry 32:659–668, 1975

Wehr TA, Goodwin FK: Rapid cycling in manic-depressives induced by tricyclic antidepressants. Arch Gen Psychiatry 36:555–559, 1979

Wehr TA, Rosenthal NE, Sack DA, et al: Antidepressant effects of sleep deprivation in bright and dim light. Acta Psychiatr Scand 72:161–165, 1985

Wehr TA, Sack DA, Rosenthal NE: Seasonal affective disorder with summer depression and winter hypomania. Am J Psychiatry 144:1602–1603, 1987

Wehr TA, Sack DA, Rosenthal NE, et al: Rapid cycling affective disorder: contributing factors and treatment responses in 51 patients. Am J Psychiatry 145:179–184, 1988

Weisler RH, Hirschfeld R, Cutler AJ, et al: Extended-release carbamazepine capsules as monotherapy in bipolar disorder: pooled results from two randomised, double-blind, placebo-controlled trials. CNS Drugs 20:219–231, 2006

Wright JB: Mania following sleep deprivation. Br J Psychiatry 163:679–680, 1993

Wu JC, Bunney WE: The biological basis of an antidepressant response to sleep deprivation and relapse: review and hypothesis. Am J Psychiatry 147:14–21, 1990

Xia G, Gajwani P, Muzina DJ, et al: Treatment-emergent mania in unipolar and bipolar depression: focus on repetitive transcranial magnetic stimulation. Int J Neuropsychopharmacol 11:119–130, 2008

Yatham LN, Kennedy SH, O'Donovan C, et al: Canadian Network for Mood and Anxiety Treatments (CANMAT) guidelines for the management of patients with bipolar disorder: update 2007. Bipolar Disord 8:721–739, 2006

Young AH, Carlsson A, Olausson B, et al: A double-blind, placebo-controlled study with acute and continuation phase of quetiapine and lithium in adults with bipolar depression (EMBOLDEN I) (610), in 55th Annual Convention and Scientific Program of the Society of Biological Psychiatry, Washington, DC, May 1–3, 2008. Biol Psychiatry 63 (suppl 7):194S, 2008

Young LT, Joffe RT, Robb JC, et al: Double-blind comparison of addition of a second mood stabilizer versus an antidepressant to an initial mood stabilizer for treatment of patients with bipolar depression. Am J Psychiatry 157:124–126, 2000

Zarate CA Jr, Tohen M, Baldessarini RJ: Clozapine in severe mood disorders. J Clin Psychiatry 56:411–417, 1995

Zarate CA Jr, Payne JL, Singh J, et al: Pramipexole for bipolar II depression: a placebo-controlled proof of concept study. Biol Psychiatry 56:54–60, 2004

Zaretsky AE, Segal ZV, Gemar M: Cognitive therapy for bipolar depression: a pilot study. Can J Psychiatry 44:491–494, 1999

Zarzar MN, Graham J, Roberts J, et al: Effectiveness and weight effects of open-label lamotrigine with and without concomitant psychotropic medications in patients with bipolar I disorder. MedGenMed 9:41, 2007

Zhang ZJ, Kang WH, Tan QR, et al: Adjunctive herbal medicine with carbamazepine for bipolar disorders: a double-blind, randomized, placebo-controlled study. J Psychiatr Res 41:360–309, 2007

Zornberg GL, Pope HG Jr: Treatment of depression in bipolar disorder: new directions for research. J Clin Psychopharmacol 13:397–408, 1993

CHAPTER 8

Longer-Term Management of Bipolar Disorders

Terence A. Ketter, M.D.

Po W. Wang, M.D.

The recurrent episodic nature of bipolar disorders and the dysfunction, morbidity, illness progression, and mortality associated with acute episodes make the prevention of new episodes one of the most important goals in the management of these conditions.

Lithium was approved by the U.S. Food and Drug Administration (FDA) for bipolar maintenance therapy in 1974 and for almost three decades was the only approved longer-term treatment for bipolar disorders. During this time, the robust efficacy of lithium in bipolar disorders, compared with its much less impressive benefits in other psychiatric conditions, led to the view that lithium had specific efficacy for bipolar disorders (Soares and Gershon 2000).

Lithium was perceived as being unique because it was effective in acute mania and maintenance treatment as well as (perhaps to a lesser extent) in acute bipolar depression. In contrast, first-generation antipsychotics could relieve mania but might exacerbate depression, and antidepressants could relieve depression but might trigger mania. Thus, first-generation antipsychotics and antidepressants were considered adjunctive unimodal agents that could provide acute symptomatic relief for one pole of bipolar disorders. Lithium was considered the only bimodal agent that could address not only acute episodes of either

251

polarity but also the disorder as a whole over time. Eventually, the term *mood stabilizer* (synonymous with *antibipolar medication*) was applied to lithium, distinguishing it from other classes of agents and emphasizing its role as *the* comprehensive treatment for bipolar disorders.

After two decades, the notion that lithium was *the* rather than *a* mood stabilizer was challenged, when in the middle 1990s divalproex was approved for the treatment of acute mania. Divalproex was not an antipsychotic, had efficacy for acute mania, and did not appear to exacerbate the depressive component of the illness. Perhaps by a process of elimination, in an effort to maintain mutually exclusive psychotropic drug categories, divalproex became referred to as a mood stabilizer. There is no consensus definition of the term *mood stabilizer,* and the FDA does not use the term. However, over time common usage of the term evolved so that agents with bipolar indications that are not antipsychotics have been referred to as mood stabilizers. As discussed later in this chapter, because of methodological limitations, the pivotal divalproex monotherapy maintenance study failed; neither divalproex nor lithium separated from placebo on the primary outcome measure and thus divalproex monotherapy has *not* been approved by the FDA for the longer-term treatment of bipolar disorders.

Similarly, carbamazepine is another agent approved for acute mania that is not an antipsychotic and does not appear to exacerbate the depressive component of the illness, but lacks randomized, double-blind, placebo-controlled evidence of maintenance efficacy, and hence lacks a longer-term indication for the management of bipolar disorders. The term *mood stabilizer* is also applied to carbamazepine.

Thus, it was not until 2003, when lamotrigine was approved, that clinicians had a sanctioned alternative to lithium for the longer-term treatment of bipolar disorders. Lamotrigine was distinctive in two important ways. First, lamotrigine appeared to "stabilize mood from below," in that it was more effective against depressive than the mood elevation aspects of the illness (Ketter and Calabrese 2002). Second, lamotrigine was the first, and remains the only, medication to receive a maintenance indication while lacking an acute indication. The latter was particularly challenging because one of the fundamental approaches to selecting treatments for the maintenance treatment phase is to utilize agents that prove themselves effective in the acute treatment phase. Nevertheless, lamotrigine became the third anticonvulsant that was not an antipsychotic that was approved to address a component (in this case maintenance treatment) of bipolar disorders without exacerbating other aspects of the illness. Thus, over time the term *mood stabilizer* was also applied to lamotrigine.

In 2004 and 2005, two agents already approved for acute mania, the second-generation antipsychotics olanzapine and aripiprazole, respectively, received FDA approval for the longer-term treatment of bipolar disorders. In addition, in 2008 quetiapine immediate-release formulation and, later, extended-release formulation (quetiapine XR) received the first adjunctive (added to lithium or divalproex) longer-term bipolar treatment indications. These developments further challenged assumptions regarding longer-term management because previously, first-generation antipsychotics were considered mere short-term adjuncts for acute mania, which needed to be discontinued as quickly as possible in order to minimize the risks of tardive dyskinesia and exacerbation of depressive symptoms in patients with bipolar disorders. Arguably, the ambivalence of the FDA in granting longer-term approvals for second-generation antipsychotics (particularly as monotherapy) is evident in the prescribing information for second-generation antipsychotics in monotherapy longer-term bipolar treatment, which emphasizes utility in the continuation treatment phase more than in the maintenance treatment phase. Moreover, at least some second-generation antipsychotics have substantial tolerability limitations that limit their utility in longer-term treatment. Thus, despite evidence of efficacy, ongoing controversy is expected regarding the roles of olanzapine, aripiprazole, and adjunctive quetiapine in the longer-term management of bipolar disorders.

Another controversial issue is the role of adjunctive antidepressants in the longer-term management of bipolar disorders. In the past, these agents were considered mere short-term adjuncts for acute bipolar depression that needed to be discontinued as quickly as possible in order to minimize the risk of exacerbation of mood elevation symptoms in patients with bipolar disorders. However, limited data suggest that the subset (perhaps 15%) of patients with excellent responses during the acute treatment phase and the continuation treatment phase may receive benefit from longer-term treatment with these agents (Altshuler et al. 2003).

Thus, four monotherapies (lithium, lamotrigine, olanzapine, and aripiprazole) and one adjunctive (added to lithium or divalproex) therapy (quetiapine/quetiapine XR) have been approved for the longer-term treatment of bipolar disorders. Two of these agents that are not antipsychotics (lithium and lamotrigine), along with divalproex and carbamazepine, are referred to as mood stabilizers. In contrast, the antipsychotics with evidence of longer-term efficacy (olanzapine, aripiprazole, quetiapine/quetiapine XR) are still called second-generation (or atypical) antipsychotics rather than mood stabilizers, despite each not only having evidence of efficacy for longer-term treatment but also having acute treatment phase indications. In addition to these advances in pharmacological longer-term treatment, emerging data suggest the adjunctive psychosocial interventions could contribute importantly to prevention of relapse and recurrence in patients with bipolar disorders.

Preceding chapters in this volume have described the management of acute manic and mixed episodes, and major depressive episodes in patients with bipolar disorders. In this chapter we focus on longer-term management of bipolar disorders, initially in the temporal order encountered clinically: first the continuation treatment phase and then the maintenance treatment phase, as described in Chapter 4 of this volume, "Multiphase Treatment Strategy for Bipolar Disorders." This is followed by a discussion of clinical implications of bipolar disorder longer-term treatment trial designs and a description of the individual approved and unapproved longer-term treatment options for bipolar disorders.

Continuation Treatment Phase

The continuation treatment phase provides a crucial bridge between the acute treatment phase and the maintenance treatment phase and shares some characteristics with each. This phase starts with either response or (ideally) remission, so that subsyndromal symptoms may be present or absent, respectively. Thus, overt or covert (partially or fully suppressed) mood symptoms are considered to be present. The continuation treatment phase ends ideally with recovery, leading to the maintenance treatment phase. The duration of this phase is the time needed to exceed the natural episode duration (Prien and Kupfer 1986), which is commonly considered to be 2–6 months in patients with bipolar disorders.

The distinction between the continuation treatment phase and the maintenance treatment phase is commonly blurred in clinical research and clinical practice (Quitkin et al. 1976). For example, contemporary longer-term registration studies in patients with bipolar disorders tend to be continuation/maintenance studies, with two stages: 1) a briefer open stabilization stage corresponding to the acute treatment phase and the early/middle part of the continuation treatment phase, and 2) a longer randomized, double-blind, placebo-controlled stage corresponding to the middle/late continuation treatment phase and the maintenance treatment phase (Figure 8–1). For example, in the olanzapine longer-term treatment registration study, patients were only euthymic for 2 weeks prior to randomization, perhaps explaining why the longer-term indication in the prescribing information for this agent appears to resemble more a description of the continuation treatment phase than the maintenance treatment phase.

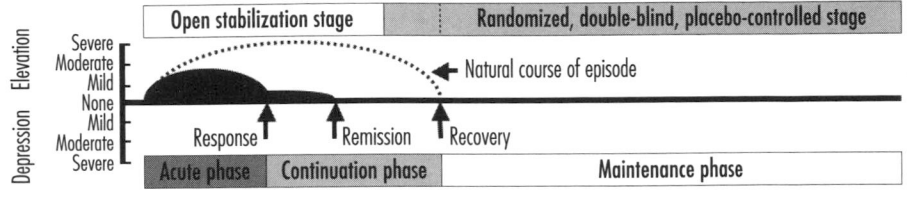

FIGURE 8–1. Contemporary randomized controlled continuation/ maintenance study paradigm.

Depending on the duration of mood stability required in the open stabilization stage, the randomized controlled stage may or may not include an early continuation treatment phase component (top, gray portion to left of dotted line) in addition to the later maintenance treatment phase component.

The therapeutic goals of the continuation treatment phase include attaining sufficient and persistent enough relief of mood symptoms to yield recovery, and preventing relapse. Medication strategies focus on balancing the dual and at times conflicting needs for efficacy and tolerability. This primarily involves striving to continue full doses of mood stabilizer(s) and adjuncts that yielded remission as tolerated. However, it may be necessary to decrease doses to relieve adverse effects or increase doses to relieve subsyndromal symptoms.

Suboptimal timing and rate of medication reduction and discontinuation can entail substantial risks. Medication reduction and/or discontinuation that is too early risks loss of remission and relapse and can undermine symptomatic recovery. Similarly, medication reduction and/or discontinuation that is too rapid risks relapse or recurrence. In contrast, attempts to decrease medication burden that are too late or slow risk nonadherence and erosion of the therapeutic alliance and can undermine functional recovery.

In longer-term treatment clinical trials that have only a brief period of stability prior to randomization, patients have not yet attained recovery, so those assigned to placebo are at high risk for relapse back into the index episode. In the survival curve, this can result in a precipitous (exponential) decrease in the percentage of patients taking placebo remaining in remission (Figure 8–2, black line). In trials with a longer period of stability prior to randomization, patients have attained recovery, so those assigned to placebo are at a risk for recurrence of a new episode, which in many instances evolves over a much longer time frame than relapse. In the survival curve, this may result in a gradual (linear) decrease in the percentage of patients taking placebo remaining in remission (Figure 8–2, gray line). Thus, as described in more detail later in this chapter, the duration of

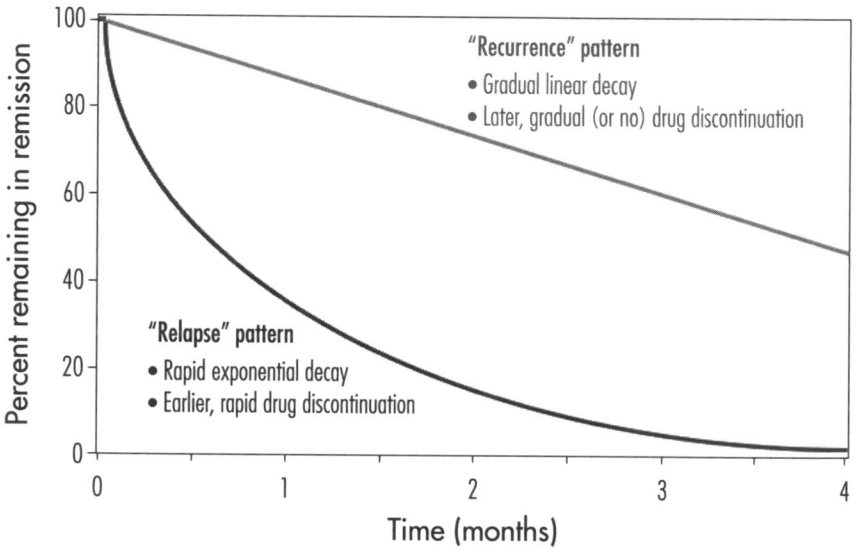

FIGURE 8–2. Relapse versus recurrence with earlier/rapid versus later/ gradual drug discontinuation.

The "relapse" pattern (black line) represents abrupt return of index episodes. The "recurrence" pattern (gray line) represents emergence of new episodes, which in many instances evolve over a much longer time frame. These types of graphs are commonly used to depict the time-to-event– based primary outcome measures (e.g., time to relapse into any mood episode) in controlled longer-term treatment trials.

stability prior to randomization influences the interpretation of longer-term treatment trials. Very brief periods of initial stability indicate that the randomized stage may have a substantial continuation treatment phase component, whereas longer periods of initial stability suggest that the randomized stage may primarily represent the maintenance treatment phase.

Maintenance Treatment Phase

The maintenance treatment phase starts with recovery, so that at least initially even subsyndromal symptoms are absent, and there is no underlying current episode. Ideally, this phase represents the vast majority of time spent in treatment, but unfortunately recurrences are common in bipolar disorders, marking an end to this phase and a return to the acute treatment phase. The duration of the maintenance treatment phase is indefinite. In view of the highly recurrent nature of bipolar disorders, North American guidelines recommend preventive treatment after the first manic episode (American Psychiatric Association 2002; Keck et al. 2004a; Suppes et al. 2005), whereas European guidelines are more conservative, with some tending to recommend preventive treatment after the second or even third manic episode (Goodwin 2003; Grunze et al. 2002).

The therapeutic goals of the maintenance treatment phase include maintaining stable mood, preventing recurrence, and facilitating a return to full function. Medication strategies focus on tolerability and include efforts to decrease medication burden by tapering down and discontinuing adjuncts that may no longer be necessary. Thus, antidepressants commonly are discontinued, but in some patients these agents may be necessary during the maintenance treatment phase to prevent depression, as described later in this chapter (Altshuler et al. 2003). It is important that any medication decreases be gradual, in order to limit the risk of recurrence. For example, rapid (less than 2 weeks) as compared with gradual (more than 2 weeks) discontinuation of lithium has been associated with more rapid and more frequent recurrence (Baldessarini et al. 1997; Faedda et al. 1993; Suppes et al. 1991). As noted briefly later in this chapter and in greater detail in Chapter 15 of this volume, "Adjunctive Psychosocial Interventions in the Management of Bipolar Disorders," psychosocial interventions during the maintenance treatment phase are an important component of preventing recurrence (Colom et al. 2003).

Clinical Implications of Longer-Term Treatment Trial Designs in Bipolar Disorder

As noted previously, longer-term treatment studies are complex, with randomized controlled stages that may assess efficacy in the continuation treatment phase as well as the maintenance treatment phase. Several features of such trials are worth considering in relationship to their clinical implications (Table 8–1).

Open Stabilization Stage

The open stabilization stage involves enrolling patients with bipolar disorder with current or recent index mood episodes. In the vast majority of studies, the index mood episode is manic, hypomanic, or mixed. Indeed, there are only two published randomized, controlled, longer-term treatment studies that enrolled currently or recently depressed patients: an older report assessing lithium compared with placebo (Prien et al. 1973b, 1974), and a more recent trial of lamotrigine compared with lithium and placebo (Calabrese et al. 2003). Thus, most of our evidence-based knowledge regarding the longer-term treatment of bipo-

TABLE 8–1.   Important features of longer-term treatment trials

Open stabilization stage	Randomized controlled stage
Polarity of most recent episode	Blind versus open treatment
Duration of open stabilization stage	Duration of randomized controlled stage
Medication(s) used to stabilize mood	Permitted adjunctive medications
Mood stabilization criteria (degree, duration)	Relapse/recurrence criteria
Rate of tapering/discontinuing medication(s)	Rate of tapering/discontinuing medication(s)
Medication(s) present immediately prior to randomization	Open adjunctive rescue treatments
Degree of enrichment	Time-to-event versus event-based measures
Completion rate	Completion rate

lar disorders is applicable to patients with current or recent mood elevation rather than depression, which is problematic because depression is far more pervasive than mood elevation in bipolar disorders (Judd et al. 2002, 2003).

The duration of the open stabilization stage impacts its clinical interpretation. If only a brief amount of time is permitted, then at the point of randomization, patients still will be in the continuation treatment phase. In addition, there may not be sufficient time for patients with more challenging illness to be stabilized, so that they will be excluded from the randomized controlled stage. Most contemporary registration studies have had open stabilization stage durations of 6–18 weeks.

The medication(s) used to stabilize mood will affect interpretation of the study. Arguably, the least biased approach would be to permit any treatment (including no treatment) prior to randomization. However, such an unbiased approach raises substantial methodological problems, increasing the risk of a failed (inconclusive) study (Bowden et al. 2000) and making clinical interpretation of the results challenging. For example, stabilizing a patient on lithium and then randomizing to divalproex does not have direct clinical relevance because the most common clinical approach to longer-term treatment is to use the medication that was effective for the acute episode. In addition, inclusion of patients who experienced resolution of the index episode without treatment permits entry of subjects with less challenging illness, increasing the placebo response rate in the randomized controlled stage, and thus the risk of a failed study.

The degree and especially the duration of mood stability required prior to randomization influence clinical interpretation. Studies of patients who are "hypostabilized" for very brief durations will have the confound of being assessments of the continuation treatment phase as well as the maintenance treatment phase, but these patients may be representative of most patients encountered in clinical practice as they will likely account for a large portion of the total number of patients enrolled in the open stabilization stage (Tohen et al. 2006). In contrast, studies of patients who are "hyperstabilized" with minimal symptoms for a very long duration will have the benefit of being true assessments of the maintenance treatment phase, but these patients will be unlikely to be representative of most patients encountered in clinical practice because they likely will only account for a small fraction of the total number of patients enrolled in the open stabilization stage (Keck et al. 2007). Longer-term treatment studies have evolved to the point of requiring 6–12 weeks of stability prior to randomization (Suppes et al. 2009; Vieta et al. 2008).

The rate of tapering/discontinuing medication both in the open stabilization stage and in the randomized controlled stage will influence interpretation because overly rapid discontinuation of medication may increase the risk of rebound episodes.

The medication present immediately prior to randomization also influences clinical interpretation. For monotherapy studies, the study drug is the only medication permitted immediately prior to randomization (aside from limited use of adjuncts), ensuring that for all randomized subjects the study drug yields adequate acute tolerability and efficacy. This creates bias in favor of the study drug over placebo but is analogous to clinical treatment, during which medications that are at least briefly well tolerated and effective are considered candidates for longer-term administration. Thus, such studies address the question "If this medication yields adequate acute tolerability and efficacy, will it have sufficient longer-term tolerability and efficacy to merit its continuation?" However, this process creates more problematic bias regarding comparisons of the study drug to active control treatments. Thus, in such studies active control treatments may be only fairly compared with placebo and even that comparison is limited by the fact that patients randomized to the active control treatment have not proved to have adequate acute tolerability and efficacy with that intervention.

The previously mentioned process of only randomizing patients with adequate acute tolerability and efficacy with the study drug is referred to as *enrichment*. *Underenriched* studies may have less bias and be more generalizable but are at greater risk for failure, whereas *overenriched* studies may entail more bias and less generalizability but less risk of failure.

The completion rate for the open stabilization phase reflects the degree of enrichment and generalizability. Thus, a higher completion rate may suggest a lower degree of enrichment and more generalizability but increased risk of a failed study. In contrast, a lower completion rate may suggest a higher degree of enrichment and less generalizability but decreased risk of a failed study. Accordingly, among contemporary randomized, double-blind, placebo-controlled monotherapy studies, the open stabilization stage completion rate for the one failed study was high at 65% (Bowden et al. 2000), whereas rates for the four successful studies were lower at 36% (Keck et al. 2006), 49% (Tohen et al. 2006), 50% (Calabrese et al. 2003), and 53% (Bowden et al. 2003).

Randomized Controlled Stage

The randomized controlled stage involves assessing preventive efficacy in completers of the open stabilization stage assigned to different treatments. Studies designed to obtain regulatory approval use double-blind methodology, with placebo control required in the United States and active control accepted in Europe. Occasional effectiveness studies that are not designed to obtain regulatory approval utilize randomized open rather than double-blind designs and thus may represent more closely clinical practice, in which clinicians and patients know what medication is being taken.

The duration of the randomized controlled stage affects its clinical interpretation. Shorter durations raise concerns that the trial is unduly confounded by assessment of the continuation treatment phase, so that longer durations are considered to assess more rigorously the maintenance treatment phase. Recent contemporary, longer-term, treatment studies have randomized controlled stage durations ranging between 6 and 24 months.

Limited use of adjunctive benzodiazepines commonly is permitted to allow greater patient retention, particularly for those randomized to placebo. Such use is commonly compared across treatment groups to assess the potential for such use to be a confounding influence.

The choice of relapse/recurrence criteria influences clinical interpretation. Such criteria can involve measures such as hospitalization or syndromal or subsyndromal symptoms as identified by mood ratings or the need to prescribe rescue medication(s). Not requiring full syndromal relapse/recurrence may permit more severely ill patients to participate safely in clinical trials.

The rate of tapering/discontinuing medication both in the randomized controlled stage and in the open stabilization stage will influence interpretation because overly rapid discontinuation of medication may increase the risk of rebound episodes.

Studies may continue to follow patients after relapse/recurrence to permit assessment of the effects of open rescue treatments (e.g., antidepressants) added to the study drug or placebo (Gyulai et al. 2003). Although data regarding the outcome of such open adjunctive treatment are not utilized in the primary assessment of maintenance efficacy, they may help inform clinicians regarding treatment of breakthrough symptoms.

The primary outcomes in longer-term treatment studies most often involve time-to-event–based measures, comparing the time from randomization to relapse/recurrence across treatments. Although such approaches yield greater statistical power, they are less meaningful to clinicians than event-based measures such as relapse/recurrence rates, which are commonly reported as secondary outcomes. In some instances, there are sufficient differences in statistical power that the time-to-event–based and event-based outcomes differ. If this occurs, most often efficacy will be more robust with the time-to-event–based approach. Indeed, this was the case with the lamotrigine registration trials (Goodwin et al. 2004), resulting in the FDA indication involving approval for use of lamotrigine to "delay the time to occurrence," in contrast to that of lithium to "prevent or diminish the intensity" of mood episodes. Curiously, in the divalproex-versus-lithium-versus-placebo longer-term treatment trial, divalproex (and lithium) failed to separate from placebo on all three time-to-event–based measures (time to manic, depressive, or any episode), although divalproex (but not lithium) separated from placebo on two of three event-based measures (premature discontinuation rates for depressive, or any, but not manic, episodes) (Bowden et al. 2000).

The completion rate for the randomized controlled stage influences clinical interpretation, with lower completion rates suggesting potentially less generalizability. Completion rates may be calculated with respect to the total number of patients enrolled or the total number entering the randomized controlled stage. Importantly, among contemporary randomized, double-blind, placebo-controlled studies, the randomized controlled stage completion rates in relationship to the number of patients enrolled have been low, ranging between 1% (for a prematurely terminated positive study) (Bowden et al. 2003) and 20% (for a failed study with a high placebo response rate) (Bowden et al. 2000), emphasizing the potentially limited generalizability of these studies.

Maintenance Treatment of Bipolar Disorders: Balancing Benefits and Risks

There are four monotherapies (lithium, lamotrigine, olanzapine, and aripiprazole) approved for longer-term treatment of bipolar disorders (Figure 8–3, left). Also, one adjunctive (added to lithium or divalproex) therapy (quetiapine/ quetiapine XR) has been approved for longer-term treatment of bipolar disorders. In addition, divalproex, although not approved for bipolar maintenance monotherapy, is commonly used both alone and in combination with other agents.

The approved longer-term treatments, as with approved treatments for other aspects of bipolar disorders, have single-digit numbers needed to treat (NNT; Figure 8–3, top, left), indicating that treating fewer than 10 patients with an approved agent compared with placebo can be expected to yield one more responder. In addition, divalproex has a single-digit NNT. The practice of evidence-based medicine entails considering not only efficacy data, that is, giving higher priorities to treatments with lower NNT, but also taking into account safety/ tolerability data, that is, giving higher priorities to treatments with higher numbers needed to harm (NNH). For example, as discussed later in this chapter, in spite of favorable NNT, the tolerability limitations of second-generation antipsychotics suggest that in many instances clinicians and patients may prefer to hold these agents in reserve for patients with inadequate efficacy or tolerability with mood stabilizers.

More detailed assessment of the preventive efficacy of various longer-term treatment options is presented in Table 8–2. Although these interventions all have single-digit NNT for episode prevention in general, they have distinctive patterns of efficacy with respect to prevention of manic as compared with depressive episodes. Thus, lithium, olanzapine, and aripiprazole have markedly lower NNT for mania as compared with depression prevention, suggesting that they may "stabilize mood from above." In contrast, lamotrigine had a lower NNT for depression as compared with mania prevention, suggesting that lamotrigine may "stabilize mood from below." Curiously, in a multicenter divalproex maintenance study, divalproex and lithium as an active comparator had lower NNT for depression compared with mania prevention (Bowden et al. 2000). However, as noted later in this chapter, this study had methodological limitations and failed in the sense that both lithium and divalproex failed to separate from placebo on the primary outcome measure, limiting interpretation of polarity of benefits. Of particular interest, adjunctive quetiapine has single-digit NNT for both ma-

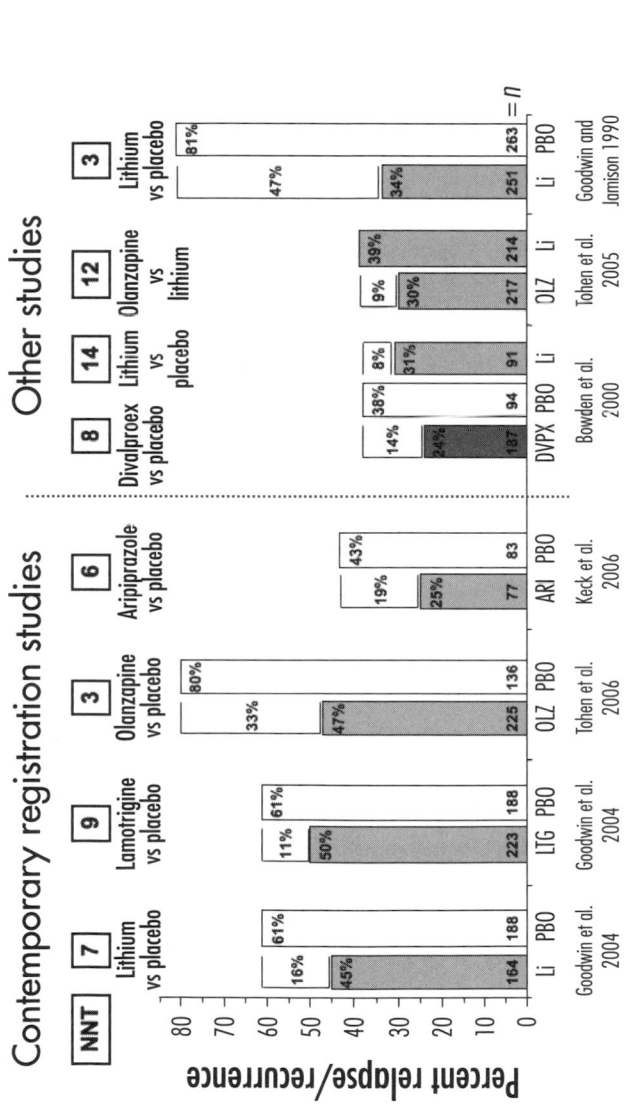

FIGURE 8–3.   Overview of bipolar monotherapy maintenance studies, numbers needed to treat (NNT), and relapse/recurrence rates.

Data from contemporary registration studies (*left*) and other studies (*right*). Approved treatments have single-digit NNTs (*left*). Divalproex is an unapproved treatment with a single-digit NNT. Lithium data from the lamotrigine registration studies (*left*) suggest less robust efficacy than pooled data from early lithium trials (*right*). ARI=aripiprazole; DVXP=divalproex; Li=lithium; LTG=lamotrigine; OLZ=olanzapine; PBO=placebo.

Source.   Data from Bowden et al. 2000; Goodwin and Jamison 1990; Goodwin et al. 2004; Keck et al. 2005; Tohen et al. 2005, 2006.

TABLE 8–2.   Numbers needed to treat (NNT) in bipolar maintenance

	Episode prevention	Mania prevention	Depression prevention
Mood stabilizers			
Lithium[a]	7	8	49
Divalproex[b]	8	22	11
Lamotrigine[a]	9	23	15
Second-generation antipsychotics			
Olanzapine[c]	3	5	12
Aripiprazole[d]	6	6	64
Quetiapine+lithium/divalproex[e]*	4	8	6

Note.   Italics indicate drug name for approved longer-term treatments. Noteworthy (single-digit) NNT are indicated in **boldface**.
*Compared with lithium/divalproex monotherapy.
[a]Goodwin et al. 2004.
[b]Bowden et al. 2000.
[c]Tohen et al. 2006.
[d]Keck et al. 2006.
[e]Suppes et al. 2008; Vieta et al. 2008.

nia and depression prevention, suggesting that it may have a balanced bimodal stabilizing action, consistent with it having acute indications for both mania and bipolar depression.

Balancing benefit and risk is arguably even more crucial during the maintenance treatment phase than during the acute treatment phase because of longer duration of the phase and the absence of an acute episode to provide motivation for adherence. Thus, clinicians need to integrate the efficacy data in Figure 8–3 and Table 8–2 with safety and tolerability data, as described later in this chapter.

Interventions for the longer-term treatment of bipolar disorders are reviewed later using the four-tier system presented in Table 8–3. This system is a hybrid approach, combining evidence-based medical information regarding efficacy and tolerability, with more empirical constructs such as familiarity and patient acceptability, to prioritize treatments in a fashion broadly consistent with North American clinical practice and treatment guidelines.

Tier I treatment options have FDA approval for the longer-term treatment of bipolar disorders and are supported by the most compelling evidence of efficacy. However, tolerability limitations of at least some Tier I treatments may

TABLE 8–3. A four-tier approach to the longer-term management of bipolar disorder

Tier	Priority	Name	Treatment options
I	High	Approved	Mood stabilizers: Lithium, lamotrigine
			Second-generation antipsychotics: olanzapine, aripiprazole, quetiapine (adjunctive)
II	High	High-priority unapproved	Other mood stabilizers: divalproex
III	Intermediate	Other	Other mood stabilizers: carbamazepine
			Other second-generation antipsychotics: olanzapine plus fluoxetine, risperidone, ziprasidone, clozapine
			Adjunctive antidepressants
			Adjunctive psychotherapy: psychoeducation, cognitive-behavioral therapy, family-focused therapy, interpersonal and social rhythm therapy
IV	Low	Novel adjuncts	Electroconvulsive therapy
			Vagus nerve stimulation

lead clinicians and patients, after comparing the risks and benefits, to consider treatments in other tiers, particularly Tier II. Indeed, in clinical practice and in some treatment guidelines, some Tier I treatments (e.g., aripiprazole) have been considered to have equal or even lower priority than some Tier II options (e.g., divalproex) (Suppes et al. 2005; Yatham et al. 2006).

Tier II treatment options lack FDA approval for the treatment of acute bipolar depression and have less compelling evidence of efficacy than Tier I options but arguably have mitigating advantages such as tolerability, familiarity, or acute indications that might make them attractive for a substantial number of patients. In clinical practice and in some treatment guidelines, some of these medications (e.g., divalproex) have been considered first-line interventions in spite of the absence of FDA indications for longer-term treatment of bipolar disorders.

Tier III treatment options lack FDA approval for the longer-term treatment of bipolar disorders and have even less compelling evidence of efficacy than Tier I or II options. In general, treatment guidelines do not consider these modalities to be first-line interventions but cite them as intermediate-priority options.

However, some Tier III options have mitigating advantages such as tolerability, familiarity, or acute indications that might make them attractive for selected patients, and in certain circumstances some of these interventions may be considered early on (e.g., psychotherapy in pregnant women). For some of these treatments (e.g., adjunctive psychotherapy), advances in research, familiarity, and/or availability may ultimately be sufficient to merit their consideration for placement in higher tiers.

Tier IV treatment options lack FDA approval for the longer-term treatment of bipolar disorders and have even more limited evidence of efficacy than Tier I, II, or III options. In general, treatment guidelines consider these modalities to be low-priority interventions. Nevertheless, some Tier IV options could prove attractive for carefully selected patients after consideration of Tier I–III treatments (e.g., patients treatment resistant or intolerant to Tier I–III treatments). For some of these treatments, advances in research ultimately may provide sufficient evidence to merit their consideration for placement in higher tiers.

Tier I: Approved Longer-Term Treatment Options for Bipolar Disorder

The approved longer-term treatments for bipolar disorders are the mood stabilizers lithium and lamotrigine and the second-generation antipsychotics olanzapine as monotherapy, aripiprazole as monotherapy, and quetiapine and quetiapine XR as adjunctive (added to lithium or divalproex) therapy. As noted previously and described in greater detail later in this chapter, these options have favorable efficacy (single-digit NNT; Figure 8–3, left), although some may also have safety/tolerability challenges. Thus, tolerability limitations of some Tier I treatments may lead clinicians and patients, after comparing the risks and benefits, to consider treatments in other tiers, particularly Tier II. This section begins with a description of clinical implications of aspects of the U.S. prescribing information for agents approved for the longer-term treatment for bipolar disorders and is followed by more detailed discussions of the individual approved agents.

Clinical Implications of U.S. Prescribing Information for Longer-Term Treatments for Bipolar Disorders

For many drugs, the U.S. prescribing information is complex and in certain instances challenging to interpret clinically. This is particularly the case for medications indicated for the longer-term treatment of bipolar disorders.

In the case of lithium, the information was relatively straightforward, representing approval to use the medicine to prevent or diminish intensity of subsequent episodes during the maintenance treatment phase, with no specific time limit. However, later approvals for additional agents became more complex.

For lamotrigine, the information indicated approval to use the medicine to delay the time to occurrence (rather than prevent or diminish intensity) of mood episodes during the maintenance treatment phase but noted that for periods extending beyond 18 months, clinicians should periodically reevaluate long-term usefulness for individual patients.

For the second-generation antipsychotic olanzapine, the information is particularly noteworthy because the approval did not specify the nature of the benefit, leaving open the possibility that the benefit was to prevent relapse back into the index episode. Moreover, the information cited the 2-week minimum duration of prerandomization open stability rather than the 12-month duration of the randomized double-blind, placebo-controlled phase of the registration trial. Thus, taken together, the information appeared to more resemble approval for the continuation treatment phase than the maintenance treatment phase.

For the second-generation antipsychotic aripiprazole, the information cited the 6-week minimum duration of prerandomization open stability, rather than the 12-week mean actual duration of prerandomization open stability or the 6-month duration of the randomized double-blind, placebo-controlled phase of the registration trial, appearing to more resemble approval for the continuation treatment phase than the maintenance treatment phase.

For the second-generation antipsychotic quetiapine (both immediate-release and extended release), the information was relatively straightforward, representing approval to use the medicine as maintenance in bipolar I disorder as adjunct therapy to lithium or divalproex, with no specific time limit. Thus, the information appeared to resemble approval for the maintenance treatment phase.

Mood Stabilizers

Mood stabilizers are considered foundational agents in the treatment of bipolar disorders. Two of these agents, lithium and lamotrigine, have been approved for the longer-term treatment of bipolar disorders. These agents appear to have distinctive and in some ways complementary efficacy and tolerability profiles. Lithium provides more robust prevention of mood elevation than depression and has an indication for acute mania but has some tolerability limitations.

Lamotrigine provides more robust prevention of depression than mood elevation and generally has very good tolerability but lacks an acute bipolar disorder
indication.

Lithium

Lithium received FDA approval for the monotherapy treatment of manic episodes of manic-depressive illness in 1970. In 1974 it became the first medication
approved for the longer-term treatment of bipolar disorders, and it remains the
best-established agent for this indication. However, in 2008, quetiapine and
quetiapine XR received adjunctive (added to lithium or divalproex) maintenance indications, as discussed in the section on adjunctive quetiapine in this
chapter. The U.S. prescribing information for lithium states in the Indication section: "Maintenance therapy prevents or diminishes the intensity of subsequent
episodes in those manic-depressive patients with a history of mania." This information differs from that of subsequently approved longer-term monotherapies because it does not mention any specific treatment duration.

The majority of the lithium maintenance trials were performed in the 1970s
(Figure 8–4). These early studies indicated robust preventive effects, with approximately two-thirds of patients taking lithium being relapse free.

Thus, in these early studies, as reviewed by Goodwin and Jamison (1990),
lithium was robustly superior to placebo (pooled NNT for overall prevention of
3), with 9 of 10 trials involving a total of 514 patients primarily after manic/
mixed episodes being positive (Baastrup et al. 1970; Coppen et al. 1971, 1973;
Cundall et al. 1972; Dunner et al. 1976c; Fieve et al. 1976; Melia 1970; Prien et al.
1973a, 1973b; Quitkin et al. 1978; Stallone et al. 1973). The sole negative trial
involved only seven patients taking lithium (Melia 1970). These trials suggested
impressive bimodal efficacy for lithium, with somewhat more robust efficacy in
preventing manic (NNT=3) compared with depressive (NNT=7) episodes.

Multiple reports from the 1980s and 1990s suggested that the effectiveness
of lithium maintenance was less robust in clinical settings compared with its efficacy in randomized trials (Dickson and Kendell 1986; Guscott and Taylor
1994; Harrow et al. 1990; Licht et al. 2001; Markar and Mander 1989; Silverstone et al. 1998), with approximately only one-third of patients maintained on
lithium having optimal symptomatic and functional outcomes (Harrow et al.
1990; Maj et al. 1998; O'Connell et al. 1991). This phenomenon may have been
driven by an efficacy-effectiveness gap for lithium maintenance because treatment of clinical patients is more complex than that for research patients (Dickson and Kendell 1986; Harrow et al. 1990; Licht et al. 2001; Markar and Mander

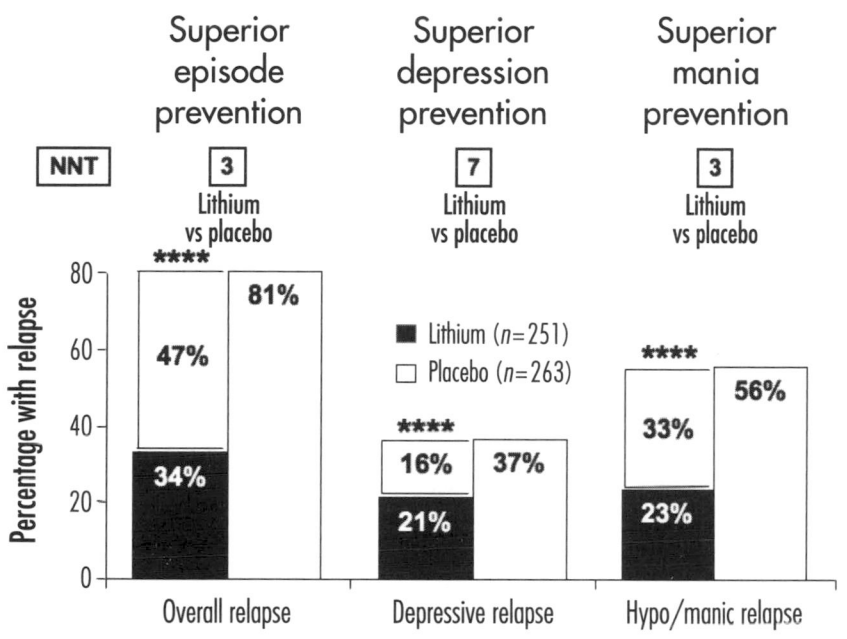

Fiαure 8–4. Summary of 10 double-blind lithium monotherapy versus placebo maintenance trials from the 1970s, numbers needed to treat (NNT), and relapse rates.

Lithium monotherapy (black bars) was superior to placebo monotherapy (white bars) in 9/10 placebo-controlled studies (involving 499/514 patients) that were primarily conducted after manic/mixed episodes. ****$P<0.0001$, versus placebo.

Source. Data from Goodwin and Jamison 1990, pp. 688–689.

1989). It was also suggested that early lithium maintenance trials were confounded by withdrawal effects because of rapid lithium discontinuation in placebo groups (Moncrieff 1995). Poor adherence was also cited as an important contributor to lithium maintenance clinical utility limitations (Guscott and Taylor 1994). Indeed, in one report in 1,594 health maintenance organization members the mean duration of lithium therapy was only 72 days (Johnson and McFarland 1996).

In contrast, a review of 11 controlled and 13 open longer-term lithium studies published between 1970 and 1996, as well as a retrospective review of 360 adherent patients without substance use disorder comorbidity who attended a Sardinian lithium clinic (that used minimal antidepressants) for at least 1 year (mean 4.6 years), suggested that lithium efficacy and effectiveness had been stable over that time period (Baldessarini and Tondo 2000). Also, in a 1-year U.S. multicenter, randomized open maintenance trial, adding lithium to treatment as usual was as effective as adding divalproex to treatment as usual in controlling mood symptoms (Revicki et al. 2005).

Subsequent randomized controlled trials also confirmed that lithium was effective in the longer-term treatment of bipolar disorder, although the findings were less robust than in early trials. Multiple factors may have contributed to this phenomenon, including more inclusive entry criteria that permitted patients with lithium-resistant illness (e.g., rapid cyclers), advances in clinical trials methodology, and potential bias (e.g., using a sample enriched for lamotrigine response in the registration studies for that agent).

Thus, the results of a recent meta-analysis (Geddes et al. 2004) involving newer (Bowden et al. 2000, 2003; Calabrese et al. 2003) as well as older (Kane et al. 1982; Prien et al. 1973a) trials were less robust, with lithium superior to placebo (pooled NNT for overall prevention of 5), with 4/5 trials involving 770 patients being positive. The sole negative trial was also negative for divalproex (Bowden et al. 2000). These trials suggested lithium had somewhat more robust efficacy in preventing manic (NNT=11) compared with depressive (NNT=14) episodes, with the response in depressive episodes just failing to attain statistical significance (Figure 8–5).

In three of these trials, which are discussed in greater detail in the lamotrigine and divalproex sections later in this chapter, lithium was an active comparator. Thus, lithium was superior to placebo for delaying overall relapse and manic relapse in two lamotrigine registration trials enriched for acute lamotrigine efficacy and tolerability (Bowden et al. 2003; Calabrese et al. 2003), whereas lithium and divalproex were no better than placebo on the primary outcome measure in a study that appeared to fail because of methodological limitations (Bowden et al. 2000).

Lithium maintenance was also assessed in additional active comparator maintenance studies that lacked placebo arms, which are discussed in greater detail in the olanzapine and carbamazepine sections later in this chapter.

For example, in one maintenance study in patients lacking a history of lithium or olanzapine resistance, these medications had comparable overall maintenance efficacy, although olanzapine appeared superior to lithium for mania prevention (Tohen et al. 2005). Also, in another maintenance trial, lithium was superior to carbamazepine overall (Greil et al. 1997), with the benefit driven by marked superiority in patients with a "classical" subtype (bipolar I without mood-incongruent delusions and without comorbidity), which overshadowed

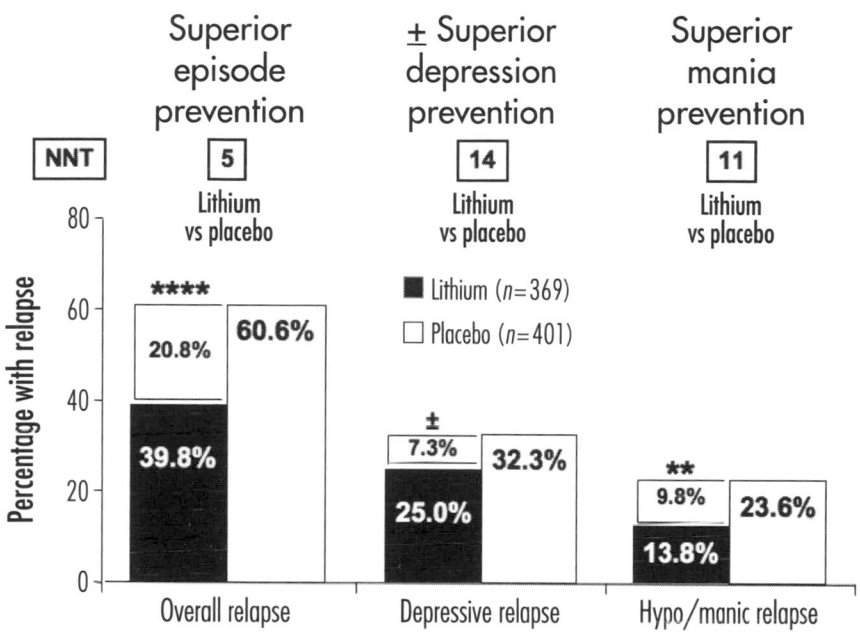

FIGURE 8–5.   Meta-analysis of five double-blind lithium monotherapy versus placebo maintenance trials between 1973 and 2003, numbers needed to treat (NNT), and relapse rates.

Lithium monotherapy (black bars) was superior to placebo monotherapy (white bars) in 4/5 controlled studies that were mostly conducted after manic/mixed episodes. $\pm P=0.063$; $**P<0.01$, $****P<0.0001$, versus placebo.

Source.   Data from Geddes et al. 2004.

a trend toward inferiority in patients with a "nonclassical" subtype (bipolar II/ not otherwise specified [NOS], mood-incongruent delusions, comorbidity) (Greil et al. 1998).

Based on having more robust effects in acute mania as compared with acute depression, it might be expected that lithium could also have more robust effects in the prevention of mania as compared with the prevention of depression. Indeed, this is consistent with an NNT analysis of 10 early lithium maintenance trials summarized by Goodwin and Jamison (1990) (Figure 8–4), a meta-analysis of five double-blind lithium monotherapy–versus–placebo maintenance trials between 1973 and 2003 (Geddes et al. 2004) (Figure 8–5), and in separate pooled analysis of lithium as an active comparator in the lamotrigine registration trials (Goodwin et al. 2004), described in the following section. Taken together, these

data indicate that lithium has more robust preventive efficacy for mania compared with depression.

This finding has been challenged (Goodwin and Jamison 2007), based on
two of the trials in the above meta-analysis being enriched for lamotrigine response (Bowden et al. 2003; Calabrese et al. 2003), and a "vote counting" analysis
of individual older studies (of varying quality). Thus, older studies mostly found
indeterminate (Fieve et al. 1976; Stallone et al. 1973), similar (Baastrup et al. 1970;
Berghofer et al. 1996; Coppen et al. 1973; Prien et al. 1973a, 1973b; Tondo et al.
1998a), or even better (Poole et al. 1978; Rybakowski et al. 1980), but only occasionally worse (Cundall et al. 1972; Dunner et al. 1976a), prevention of depression, compared with mania with lithium. Interpretation of such data is limited
by the varying quality of the studies, and the tendency of vote counting of underpowered studies to miss significant differences that can be detected in meta-
analysis.

Curiously, in a multicenter divalproex maintenance study, lithium as an active comparator (as well as the primary study drug divalproex) had a lower
NNT for depression prevention compared with mania prevention (Bowden et
al. 2000). However, as noted later in this chapter, this study had methodological
limitations and failed in the sense that both lithium and divalproex failed to separate from placebo on the primary outcome measure.

Lithium maintenance treatment may decrease suicidality (suicide attempts
and completed suicides). Thus, lithium (mean duration 6.4 years) use in a mood
disorder clinic was associated with a significantly lower incidence of suicidality
in patients with bipolar disorder followed for a total of over 5,200 patient-years
(Tondo et al. 1998b). Naturalistic lithium discontinuation yielded a rebound
increase in suicidality during the following year, which was greater than either
the period prior to initiation of lithium treatment or the subsequent period after the first year following discontinuation. In another study, Goodwin et al. (2003)
found that the risk of suicide was lower with lithium compared with divalproex
in over 20,000 patients with bipolar disorder.

Taken together, this information suggests that lithium remains an efficacious maintenance treatment for patients with bipolar disorders but is somewhat less effective in preventing depression compared with mania and in clinical
populations, in which the major unmet need is for well-tolerated maintenance
treatments that adequately address the depressive component of bipolar disorder. Indeed, this may have contributed to lamotrigine overtaking lithium as the
most prescribed mood stabilizer in the United States.

Despite limitations in groups of patients, it became clear that specific individuals had excellent responses. Thus, clinical markers of lithium acute and prophylactic responses have been extensively explored. For example, lithium responsiveness has been associated with euphoric mania (Bowden et al. 1994; Keller et al. 1986; Prien et al. 1988; Secunda et al. 1985), classical subtype (bipolar I without mood-incongruent delusions and without comorbidity) (Greil et al. 1998), an episode sequence of mania followed by depression followed by well interval (Maj et al. 1989), fewer prior episodes (Gelenberg et al. 1989; Swann et al. 2000), complete recovery between episodes (Grof et al. 1993), a personal history of lithium response (Bowden et al. 1994; Tondo et al. 1997), and a family history of bipolar disorder or lithium response (Maj et al. 1984; Mendlewicz et al. 1973).

In contrast, rapid cycling (Dunner and Fieve 1974; Dunner et al. 1976b; Goodnick et al. 1987; Maj et al. 1998; Okuma 1993), dysphoric manic or mixed episodes (Bowden et al. 1994, 2005; Keller et al. 1986; Prien et al. 1988; Secunda et al. 1985; Swann et al. 1997), a history of at least three prior episodes (Gelenberg et al. 1989; Swann et al. 2000), nonclassical subtype (bipolar II/NOS, mood-incongruent delusions, comorbidity) (Greil et al. 1998), episode sequence of depression followed by mania followed by well interval (Maj et al. 1989), severe mania (Garfinkel et al. 1980; Swann et al. 1986), and secondary mania (Himmelhoch and Garfinkel 1986; Kahn et al. 1988; Sovner 1989; Stoll et al. 1994) portend poorer responses to lithium. Adolescents (Carlson et al. 1977; Strober et al. 1988) and patients with comorbid substance abuse (Pond et al. 1981), or a personal history of nonresponse to lithium (Bowden et al. 1994) are also less likely to do well on lithium. Also, occasionally, patients stabilized on lithium for extended periods of time may become lithium resistant after discontinuing the agent and then suffering a relapse (Maj et al. 1995; Post et al. 1992).

However, there is substantial variability in research methodology and findings regarding clinical markers of lithium responsiveness. A recent very conservative meta-analysis found only a few strongly suggestive clinical markers of lithium prophylactic responsiveness (Kleindienst et al. 2005) (Table 8–4, top).

Better responses were associated with 1) later onset (10 studies, 1,138 patients) (Coryell et al. 2000; Dunner and Fieve 1974; Kato et al. 2000; Maj et al. 1986; Okuma 1993; Sarantidis and Waters 1981; Schurhoff et al. 2000; Tondo et al. 2001; Yang 1985; Yazici et al. 1999) and 2) episode sequence of mania then depression then well interval (seven studies, 904 patients) (Faedda et al. 1991; Grof et al. 1987; Haag et al. 1986; Kukopulos and Reginaldi 1980; Kukopulos et al. 1980; Maj 1990; Maj et al. 1989; Okuma 1993; Tondo et al. 2001).

TABLE 8–4. Potential clinical markers of lithium maintenance response

Marker	Better response	Poorer response
Confirmed by meta-analysis		
Onset age	Later	Earlier
Number of hospitalizations	Lower	Higher
Episode sequence	Mania-depression-interval	Depression-mania-interval
Episode pattern	Noncontinuous	Continuous
Not confirmed by meta-analysis		
Bipolar subtype (I versus II)	No difference	No difference
Illness duration	Shorter	Longer
Index episode polarity	Manic	Mixed
Index episode severity	Less severe	More severe
Index episode psychosis	Nonpsychotic	Psychotic
Index episode psychosis	Mood-congruent	Mood-incongruent
Number of prior episodes	Fewer	More
Episode type	Monophasic	Biphasic, multiphasic
Episode frequency	Lower/non–rapid cycling	Higher/rapid cycling
Comorbid alcohol/substance abuse	Absent	Present
Comorbid personality disorder	Absent	Present
Not tested with meta-analysis		
Family history of bipolar disorder	Positive	Negative
Remission completeness	Subsyndromal symptoms	No subsyndromal symptoms

Source. Adapted from Kleindienst et al. 2005.

Poorer responses were associated with 1) episode sequence of depression, then mania, then well interval (eight studies, 1,151 patients) (Maj et al. 1998; see also studies cited in paragraph above, first point), 2) a continuous-cycling pattern (the frequent absence of well intervals between episodes; four studies, 404 patients) (Faedda et al. 1991; Haag et al. 1986; Maj 1990; Maj et al. 1989), and 3) more prior hospitalizations (four studies, 677 patients) (Maj et al. 1996, 1998; O'Connell et al. 1991; Yazici et al. 1999).

In contrast, 37 other potential clinical markers of lithium prophylactic response were not confirmed (Kleindienst et al. 2005). These included several of considerable interest such as bipolar subtype, illness duration, index episode features, number of prior episodes, rapid cycling, and alcohol/substance use disorder and personality disorder comorbidities. Some important markers that were not assessed were family history of bipolar disorder, family history of lithium response, and degree of remission between episodes.

The U.S. prescribing information includes a boxed warning that lithium toxicity is closely related to serum lithium concentrations and can occur at dosages yielding close to therapeutic levels. Common dosage-related adverse effects with lithium include renal (polyuria, polydipsia), metabolic (weight gain), central nervous system (CNS) (sedation, tremor, ataxia, lethargy, decreased coordination, and cognitive problems), gastrointestinal (nausea, vomiting, diarrhea), and dermatological (hair loss, acne) problems, and edema (Gelenberg 1988). Lithium-induced CNS adverse effects can be important reasons for poor adherence (Gitlin et al. 1989). Thus, other mood stabilizers such as divalproex and particularly lamotrigine may be better tolerated than lithium. In contrast, lithium may have a favorable adverse effect profile compared with antipsychotics such as olanzapine, aripiprazole, and quetiapine. Lithium has noteworthy drug interactions with medications that affect its renal excretion. Additional information regarding lithium is provided in Chapter 13 of this volume, "Mood Stabilizers and Antipsychotics."

Despite the extensive clinical trials data regarding the efficacy of lithium maintenance treatment, there remains uncertainty regarding optimal serum concentrations. This is a particularly crucial issue because poor outcomes are related to nonadherence, which is related to adverse effects, which in turn are related to higher serum concentrations.

In an influential U.S. randomized, double-blind, controlled study, longer-term treatment with lithium with serum concentrations of 0.8–1.0 mEq/L compared with 0.4–0.6 mEq/L was more poorly tolerated but more effective at preventing syndromal relapse (Gelenberg et al. 1989) as well as subsyndromal symptoms and their progression to syndromal relapse (Keller et al. 1992), yielding better functional outcome primarily through relapse prevention (Solomon et al. 1996). However, a subsequent reanalysis of these data found that inefficacy with lower serum concentrations was primarily in individuals who had previously required higher serum concentrations (Perlis et al. 2002). In contemporary randomized controlled maintenance studies (which may emphasize efficacy), mean serum lithium concentrations have tended to be in the 0.8–1.0 mEq/L range (Bowden et al. 2000; Calabrese et al. 2003; Tohen et al. 2005). A recent review suggested that lithium serum concentrations between 0.8 and 1.2 mEq/L yield more robust mania prevention but more adverse effects, whereas concentrations between 0.5 and 0.8 mEq/L may yield similar overall prevention and possibly superior depression prevention as well as better tolerability (Severus et al. 2008). This review emphasized the importance of individualizing dosage based on efficacy and tolerability, and suggested that optimal initial maintenance target serum concentrations ranged between 0.6 and 0.8 mEq/L.

The U.S. prescribing information for lithium recommends targeting serum lithium concentrations for maintenance therapy of 0.6–1.2 mEq/L, which are usually achieved with divided dosages totaling 900–1,200 mg/day. These are substantially lower than the 1.0–1.5 mEq/L concentrations with a dosage of 1,800 mg/day recommended for acute mania. In euthymic or depressed bipolar disorder outpatients, lithium commonly is started at 300 mg/day taken at bedtime. Because lithium has a half-life of approximately 1 day, the dosage may be increased every 3–5 days in 300-mg/day increments as necessary and tolerated. Clinicians and patients commonly endeavor to have most of, or, if possible, the entire, lithium dose taken at bedtime to enhance convenience and to have peak lithium serum concentrations and hence the major burden of adverse effects occur during sleep. Twelve-hour trough serum lithium concentrations may be checked upon reaching 900 mg/day for 5 days, initially targeting 0.8 mEq/L. However, in patients who fail to tolerate 0.8 mEq/L, lithium serum concentrations as low as 0.5–0.6 mEq/L may still yield benefit, particularly if lithium is combined with other medications.

In summary, lithium is the traditional bipolar disorder maintenance treatment option and appears to provide more robust prevention of mania compared with depression. Although adverse effects with this agent may be challenging, conservative dosing can enhance tolerability. Clinicians and patients may deem this agent to have inferior tolerability compared with lamotrigine and divalproex but superior tolerability compared with antipsychotics.

Lamotrigine

In 2003, lamotrigine became the second medication approved by the FDA for the longer-term treatment of bipolar disorders, and by 2006, despite lacking an acute indication, was the most commonly prescribed mood stabilizer. The U.S. prescribing information for lamotrigine states the following in the Indication section:

> [Lamotrigine] is indicated for the maintenance treatment of bipolar I disorder to delay the time to occurrence of mood episodes (depression, mania, hypomania, mixed episodes) in patients treated for acute episodes with standard therapy.... The physician who elects to use [lamotrigine] for periods extending beyond 18 months should periodically reevaluate the long-term usefulness of the drug for the individual patient.

And in the Clinical Studies section it states:

> [B]enefit for [lamotrigine] over placebo in delaying the time to occurrence of both depression and mania, although the finding was more robust for depression.

This information substantively differed from that for lithium in that it 1) mentioned a specific treatment duration (18 months, the duration of the randomized double-blind, placebo-controlled stages of the registration trials) after which clinicians should periodically reevaluate usefulness, 2) claimed that lamotrigine "delay[ed] the time to occurrence" rather than "prevent[ed] or diminish[ed] the intensity" of mood episodes, and 3) acknowledged particular benefit with respect to delaying depressive recurrences.

The two 18-month, multicenter, double-blind, placebo-controlled and lithium-controlled lamotrigine maintenance therapy registration studies had several innovative features compared with prior longer-term treatment studies. Thus, there were two separate but similarly designed studies, one after recent mood elevation episodes (Bowden et al. 2003) and, importantly, one after depressive episodes (Calabrese et al. 2003). The latter type of data, although critically important, to that date had been very seldom encountered. The similar study designs facilitated a planned pooled analysis (Goodwin et al. 2004). In these studies, the samples were enriched for lamotrigine response. Thus, in the 8- to 16-week open stabilization stage, patients were transitioned from prior medication(s) to lamotrigine monotherapy, on which they needed to remain stable (Clinical Global Impression [CGI] severity score≤3) for 4 continuous weeks prior to randomization, at which point they were assigned to lamotrigine, lithium, or placebo. The studies had the same primary outcome measure, time to intervention caused by an impending mood episode rather than relapse/recurrence defined by emergence of a syndromal episode.

Because the results of the two lamotrigine maintenance registration studies were similar (Bowden et al. 2003; Calabrese et al. 2003), the results of the planned pooled analyses are presented (Goodwin et al. 2004).

On the time-to-event–based primary outcome measure (time to intervention for any mood episode), lamotrigine and lithium were superior to placebo and did not differ from one another. On the polarity-specific time-to-event–based secondary outcome measures, lamotrigine (but not lithium) was superior to placebo for time to intervention for depression, whereas lamotrigine and lithium were both superior to placebo for time to intervention for mania. Lamotrigine was equivalent to lithium for delaying depression, whereas lithium was superior to lamotrigine for delaying mania. Thus, lithium demonstrated efficacy in overall episode and manic episode prevention despite the sample being enriched for lamotrigine acute tolerability and efficacy.

On additional secondary event-based outcome measures (i.e., relapse rates), the findings were less robust but had the same pattern. Lamotrigine was superior to placebo for overall episode prevention (NNT=9), with the benefit driven by depression prevention (NNT=15) (Figure 8–6, black bars). Lithium was superior to placebo for overall episode prevention (NNT=7), with the benefit driven by mania prevention (NNT=8) (Figure 8–6, gray bars).

Adverse event discontinuation rates were 8.2% with lamotrigine, 18% with lithium, and 7.9% with placebo, with the rate with lithium being significantly higher than with lamotrigine or placebo (Figure 8–7, middle). Thus, compared with placebo, the NNH for adverse event discontinuation with lamotrigine was 313 and with lithium was 10. Lithium (but not lamotrigine) yielded higher rates of nausea, diarrhea, tremor, and somnolence compared with placebo.

In addition, at 52 weeks lithium yielded significant weight gain compared with lamotrigine because the mean changes in weight were −1.2 kg with lamotrigine, +2.2 kg with lithium, and +0.2 kg with placebo (Sachs et al. 2006). These differences were primarily occurring in the 155 obese patients, in whom mean changes in weight were −4.2 kg with lamotrigine, +6.1 with lithium, and −0.6 kg with placebo (Bowden et al. 2006). However, the incidence of clinically significant (≥7%) weight gain at 52 weeks was statistically similar with lamotrigine (10.9%), lithium (11.8%), and placebo (7.6%) (Figure 8–7, right) (Sachs et al. 2006).

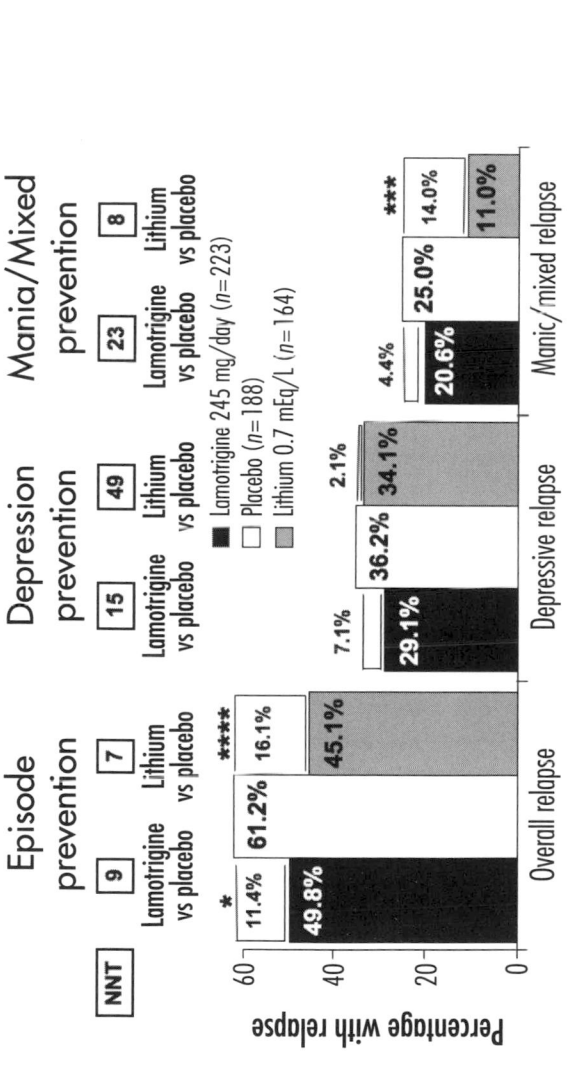

FIGURE 8–6. Comparison of 18-month double-blind lamotrigine monotherapy versus lithium monotherapy versus placebo maintenance, numbers needed to treat (NNT), and relapse rates.

Lamotrigine monotherapy (black bars) and lithium monotherapy (gray bars) were superior to placebo monotherapy (white bars) in pooled data from two controlled studies that were conducted after manic/mixed and depressive episodes, respectively. *$P<0.05$; ***$P<0.001$; ****$P<0.0001$ versus placebo.

Source. Data from Goodwin et al. 2004.

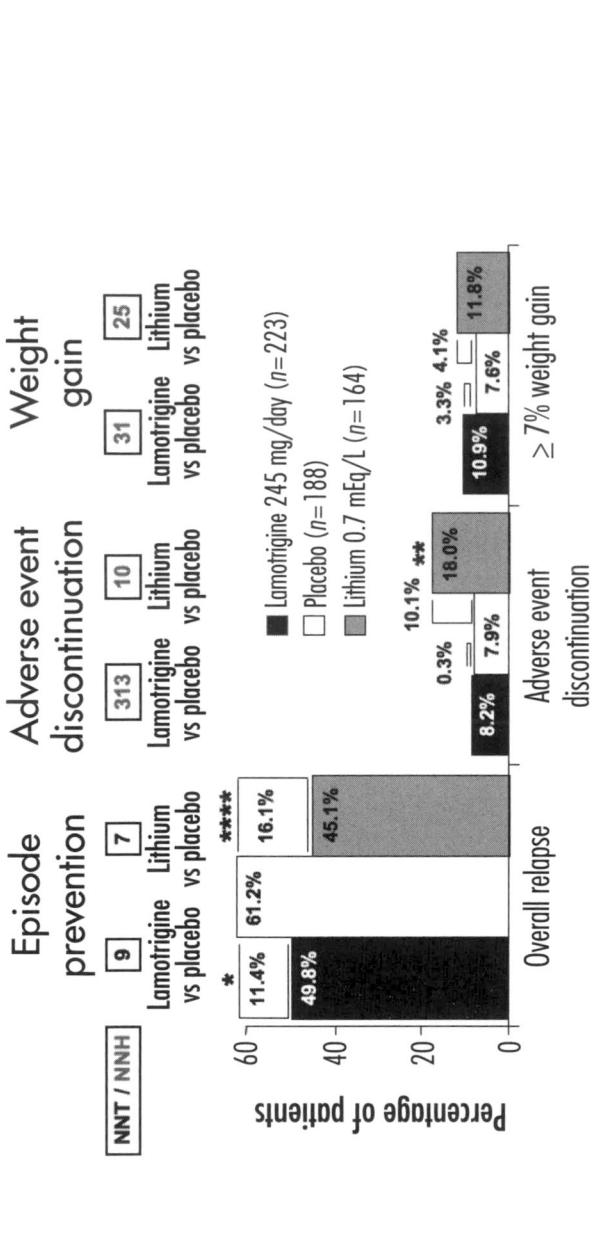

Figure 8–7.   Comparison of 18-month double-blind lamotrigine monotherapy versus lithium monotherapy versus placebo maintenance, numbers needed to treat (NNT), numbers needed to harm (NNH), and relapse, adverse event discontinuation, and weight gain rates.

Lamotrigine monotherapy (black bars) compared with lithium monotherapy (gray bars) was similarly effective but better tolerated. *P<0.05; **P<0.01; ****P<0.0001, versus placebo.

Source.   Data from Goodwin et al. 2004.

In the open stabilization stage, the incidence of any rash was 0.8% (11/1,305), which included two noteworthy rashes. One was a case of Stevens-Johnson syndrome classified as nonserious because it did not require hospitalization, and the other was a case of severe maculopapular nonpruritic facial rash classified as serious because it did require hospitalization. Both resolved uneventfully with lamotrigine discontinuation. In the randomized controlled stage, the incidence of rash was 5% with lamotrigine, 7% with lithium, and 5% with placebo.

There are limited data regarding baseline markers of lamotrigine maintenance response. Baseline markers of lamotrigine compared with lithium response appear in some ways overlapping and in other ways complementary.

In a post hoc analysis of the lamotrigine maintenance registration studies, in 280 patients taking lamotrigine, index mixed episodes and having 3 or more depressions in the prior 2 years increased the risk of relapse (Ketter et al. 2003). Index mixed episodes also tended to predict relapse for patients taking placebo ($n=191$), whereas illness onset before age 20 years predicted relapse for patients taking lithium ($n=167$).

Another study assessed 164 subjects from 21 families of probands with bipolar I disorder or bipolar II disorder who had maintenance treatment responses to lamotrigine ($n=7$) or lithium ($n=14$) (Passmore et al. 2003). The probands differed with respect to clinical course (rapid cycling in the lamotrigine responder group, episodic in the lithium responder group) and comorbidity (panic attacks and substance abuse in the lamotrigine responder group). The relatives of lamotrigine responders had higher prevalence of schizoaffective disorder, major depression, and panic attacks, whereas relatives of lithium responders had significantly higher risk of having bipolar disorder.

The U.S. prescribing information for lamotrigine includes a boxed warning regarding the risk of serious rashes requiring hospitalization, which have included Stevens-Johnson syndrome, in 0.08% and 0.13% of adult mood disorder patients receiving monotherapy and adjunctive therapy, respectively. In mid-2008 the FDA released an alert regarding increased risk of suicidality (suicidal behavior or ideation) in patients with epilepsy as well as psychiatric disorders for eleven anticonvulsants (including lamotrigine). Lamotrigine can cause CNS (headache, somnolence, insomnia, dizziness, tremor) and gastrointestinal (nausea, diarrhea) (Bowden et al. 2003; Calabrese et al. 1999, 2000, 2003) adverse effects. In most instances these problems attenuate or resolve with time or lamotrigine dosage adjustment, but occasionally patients may require lamotrigine discontinuation. Indeed, in view of its generally very good tolerability, clinicians and patients may prefer lamotrigine compared with other longer-term treatment options.

Lamotrigine dosage is initially titrated *very slowly* to decrease the risk of rash. When lamotrigine is given without valproate, the prescribing information recommends starting lamotrigine at 25 mg/day for 2 weeks, then increasing to 50 mg/day for the next 2 weeks, then increasing to 100 mg/day for 1 week, and then increasing to 200 mg/day in a single daily dose, with dosages exceeding 200 mg/day not recommended unless concurrent hormonal contraceptives (which decrease serum lamotrigine concentrations) are administered (*Physicians' Desk Reference* 2008). The FDA did not recommend dosages over 200 mg/day because in the registration trials 400 mg/day, although effective, was no more effective than 200 mg/day. Nevertheless, even in the absence of hormonal contraceptive, selected patients may benefit from further gradual lamotrigine titration to final dosages as high as 500 mg/day. Even more gradual titration, starting with 25 mg/day for 2 weeks, then increasing to 50 mg/day for the next 2 weeks, and then increasing as necessary and tolerated weekly by 25 mg/day, may further decrease the risk of rash (Ketter et al. 2005). When lamotrigine is added to valproate (which doubles serum lamotrigine concentrations), the previous recommended doses are halved, and when lamotrigine is given with carbamazepine (which halves serum lamotrigine concentrations), these recommended doses may be doubled. Additional information regarding lamotrigine is provided in Chapter 13 of this volume.

In summary, lamotrigine is a newer bipolar disorder maintenance treatment option with a novel pharmacological profile in that it is uncommonly well tolerated and provides more robust prevention of depression compared with mania, although it lacks an acute bipolar disorder indication. Clinicians and patients may deem this agent to have superior tolerability compared with other mood stabilizers such as divalproex as well as compared with antipsychotics and thus be an attractive treatment option.

Second-Generation Antipsychotics

Second-generation antipsychotics are commonly used in acute mania and increasingly used for other aspects of the management of bipolar disorders, including longer-term therapy.

Olanzapine

In 2004, olanzapine became the third medication approved by the FDA for the longer-term treatment of bipolar disorders. This was a significant milestone because in the past antipsychotics were considered adjuncts for the acute treatment phase rather than longer-term treatments. The U.S. prescribing information for olanzapine states the following in the Indication section:

> The benefit of maintaining bipolar patients on monotherapy with oral [olanzapine] after achieving a responder status for an average duration of two weeks was demonstrated in a controlled trial. The physician who elects to use [olanzapine] for extended periods should periodically reevaluate the long-term risks and benefits of the drug for the individual patient.

Thus, the information appeared to more resemble the continuation treatment phase than the maintenance treatment phase.

The olanzapine longer-term treatment registration trial was a multicenter, randomized, double-blind, placebo-controlled study of patients with bipolar I disorder with a recent manic or mixed episode (Tohen et al. 2006). Olanzapine was superior to placebo on the time-to-event–based primary outcome measure (time to symptomatic relapse into any episode) (Figure 8–8, left), and on the three polarity-specific time-to-event–based secondary outcome measures (time to symptomatic relapse into 1) manic episode, 2) depressive episode, and 3) mixed episode). The brief period of stability prior to randomization and the early very rapid (exponential) decline in the proportion of patients remaining well (Figure 8–8, left) raised the possibility that patients were relapsing into the index episode and that the study involved a substantial continuation treatment phase component. Excluding any relapses during the first 8 weeks in part addressed such concerns, yielding a more gradual (linear) decline in the proportion of patients remaining well (Figure 8–8, right), with olanzapine still being superior to placebo on the time to symptomatic relapse into any episode, consistent with the study also having a maintenance treatment phase component.

Olanzapine appeared to have preventive efficacy in a broad spectrum of patients. Thus, subgroup analyses revealed that time to symptomatic relapse was longer with olanzapine compared with placebo in patients with both manic and mixed index episodes, both psychotic and nonpsychotic index episodes, and with and without rapid cycling. Indeed, none of these factors appeared to influence time to relapse.

On additional secondary event-based outcome measures (i.e., relapse rates), the findings were less robust but had the same pattern. Olanzapine was superior to placebo for overall episode prevention (NNT=3), with the benefit driven by mania/mixed episode prevention (NNT=5) (Figure 8–9, black bars). Olanza-

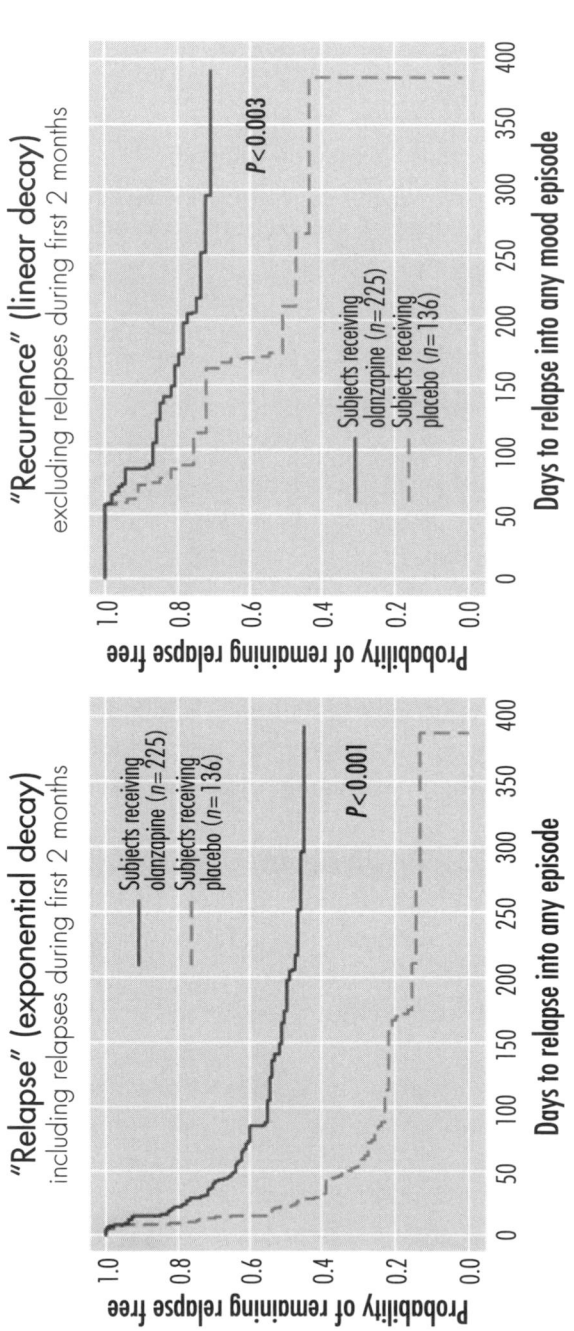

FIGURE 8–8.   Comparison of 12-month double-blind olanzapine monotherapy versus placebo maintenance.

Olanzapine compared with placebo after manic/mixed episodes was superior in the time-to-event–based analysis for overall episode prevention. Patients were stabilized on open olanzapine before randomization (mean 16.3 days). The relapse criteria were hospitalization or Young Mania Rating Scale or Hamilton Rating Scale for Depression–21 ≥15. (*Left*) Note the rapid (exponential) decrease in probability of remaining well (particularly for the placebo group), resembling the "relapse" pattern in Figure 8–2. (*Right*) Note the gradual (more linear) decrease in probability of remaining well, resembling the "recurrence" pattern in Figure 8–2.

Source.   Adapted and reproduced from Tohen M, Calabrese JR, Sachs GS, et al.: "Randomized, Placebo-Controlled Trial of Olanzapine as Maintenance Therapy in Patients With Bipolar I Disorder Responding to Acute Treatment With Olanzapine." *American Journal of Psychiatry* 163:247–256, 2006. Used with permission.

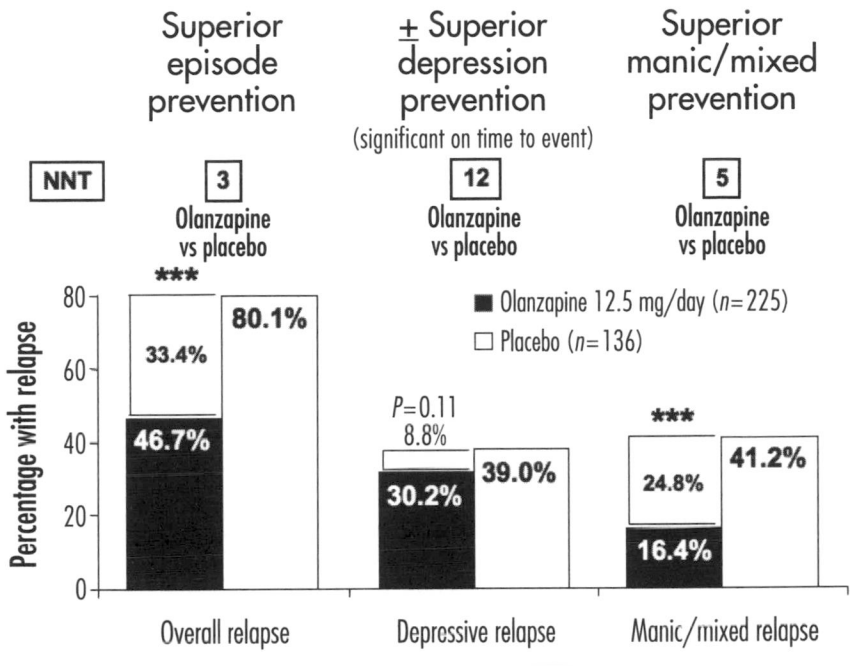

FIGURE 8–9. **Comparison of 12-month double-blind olanzapine monotherapy versus placebo maintenance, numbers needed to treat (NNT), and relapse rates.**

Olanzapine monotherapy (black bars) compared with placebo monotherapy (white bars) after manic/mixed episodes was superior in the time-to-event–based analyses for overall, depressive, and manic/mixed prevention, but in the event-based analysis in this figure failed to attain significance for prevention of depressive relapse. ***$P<0.001$, versus placebo.

Source. Data from Tohen et al. 2006.

pine was numerically but nonsignificantly superior to placebo for depressive episode prevention (NNT=12).

In the randomized controlled stage, overall tolerability with olanzapine was poorer than with placebo. Specifically, adverse event discontinuation rates were 7.6% with olanzapine and 0% with placebo (Figure 8–10, middle). Thus, compared with placebo, the NNH for adverse event discontinuation with olanzapine was 14. Mean weight change was +1 kg with olanzapine and −2 kg with placebo. Clinically significant (≥7%) weight gain was seen in 16.1% with olanzapine and 2.3% with placebo, so that the NNH for clinically significant weight gain with olanzapine compared with placebo was 8 (Figure 8–10, right). Importantly, in

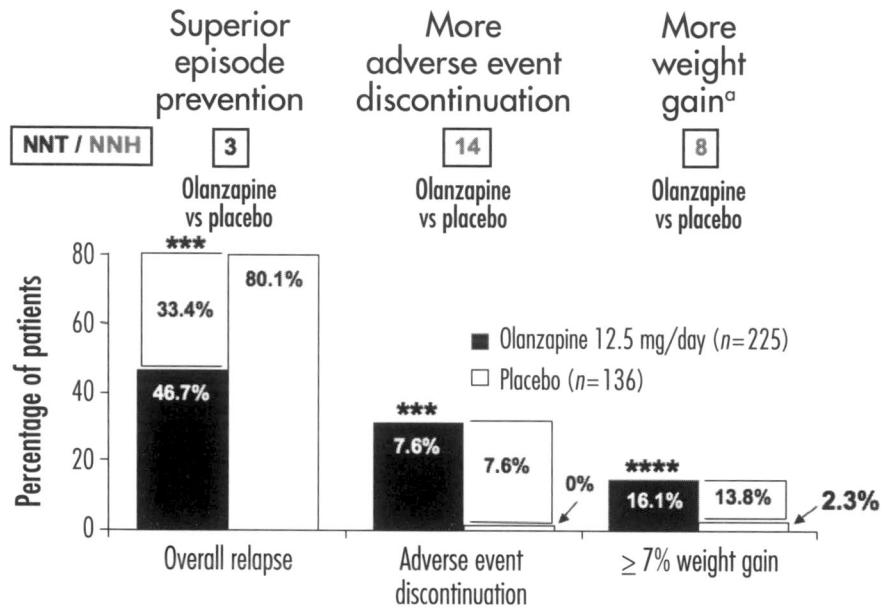

FIGURE 8–10.   Comparison of 12-month double-blind olanzapine monotherapy versus placebo maintenance, numbers needed to treat (NNT), numbers needed to harm (NNH), and relapse, adverse event discontinuation, and weight gain rates.

Olanzapine monotherapy (black bars) compared with placebo monotherapy (white bars) was more effective but more poorly tolerated. ***$P<0.001$; ****$P<0.0001$, versus placebo.
[a]But 35% of patients had a ≥7% weight gain with olanzapine during the open stabilization stage.

Source.   Data from Tohen et al. 2006.

the open stabilization stage, olanzapine yielded clinically significant weight gain in 35% of patients.

An additional 12-month, multicenter, randomized, double-blind, active-controlled study compared olanzapine and lithium in patients with bipolar I disorder with a recent manic or mixed episode and no history of intolerance or inefficacy with olanzapine or lithium (Tohen et al. 2005). Exclusion of treatment-resistant and treatment-intolerant patients yielded a sample with substantially fewer mixed index episodes and less rapid cycling than the previously mentioned olanzapine compared with placebo maintenance trial.

Thus, the randomized sample included only 6.3% with mixed episodes, 26% with psychotic index episodes, and only 3% with rapid cycling. In the randomized double-blind controlled stage either olanzapine or lithium was tapered and discontinued over 4 weeks.

Olanzapine was similar (albeit with a $P=0.07$ trend toward being superior) to lithium on the time-to-event–based primary outcome measure (time to symptomatic relapse into any episode). On the three polarity-specific time-to-event–based secondary outcome measures, olanzapine was similar to lithium for time to symptomatic relapse into depressive episodes but superior for time to symptomatic relapse into manic episodes and mixed episodes.

On additional secondary event-based outcome measures (i.e., relapse rates), the findings were less robust but had the same pattern. Olanzapine was similar (albeit with a $P=0.055$ trend toward being superior) to lithium for overall episode prevention (NNT=12) and superior for mania/mixed episode prevention (NNT=8) (Figure 8–11, black bars). Lithium was numerically but nonsignificantly superior to lithium for depressive episode prevention (NNT= 20).

In the randomized controlled stage, overall tolerability with olanzapine was similar to that of lithium. Specifically, adverse event discontinuation rates were 18.9% with olanzapine and 25.7% with lithium (Figure 8–12, middle). Thus, compared with olanzapine, the NNH for adverse event discontinuation with lithium was 15. Olanzapine compared with lithium yielded higher rates of depression and hypersomnia and lower rates of insomnia, mania, and nausea. Mean weight change was +1.8 kg with olanzapine and −1.4 kg with lithium. Clinically significant (≥7%) weight gain was seen in 29.8% with olanzapine and 9.8% with lithium, so that the NNH for clinically significant weight gain with olanzapine compared with lithium was 5 (Figure 8–12, right). Importantly, in the open stabilization phase, lithium plus olanzapine yielded clinically significant weight gain in 27.8% of patients.

In addition, two longer-term extensions of olanzapine monotherapy and combination therapy acute mania trials have been published. Because they are extensions of acute studies, these reports provide more limited data regarding recurrence (Tohen et al. 2003a, 2004b).

There are limited data regarding baseline markers of maintenance response to olanzapine. In a post hoc analysis of pooled data involving 779 patients in the previously mentioned olanzapine-versus-placebo (Tohen et al. 2006) and olanzapine-versus-lithium (Tohen et al. 2005) maintenance studies, considering all treatments collectively, earlier relapse was related to rapid-cycling course, mixed index episode, having more than one mood episode in the prior year, age at onset of 20 years or greater, having a first-degree relative with bipolar disorder, female gender, and not being hospitalized for bipolar disorder in the prior year

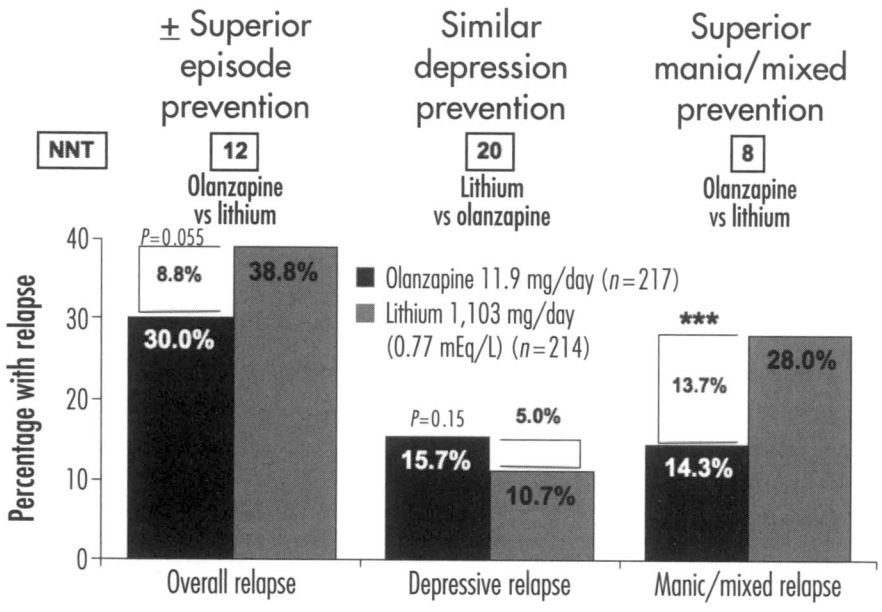

FIGURE 8–11.   Comparison of 12-month double-blind olanzapine versus lithium monotherapy maintenance, numbers needed to treat (NNT), and relapse rates.

Olanzapine monotherapy (black bars) compared with lithium monotherapy (gray bars) after manic/mixed episodes was superior for prevention of manic/mixed episodes and similar for prevention of depressive episodes. Patients were stabilized on open olanzapine plus lithium before randomization (mean 20.2 days). The relapse criteria were Young Mania Rating Scale or Hamilton Rating Scale for Depression ≥15. ***P<0.001, versus placebo.

Source.   Data from Tohen et al. 2005.

(Tohen et al. 2004a). History of rapid cycling and mixed index episode were the strongest predictors of earlier relapse. An important limitation of this study was that all treatments were considered collectively rather than individually.

The U.S. prescribing information for olanzapine includes a boxed warning regarding the increased risk of mortality (primarily cardiovascular or infectious) in elderly patients with dementia-related psychosis (a second-generation antipsychotic class warning). The FDA has stipulated changes in the olanzapine prescribing information to include a warning of the risk of hyperglycemia and diabetes mellitus. Olanzapine can also yield weight gain and cholesterol and triglyceride elevations. Other warnings in the prescribing information include the risks of cerebrovascular adverse events, including stroke, in elderly patients

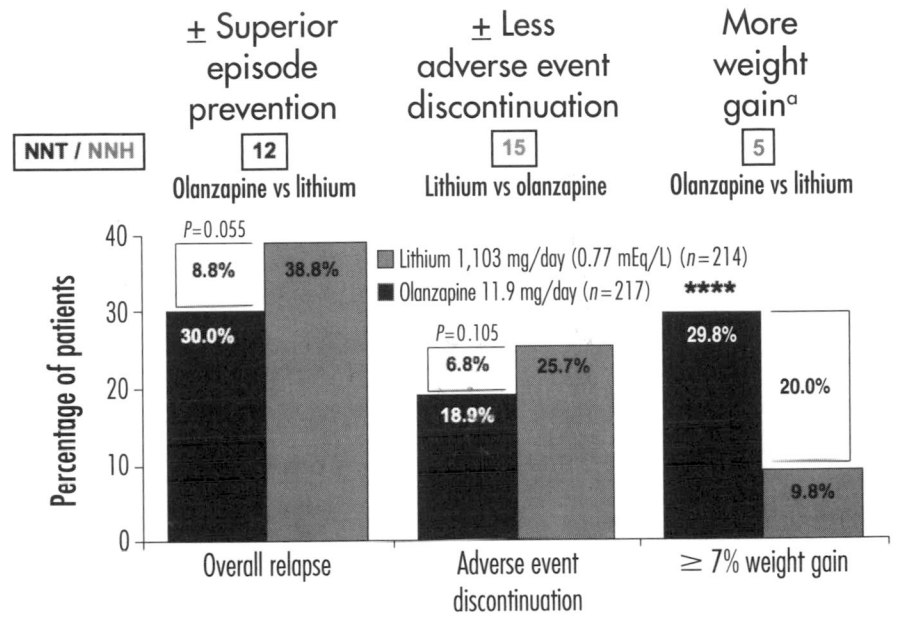

FIGURE 8–12. Comparison of 12-month double-blind olanzapine versus lithium monotherapy maintenance, numbers needed to treat (NNT), numbers needed to harm (NNH), and relapse, adverse event discontinuation, and weight gain rates.

Olanzapine monotherapy (black bars) compared with lithium monotherapy (gray bars) tended to be more effective but yielded more weight gain. ****$P<0.0001$, versus olanzapine.
[a]Importantly, in the prior open stabilization stage, the olanzapine plus lithium combination yielded clinically significant weight gain ($\geq7\%$) in 27.8% of patients.

Source. Data from Tohen et al. 2005.

with dementia-related psychosis (a warning shared with risperidone and aripiprazole); neuroleptic malignant syndrome; and tardive dyskinesia. Other adverse effects include orthostatic hypotension, syncope (in 0.6% of patients), seizures (in 0.9% of patients), hyperprolactinemia, and benign transaminase elevations (in 0.2% of patients) (Conley and Meltzer 2000).

Olanzapine has some drug-drug interactions because certain enzyme inducers such as carbamazepine can decrease and some enzyme inhibitors such as fluvoxamine may increase serum olanzapine concentrations. Additional information regarding olanzapine is provided in Chapter 13 of this volume.

The U.S. prescribing information notes that olanzapine dosages ranged between 5 mg/day and 20 mg/day in the pivotal longer-term treatment study and does not provide information regarding initiation of olanzapine in euthymic patients. Given the risk of adverse effects, it is prudent to start olanzapine in euthymic patients in a gradual fashion similar to initiation in depressed patients rather than the rapid initiation used in manic patients. In a large controlled acute bipolar depression study, olanzapine monotherapy was started at 5 mg/day and could be increased daily by 5 mg/day to as high as 20 mg/day, with a mean final dosage of 10 mg/day (Tohen et al. 2003b). As that approach yielded sedation in 28.1% of depressed bipolar patients, in order to limit adverse effects, clinicians may prefer to titrate more conservatively, starting olanzapine at 2.5 mg/day at bedtime and increasing every 4–7 days as necessary and tolerated by 2.5 mg/day, initially targeting a dosage of 12.5 mg/day (the mean dosage in the pivotal olanzapine maintenance trial) at bedtime. Patients who tolerate but fail to respond to 12.5 mg/day may benefit from continuing to gradually increase olanzapine every 4–7 days as necessary and tolerated by 2.5 mg/day to as high as 20 mg/day. Lower final dosages may be necessary in combination therapy. For example, in a controlled adjunctive olanzapine (added to lithium or divalproex) longer-term trial, the mean modal olanzapine dosage was 8.6 mg/day (Tohen et al. 2004b).

In summary, olanzapine is a newer bipolar disorder longer-term treatment option that appears to provide more robust prevention of mania compared with depression. Adverse effects with this agent may be challenging, and clinicians and patients may deem this agent to have inferior tolerability not only compared with mood stabilizers such as lamotrigine and divalproex but also compared with some other antipsychotics such as aripiprazole. Indeed, the FDA longer-term olanzapine indication appears to focus on its use in the continuation treatment phase.

Aripiprazole

Aripiprazole received FDA approval for the treatment of acute manic or mixed episodes associated with bipolar disorder as monotherapy in adults in 2004 and in children and adolescents ages 10–17 years in 2008. In 2005 aripiprazole became the fourth medication (and second antipsychotic) approved by the FDA for the longer-term treatment of bipolar disorders. The U.S. prescribing information for aripiprazole states the following in the Indication section:

> [Aripiprazole] is indicated for acute and maintenance treatment of manic and mixed episodes associated with bipolar I disorder with or without psychotic features.

In the Dosage and Administration section it states:

While it is generally agreed that treatment beyond acute response in mania is desirable, both for maintenance of the initial treatment response and for prevention of new manic episodes, there are no systematically obtained data to support the use of aripiprazole in such longer-term treatment (beyond 6 weeks). Physicians who elect to use [aripiprazole] for extended periods, that is, longer than 6 weeks, should periodically reevaluate the long-term usefulness of the drug for the individual patient.

And in the Clinical Studies section it states:

[Aripiprazole] was superior to placebo on time to and number of combined affective relapses (manic plus depressive)....There is insufficient data to know whether [aripiprazole] is effective in delaying the time to occurrence of depression in patients with bipolar I disorder.

This information appears to reflect the FDA's reservations regarding approving antipsychotics for longer-term treatment in bipolar disorders, citing the 6-week minimum duration of open stability prior to randomization rather than the 6-month duration of the randomized, double-blind, placebo-controlled phase of the registration trial.

The aripiprazole longer-term treatment registration trial was a multicenter, randomized, double-blind, placebo-controlled study of patients with bipolar I disorder with a recent manic or mixed episode (Keck et al. 2006).

Aripiprazole was superior to placebo on the time-to-event–based primary outcome measure (time to symptomatic relapse into any episode). On the polarity-specific, time-to-event–based secondary outcome measures, aripiprazole was superior to placebo for time to symptomatic relapse into manic episodes but not depressive episodes. In this study, there were relatively few patients with mixed index episodes or rapid cycling, a substantial (mean 12.7 weeks) period of prerandomization stability, and, although aripiprazole was abruptly discontinued in view of its long half-life, serum concentrations were assumed to have gradually declined. These factors may have contributed to the decline in the proportion of patients remaining well being gradual (linear) rather than rapid (exponential), in contrast to the previously mentioned olanzapine-versus-placebo maintenance trial. Despite the sustained mean period of actual stability prior to randomization (12.7 weeks), gradual (linear) decline in the proportion of patients remaining well, and the 6-month randomized controlled stage, the

U.S. prescribing information focuses on the 6-week minimum duration of pre-randomization stability, perhaps reflecting reluctance to recommend antipsychotics for the maintenance treatment phase.

When additional secondary event-based outcome measures (i.e., relapse rates) were considered, the findings had the same pattern. Aripiprazole was superior to placebo for overall episode prevention (NNT=6) and mania/mixed episode prevention (NNT=8), but not depressive episode prevention (NNT=64) (Figure 8–13, black bars).

In the randomized controlled stage, overall tolerability with aripiprazole was comparable to that with placebo. Specifically, adverse event discontinuation rates

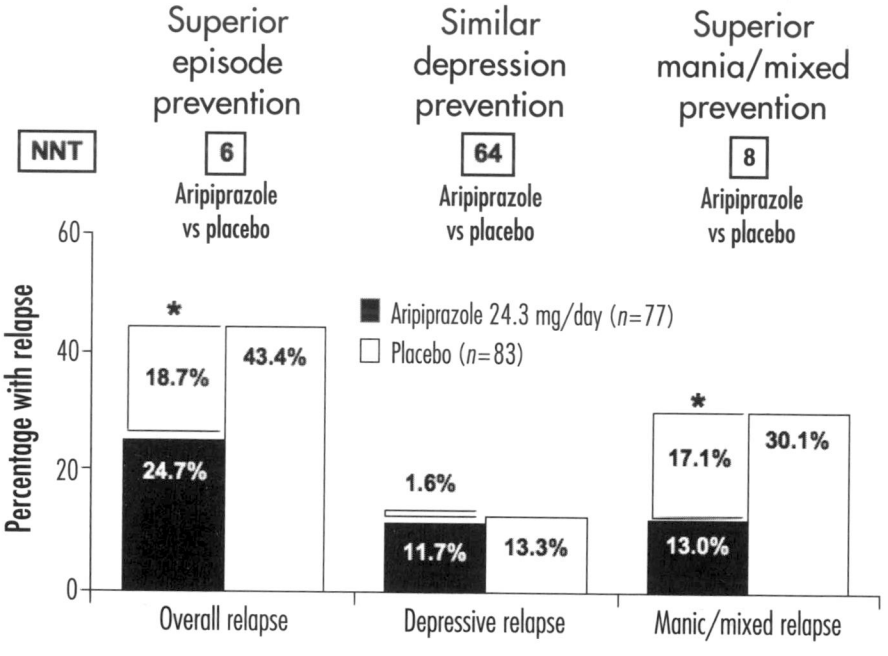

FIGURE 8–13.   Comparison of 26-week double-blind aripiprazole versus placebo continuation/maintenance monotherapy, numbers needed to treat (NNT), and relapse rates.

Aripiprazole monotherapy (black bars) compared with placebo monotherapy (white bars) after manic/mixed episodes was superior in the time-to-event–based analyses for prevention of manic but not depressive episodes. Patients were stabilized on open aripiprazole before randomization (mean 12.7 weeks). The relapse criteria were hospitalization or medication added. *$P<0.05$, versus placebo.

Source.   Data from Keck et al. 2006.

were 10.4% with aripiprazole and 19.3% with placebo (Figure 8–14, middle). Thus, compared with aripiprazole, the NNH for adverse event discontinuation with placebo was 12. Aripiprazole yielded rates of tremor, akathisia, vaginitis, and extremity pain that were higher than with placebo. Mean weight change was +0.5 kg with aripiprazole and –1.7 kg with placebo. Clinically significant (≥7%) weight gain was seen in 12.5% with aripiprazole and 0% with placebo, so that the NNH for clinically significant weight gain with aripiprazole compared with placebo was 8 (Figure 8–14, right).

A subsequent article describing an up to 74-week, double-blind, placebo-controlled extension of the previous 26-week trial, thus extending the total double-blind, placebo-controlled evaluation time to up to 100 weeks, had similar findings (Keck et al. 2007). Aripiprazole was superior to placebo for time to

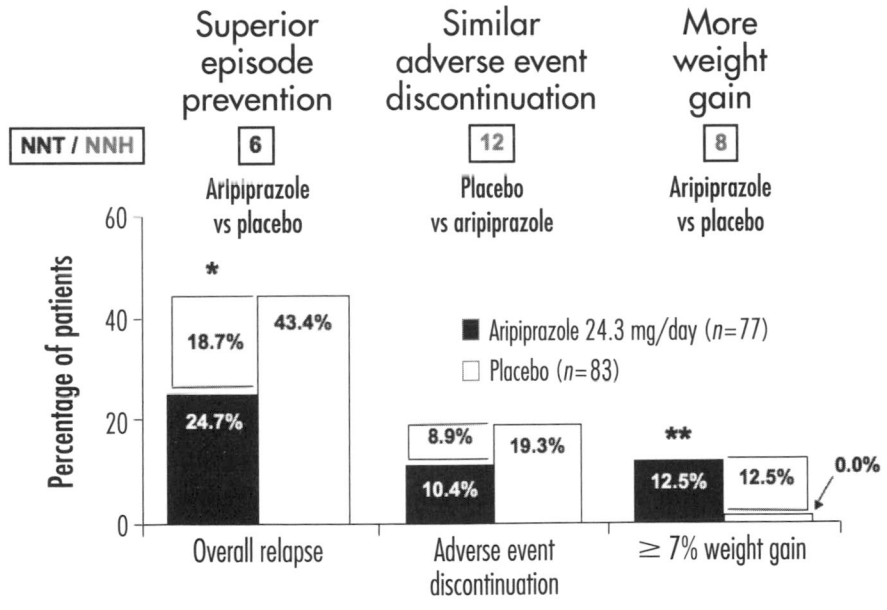

FIGURE 8–14.   Comparison of 26-week double-blind aripiprazole versus placebo continuation/maintenance monotherapy, numbers needed to treat (NNT), numbers needed to harm (NNH), and relapse, adverse event discontinuation, and weight gain rates.

Aripiprazole monotherapy (black bars) compared with placebo monotherapy (white bars) had superior efficacy but yielded more adverse event discontinuations and weight gain. *P<0.05; **P<0.01, versus placebo.

Source.   Data from Keck et al. 2006.

symptomatic relapse into any episode, and into manic episodes but not into depressive episodes, and for overall episode prevention (32.5% vs. 51.8%, $P<0.02$, NNT=6) and manic/mixed/unknown polarity episode prevention (18.2% vs. 36.1%, $P<0.02$, NNT=6) but not depressive episode prevention (14.3% vs. 15.7%, NNT=73).

The U.S. prescribing information for aripiprazole includes boxed warnings regarding the increased risks of 1) mortality (primarily cardiovascular or infectious) in elderly patients with dementia-related psychosis (a second-generation antipsychotic class warning), and 2) suicidality with use of antidepressant drugs in patients up to age 24 years (based on an antidepressant class warning). The FDA has stipulated that the aripiprazole U.S. prescribing information include the risks of hyperglycemia and diabetes mellitus, but the report of a recent consensus development conference suggests the risks of obesity, diabetes, and hyperlipidemia with this agent are similar to those with ziprasidone and less than with other second-generation antipsychotics (*Physicians' Desk Reference* 2008). Other warnings in the prescribing information include the risks of cerebrovascular adverse events, including stroke, in elderly patients with dementia; neuroleptic malignant syndrome; and tardive dyskinesia.

Perhaps because of partial agonist effects at dopamine receptors, nausea and vomiting can occur in some patients if aripiprazole is initiated aggressively. Tolerability may be enhanced in patients at risk for gastrointestinal or other adverse effects if aripiprazole is initiated gradually. Weight gain is less and akathisia is more of a concern with aripiprazole compared with olanzapine, quetiapine, and risperidone. Adjunctive lorazepam used in clinical trials may have decreased problems with akathisia.

Aripiprazole has some drug-drug interactions because enzyme inducers such as carbamazepine can decrease, and some enzyme inhibitors such as macrolide antibiotics may increase, serum aripiprazole concentrations. Additional information regarding aripiprazole is provided in Chapter 13 of this volume.

The U.S. prescribing information notes that the dosages of aripiprazole were 15 mg/day or 30 mg/day in the pivotal longer-term treatment study and does not provide information regarding initiation of aripiprazole in euthymic patients. Given the risk of adverse effects, it is prudent to start aripiprazole in euthymic patients in a gradual fashion similar to initiation in depressed patients, rather than the rapid initiation used in manic patients. In the (negative) controlled acute bipolar depression trials, aripiprazole was started at 10 mg/day (5 mg twice daily), and dosage could be adjusted weekly by 5 mg/day, with final dosages ranging from 5 mg/day to 30 mg/day and a pooled mean dosage of

16.5 mg/day. However, this approach yielded adverse effects such as akathisia, insomnia, and nausea, with rates ranging between approximately 14% and 28% of patients. Thus, clinicians may wish to initiate aripiprazole even more gradually in order to limit adverse effects, starting with 2 mg each morning and increasing as necessary and tolerated every 4–7 days by 2 mg/day, initially targeting a dosage of 15 mg/day. Patients who tolerate but fail to respond to 15 mg/day may benefit from continuing to gradually increase aripiprazole every 4–7 days as necessary and tolerated by 2 mg/day to as high as 30 mg/day (24.3 mg/day was the mean dosage in the pivotal maintenance trial). Occasional patients may find aripiprazole sedating, requiring shifting the medication to bedtime.

In summary, aripiprazole is a newer bipolar disorder longer-term treatment option that appears to provide more robust prevention of mania compared with depression. Adverse effects with this agent may be challenging, and clinicians and patients may deem this agent to have inferior tolerability compared with mood stabilizers such as lamotrigine and divalproex but superior tolerability compared with olanzapine. Indeed, the FDA longer-term aripiprazole indication appears to focus on its use in the continuation treatment phase.

Adjunctive Quetiapine

Based on controlled trials indicating that quetiapine immediate-release formulation added to lithium or valproate was effective in bipolar maintenance treatment (Suppes et al. 2009; Vieta et al. 2008), quetiapine (and by inference, quetiapine XR) received an indication for adjunctive longer-term treatment of bipolar disorder in 2008. The U.S. prescribing information states in the Indications section, "Quetiapine is indicated for the…maintenance treatment of bipolar I disorder as adjunct therapy to lithium or divalproex."

There have been two recent multicenter, randomized, double-blind, placebo-controlled adjunctive quetiapine immediate-release formulation (added to lithium or divalproex) longer-term treatment studies of patients with bipolar I disorder with recent manic, mixed, or depressive episodes with or without psychotic features (Suppes et al. 2009; Vieta et al. 2008). Because the findings were similar for the two studies, pooled results are described.

Quetiapine was superior to placebo on the time-to-event–based primary outcome measure (time to relapse into any episode). The effect of quetiapine was independent of any specific subgroup such as assigned mood stabilizer, sex, age, race, most recent bipolar episode, or rapid-cycling course. On the polarity-specific time-to-event–based secondary outcome measures, quetiapine was superior to placebo for time to relapse into manic episodes as well as depressive episodes. In this study, there was a substantial (at least 12 weeks) period of pre-randomization stability, but quetiapine was relatively rapidly discontinued. This rapid discontinuation may have contributed to the decline in the proportion of patients remaining well being relatively rapid in the adjunctive placebo group.

On additional secondary event-based outcome measures (i.e., relapse rates), the findings had the same pattern. Quetiapine was superior to placebo for overall episode prevention (NNT=4), depressive episode prevention (NNT=6), and manic episode prevention (NNT=8) (Figure 8–15, black bars).

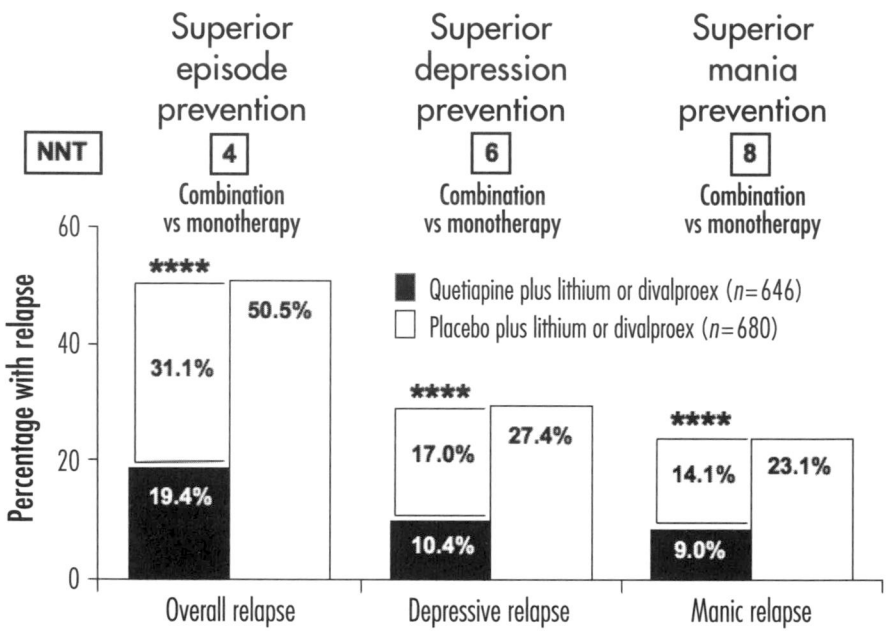

FIGURE 8–15.   Comparison of 24-month quetiapine versus placebo added to lithium or divalproex bipolar I disorder maintenance, numbers needed to treat (NNT), and relapse rates.

Combination therapy (black bars) compared with monotherapy (white bars) after manic, mixed, or depressed episodes was superior for prevention of both manic and depressive episodes. Patients were stabilized on open quetiapine plus lithium or divalproex for at least 12 weeks and on average 15 weeks before randomization. Duration of randomized treatment (mean±standard deviation): quetiapine=213.3±183.5 days; placebo=152.4±163.2 days. Mean quetiapine dosage 508 mg/day; mean serum lithium concentration 0.7 mEq/L; mean serum valproate concentration 71 μg/mL. ****$P<0.0001$, versus placebo.

Source.   Data from Suppes et al. 2008; Vieta et al. 2008.

In the open stabilization phase for the pooled trials, 9.7% of patients discontinued due to adverse events. Clinically significant (≥7%) weight gain was seen in 23.6% of patients, while sedation was seen in 23.4% of patients. In the randomized controlled stage, adjunctive quetiapine compared with adjunctive placebo yielded sedation/somnolence, weight gain, and metabolic changes. Sedation/somnolence was seen in 6.3% with adjunctive quetiapine and 1.6% with adjunctive placebo, so that the NNH for sedation/somnolence with adjunctive quetiapine compared with adjunctive placebo was 22 (Figure 8–16, center). Mean weight change was +0.5 kg with adjunctive quetiapine and −1.9 kg with adjunctive placebo. Clinically significant (≥7%) weight gain was seen in 7.7% with adjunctive quetiapine and 2.1% with adjunctive placebo, so that the NNH for clinically significant weight gain with adjunctive quetiapine compared with adjunctive pla-

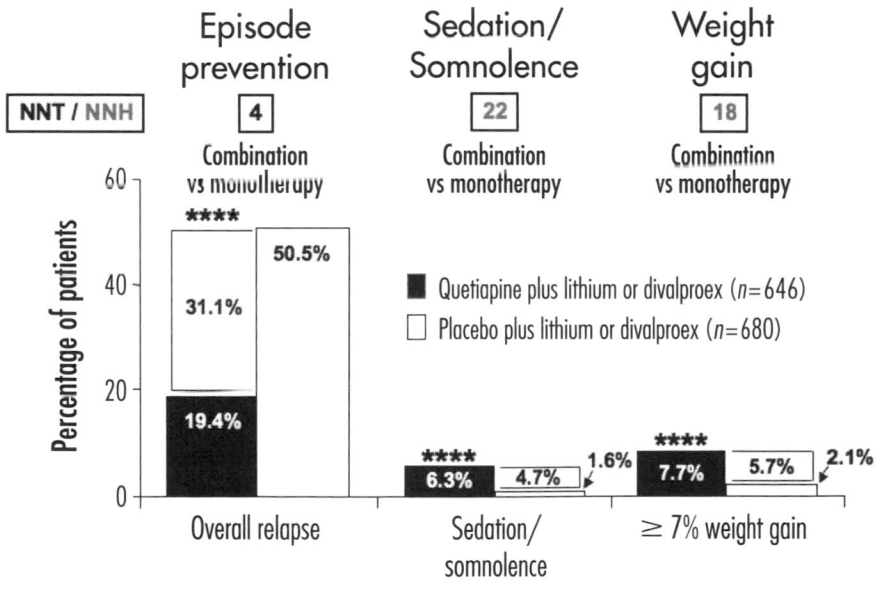

FIGURE 8–16. Comparison of 24-month quetiapine versus placebo added to lithium or divalproex bipolar I disorder maintenance, numbers needed to treat (NNT), numbers needed to harm (NNH), and relapse, sedation/somnolence, and weight gain rates.

Adjunctive quetiapine (black bars) compared with adjunctive placebo (white bars) had superior efficacy but yielded more sedation/somnolence and weight gain. Mean quetiapine dosage was 508 mg/day, mean serum lithium concentration was 0.7 mEq/L, and mean serum valproate concentration was 71 µg/mL. ****P<0.0001, versus placebo.

Source.   Data from Suppes et al. 2008; Vieta et al. 2008.

cebo was 18 (Figure 8–16, right). Metabolic changes (increased fasting blood glucose and triglycerides) were seen with adjunctive quetiapine compared with adjunctive placebo. The incidence density of at least one emergent fasting blood glucose≥126 mg/dL was greater with adjunctive quetiapine (10.7%, 18 per 100 patient-years) compared with adjunctive placebo (4.6%, 9.5 per 100 patient-years), so that the NNH for at least one emergent fasting blood glucose≥126 mg/dL with adjunctive quetiapine compared with adjunctive placebo was 17.

The U.S. prescribing information for quetiapine includes boxed warnings regarding the increased risks of 1) mortality (primarily cardiovascular or infectious) in elderly patients with dementia-related psychosis (a second-generation antipsychotic class warning), and 2) suicidality with use of antidepressant drugs in patients up to age 24 years (based on an antidepressant class warning). The FDA has stipulated changes in the quetiapine prescribing information to reflect the risks of hyperglycemia and diabetes mellitus, and the report of a recent consensus development conference suggests the risks of obesity, diabetes, and hyperlipidemia with this agent are intermediate, being less than with clozapine and olanzapine but more than with ziprasidone and aripiprazole (*Physicians' Desk Reference* 2008). Other warnings in the prescribing information include the risks of neuroleptic malignant syndrome and tardive dyskinesia. Other risks include syncope (in 1% of patients), seizures (in 0.5% of patients), hypothyroidism, and benign transaminase elevations (in 6% of patients).

Quetiapine has some drug-drug interactions because certain enzyme inducers such as carbamazepine can decrease and some enzyme inhibitors such as macrolide antibiotics may increase serum quetiapine concentrations. In addition, combining quetiapine with antiarrhythmic medications is not recommended because of the concerns regarding the potential for additive cardiac conduction delays. Additional information regarding quetiapine is provided in Chapter 13 of this volume.

The U.S. prescribing information for the longer-term adjunctive use of quetiapine and quetiapine XR recommends continuing the dosage necessary to maintain symptom remission, and states that dosages of 400–800 mg/day were used in the quetiapine immediate-release registration studies. The information does not provide recommendations for initiating quetiapine in euthymic patients. Given the risk of adverse effects, it is prudent to start quetiapine in euthymic patients in a gradual fashion similar to initiation in depressed patients, rather than the rapid initiation used in manic patients. The U.S. prescribing information recommends starting quetiapine and quetiapine XR in bipolar depression at 50 mg the first evening, increased to 100 mg by the second night, to

200 mg by the third night, and to 300 mg/day by the fourth night. In some patients, the recommended titration may not be tolerated (most often because of sedation), so that more gradual increases (e.g., starting with 25 mg at bedtime and increasing daily by 25 mg/day) will be necessary. Smaller, less frequent dosage increases that are judiciously timed (e.g., on Friday and Saturday evenings to avoid affecting work or school performance) may yield fewer adverse effects with less functional impairment. Occasional patients may tolerate and benefit from dosages as high as 600 mg/day. Across the two adjunctive quetiapine maintenance studies, the mean final dosage was just over 500 mg/day.

In summary, adjunctive quetiapine and quetiapine XR (combined with lithium or divalproex) are approved bipolar disorder longer-term treatment options that appear to be novel in that they may provide similarly robust prevention of mania and depression. However, adverse effects with these agents may be challenging, and clinicians and patients may deem them to have inferior tolerability not only compared with mood stabilizers such as lithium, lamotrigine and divalproex but also compared with some other antipsychotics such as aripiprazole.

Tier II: High-Priority Unapproved Longer-Term Treatment Options for Bipolar Disorder

As noted previously, safety and tolerability limitations of some Tier I approved treatments for the longer-term treatment of bipolar disorders such as olanzapine, aripiprazole, and adjunctive quetiapine may lead clinicians and patients to consider other options. When assessing alternative treatments, one approach is to consider medications such as divalproex that have substantive familiarity and/or evidence of efficacy in the longer-term treatment of bipolar disorders. Divalproex lacks a longer-term bipolar treatment indication because the pivotal maintenance trial failed, apparently because of methodological limitations. Nevertheless, divalproex has widespread familiarity and is ranked highly in multiple treatment guidelines (American Psychiatric Association 2002; Goodwin 2003; Grunze et al. 2002; Keck et al. 2004a; Suppes et al. 2005; Yatham et al. 2006).

Divalproex

Divalproex monotherapy lacks a bipolar disorder longer-term treatment indication. Thus, the U.S. prescribing information states,

> The safety and effectiveness of [divalproex] for long-term use in mania, i.e.,
> more than 3 weeks, has not been systematically evaluated in controlled clinical

trials. Therefore, physicians who elect to use [divalproex] for extended periods should continually reevaluate the long-term usefulness of the drug for the individual patient.

However, in 2008, quetiapine and quetiapine XR received adjunctive (added to divalproex or lithium) indications, as discussed in the section on adjunctive quetiapine earlier in this chapter.

The divalproex monotherapy longer-term treatment pivotal trial was a multicenter, randomized, double-blind, placebo-controlled and lithium-controlled study of patients with bipolar I disorder with a recent manic (but not mixed) episode (Bowden et al. 2000).

Divalproex, lithium, and placebo did not differ significantly from one another on the time-to-event–based primary outcome measure (time to any relapse) and on the two polarity-specific time-to-event–based secondary outcome measures (time to manic and time to depressive relapse), although divalproex tended to be superior to lithium on time to any relapse ($P=0.06$) and time to depressive relapse ($P=0.08$). Thus, the trial was deemed a failed study and did not result in FDA approval for divalproex for the longer-term treatment of bipolar disorder. Failure may have been because of methodological limitations, including lack of enrichment undermining statistical power (as discussed further later in this chapter) as well as the sample involving less severely ill patients, as mixed index episodes were excluded, only 18% were hospitalized for the index episode, and some index episodes resolved without treatment. Indeed, the placebo relapse rate in this study was lower than that seen in other contemporary maintenance trials (Figure 8–3).

Nevertheless, findings of additional secondary event-based outcome measures (i.e., relapse rates) were noteworthy. Using a relapse criterion of premature discontinuation because of mood episode, divalproex was superior to placebo for overall episode prevention (NNT=8) and depressive episode prevention (NNT=11) but not manic episode prevention (NNT=22) (Figure 8–17, black bars). In contrast, lithium was similar to placebo for overall episode prevention (NNT=14), depressive episode prevention (NNT=17), and manic episode prevention (NNT=69).

In the randomized controlled stage, overall tolerability with divalproex and lithium was poorer than with placebo. Specifically, adverse event discontinuation rates were 13.4% with divalproex, 22% with lithium, and 3.2% with placebo (Figure 8–18, middle). Thus, compared with placebo, the NNH for adverse event discontinuation with divalproex was 10 and with lithium was 6. Dival-

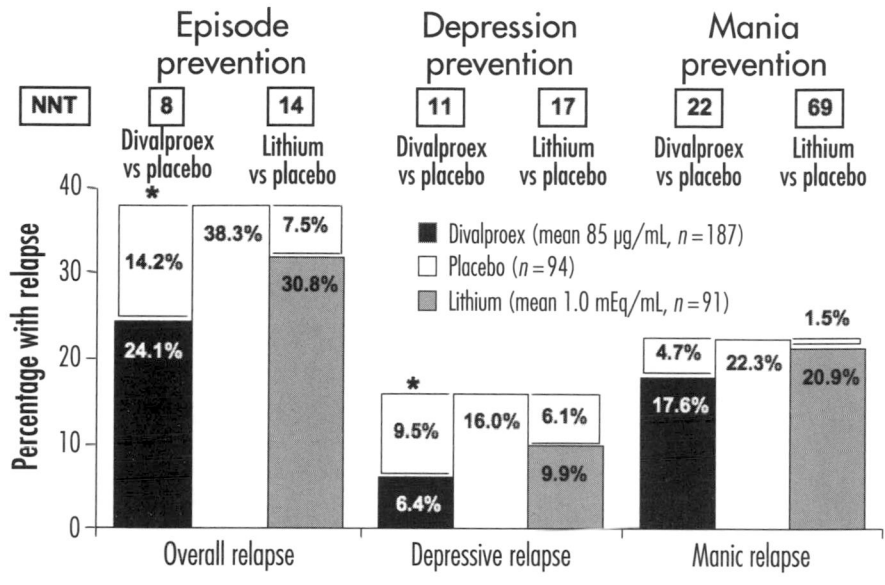

FIGURE 8–17. **Comparison of 12-month double-blind divalproex monotherapy versus lithium monotherapy versus placebo maintenance, numbers needed to treat (NNT), and relapse rates.**

Divalproex monotherapy (black bars), lithium monotherapy (gray bars), and placebo monotherapy (white bars) after manic/mixed episodes were equivalent on the primary time-to-event–based outcome measure (time to recurrence of any mood episode). Patients were stabilized on open treatment for two consecutive visits at least 6 days apart. *$P<0.02$ versus placebo. The relapse criterion was premature discontinuation because of mood episode.

Source. Data from Bowden et al. 2000.

proex yielded rates of tremor and alopecia that were higher than with placebo. Lithium yielded rates of diarrhea, nausea, and tremor that were higher than with placebo. Weight gain was seen in 20.9% with divalproex, 13.2% with lithium, and 7.5% with placebo, so that compared with placebo, the NNH for weight gain was 8 with divalproex and 18 with lithium (Figure 8–18, right).

A subsequent report described post hoc analyses indicating that divalproex may prevent depressive relapse, particularly in patients initially stabilized with open divalproex, and in patients with prior hospitalizations (Gyulai et al. 2003). Also, among patients with breakthrough depression treated with adjunctive paroxetine or sertraline, fewer patients taking maintenance divalproex compared with placebo discontinued early because of depression.

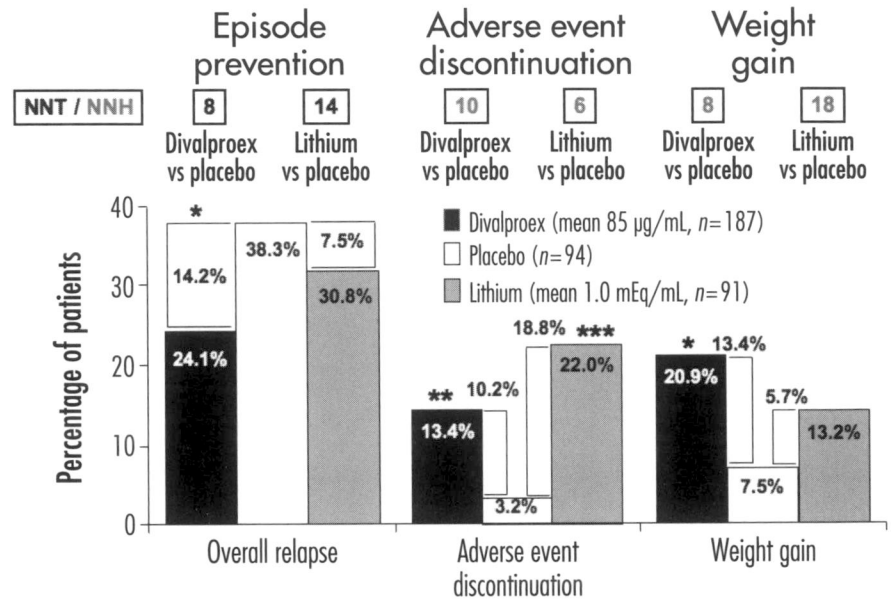

FIGURE 8–18.   Comparison of 12-month double-blind divalproex mono-therapy versus lithium monotherapy versus placebo maintenance, numbers needed to treat (NNT), numbers needed to harm (NNH), and relapse, adverse event discontinuation, and weight gain rates.

Divalproex monotherapy (black bars) compared with placebo monotherapy (white bars) had superior efficacy but yielded more adverse event discontinuations and weight gain. *$P<0.05$, **$P<0.01$, ***$P<0.001$ versus placebo.

Source.   Data from Bowden et al. 2000.

Another subsequent report described post hoc analyses of the effects of enrichment (McElroy et al. 2008). Thus, in patients initially stabilized with open divalproex, divalproex was superior to lithium and placebo for overall episode prevention. In contrast, in patients initially stabilized with open lithium, divalproex, lithium, and placebo all yielded similar overall episode prevention.

There are limited data regarding divalproex maintenance response prediction. Baseline markers of divalproex compared with lithium acute response appear in some ways overlapping and in other ways complementary. Many patients with poor response to lithium may respond to divalproex, which is effective acutely in pure (Bowden et al. 1994), mixed (Calabrese et al. 1993; Freeman et al. 1992), or dysphoric mania (Freeman et al. 1992; Swann et al. 1997), and in patients with a history of at least three prior episodes (Swann et al. 2000). Moreover, adolescents (Papatheodorou and Kutcher 1993); patients with rapid-cycling (Bowden et al. 1994; Calabrese et al. 1993) or secondary (Kahn et al. 1988; Sovner 1989; Stoll et al. 1994) bipolar disorder, or bipolar disorder combined with concurrent substance abuse (Brady et al. 1995); and patients unresponsive to or who cannot tolerate lithium (Bowden et al. 1994) may respond to divalproex acutely.

The U.S. prescribing information for divalproex includes boxed warnings regarding the risks of 1) hepatotoxicity, 2) teratogenicity, and 3) pancreatitis. Divalproex is generally discontinued if hepatic indices rise above three times the upper limit of normal. Other warnings include the risks of hyperammonemic encephalopathy in patients with urea cycle disorders, somnolence in the elderly, and thrombocytopenia. In mid-2008 the FDA released an alert regarding increased risk of suicidality (suicidal behavior or ideation) in patients with epilepsy as well as psychiatric disorders for eleven anticonvulsants (including divalproex). Divalproex tends to be somewhat better tolerated than lithium or carbamazepine, with CNS and gastrointestinal problems being the most common adverse effects.

Valproate has some drug interactions because it can inhibit metabolism of other drugs, including lamotrigine and the active carbamazepine epoxide metabolite. Moreover, valproate is susceptible to enzyme inducers, so that carbamazepine decreases valproate serum concentrations. Additional information regarding valproate is provided in Chapter 13 of this volume.

Divalproex lacks FDA approval for bipolar maintenance treatment, so the U.S. prescribing information does not provide dosing recommendations for this application. Given the risk of adverse effects, it is prudent to start divalproex in euthymic patients in a gradual fashion similar to initiation in depressed patients, rather than the rapid initiation used in manic patients. Thus, in euthymic bipolar patients, divalproex may be started at 250 mg/day, dosing at bedtime. Dosages may be increased as necessary and tolerated every 4–7 days, with an initial target dosage of 750 mg/day before blood levels are checked. This titration is considerably slower than that seen in acute mania and strives to decrease the risk of adverse effects, which are more common in depressed compared with manic patients. Based on the available literature, blood levels of at least 85 µg/mL may have better efficacy than lower blood levels.

In summary, divalproex is a bipolar disorder longer-term treatment option that is commonly used, despite lacking an FDA indication for bipolar maintenance. Although adverse effects with this agent may be challenging, conservative dosing can enhance tolerability. Clinicians and patients may deem this agent to have inferior tolerability compared with lamotrigine but superior tolerability compared with lithium and antipsychotics.

Tier III: Intermediate-Priority Unapproved Longer-Term Treatment Options for Bipolar Disorder

The longer-term management of bipolar disorder is sufficiently challenging that clinical need commonly outstrips the previously mentioned evidence-based treatment options. In this section we consider other treatment options with more limited evidence of efficacy than the previously mentioned Tier I and Tier II treatments. These alternatives include other mood stabilizers (carbamazepine), other second-generation antipsychotics (risperidone, ziprasidone, and clozapine), the olanzapine plus fluoxetine combination, adjunctive antidepressants, and adjunctive psychotherapy. Agents with proven efficacy and indications for acute mania (such as carbamazepine, risperidone, and ziprasidone) and acute bipolar depression (such as the olanzapine plus fluoxetine combination) might ultimately prove to have utility in longer-term treatment, but the evidence supporting such use is insufficient for them to carry a high priority. In general, treatment guidelines do not consider these modalities to be first-line interventions but cite them as intermediate-priority options (American Psychiatric Association 2002; Goodwin 2003; Grunze et al. 2002; Keck et al. 2004a; Suppes et al. 2005; Yatham et al. 2006). However, some Tier III options have mitigating advantages such as acute indications or tolerability that might make them attractive for selected patients, and in certain circumstances some of these interventions may be considered early on (e.g., psychotherapy in pregnant women). For some of these treatments (e.g., adjunctive psychotherapy) advances in research, familiarity, and/or availability may ultimately be sufficient to merit their consideration for placement in higher tiers.

Other Mood Stabilizers

The other mood stabilizer, carbamazepine, unlike lithium, lamotrigine, and divalproex, has less of an evidence base supporting its use in bipolar maintenance treatment and, unlike lithium and lamotrigine, lacks an indication for longer-term treatment in bipolar disorders. Nevertheless, limited systematic data support its consideration as an alternative treatment.

Carbamazepine

Carbamazepine lacks a bipolar disorder longer-term treatment indication. Thus, the U.S. prescribing information states,

> The effectiveness of [carbamazepine] for longer-term use and for prophylactic use in mania has not been systematically evaluated in controlled clinical trials. Therefore, physicians who elect to use [carbamazepine] for extended periods should periodically reevaluate the long-term risks and benefits of the drug for the individual patient.

In view of its having efficacy and an FDA indication for the treatment of acute mania, it is possible carbamazepine also may have efficacy in longer-term treatment, and limited randomized controlled maintenance data suggest carbamazepine may be either somewhat inferior or comparable to lithium. Thus, in a 30-month multicenter, randomized open bipolar maintenance study, carbamazepine was inferior to lithium overall (Greil et al. 1997), with the difference driven by marked inferiority in patients with a classical subtype (bipolar I without mood-incongruent delusions and without comorbidity), which overshadowed a trend toward superiority in patients with a nonclassical subtype (bipolar II/NOS, mood-incongruent delusions, comorbidity) (Greil et al. 1998).

A 2-year, randomized, double-blind study in 94 bipolar disorder (76.6% bipolar I disorder, 23.4% bipolar II disorder) patients with no more than 6 months of prior treatment found similar overall relapse rates with carbamazepine and lithium, but with lithium most relapses occurred during the first 3 months in patients who were "acutely randomized" rather than "prophylactically randomized" (Hartong et al. 2003).

In a 12-month, randomized, double-blind, crossover trial, in 52 patients with bipolar I disorder, carbamazepine and lithium yielded similar outcomes, with the carbamazepine plus lithium combination yielding better outcomes (nonsignificantly overall, and significantly in rapid cyclers) (Denicoff et al. 1997).

There are limited data regarding carbamazepine acute and maintenance response prediction. Baseline markers of carbamazepine compared with lithium response appear in some ways overlapping and in other ways complementary. Clinical markers of response to carbamazepine are similar in some respects to those for response to divalproex; that is, patients with nonclassical presentations (Greil et al. 1998), secondary mood disorders (Himmelhoch and Garfinkel 1986), or lithium resistance or intolerance (Okuma et al. 1979; Post et al. 1987) may respond to carbamazepine. However, findings have been less consistent with regard to the predictive value of a rapid-cycling pattern (Dilsaver et al. 1993; Joyce 1988; Okuma 1993; Post et al. 1987), dysphoric mania (Lusznat et al. 1988; Post et al. 1989), and severe mania (Post et al. 1987; Small et al. 1991).

The most common dosage-related adverse effects with carbamazepine involve CNS (diplopia, blurred vision, fatigue, sedation, dizziness, and ataxia) or gastrointestinal system (nausea, vomiting) problems. The U.S. prescribing information includes boxed warnings regarding the risks of serious dermatological reactions and the HLA-B*1502 allele, as well as aplastic anemia and agranulocytosis. Carbamazepine is also associated with common benign leukopenia, which in rare instances may be an early indication of serious blood dyscrasia. Other warnings in the prescribing information include the risks of teratogenicity and increased intraocular pressure caused by mild anticholinergic activity. In mid-2008 the FDA released an alert regarding increased risk of suicidality (suicidal behavior or ideation) in patients with epilepsy as well as psychiatric disorders for 11 anticonvulsants (including carbamazepine).

Carbamazepine drug interactions can yield carbamazepine toxicity (e.g., when erythromycin or valproate is added to carbamazepine) and inefficacy of other medications (e.g., hormonal contraceptives and multiple psychotropic drugs, including several newer anticonvulsants and second-generation antipsychotics). Additional information regarding carbamazepine is provided in Chapter 13 of this volume.

Carbamazepine lacks FDA approval for bipolar maintenance treatment, so the U.S. prescribing information does not provide dosing recommendations for this application. Given the risk of adverse effects, it is prudent to start carbamazepine in euthymic patients in a gradual fashion similar to initiation in depressed patients rather than the rapid initiation used in manic patients. In outpatients with acute bipolar depression, carbamazepine is generally started at 200 mg/day, given at bedtime, and increased every 3–7 days by 200 mg/day. This titration is considerably slower than that seen in acute mania and strives to decrease the risk of adverse effects, which are more common in depressed as compared with manic patients. Even more gradual titration may be achieved by starting with 100 mg/day and increasing every 3–7 days by 100 mg/day increments. The target dosage is generally 600–1,200 mg/day, with blood levels commonly in the range of 4–12 µg/mL.

In summary, carbamazepine is a bipolar disorder longer-term alternative treatment option that lacks an FDA indication for bipolar maintenance. Adverse effects and drug interactions with this agent may be challenging, but some patients may experience adequate tolerability compared with treatment with mood stabilizers such as lithium and divalproex or compared with treatment with antipsychotics.

Other Second-Generation Antipsychotics

The other second-generation antipsychotics—olanzapine plus fluoxetine combination, risperidone, ziprasidone, and clozapine—lack FDA indications for the longer-term treatment of bipolar disorder. Nevertheless, limited data suggest these agents may be worth considering as alternative treatments.

Olanzapine Plus Fluoxetine Combination

The combination of olanzapine plus fluoxetine was approved for acute bipolar depression in 2003 but lacks a bipolar maintenance indication. Thus, the U.S. prescribing information for the olanzapine plus fluoxetine combination states the following in the "Indications and Usage" section:

> Unlike with unipolar depression, there are no established guidelines for the length of time patients with bipolar disorder experiencing a major depressive episode should be treated with agents containing antidepressant drugs. The effectiveness of [olanzapine plus fluoxetine] for maintaining antidepressant response in this patient population beyond 8 weeks has not been established in controlled clinical studies. Physicians who elect to use [olanzapine plus fluoxetine] for extended periods should periodically reevaluate the benefits and long-term risks of the drug for the individual patient.

A 24-week, open-label extension (Corya et al. 2006) of the 8-week, controlled trial (Tohen et al. 2003b) described in Chapter 7 of this volume, "Management of Acute Major Depressive Episodes in Bipolar Disorders," provided very limited data regarding the potential efficacy and tolerability of longer-term administration of the olanzapine plus fluoxetine combination. The design of this study made interpretation challenging.

A recent 25-week, multicenter, randomized, double-blind, head-to-head comparison of the olanzapine plus fluoxetine combination and lamotrigine, in spite of lacking a placebo arm, may help inform clinicians and patients wishing to assess the benefit-to-risk ratio of these interventions in the longer-term treatment of bipolar disorders (Brown et al. 2005). This study was an extension of the 7-week comparison of these agents described in Chapter 7 of this volume (Brown et al. 2006). In the extension study, as in the acute study, the olanzapine plus fluoxetine combination was somewhat more effective but somewhat poorly tolerated. The olanzapine plus fluoxetine combination compared with lamotrigine yielded somnolence, increased appetite, dry mouth, sedation, weight gain, and tremor, and incidence of treatment-emergent cholesterol of 240 or higher (15.9% vs. 3.7%, NNH=9) and clinically significant (≥7%) weight gain (33.8% vs. 2.1%, NNH=4).

The olanzapine plus fluoxetine combination lacks FDA approval for longer-term treatment of bipolar disorder, so the U.S. prescribing information does not provide dosing recommendations for this application. In order to limit adverse effects, in euthymic bipolar disorder patients this treatment may be started in a fashion similar to that in acute bipolar depression as described in Chapter 7 of this volume. The limited data presented above suggest that longer-term dosages may be similar to those used in acute bipolar depression. As discussed later in this chapter, the longer-term administration of antidepressants in patients with bipolar disorders is controversial.

In summary, although the olanzapine plus fluoxetine combination is indicated for acute bipolar depression, placebo-controlled trials are needed to establish the benefits of continuing this intervention in responders. The olanzapine plus fluoxetine combination has safety and tolerability challenges such as sedation, weight gain, and metabolic problems that may limit its utility, particularly in longer-term treatment.

Risperidone

Risperidone received FDA approval for the treatment of acute mania in 2003 but currently lacks a bipolar maintenance indication. Thus, the U.S. prescribing information for risperidone states the following in the Dosage and Administration section:

> There is no body of evidence available from controlled trials to guide a clinician in the longer-term management of a patient who improves during treatment of an acute manic episode with [risperidone]. While it is generally agreed that pharmacological treatment beyond an acute response in mania is desirable, both for maintenance of the initial treatment response and for prevention of new manic episodes, there are no systematically obtained data to support the use of [risperidone] in such longer-term treatment (i.e., beyond 3 weeks). The physician who elects to use [risperidone] for extended periods should periodically reevaluate the long-term usefulness of the drug for the individual patient.

There are limited data regarding the longer-term use of risperidone in the management of bipolar disorders. In a 6-month, multicenter, open study in 358 (299 bipolar I disorder, 45 bipolar II disorder, 14 bipolar disorder NOS) patients with bipolar disorder, risperidone was added to mood stabilizers, as well as antidepressants, in approximately 10% of the patients, with encouraging results (Vieta et al. 2001).

Small open naturalistic (i.e., not randomized) studies suggested longer-term adjunctive risperidone compared with adjunctive olanzapine yielded similar efficacy but less weight gain (Ghaemi et al. 2004; McIntyre et al. 2004).

In 2003, a risperidone long-acting injectable (RLAI) formulation was approved for the treatment of schizophrenia, but it has not been approved for bipolar disorder. Such a formulation could have utility in longer-term treatment, particularly in patients with adherence and/or tolerability problems with the oral formulation. Several small open trials suggested longer-term RLAI might be well tolerated and yield benefit in patients with bipolar disorder (Han et al. 2007; Malempati et al. 2008; Savas et al. 2006).

In addition, a recent controlled trial suggested that adjunctive RLAI (25–50 mg every 2 weeks) added to treatment as usual might help delay relapse in patients with frequently relapsing bipolar disorder (four or more mood episodes requiring treatment in the prior year) (MacFadden et al. 2008). This trial is discussed in more detail in Chapter 9 of this volume, "Management of Rapid-Cycling Bipolar Disorders."

Risperidone monotherapy lacks FDA approval for longer-term treatment of bipolar disorder, so the U.S. prescribing information does not provide dosing recommendations for this application. In order to limit adverse effects, oral risperidone in euthymic bipolar disorder patients may be started at 0.25–0.5 mg/day and increased as necessary and tolerated every 4–7 days by 0.25–0.5 mg/day, with an initial target dosage of 1–2 mg/day. RLAI may be initiated at 25 mg intramuscularly every 2 weeks, overlapping with oral risperidone or another oral antipsychotic, and increased monthly as necessary and tolerated to as high as 50 mg intramuscularly every 2 weeks.

In summary, controlled trials are necessary to assess the utility of oral risperidone in the longer-term treatment of bipolar disorders. The RLAI formulation ultimately may prove to have utility in patients with adherence or tolerability problems with oral antipsychotics. However, extrapyramidal symptoms, sedation, and weight gain may limit the utility of risperidone in longer-term treatment.

Ziprasidone

Ziprasidone received FDA approval for the treatment of acute mania in 2004 but currently lacks acute bipolar depression and bipolar maintenance indications. Thus, the U.S. prescribing information for ziprasidone states the following in the Indications and Usage section:

> The effectiveness of ziprasidone for longer-term use and for prophylactic use in mania has not been systematically evaluated in controlled clinical trials. Therefore, physicians who elect to use ziprasidone for extended periods should periodically reevaluate the long-term risks and benefits of the drug for the individual patient.

And in the Dosage and Administration section it states:

> There is no body of evidence available from controlled trials to guide a clinician in the longer-term management of a patient who improves during treatment of mania with ziprasidone. While it is generally agreed that pharmacological treatment beyond an acute response in mania is desirable, both for maintenance of the initial treatment response and for prevention of new manic episodes, there are no systematically obtained data to support the use of ziprasidone in such longer-term treatment (i.e., beyond 3 weeks).

Open extensions of 3-week, randomized, double-blind, placebo-controlled ziprasidone monotherapy and adjunctive therapy (added to lithium) acute mania studies suggested ongoing improvement compared with acute baseline (Keck et al. 2004b; Warrington et al. 2007; Weisler et al. 2004).

Ziprasidone monotherapy lacks FDA approval for bipolar maintenance treatment, so the U.S. prescribing information does not provide dosing recommendations for this application. In order to limit adverse effects (particularly akathisia at low dosages), ziprasidone in euthymic bipolar disorder patients may be started at 80 mg/day at dinner or at bedtime with a snack and increased as necessary and tolerated daily by 20 mg/day, with an initial target dosage of 160 mg/day, which is the recommended maximum dosage in the U.S. prescribing information (Wang et al. 2008). In patients who tolerate but fail to respond to 160 mg/day, continuing to increase ziprasidone as necessary and tolerated daily by 20 mg/day to as high as 240–320 mg/day may yield additional benefit. Higher dosages tend to yield sedation and appetite suppression. If akathisia develops with the first-day 80-mg/day dosage, abruptly increasing to 160 mg/day, and if appropriate adding or increasing the dosage of a benzodiazepine, may offer benefit. If sedation develops with the first-day dosage of 80 mg/day, decreasing daily by 20 mg/day (monitoring carefully for akathisia) or decreasing dosage of concurrent sedating medications may yield benefit. Attaining a ziprasidone dosage of at least 160 mg/day before beginning to taper other agents may help avoid akathisia when crossing over from another second-generation antipsychotic to ziprasidone. It is important that ziprasidone be ingested with food, which doubles ziprasidone absorption.

In summary, controlled trials are necessary to assess the utility of ziprasidone in the longer-term treatment of bipolar disorders. Although initiation may be complex, and some patients may experience akathisia, the relative lack of problems with weight gain and metabolic complications may make longer-term ziprasidone worth considering in patients who have an acute response to ziprasidone or fail to tolerate longer-term treatment with other agents because of weight gain and/or metabolic problems.

Clozapine

Clozapine lacks any indication for bipolar disorder. Uncontrolled reports (for reviews, see Frye et al. 1998; Zarate et al. 1995) and two controlled trials (Barbini et al. 1997; Suppes et al. 1999) suggest that clozapine might have efficacy in bipolar disorders. In published reports, mean clozapine dosages in patients with bipolar disorder ranged between approximately 125 and 550 mg/day.

It appears that in aggregate, clozapine may have less therapeutic potential in depressive as compared with manic/mixed states.

There has been only one published controlled trial of clozapine in the longer-term treatment of bipolar disorder. In a 1-year, randomized, open trial in patients with treatment-resistant bipolar I disorder and schizoaffective disorder, bipolar type, 19 patients receiving clozapine plus treatment as usual compared with 19 patients receiving treatment as usual without clozapine had better outcomes (Suppes et al. 1999). Mean clozapine dosage was lower in bipolar I disorder (234 mg/day) than in schizoaffective disorder, bipolar type (623 mg/day), patients, and only 3/19 (16%) clozapine patients discontinued because of adverse effects.

Clozapine lacks FDA approval for bipolar maintenance treatment, so the U.S. prescribing information does not provide dosing recommendations for this application. Clozapine dosages in patients with mood disorders tend to be considerably lower than in patients with schizophrenia. In order to limit adverse effects (particularly sedation), clozapine in euthymic bipolar disorder patients may be started at 12.5 mg/day at bedtime, and increased as necessary and tolerated every 4–7 days by 12.5 mg/day, with an initial target dosage of 100 mg/day. In patients who tolerate but fail to respond to 100 mg/day, continuing to increase as necessary and tolerated by 12.5 mg/day every 4–7 days to as high as

300 mg/day, which is one-third of the recommended maximum dosage for patients with schizophrenia in the U.S. prescribing information, may yield additional benefit. Occasionally patients with bipolar disorder may need and tolerate dosages higher than 300 mg/day.

In summary, in view of the challenging adverse effect profile of this agent, clozapine is usually held in reserve for patients with treatment-resistant illness. Additional controlled trials of clozapine in the longer-term treatment of bipolar disorder are needed to inform clinical practice.

Adjunctive Antidepressants

The use of adjunctive antidepressants in the longer-term treatment of bipolar disorder is even more controversial than in the treatment of acute bipolar depression. These agents have been seen by some investigators as temporary adjuncts for administration during acute bipolar depression and best avoided in the longer term because of inefficacy and tolerability (i.e., treatment-emergent affective switch) concerns. Indeed, a review of seven controlled trials involving 363 bipolar disorder (256 bipolar I disorder and 107 bipolar II disorder) patients (Amsterdam et al. 1998; Kane et al. 1982; Prien et al. 1973b, 1984; Quitkin et al. 1981; Sachs et al. 1994; Wehr and Goodwin 1979) indicated that adding antidepressants to lithium did not confer enhanced prevention of depression and that antidepressant monotherapy and perhaps adding an antidepressant to lithium increased treatment-emergent affective switch (Ghaemi et al. 2001).

Nevertheless, it may be that a minority of patients could benefit from longer-term adjunctive antidepressants. In a naturalistic (i.e., not randomized) effectiveness study of Stanley Foundation Bipolar Network patients receiving adjunctive antidepressants for new-onset major depressive episodes, only a small subset (15%, 84/549) achieved durable remission (6 consecutive weeks with CGI severity scores indicating no more than mild subsyndromal symptoms) (Altshuler et al. 2003). However, in this subset of patients, continuing antidepressants more than 6 months compared with less than 6 months was associated with a lower rate of depressive relapse (36% vs. 70%) with no increase in treatment-emergent affective switch.

In summary, longer-term administration of adjunctive antidepressants in patients with bipolar disorder is controversial. In many instances, these agents may have even short-term inefficacy and tolerability problems that limit their utility. However, in the small minority of patients who experience adequate acute relief of depression without treatment-emergent affective switch, continuing these agents in longer-term therapy may be worth considering. Controlled trials of adjunctive antidepressants in the longer-term treatment of bipolar disorder are needed to provide an evidence base necessary to inform clinical practice.

Adjunctive Psychotherapy

Emerging data from controlled trials indicate the increasing importance of adjunctive psychosocial interventions in the management of bipolar disorders, as discussed in detail in Chapter 15 of this volume. The most studied psychosocial interventions in patients with bipolar disorders have been psychoeducation (Colom et al. 2003), cognitive-behavioral therapy (Lam et al. 2003), family-focused therapy (FFT) (Miklowitz et al. 2003), and interpersonal and social rhythm therapy (IPSRT) (Frank et al. 2005).

These treatments may have illness phase–specific features, with optimal time of administration being during euthymia or depression as opposed to during mania, and greater acute and preventive effects against depressive as compared with the mood elevation aspects of the illness (Swartz and Frank 2001). Thus, some data suggest that psychoeducation (Colom et al. 2003), FFT (Miklowitz et al. 2003), and IPSRT (Frank et al. 2005) may have greater ability to prevent depressive as compared with mood elevation symptoms. However, other data suggest psychoeducation (Perry et al. 1999) and cognitive-behavioral therapy (Lam et al. 2003) may have greater ability to prevent mood elevation as compared with depressive symptoms.

It is particularly noteworthy that adjunctive psychosocial interventions compared with control conditions yield single-digit NNTs comparable to FDA-approved pharmacotherapies for bipolar disorder (Figure 8–19). These and other psychotherapy studies are discussed in Chapter 15 of this volume.

Some treatment settings (particularly within large organizations) may benefit from the development of comprehensive case management programs that incorporate psychoeducation, evidence-based pharmacotherapy, and increased access to care. Indeed, randomized controlled trials indicate that such chronic disease management programs may enhance outcomes of longer-term treatment (Bauer et al. 2006; Simon et al. 2006).

In summary, these data indicate an increasingly important role for adjunctive psychosocial interventions in the longer-term management of bipolar disorder, which has already been acknowledged in multiple treatment guidelines (American Psychiatric Association 2002; Goodwin 2003; Keck et al. 2004a; Yatham et al. 2006).

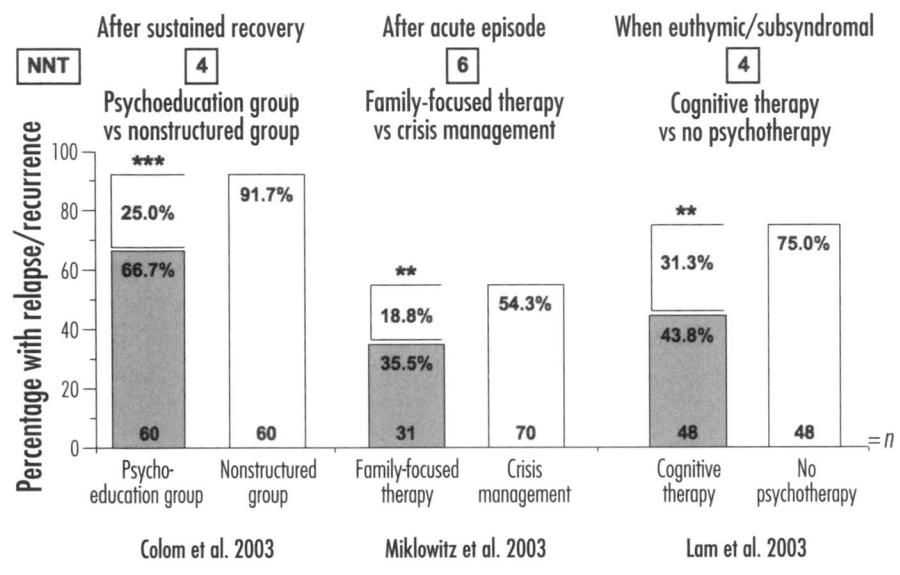

FIGURE 8–19.   Overview of adjunctive psychosocial maintenance studies, numbers needed to treat (NNT), and relapse/recurrence rates.

Randomized controlled trials demonstrated lower relapse/recurrence rates with adjunctive psychoeducation group compared with unstructured group (*left*) (Colom et al. 2003), family-focused therapy compared with crisis management (second from left) (Miklowitz et al. 2003), and cognitive-behavioral therapy group compared with no adjunctive psychotherapy (*right*) (Lam et al. 2003). The NNT for adjunctive psychotherapy were comparable with the single-digit NNT seen with U.S. Food and Drug Administration–approved pharmacotherapies across phases of bipolar disorders. **P<0.01, ***P<0.001 versus control.

Source.   Data from Colom et al. 2003, Lam et al. 2003, Miklowitz et al. 2003.

Tier IV: Novel Adjunctive Treatments

Treatment resistance or intolerance is sufficiently common in patients with bipolar disorders that even the previously mentioned armamentarium is insufficient to meet clinical needs. In this section we describe novel adjunctive treatments with even more limited evidence of efficacy than the previously mentioned treatments. These treatments include electroconvulsive therapy (ECT) and vagus nerve stimulation (VNS). In general, as noted earlier, treatment guidelines consider these modalities to be low-priority interventions (American Psychiatric Association 2002; Goodwin 2003; Grunze et al. 2002; Keck et al. 2004a; Suppes et al. 2005; Yatham et al. 2006). Nevertheless, some Tier IV options could prove attractive for carefully selected patients after consideration of Tier I–III treatments (e.g., patients treatment resistant or intolerant to Tier I–III treatments). For some of these treatments, advances in research may ultimately provide sufficient evidence to merit their consideration for placement in higher tiers.

Electroconvulsive Therapy

As reviewed by Vaidya et al. (2003), limited case reports and case series describe maintenance ECT efficacy in mixed samples of bipolar and unipolar patients (Loo et al. 1991; Vanelle et al. 1994). However, some patients may have better outcomes with mood stabilizer combinations than with maintenance ECT (Jaffe et al. 1991).

In the first randomized controlled trial of continuation ECT in unipolar depression, 37% (33/89) of patients relapsed, which was statistically similar to the relapse rate with nortriptyline plus lithium continuation therapy (32%, 30/95) (Kellner et al. 2006).

Concerns based on case reports regarding the risks of delirium, seizures, and prolonged apnea resulted in recommendations that lithium not be combined with ECT (Small and Milstein 1990). As advocated in multiple treatment guidelines (American Psychiatric Association 2002; Goodwin 2003; Grunze et al. 2002; Suppes et al. 2005; Yatham et al. 2006), maintenance ECT is generally held in reserve for patients intolerant of or refractory to pharmacotherapy because of the risk of interruption of function related to cognitive adverse effects, stigma, consent challenges, and logistical concerns such as coordination of care and aftercare.

Adjunctive Vagus Nerve Stimulation

VNS involves surgical implantation of an electronic device similar to a pacemaker with an electrode connecting it to the left vagus nerve and delivering low-frequency, chronic intermittent-pulsed electrical signals to the left vagus nerve, yielding deep brain and limbic cortical stimulation. VNS was approved for the adjunctive treatment of medically refractory partial-onset seizures in adults and adolescents over 12 years of age in 1997 and in 2005 was approved by the FDA for the adjunctive long-term treatment of chronic or recurrent depression resistant to four or more antidepressants in adults but not for rapid-cycling bipolar disorder. Given the invasiveness and expense, VNS is commonly considered a longer-term treatment. Limited data support this view.

In a 12-month, multicenter, open, uncontrolled, extension study of the pivotal trial in unipolar ($n=185$) and bipolar ($n=20$) patients, VNS plus treatment as usual yielded a final Hamilton Rating Scale for Depression response ($\geq 50\%$

decrease) rate of 27% (Rush et al. 2005). In these VNS studies, patients with bipolar disorders accounted for approximately 10% of participants, but patients with a history of psychosis or rapid-cycling bipolar disorder were excluded. Adjunctive VNS was generally well tolerated, but treatment-emergent affective switch occurred sporadically.

The cost and invasiveness of VNS and the relatively modest efficacy raise cost-benefit concerns. Indeed, patients commonly find their insurance companies deny reimbursement for VNS.

Conclusion

Since 2003 there has been substantial expansion of the therapeutic options for the longer-term treatment of bipolar disorders. Three mood stabilizers (lithium, lamotrigine, and divalproex) commonly are used for bipolar maintenance treatment. Lithium, although no longer the sole approved treatment, remains an important option. Lamotrigine is a novel treatment in that it addresses depressive more than mood elevation aspects of the illness, has uncommonly good tolerability, and, although having a longer-term indication, lacks an acute indication. Divalproex, although lacking a longer-term bipolar treatment indication, has limited controlled data to support this practice. In contrast, carbamazepine, because there is less compelling evidence of efficacy and greater complexity of treatment, is considered an alternative rather than a first-line therapy.

The role of second-generation antipsychotics in the longer-term treatment of bipolar disorders is evolving. Although two of these agents (olanzapine and aripiprazole) have longer-term monotherapy indications, their U.S. prescribing information emphasizes the continuation treatment phase rather than the maintenance treatment phase. In contrast, the U.S. prescribing information for adjunctive (added to lithium or divalproex) quetiapine and quetiapine XR for longer-term bipolar treatment emphasizes the maintenance treatment phase. Safety and tolerability concerns such as sedation, weight gain, and metabolic problems may limit the longer-term utility of second-generation antipsychotics. The longer-term administration of adjunctive antidepressants in patients with bipolar disorders is controversial, but a minority of patients may benefit from this approach. An increasing amount of controlled data supports the use of adjunctive psychotherapy in the longer-term treatment of bipolar disorders.

It is anticipated that in the coming years, additional controlled trials will provide new treatment options and hopefully resolution of some of the current controversies regarding the longer-term management of bipolar disorders.

Case Study: Longer-Term Management of Bipolar Disorders

Ms. Jones was a 39-year-old married professional woman who presented after a 6-day hospitalization for an acute pure (not mixed) manic episode with psychotic features. This had been her first affective episode, and she denied any history of prior psychiatric or substance abuse problems. She admitted to a history of migraine headaches, but her medical history was otherwise negative. Aside from a nephew who had been treated for depression, her family history was negative for psychiatric or substance abuse problems.

At the initial visit (posthospital week 1), she was taking olanzapine 15 mg at bedtime and zolpidem 10 mg at bedtime. She had improved substantially during hospitalization, with attenuation of euphoria, grandiose and religious delusions, decreased need for sleep, distractibility, and excessive goal-directed activity. She was beginning to obtain some distance from her delusions and denied any hallucinations. She appeared to be tolerating treatment well and denied sedation, excessive appetite, or weight gain, and weighed 118 lb. on a 5-foot 4-inch frame. Olanzapine was continued at 15 mg at bedtime, but zolpidem was decreased to as-needed usage.

The following week (posthospital week 2), she had improved further and did not require any zolpidem. She denied sedation but reported increased appetite, although her weight remained 118 lb. She was counseled regarding the risks of sedation, weight gain, and metabolic problems with olanzapine (which was continued at 15 mg at bedtime) and the importance of diet and exercise.

The following week (posthospital week 3), she complained of pervasive anhedonia, fatigue, decreased concentration, increased appetite, and psychomotor retardation and thus met criteria for a major depressive episode. She complained of sedation and her weight was 121 lb. On her own initiative she had decreased olanzapine to 7.5 mg at bedtime for 2 days. She was counseled regarding the phenomenon of postmania depression and its symptomatic overlap with adverse effects of medications. She agreed to a more gradual taper of olanzapine— that is, taking 12.5 mg/day for 4 days and then 10 mg/day.

The following week (posthospital week 4), she noted some mood improvement and did not meet criteria for a major depressive episode, but still complained of pervasive fatigue, decreased concentration, and increased appetite. She complained of sedation, and her weight was 123 lb. She had complied with the recommended olanzapine dosing and was thus taking 10 mg at bedtime. She agreed to decrease olanzapine to 7.5 mg at bedtime.

Two weeks later (posthospital week 6), she noted further gradual mood improvement but still complained of pervasive fatigue, decreased concentration, increased appetite, and sedation, and her weight was 125 lb. She had complied with the recommended olanzapine dosing and was thus taking 7.5 mg at bedtime. She agreed to decrease olanzapine to 5 mg at bedtime. She was counseled regarding the need for a different maintenance treatment (because it appeared she would not be able to tolerate longer-term olanzapine). In view of the risk of weight gain and sedation with most approved maintenance therapies, she agreed to a trial of lamotrigine because of its uncommonly good tolerability profile and in spite of its limited efficacy in the prevention of manic episodes. She was advised of the risk of serious rash with lamotrigine.

Two weeks later (posthospital week 8), she noted further gradual mood improvement, with relief of fatigue, normal appetite, and no sedation, and her weight was 122 lb. She was taking olanzapine 5 mg at bedtime and lamotrigine 25 mg in the morning. She agreed to continue olanzapine 5 mg at bedtime and to continue to gradually increase lamotrigine.

Two weeks later (posthospital week 10), in the setting of occupational stress, she had subsyndromal depressive symptoms but denied fatigue or sedation. She complained of increased appetite managed with diet and exercise, and her weight was 121 lb. She was taking olanzapine 5 mg at bedtime and lamotrigine 50 mg in the morning. She agreed to continue olanzapine 5 mg at bedtime and to continue to gradually increase lamotrigine.

Two weeks later (posthospital week 12), her mood was euthymic, with no fatigue or sedation. She complained of increased appetite, and in spite of diet and exercise her weight was 125 lb. She was taking olanzapine 5 mg at bedtime and lamotrigine 100 mg in the morning. She agreed to decrease olanzapine to 2.5 mg at bedtime and to continue to gradually increase lamotrigine.

One month later (posthospital week 16), her mood was euthymic, with no fatigue or sedation. Again, she complained of increased appetite, and in spite of diet and exercise her weight was 128 lb. She was taking olanzapine 2.5 mg at bedtime and lamotrigine 200 mg in the morning. She agreed to decrease olanzapine to 1.25 mg at bedtime and to continue lamotrigine 200 mg/day.

Six weeks later (posthospital week 22), her mood was euthymic, with no fatigue or sedation. Her appetite was normal, and her weight was 121 lb. On her own initiative she had discontinued olanzapine. She was taking lamotrigine 200 mg in the morning. She agreed to continue lamotrigine 200 mg/day.

Subsequently, she has been maintained on lamotrigine 200 mg/day with excellent compliance and has been euthymic for 3 years, with no fatigue, sedation, or appetite problems. With ongoing attention to diet and exercise, she has maintained her weight in the 113- to 116-lb range.

In summary, this middle-aged woman with bipolar I disorder had a good antimanic response to olanzapine but was unable to tolerate this medication for longer-term treatment because of weight gain of 10 lb. (8.5% of her original weight) in the 4 months after hospitalization. She was sufficiently distressed by this problem (as well as sedation and fatigue early in treatment) that it threatened adherence. She was gradually uneventfully cross-tapered from olanzapine to lamotrigine 200 mg/day, with the latter providing excellent tolerability and stable mood for 3 years. She has multiple markers of good prognosis: intermediate (rather than very early or late) age at onset, pure manic (rather than mixed) index episode, limited number of episodes (one mania, and one postmanic depression), lack of comorbid psychiatric and medical disorders, supportive family, good occupational adjustment, careful attention to diet and exercise, and prolonged recovery. These may attenuate the risk of breakthrough mania with lamotrigine monotherapy. Her family is aware of prodromal symptoms of mood elevation and, should these occur, the need to rapidly intervene with an effective antimanic agent.

References

Altshuler L, Suppes T, Black D, et al: Impact of antidepressant discontinuation after acute bipolar depression remission on rates of depressive relapse at 1-year follow-up. Am J Psychiatry 160:1252–1262, 2003

American Psychiatric Association: Practice guideline for the treatment of patients with bipolar disorder (revision). Am J Psychiatry 159:1–50, 2002

Amsterdam JD, Garcia-Espana F, Fawcett J, et al: Efficacy and safety of fluoxetine in treating bipolar II major depressive episode. J Clin Psychopharmacol 18:435–440, 1998

Baastrup PC, Poulsen JC, Schou M, et al: Prophylactic lithium: double blind discontinuation in manic-depressive and recurrent-depressive disorders. Lancet 2: 326–330, 1970

Baldessarini RJ, Tondo L: Does lithium treatment still work? Evidence of stable responses over three decades. Arch Gen Psychiatry 57:187–190, 2000

Baldessarini RJ, Tondo L, Floris G, et al: Reduced morbidity after gradual discontinuation of lithium treatment for bipolar I and II disorders: a replication study. Am J Psychiatry 154:551–553, 1997

Barbini B, Scherillo P, Benedetti F, et al: Response to clozapine in acute mania is more rapid than that of chlorpromazine. Int Clin Psychopharmacol 12:109–112, 1997

Bauer MS, McBride L, Williford WO, et al: Collaborative care for bipolar disorder, part II: impact on clinical outcome, function, and costs. Psychiatr Serv 57:937–945, 2006

Berghofer A, Kossmann B, Muller-Oerlinghausen B: Course of illness and pattern of recurrences in patients with affective disorders during long-term lithium prophylaxis: a retrospective analysis over 15 years. Acta Psychiatr Scand 93:349–354, 1996

Bowden CL, Brugger AM, Swann AC, et al: Efficacy of divalproex vs lithium and placebo in the treatment of mania. The Depakote Mania Study Group. JAMA 271:918–924, 1994

Bowden CL, Calabrese JR, McElroy SL, et al: A randomized, placebo-controlled 12-month trial of divalproex and lithium in treatment of outpatients with bipolar

I disorder. Divalproex Maintenance Study Group. Arch Gen Psychiatry 57:481–489, 2000

Bowden CL, Calabrese JR, Sachs G, et al: A placebo-controlled 18-month trial of lamotrigine and lithium maintenance treatment in recently manic or hypomanic patients with bipolar I disorder. Arch Gen Psychiatry 60:392–400, 2003

Bowden CL, Collins MA, McElroy SL, et al: Relationship of mania symptomatology to maintenance treatment response with divalproex, lithium, or placebo. Neuropsychopharmacology 30:1932–1939, 2005

Bowden CL, Calabrese JR, Ketter TA, et al: Impact of lamotrigine and lithium on weight in obese and nonobese patients with bipolar I disorder. Am J Psychiatry 163:1199–1201, 2006

Brady KT, Sonne SC, Anton R, et al: Valproate in the treatment of acute bipolar affective episodes complicated by substance abuse: a pilot study. J Clin Psychiatry 56:118–121, 1995

Brown E, Dunner D, Adams D, et al: Olanzapine/fluoxetine combination versus lamotrigine in the long-term treatment of bipolar I depression (80). Neuropsychopharmacology 30 (suppl 1):S108–S109, 2005

Brown EB, McElroy SL, Keck PE Jr, et al: A 7-week, randomized, double-blind trial of olanzapine/fluoxetine combination versus lamotrigine in the treatment of bipolar I depression. J Clin Psychiatry 67:1025–1033, 2006

Calabrese JR, Woyshville MJ, Kimmel SE, et al: Predictors of valproate response in bipolar rapid cycling. J Clin Psychopharmacol 13:280–283, 1993

Calabrese JR, Bowden CL, Sachs GS, et al: A double-blind placebo-controlled study of lamotrigine monotherapy in outpatients with bipolar I depression. Lamictal 602 Study Group. J Clin Psychiatry 60:79–88, 1999

Calabrese JR, Suppes T, Bowden CL, et al: A double-blind, placebo-controlled, prophylaxis study of lamotrigine in rapid-cycling bipolar disorder. Lamictal 614 Study Group. J Clin Psychiatry 61:841–850, 2000

Calabrese JR, Bowden CL, Sachs G, et al: A placebo-controlled 18-month trial of lamotrigine and lithium maintenance treatment in recently depressed patients with bipolar I disorder. J Clin Psychiatry 64:1013–1024, 2003

Carlson GA, Davenport YB, Jamison K: A comparison of outcome in adolescent- and later-onset bipolar manic-depressive illness. Am J Psychiatry 134:919–922, 1977

Colom F, Vieta E, Martinez-Aran A, et al: A randomized trial on the efficacy of group psychoeducation in the prophylaxis of recurrences in bipolar patients whose disease is in remission. Arch Gen Psychiatry 60:402–407, 2003

Conley RR, Meltzer HY: Adverse events related to olanzapine. J Clin Psychiatry 61 (suppl 8):26–30, 2000

Coppen A, Noguera R, Bailey J, et al: Prophylactic lithium in affective disorders. Controlled trial. Lancet 2:275–279, 1971

Coppen A, Peet M, Bailey J, et al: Double-blind and open prospective studies on lithium prophylaxis in affective disorders. Psychiatr Neurol Neurochir 76:501–510, 1973

Corya SA, Perlis RH, Keck PE Jr, et al: A 24-week open-label extension study of olanzapine-fluoxetine combination and olanzapine monotherapy in the treatment of bipolar depression. J Clin Psychiatry 67:798–806, 2006

Coryell W, Akiskal H, Leon AC, et al: Family history and symptom levels during treatment for bipolar I affective disorder. Biol Psychiatry 47:1034–1042, 2000

Cundall RL, Brooks PW, Murray LG: A controlled evaluation of lithium prophylaxis in affective disorders. Psychol Med 2:308–311, 1972

Denicoff KD, Smith-Jackson EE, Disney ER, et al: Comparative prophylactic efficacy of lithium, carbamazepine, and the combination in bipolar disorder. J Clin Psychiatry 58:470–478, 1997

Dickson WE, Kendell RE: Does maintenance lithium therapy prevent recurrences of mania under ordinary clinical conditions? Psychol Med 16:521–530, 1986

Dilsaver SC, Swann AC, Shoaib AM, et al: The manic syndrome: factors which may predict a patient's response to lithium, carbamazepine and valproate. J Psychiatry Neurosci 18:61–66, 1993

Dunner DL, Fieve RR: Clinical factors in lithium carbonate prophylaxis failure. Arch Gen Psychiatry 30:229–233, 1974

Dunner DL, Dwyer T, Fieve RR: Depressive symptoms in patients with unipolar and bipolar affective disorder. Compr Psychiatry 17:447–451, 1976a

Dunner DL, Fleiss JL, Fieve RR: The course of development of mania in patients with recurrent depression. Am J Psychiatry 133:905–908, 1976b

Dunner DL, Stallone F, Fieve RR: Lithium carbonate and affective disorders, V: a double-blind study of prophylaxis of depression in bipolar illness. Arch Gen Psychiatry 33:117–120, 1976c

Faedda GL, Baldessarini RJ, Tohen M, et al: Episode sequence in bipolar disorder and response to lithium treatment. Am J Psychiatry 148:1237–1239, 1991

Faedda GL, Tondo L, Baldessarini RJ, et al: Outcome after rapid vs gradual discontinuation of lithium treatment in bipolar disorders. Arch Gen Psychiatry 50:448–455, 1993

Fieve RR, Kumbaraci T, Dunner DL: Lithium prophylaxis of depression in bipolar I, bipolar II, and unipolar patients. Am J Psychiatry 133:925–929, 1976

Frank E, Kupfer DJ, Thase ME, et al: Two-year outcomes for interpersonal and social rhythm therapy in individuals with bipolar I disorder. Arch Gen Psychiatry 62:996–1004, 2005

Freeman TW, Clothier JL, Pazzaglia P, et al: A double-blind comparison of valproate and lithium in the treatment of acute mania. Am J Psychiatry 149:108–111, 1992

Frye MA, Ketter TA, Altshuler LL, et al: Clozapine in bipolar disorder: treatment implications for other atypical antipsychotics. J Affect Disord 48:91–104, 1998

Garfinkel PE, Stancer HC, Persad E: A comparison of haloperidol, lithium carbonate and their combination in the treatment of mania. J Affect Disord 2:279–288, 1980

Geddes JR, Burgess S, Hawton K, et al: Long-term lithium therapy for bipolar disorder: systematic review and meta-analysis of randomized controlled trials. Am J Psychiatry 161:217–222, 2004

Gelenberg AJ: Lithium efficacy and adverse effects. J Clin Psychiatry 49(suppl):8–11, 1988

Gelenberg AJ, Kane JM, Keller MB, et al: Comparison of standard and low serum levels of lithium for maintenance treatment of bipolar disorder. N Engl J Med 321:1489–1493, 1989

Ghaemi SN, Lenox MS, Baldessarini RJ: Effectiveness and safety of long-term antidepressant treatment in bipolar disorder. J Clin Psychiatry 62:565–569, 2001

Ghaemi SN, Hsu DJ, Rosenquist KJ, et al: Long-term observational comparison of risperidone and olanzapine in bipolar disorder. Ann Clin Psychiatry 16:69–73, 2004

Gitlin MJ, Cochran SD, Jamison KR: Maintenance lithium treatment: side effects and compliance. J Clin Psychiatry 50:127–131, 1989

Goodnick PJ, Fieve RR, Schlegel A, et al: Predictors of interepisode symptoms and relapse in affective disorder patients treated with lithium carbonate. Am J Psychiatry 144:367–369, 1987

Goodwin FK, Fireman B, Simon GE, et al: Suicide risk in bipolar disorder during treatment with lithium and divalproex. JAMA 290:1467–1473, 2003

Goodwin FR, Jamison K: Manic-Depressive Illness. New York, Oxford University Press, 1990

Goodwin FR, Jamison K: Manic-Depressive Illness: Bipolar Disorders and Recurrent Depression, 2nd Edition. New York, Oxford University Press, 2007

Goodwin GM: Evidence-based guidelines for treating bipolar disorder: recommendations from the British Association for Psychopharmacology. J Psychopharmacol 17:149–173, 2003

Goodwin GM, Bowden CL, Calabrese JR, et al: A pooled analysis of 2 placebo-controlled 18-month trials of lamotrigine and lithium maintenance in bipolar I disorder. J Clin Psychiatry 65:432–441, 2004

Greil W, Ludwig-Mayerhofer W, Erazo N, et al: Lithium versus carbamazepine in the maintenance treatment of bipolar disorders—a randomised study. J Affect Disord 43:151–161, 1997

Greil W, Kleindienst N, Erazo N, et al: Differential response to lithium and carbamazepine in the prophylaxis of bipolar disorder. J Clin Psychopharmacol 18:455–460, 1998

Grof E, Haag M, Grof P, et al: Lithium response and the sequence of episode polarities: preliminary report on a Hamilton sample. Prog Neuropsychopharmacol Biol Psychiatry 11:199–203, 1987

Grof P, Alda M, Grof E, et al: The challenge of predicting response to stabilising lithium treatment. The importance of patient selection. Br J Psychiatry Suppl (21):16–19, 1993

Grunze H, Kasper S, Goodwin G, et al: World Federation of Societies of Biological Psychiatry (WFSBP) guidelines for biological treatment of bipolar disorders. Part I: treatment of bipolar depression. World J Biol Psychiatry 3:115–124, 2002

Guscott R, Taylor L: Lithium prophylaxis in recurrent affective illness: efficacy, effectiveness and efficiency. Br J Psychiatry 164:741–746, 1994

Gyulai L, Bowden CL, McElroy SL, et al: Maintenance efficacy of divalproex in the prevention of bipolar depression. Neuropsychopharmacology 28:1374–1382, 2003

Haag H, Heidorn A, Haag M, et al: Response to stabilising lithium therapy and sequence of affective polarity. Pharmacopsychiatry 19:278–279, 1986

Han C, Lee MS, Pae CU, et al: Usefulness of long-acting injectable risperidone during 12-month maintenance therapy of bipolar disorder. Prog Neuropsychopharmacol Biol Psychiatry 31:1219–1223, 2007

Harrow M, Goldberg JF, Grossman LS, et al: Outcome in manic disorders: a naturalistic follow-up study. Arch Gen Psychiatry 47:665–671, 1990

Hartong EG, Moleman P, Hoogduin CA, et al: Prophylactic efficacy of lithium versus carbamazepine in treatment-naive bipolar patients. J Clin Psychiatry 64:144–151, 2003

Himmelhoch JM, Garfinkel ME: Sources of lithium resistance in mixed mania. Psychopharmacol Bull 22:613–620, 1986

Jaffe RL, Rives W, Dubin WR, et al: Problems in maintenance ECT in bipolar disorder: replacement by lithium and anticonvulsants. Convuls Ther 7:288–294, 1991

Johnson RE, McFarland BH: Lithium use and discontinuation in a health maintenance organization. Am J Psychiatry 153:993–1000, 1996

Joyce PR: Carbamazepine in rapid cycling bipolar affective disorder. Int Clin Psychopharmacol 3:123–129, 1988

Judd LL, Akiskal HS, Schettler PJ, et al: The long-term natural history of the weekly symptomatic status of bipolar I disorder. Arch Gen Psychiatry 59:530–537, 2002

Judd LL, Akiskal HS, Schettler PJ, et al: A prospective investigation of the natural history of the long-term weekly symptomatic status of bipolar II disorder. Arch Gen Psychiatry 60:261–269, 2003

Kahn D, Stevenson E, Douglas CJ: Effect of sodium valproate in three patients with organic brain syndromes. Am J Psychiatry 145:1010–1011, 1988

Kane JM, Quitkin FM, Rifkin A, et al: Lithium carbonate and imipramine in the prophylaxis of unipolar and bipolar II illness: a prospective, placebo-controlled comparison. Arch Gen Psychiatry 39:1065–1069, 1982

Kato T, Inubushi T, Kato N: Prediction of lithium response by 31P-MRS in bipolar disorder. Int J Neuropsychopharmacol 3:83–85, 2000

Keck PE Jr, Perlis RH, Otto MW, et al: The expert consensus guideline series: medication treatment of bipolar disorder 2004. Postgrad Med Spec No:1–120, 2004a

Keck PE Jr, Potkin SG, Giller E Jr, et al: Ziprasidone's long-term efficacy and safety in bipolar disorder (NR745). Abstract presented at the 157th annual meeting of the American Psychiatric Association, New York, May 1–6, 2004b, p 280

Keck PE Jr, Calabrese JR, McQuade RD, et al: A randomized, double-blind, placebo-controlled 26-week trial of aripiprazole in recently manic patients with bipolar I disorder. J Clin Psychiatry 67:626–637, 2006

Keck PE Jr, Calabrese JR, McIntyre RS, et al: Aripiprazole monotherapy for maintenance therapy in bipolar I disorder: a 100-week, double-blind study versus placebo. J Clin Psychiatry 68:1480–1491, 2007

Keller MB, Lavori PW, Coryell W, et al: Differential outcome of pure manic, mixed/cycling, and pure depressive episodes in patients with bipolar illness. JAMA 255:3138–3142, 1986

Keller MB, Lavori PW, Kane JM, et al: Subsyndromal symptoms in bipolar disorder: a comparison of standard and low serum levels of lithium. Arch Gen Psychiatry 49:371–376, 1992

Kellner CH, Knapp RG, Petrides G, et al: Continuation electroconvulsive therapy vs pharmacotherapy for relapse prevention in major depression: a multisite study from the Consortium for Research in Electroconvulsive Therapy (CORE). Arch Gen Psychiatry 63:1337–1344, 2006

Ketter TA, Calabrese JR: Stabilization of mood from below versus above baseline in bipolar disorder: a new nomenclature. J Clin Psychiatry 63:146–151, 2002

Ketter T, Bowden C, Suppes T, et al: Predictors of response to lithium and lamotrigine prophylaxis in bipolar I disorder (P106). Bipolar Disord 5 (suppl 1):60, 2003

Ketter TA, Wang PW, Chandler RA, et al: Dermatology precautions and slower titration yield low incidence of lamotrigine treatment–emergent rash. J Clin Psychiatry 66:642–645, 2005

Kleindienst N, Engel R, Greil W: Which clinical factors predict response to prophylactic lithium? A systematic review for bipolar disorders. Bipolar Disord 7:404–417, 2005

Kukopulos A, Reginaldi D: Recurrences of manic-depressive episodes during lithium treatment, in Handbook of Lithium Therapy. Edited by Johnson FN. Lancaster, UK, MTP Press, 1980, pp 109–117

Kukopulos A, Reginaldi D, Laddomada P, et al: Course of the manic-depressive cycle and changes caused by treatment. Pharmakopsychiatr Neuropsychopharmakol 13:156–167, 1980

Lam DH, Watkins ER, Hayward P, et al: A randomized controlled study of cognitive therapy for relapse prevention for bipolar affective disorder: outcome of the first year. Arch Gen Psychiatry 60:145–152, 2003

Licht RW, Vestergaard P, Rasmussen NA, et al: A lithium clinic for bipolar patients: 2-year outcome of the first 148 patients. Acta Psychiatr Scand 104:387–390, 2001

Loo H, Galinowski A, De Carvalho W, et al: Use of maintenance ECT for elderly depressed patients (letter). Am J Psychiatry 148:810, 1991

Lusznat RM, Murphy DP, Nunn CM: Carbamazepine vs lithium in the treatment and prophylaxis of mania. Br J Psychiatry 153:198–204, 1988

MacFadden W, Haskins T, Kujawa M, et al: Adjunctive risperidone long-acting inject-able is effective in delaying relapse to a mood episode in patients with frequently re-lapsing bipolar disorder (584). Abstract presented at the 55th Annual Convention and Scientific Program of the Society of Biological Psychiatry, Washington, DC, May 1–3, 2008. Biol Psychiatry 63 (suppl 7):186S, 2008

Maj M: Clinical prediction of response to lithium prophylaxis in bipolar patients: the importance of the previous pattern of course of the illness. Clin Neuropharmacol 13 (suppl 1):S66–S70, 1990

Maj M, Del Vecchio M, Starace F, et al: Prediction of affective psychoses response to lith-ium prophylaxis: the role of socio-demographic, clinical, psychological and bio-logical variables. Acta Psychiatr Scand 69:37–44, 1984

Maj M, Starace F, Nolfe G, et al: Minimum plasma lithium levels required for effective prophylaxis in DSM III bipolar disorder: a prospective study. Pharmacopsychiatry 19:420–423, 1986

Maj M, Pirozzi R, Starace F: Previous pattern of course of the illness as a predictor of re-sponse to lithium prophylaxis in bipolar patients. J Affect Disord 17:237–241, 1989

Maj M, Pirozzi R, Magliano L: Nonresponse to reinstituted lithium prophylaxis in pre-viously responsive bipolar patients: prevalence and predictors. Am J Psychiatry 152:1810–1811, 1995

Maj M, Pirozzi R, Magliano L: Late non-response to lithium prophylaxis in bipolar pa-tients: prevalence and predictors. J Affect Disord 39:39–42, 1996

Maj M, Pirozzi R, Magliano L, et al: Long-term outcome of lithium prophylaxis in bi-polar disorder: a 5-year prospective study of 402 patients at a lithium clinic. Am J Psychiatry 155:30–35, 1998

Malempati RN, Bond DJ, Yatham LN: Depot risperidone in the outpatient manage-ment of bipolar disorder: a 2-year study of 10 patients. Int Clin Psychopharmacol 23:88–94, 2008

Markar HR, Mander AJ: Efficacy of lithium prophylaxis in clinical practice. Br J Psychi-atry 155:496–500, 1989

McElroy SL, Bowden CL, Collins MA, et al: Relationship of open acute mania treatment to blinded maintenance outcome in bipolar I disorder. J Affect Disord 107:127–133, 2008

McIntyre RS, Mancini DA, Srinivasan J, et al: The antidepressant effects of risperidone and olanzapine in bipolar disorder. Can J Clin Pharmacol 11:e218–e226, 2004

Melia PI: Prophylactic lithium: a double-blind trial in recurrent affective disorders. Br J Psychiatry 116:621–624, 1970

Mendlewicz J, Fieve RR, Stallone F: Relationship between the effectiveness of lithium therapy and family history. Am J Psychiatry 130:1011–1013, 1973

Miklowitz DJ, George EL, Richards JA, et al: A randomized study of family focused psy-choeducation and pharmacotherapy in the outpatient management of bipolar dis-order. Arch Gen Psychiatry 60:904–912, 2003

Moncrieff J: Lithium revisited: a re-examination of the placebo-controlled trials of lithium prophylaxis in manic-depressive disorder. Br J Psychiatry 167:569–573, 1995

O'Connell RA, Mayo JA, Flatow L, et al: Outcome of bipolar disorder on long-term treatment with lithium. Br J Psychiatry 159:123–129, 1991

Okuma T: Effects of carbamazepine and lithium on affective disorders. Neuropsychobiology 27:138–145, 1993

Okuma T, Inanaga K, Otsuki S, et al: Comparison of the antimanic efficacy of carbamazepine and chlorpromazine: a double-blind controlled study. Psychopharmacology (Berl) 66:211–217, 1979

Papatheodorou G, Kutcher SP: Divalproex sodium treatment in late adolescent and young adult acute mania. Psychopharmacol Bull 29:213–219, 1993

Passmore MJ, Garnham J, Duffy A, et al: Phenotypic spectra of bipolar disorder in responders to lithium versus lamotrigine. Bipolar Disord 5:110–114, 2003

Perlis RH, Sachs GS, Lafer B, et al: Effect of abrupt change from standard to low serum levels of lithium: a reanalysis of double-blind lithium maintenance data. Am J Psychiatry 159:1155–1159, 2002

Perry A, Tarrier N, Morriss R, et al: Randomised controlled trial of efficacy of teaching patients with bipolar disorder to identify early symptoms of relapse and obtain treatment. BMJ 318:149–153, 1999

Physicians' Desk Reference, 62nd Edition. Montvale, NJ, Thomson Healthcare, 2008

Pond SM, Becker CE, Vandervoort R, et al: An evaluation of the effects of lithium in the treatment of chronic alcoholism, I: clinical results. Alcohol Clin Exp Res 5:247–251, 1981

Poole AJ, James HD, Hughes WC: Treatment experiences in the lithium clinic at St Thomas Hospital. J R Soc Med 71:890–894, 1978

Post RM, Uhde TW, Roy-Byrne PP, et al: Correlates of antimanic response to carbamazepine. Psychiatry Res 21:71–83, 1987

Post RM, Rubinow DR, Uhde TW, et al: Dysphoric mania: clinical and biological correlates. Arch Gen Psychiatry 46:353–358, 1989

Post RM, Leverich GS, Altshuler L, et al: Lithium-discontinuation-induced refractoriness: preliminary observations. Am J Psychiatry 149:1727–1729, 1992

Prien RF, Kupfer DJ: Continuation drug therapy for major depressive episodes: how long should it be maintained? Am J Psychiatry 143:18–23, 1986

Prien RF, Caffey EM Jr, Klett CJ: Prophylactic efficacy of lithium carbonate in manic-depressive illness. Report of the Veterans Administration and National Institute of Mental Health collaborative study group. Arch Gen Psychiatry 28:337–341, 1973a

Prien RF, Klett CJ, Caffey EM Jr: Lithium carbonate and imipramine in prevention of affective episodes: a comparison in recurrent affective illness. Arch Gen Psychiatry 29:420–425, 1973b

Prien RF, Klett CJ, Caffey EM Jr: Lithium prophylaxis in recurrent affective illness. Am J Psychiatry 131:198–203, 1974

Prien RF, Kupfer DJ, Mansky PA, et al: Drug therapy in the prevention of recurrences in unipolar and bipolar affective disorders. Report of the NIMH collaborative study group comparing lithium carbonate, imipramine, and a lithium carbonate–imipramine combination. Arch Gen Psychiatry 41:1096–1104, 1984

Prien RF, Himmelhoch JM, Kupfer DJ: Treatment of mixed mania. J Affect Disord 15:9–15, 1988

Quitkin F, Rifkin A, Klein DF: Prophylaxis of affective disorders: current status of knowledge. Arch Gen Psychiatry 33:337–341, 1976

Quitkin F, Rifkin A, Kane J, et al: Prophylactic effect of lithium and imipramine in unipolar and bipolar II patients: a preliminary report. Am J Psychiatry 135:570–572, 1978

Quitkin FM, Kane J, Rifkin A, et al: Prophylactic lithium carbonate with and without imipramine for bipolar 1 patients: a double-blind study. Arch Gen Psychiatry 38:902–927, 1981

Revicki DA, Hirschfeld RM, Ahearn EP, et al: Effectiveness and medical costs of divalproex versus lithium in the treatment of bipolar disorder: results of a naturalistic clinical trial. J Affect Disord 86:183–193, 2005

Rush AJ, Sackeim HA, Marangell LB, et al: Effects of 12 months of vagus nerve stimulation in treatment-resistant depression: a naturalistic study. Biol Psychiatry 58:355–363, 2005

Rybakowski J, Chlopocka-Wozniak M, Kapelski Z, et al: The relative prophylactic efficacy of lithium against manic and depressive recurrences in bipolar patients. Int Pharmacopsychiatry 15:86–90, 1980

Sachs G, Lafer B, Stoll AL, et al: A double-blind trial of bupropion versus desipramine for bipolar depression. J Clin Psychiatry 55:391–393, 1994

Sachs G, Bowden C, Calabrese JR, et al: Effects of lamotrigine and lithium on body weight during maintenance treatment of bipolar I disorder. Bipolar Disord 8:175–181, 2006

Sarantidis D, Waters B: Predictors of lithium prophylaxis effectiveness. Prog Neuropsychopharmacol 5:507–510, 1981

Savas HA, Yumru M, Ozen ME: Use of long-acting risperidone in the treatment of bipolar patients. J Clin Psychopharmacol 26:530–531, 2006

Schurhoff F, Bellivier F, Jouvent R, et al: Early and late onset bipolar disorders: two different forms of manic-depressive illness? J Affect Disord 58:215–221, 2000

Secunda SK, Katz MM, Swann A, et al: Mania: diagnosis, state measurement and prediction of treatment response. J Affect Disord 8:113–121, 1985

Severus WE, Kleindienst N, Seemuller F, et al: What is the optimal serum lithium level in the long-term treatment of bipolar disorder—a review? Bipolar Disord 10:231–237, 2008

Silverstone T, McPherson H, Hunt N, et al: How effective is lithium in the prevention of relapse in bipolar disorder? A prospective naturalistic follow-up study. Aust NZ J Psychiatry 32:61–66, 1998

Simon GE, Ludman EJ, Bauer MS, et al: Long-term effectiveness and cost of a systematic care program for bipolar disorder. Arch Gen Psychiatry 63:500–508, 2006

Small JG, Milstein V: Lithium interactions: lithium and electroconvulsive therapy. J Clin Psychopharmacol 10:346–350, 1990

Small JG, Klapper MH, Milstein V, et al: Carbamazepine compared with lithium in the treatment of mania. Arch Gen Psychiatry 48:915–921, 1991

Soares JC, Gershon S: The psychopharmacologic specificity of the lithium ion: origins and trajectory. J Clin Psychiatry 61:16–22, 2000

Solomon DA, Ristow WR, Keller MB, et al: Serum lithium levels and psychosocial function in patients with bipolar I disorder. Am J Psychiatry 153:1301–1307, 1996

Sovner R: The use of valproate in the treatment of mentally retarded persons with typical and atypical bipolar disorders. J Clin Psychiatry 50(suppl):40–43, 1989

Stallone F, Shelley E, Mendlewicz J, et al: The use of lithium in affective disorders, 3: a double-blind study of prophylaxis in bipolar illness. Am J Psychiatry 130:1006–1010, 1973

Stoll AL, Banov M, Kolbrener M, et al: Neurologic factors predict a favorable valproate response in bipolar and schizoaffective disorders. J Clin Psychopharmacol 14:311–313, 1994

Strober M, Morrell W, Burroughs J, et al: A family study of bipolar I disorder in adolescence: early onset of symptoms linked to increased familial loading and lithium resistance. J Affect Disord 15:255–268, 1988

Suppes T, Baldessarini RJ, Faedda GL, et al: Risk of recurrence following discontinuation of lithium treatment in bipolar disorder. Arch Gen Psychiatry 48:1082–1088, 1991

Suppes T, Webb A, Paul B, et al: Clinical outcome in a randomized 1-year trial of clozapine versus treatment as usual for patients with treatment-resistant illness and a history of mania. Am J Psychiatry 156:1164–1169, 1999

Suppes T, Dennehy EB, Hirschfeld RM, et al: The Texas Implementation of Medication Algorithms: update to the algorithms for treatment of bipolar I disorder. J Clin Psychiatry 66:870–886, 2005

Suppes T, Vieta E, Liu S, et al: Maintenance treatment for patients with bipolar I disorder: results from a North American study of quetiapine in combination with lithium or divalproex (trial 127). Am J Psychiatry 166:476–488, 2009

Swann AC, Secunda SK, Katz MM, et al: Lithium treatment of mania: clinical characteristics, specificity of symptom change, and outcome. Psychiatry Res 18:127–141, 1986

Swann AC, Bowden CL, Morris D, et al: Depression during mania: treatment response to lithium or divalproex. Arch Gen Psychiatry 54:37–42, 1997

Swann AC, Bowden CL, Calabrese JR, et al: Mania: differential effects of previous depressive and manic episodes on response to treatment. Acta Psychiatr Scand 101:444–451, 2000

Swartz HA, Frank E: Psychotherapy for bipolar depression: a phase-specific treatment strategy? Bipolar Disord 3:11–22, 2001

Tohen M, Ketter TA, Zarate CA, et al: Olanzapine versus divalproex sodium for the treatment of acute mania and maintenance of remission: a 47-week study. Am J Psychiatry 160:1263–1271, 2003a

Tohen M, Vieta E, Calabrese J, et al: Efficacy of olanzapine and olanzapine-fluoxetine combination in the treatment of bipolar I depression. Arch Gen Psychiatry 60:1079–1088, 2003b

Tohen MF, Bowden CL, Calabrese JR, et al: Predictors of time to relapse in bipolar I disorder (NR800). Abstract presented at the 157th annual meeting of the American Psychiatric Association, New York, May 1–6, 2004a, p 301

Tohen M, Chengappa KN, Suppes T, et al: Relapse prevention in bipolar I disorder: 18-month comparison of olanzapine plus mood stabiliser v. mood stabiliser alone. Br J Psychiatry 184:337–345, 2004b

Tohen M, Greil W, Calabrese JR, et al: Olanzapine versus lithium in the maintenance treatment of bipolar disorder: a 12-month, randomized, double-blind, controlled clinical trial. Am J Psychiatry 162:1281–1290, 2005

Tohen M, Calabrese JR, Sachs GS, et al: Randomized, placebo-controlled trial of olanzapine as maintenance therapy in patients with bipolar I disorder responding to acute treatment with olanzapine. Am J Psychiatry 163:247–256, 2006

Tondo L, Baldessarini RJ, Floris G, et al: Effectiveness of restarting lithium treatment after its discontinuation in bipolar I and bipolar II disorders. Am J Psychiatry 154:548–550, 1997

Tondo L, Baldessarini RJ, Hennen J, et al: Lithium maintenance treatment of depression and mania in bipolar I and bipolar II disorders. Am J Psychiatry 155:638–645, 1998a

Tondo L, Baldessarini RJ, Hennen J, et al: Lithium treatment and risk of suicidal behavior in bipolar disorder patients. J Clin Psychiatry 59:405–414, 1998b

Tondo L, Baldessarini RJ, Floris G: Long-term clinical effectiveness of lithium maintenance treatment in types I and II bipolar disorders. Br J Psychiatry Suppl 41:S184–S190, 2001

Vaidya NA, Mahableshwarkar AR, Shahid R: Continuation and maintenance ECT in treatment-resistant bipolar disorder. J ECT 19:10–16, 2003

Vanelle JM, Loo H, Galinowski A, et al: Maintenance ECT in intractable manic-depressive disorders. Convuls Ther 10:195–205, 1994

Vieta E, Goikolea JM, Corbella B, et al: Risperidone safety and efficacy in the treatment of bipolar and schizoaffective disorders: results from a 6-month, multicenter, open study. J Clin Psychiatry 62:818–825, 2001

Vieta E, Suppes T, Eggens I, et al: Efficacy and safety of quetiapine in combination with lithium or divalproex for maintenance of patients with bipolar I disorder (international trial 126). J Affect Disord 109:251–263, 2008

Wang PW, Keller KL, Hill S, et al: Effectiveness of open adjunctive ziprasidone in obese and overweight bipolar disorder patients (606). Biol Psychiatry 63 (suppl 7):193S–194S, 2008

Warrington L, Lombardo I, Loebel A, et al: Ziprasidone for the treatment of acute manic or mixed episodes associated with bipolar disorder. CNS Drugs 21:835–849, 2007

Wehr TA, Goodwin FK: Rapid cycling in manic-depressives induced by tricyclic antidepressants. Arch Gen Psychiatry 36: 555–559, 1979

Weisler RH, Warrington L, Dunn J, et al: Adjunctive ziprasidone in bipolar mania: short-term and long-term data (NR358). Abstract presented at the 157th annual meeting of the American Psychiatric Association, New York, May 1–6, 2004, pp 132–133

Yang YY: Prophylactic efficacy of lithium and its effective plasma levels in Chinese bipolar patients. Acta Psychiatr Scand 71:171–175, 1985

Yatham LN, Kennedy SH, O'Donovan C, et al: Canadian Network for Mood and Anxiety Treatments (CANMAT) guidelines for the management of patients with bipolar disorder: update 2007. Bipolar Disord 8:721–739, 2006

Yazici O, Kora K, Ucok A, et al: Predictors of lithium prophylaxis in bipolar patients. J Affect Disord 55:133–142, 1999

Zarate CA Jr, Tohen M, Baldessarini RJ: Clozapine in severe mood disorders. J Clin Psychiatry 56:411–417, 1995

Management of Rapid-Cycling Bipolar Disorders

Terence A. Ketter, M.D.

Po W. Wang, M.D.

Defined by Dunner and Fieve (1974) as the occurrence of at least four mood episodes within a 12-month period, rapid cycling was first included as a bipolar disorder course specifier 20 years later in the *Diagnostic and Statistical Manual of Mental Disorders*, 4th Edition (American Psychiatric Association 1994; Bauer et al. 1994), and was continued unaltered in the *Diagnostic and Statistical Manual of Mental Disorders*, 4th Edition, Text Revision (DSM-IV-TR; American Psychiatric Association 2000). This cycle frequency is accompanied by distinctive phenomenology and treatment response characteristics.

According to the DSM-IV-TR definition of rapid cycling, episodes must be demarcated by remissions lasting at least 2 months or by switches into episodes of opposite polarity. Broader definitions of rapid cycling have suggested including episodes and/or intervening periods that do not always meet DSM-IV-TR episode duration or remission criteria (Maj et al. 1999). Thus, non-DSM-IV-TR terms have been proposed to describe affective oscillations occurring within days to weeks (ultra-rapid cycling) and within single days (ultradian cycling) (Kramlinger and Post 1996). Patients with ultradian cycling may meet DSM-IV-TR criteria for mixed episodes.

In this chapter, we review the epidemiology, clinical characteristics, and treatment of rapid-cycling bipolar disorders, with special emphasis on evidence-based, practical, clinical information.

Epidemiology

The prevalence of rapid cycling in patients with bipolar disorders in clinical studies most often ranges between approximately 15% and 20% (Dunner and Fieve 1974; Kupka et al. 2003; Maj et al. 1994, 1999; Schneck et al. 2004) but in some studies has been as high as 55% (Cowdry et al. 1983). In Kupka et al.'s (2003) meta-analysis of eight studies (Avasthi et al. 1999; Baldessarini et al. 2000; Coryell et al. 1992; Cowdry et al. 1983; Kukopulos et al. 1980; Maj et al. 1989, 1999; Nurnberger et al. 1988), the prevalence of rapid cycling was 16.3% (335/2,054). Rapid cycling has been consistently associated with female gender but not with other demographic parameters (Bauer et al. 1994; Kupka et al. 2003; Schneck et al. 2004). Thus, in a meta-analysis of 16 studies (Kupka et al. 2003), female gender was more common among individuals with rapid cycling (66%, 613/929) than those with non–rapid cycling (53%, 1,304/2,465) (Figure 9–1, leftmost graph). As discussed in Chapter 11, "Management of Bipolar Disorders in Women," the overrepresentation of women with rapid cycling may be related to central actions of female gonadal steroids.

Clinical Characteristics

Rapid cycling has been associated with increased depressive morbidity (Calabrese et al. 2001; Coryell et al. 2003) and possibly with bipolar II disorder (Baldessarini et al. 2000; Coryell et al. 1992; Kukopulos et al. 1980; Maj et al. 1999; Wu and Dunner 1993). In a meta-analysis of 11 studies (Kupka et al. 2003), the prevalence of rapid cycling in bipolar II disorder (43%, 345/802) was higher than in bipolar I disorder (31%, 584/1,884) (Figure 9–1, second set of bars from left), but was lower (Kupka et al. 2005) or similar (Schneck et al. 2004) in subsequent large studies. There may be gender effects on relationships between rapid cycling and other constructs, such as bipolar illness subtype and episode frequency. For example, in women, rapid cycling may be associated with bipolar II disorder (Schneck et al. 2004) and may be associated with having eight or more episodes per year (Kupka et al. 2005).

Other possible associations with rapid cycling—such as early age at onset (Bowden et al. 1999; Coryell et al. 2003), index depressive episodes (Avasthi et al. 1999), history of suicide attempts (Wehr et al. 1988), anxiety disorders (Kauer-

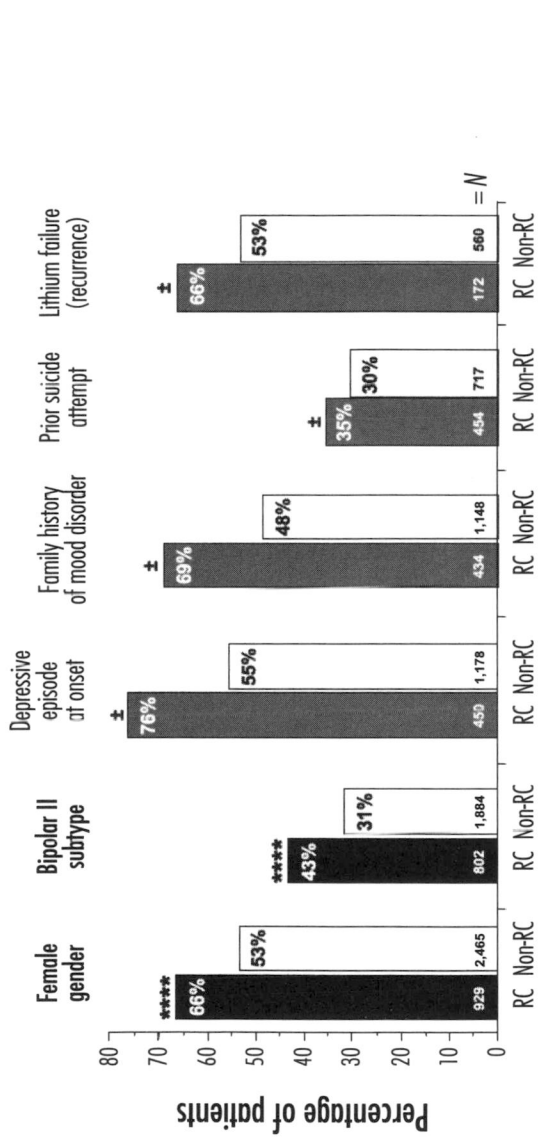

FIGURE 9–1. Increased female gender and bipolar II disorder in rapid-cycling bipolar disorder meta-analysis.

Other possible associations with rapid cycling (gray bars) were less consistent. RC=rapid cycling; Non-RC=non–rapid cycling. ****P<0.0001 significant; ±P=nonsignificant trend (after Hochberg adjustment) versus non–rapid cycling.

Source.   Data from Kupka et al. 2003.

Sant'Anna et al. 2007), thyroid disorders (Bauer et al. 1990), alcohol/substance abuse (McKowen et al. 2005), and prior antidepressant administration (Kukopulos et al. 1983)—have been less consistent (Kupka et al. 2003) (Figure 9–1, four gray graphs on right).

From the perspectives of phenomenology (Coryell et al. 1992; Kupka et al. 2005; Schneck et al. 2004) and family history (Coryell et al. 1992; Nurnberger et al. 1988; Wehr et al. 1988), rapid cycling appears to be on a continuum with rather than categorically distinct from other forms of bipolar disorders. Hence, a dimensional model may be more appropriate than the current categorical approach to rapid cycling.

Post et al. (1986, 1988) proposed that in some patients, rapid cycling may occur later in the course of bipolar disorder as a result of illness progression, characterized by progressively shorter well intervals and progressively more severe episodes (Post et al. 1988). In one analysis, approximately one-half (52%, 24/46) of treatment-resistant patients demonstrated a "sensitization pattern," with progressively shorter well intervals (Roy-Byrne et al. 1985). However, illness progression may not be the only course leading to rapid cycling. Indeed, limited data suggest that rapid cycling may occur at the time of bipolar illness onset in a minority of individuals (30%, 36/122) (Kukopulos et al. 1983).

Four naturalistic studies suggest that rapid cycling may persist on average in approximately 40% of patients (Bauer et al. 1994; Koukopoulos et al. 2003; Kupka et al. 2005; Wehr et al. 1988) (Figure 9–2, black bars on left). However, three other naturalistic studies suggest that rapid cycling may persist on average in only approximately 10% of patients (Coryell et al. 2003; Maj et al. 1994; Schneck et al. 2008; Figure 9–2, gray bars on right). Methodological differences (e.g., patient selection, intensity of longitudinal monitoring) might have contributed to varying findings. However, treatment differences also might have contributed importantly to differential outcomes, indicating the importance of efforts to optimize therapeutic interventions.

Treatment of Rapid-Cycling Bipolar Disorder

A Clinical Challenge

Patients with rapid-cycling bipolar disorder commonly struggle with illness with a large depressive component, accompanied by suboptimal efficacy with lithium, divalproex, carbamazepine, and antidepressants, with antidepressants commonly also yielding treatment-emergent affective switch and/or cycle acceleration. Clinical trials of the acute treatment phase commonly fail to adequately

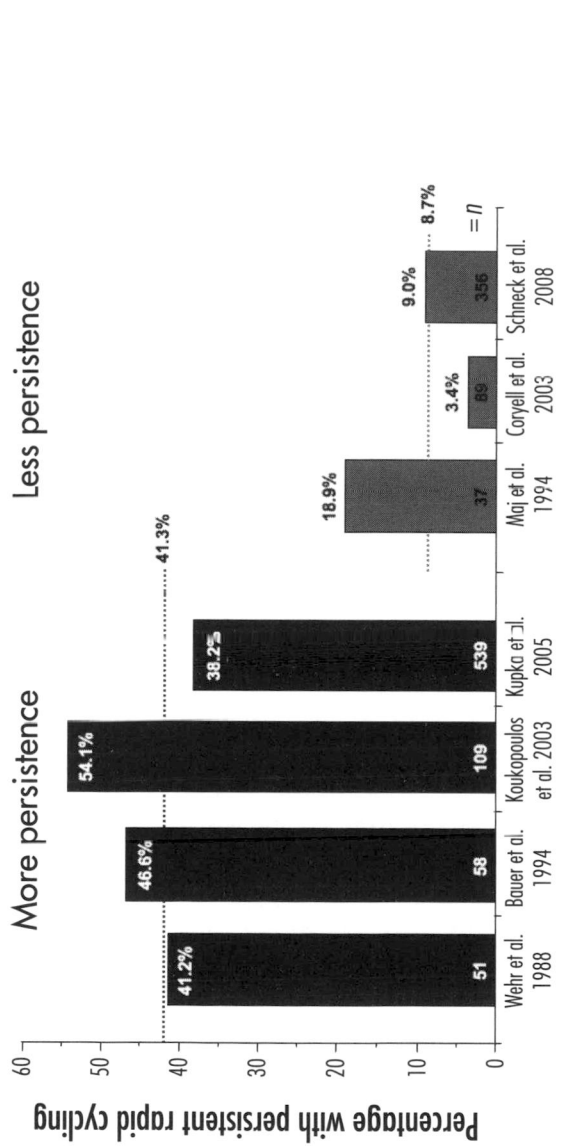

FIGURE 9–2. **Variable rates of persistence of rapid cycling.**

Four observational studies (Bauer et al. 1994; Koukopoulos et al. 2003; Kupka et al. 2005; Wehr et al. 1988) found that in a total of 757 subjects, rapid cycling persisted on average in approximately 40% of patients (*left*, black bars). However, three other observational studies (Coryell et al. 2003; Maj et al. 1994; Schneck et al. 2008) found that in a total of 482 subjects, rapid cycling persisted on average in only approximately 10% of patients (*right*, gray bars).

address the outcomes of patients with rapid cycling, as in many cases response may be feigned by cycling out of the index episode during the acute trial. Thus, the most meaningful clinical trials for patients with rapid cycling involve longer-term treatment. Indeed, Schneck (2006) suggested that outcomes of interventions in patients with rapid cycling ought to be evaluated over approximately 4 months or three cycle lengths, using systematic mood charting. Although rapid-cycling patients may be included in the general type of longer-term treatment trials (as discussed in Chapter 8, "Longer-Term Management of Bipolar Disorders"), patients with more than six episodes are commonly excluded from such general studies. In this chapter, we discuss the management of patients with rapid cycling, emphasizing data from randomized controlled trials.

In early studies, rapid cycling appeared to be related to lithium resistance (Dunner and Fieve 1974), but later work suggested that rapid cycling was also associated with resistance to other agents, such as carbamazepine (Okuma 1993) and even valproate combined with lithium (Calabrese et al. 2005b). Antidepressant treatment has been suggested to yield more frequent mood episodes in some studies (Kukopulos et al. 1983; Wehr et al. 1988), but not in others (Coryell et al. 1992, 2003), with the latter suggesting that frequent depressive episodes may lead to more antidepressant administration.

Balancing Benefits and Risks

No medication has yet been approved for treatment of rapid-cycling bipolar disorders. In clinical practice, mood stabilizers and second-generation antipsychotics are commonly used, and although providers may strive to avoid adjunctive antidepressants, the common occurrence of treatment-resistant depressive symptoms results in substantial rates of utilization of these agents despite concerns regarding efficacy and tolerability.

Systematic approaches to the management of rapid-cycling bipolar disorder have been advocated. For example, the Systematic Treatment Enhancement Program for Bipolar Disorder (STEP-BD) study used a three-stage management pathway that strove to minimize or eliminate antidepressant exposure and to focus on mood stabilizers and second-generation antipsychotics, and that permitted sufficient time for individual interventions to be assessed (Table 9–1) (Sachs 2004; Schneck 2006).

In the following sections, we review interventions for the treatment of rapid-cycling bipolar disorders. Categories of treatments are grouped similarly to those in the STEP-BD algorithm—that is, mood stabilizers, second-generation

TABLE 9–1.   Systematic Treatment Enhancement Program for Bipolar Disorder (STEP-BD) three-stage rapid-cycling management pathway

1. Identify, and minimize or eliminate, pro-cycling factors (e.g., antidepressants, stimulants, caffeine, sympathomimetics, steroids, alcohol or substance abuse, medical illnesses, and circadian rhythm disturbance). Gradually taper (approximately 25% per month) antidepressants, rather than abruptly discontinuing them.
2. If cycling persists, first optimize, and later if necessary add, mood stabilizers (e.g., lithium, lamotrigine, divalproex) and/or second-generation antipsychotics (e.g., olanzapine, aripiprazole, quetiapine), emphasizing agents with evidence of utility in bipolar maintenance treatment. Assess efficacy over approximately 4 months or three cycle lengths, using systematic mood charting. Several iterations may be necessary, yielding two-drug and even three-drug combinations.
3. If cycling still persists, invoke novel treatments (e.g., levothyroxine, electroconvulsive therapy, nimodipine, omega-3 fatty acids, light therapy) with less evidence than those used in stage 2.

Source.   Adapted from Sachs 2004.

antipsychotics, and other adjunctive therapies (e.g., antidepressants, novel interventions).

Mood Stabilizers

Mood stabilizers are considered foundational agents in the treatment of bipolar disorders. These agents appear to have distinctive, and in some instances complementary, efficacy and tolerability profiles. Lithium has long been considered to yield limited efficacy in rapid-cycling bipolar disorder. Although divalproex and carbamazepine were initially considered to be more effective than lithium in patients with rapid cycling, subsequent data suggested that carbamazepine was less effective in rapid-cycling compared with non-rapid-cycling patients, and had comparable efficacy to lithium in both rapid-cycling and non-rapid-cycling patients. More recent randomized controlled data indicated that divalproex had similar efficacy to lithium in rapid-cycling bipolar disorder. Recent randomized controlled data suggest that lamotrigine may have efficacy in rapid-cycling bipolar II disorder.

Lithium

For over 30 years, concerns have been raised that lithium may yield suboptimal efficacy in patients with rapid cycling (Dunner and Fieve 1974). In patients with rapid-cycling, as compared with non-rapid-cycling, bipolar disorder, lithium prophylaxis commonly yields lower rates of both full response and partial response, although occasional studies fail to demonstrate this finding (Baldessarini et al. 2000). In an eight-study (Baldessarini et al. 2000; Denicoff et al. 1997; Dunner et al. 1977; Fujiwara et al. 1998; Koukopoulos et al. 1995; Maj et al. 1989; Okuma 1993; Walden et al. 2000) meta-analysis (Tondo et al. 2003), the rate of lithium (as monotherapy or combination therapy) *partial* prophylactic response (improvement) was lower in patients with rapid-cycling bipolar disorder than in those with non-rapid-cycling bipolar disorder (48%, 130/273 vs. 63%, 467/744, number needed to harm [NNH]=7) (Figure 9–3, left). Similarly, in a six-study (Baldessarini et al. 2000; Dunner and Fieve 1974; Dunner et al. 1977; Okuma 1993; Walden et al. 2000; Wehr et al. 1988) meta-analysis (Tondo et al. 2003), the rate of lithium (as monotherapy or combination therapy) *full* prophylactic response (complete mood episode prevention) was lower in patients with rapid-cycling bipolar disorder than in those with non-rapid-cycling bipolar disorder (16%, 33/202 vs. 36%, 150/415, NNH=6, not illustrated).

Lithium prophylaxis failure in rapid cyclers may be due to a relative inability to prevent depressive as opposed to mood elevation episodes (Calabrese et al. 2001). However, concurrent antidepressants may yield poorer lithium prophylactic responses in rapid cyclers (Baldessarini et al. 2000; Kukopulos et al. 1980, 1983; Wehr et al. 1988).

Patients with rapid-cycling bipolar disorders, as compared with those with non-rapid-cycling bipolar disorders, appear to have poorer responses to treatments in general rather than to lithium selectively. In a meta-analysis of 16 studies (Tondo et al. 2003), prophylactic response rates with lithium, carbamazepine, and lamotrigine, administered alone or with other agents, were similarly poorer in patients with rapid-cycling bipolar disorder than in those with non-rapid-cycling bipolar disorder. This pattern did not appear with divalproex, perhaps because only one small study has assessed this medication in both rapid-cycling and non-rapid-cycling patients. In addition, for mood stabilizers considered collectively (Tondo et al. 2003), in patients with rapid-cycling bipolar disorder compared with those with non-rapid-cycling bipolar disorder, pooled response rates were lower for both *partial* prophylactic response (49%, 237/480 vs. 64%, 564/878, NNH=7) (Figure 9–3, right) and *full* prophylactic response (complete mood episode prevention) (24%, 121/505 vs. 37%, 165/452, NNH=8, not illustrated).

Very few randomized controlled pharmacotherapy trials have been done exclusively in rapid-cycling patients. A 20-month, double-blind, randomized controlled trial found that lithium monotherapy compared with divalproex

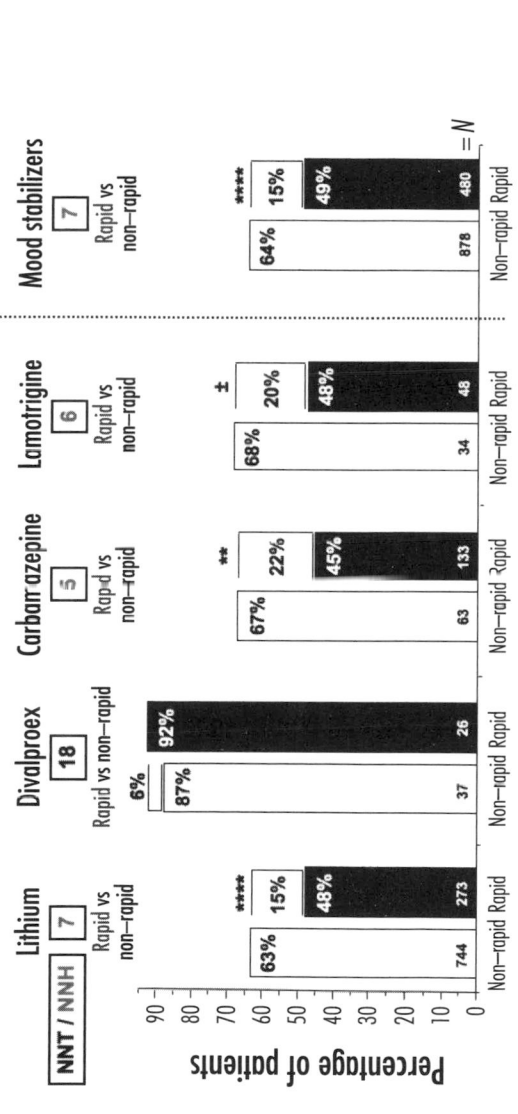

FIGURE 9–3. **Overview of rapid-cycling bipolar disorder treatment studies, numbers needed to harm (NNH) for lower partial prophylactic response (improvement) rates, and numbers needed to treat (NNT) for higher partial prophylactic response (improvement) rate in rapid compared with non–rapid cycling.**

Rapid-cycling patients (black bars) compared with non–rapid-cycling patients (white bars) had 15%–22% lower partial prophylactic response rates for lithium, carbamazepine, and lamotrigine (but not divalproex). Medications were administered as either monotherapies or combination therapies. Partial prophylactic response definitions varied across studies, reflecting varying degrees of improvement. Study durations varied. Divalproex data need to be considered with caution because they were from a single small study. Attempts to compare treatments across studies need to be considered with substantial caution—across studies, in both rapid-cycling and non–rapid-cycling patients, lithium, carbamazepine, and lamotrigine had efficacy that was similar to one another but inferior to divalproex. However, a subsequent randomized controlled trial indicated that lithium and divalproex had similar efficacy in rapid cycling (Figure 9–4). ±P=0.11, ∗∗P<0.01, ∗∗∗∗P<0.0001 versus non–rapid cycling.

Source. Data from Tondo et al. 2003.

monotherapy had similar efficacy but somewhat poorer tolerability in recently hypomanic or manic patients with bipolar I disorder or bipolar II disorder (Calabrese et al. 2005b). The 12- to 24-week open stabilization phase of this study highlighted the clinical challenge of treating rapid-cycling bipolar disorder, because only approximately one in four patients achieved the persistent bimodal response to combined treatment with lithium and divalproex required to go on to the randomized controlled phase, with depression refractory to this combination commonly occurring.

During the 20-week, double-blind, randomized controlled phase, attrition was also high, with only 16% (5/32) of patients taking lithium and 29% (8/28) of patients taking divalproex completing the phase. Lithium (mean dosage 1,359 mg/day, mean serum level 0.92 mEq/L) and divalproex (mean dosage 1,571 mg/day, mean serum level 77 µg/mL) were similar with respect to the time-to-event–based primary outcome measure (time to intervention for a mood episode) and the polarity-specific time-to-event–based secondary outcome measures (time to intervention for a depressive or manic episode). On additional secondary event-based outcome measures (i.e., relapse rates), the findings had the same pattern. Divalproex was nonsignificantly superior to lithium for overall episode prevention (number needed to treat [NNT]=16), depressive episode prevention (NNT=18), and manic episode prevention (NNT=224) (Figure 9–4).

Lithium compared with divalproex yielded a statistically similar rate of adverse event discontinuation, but significantly higher rates of polyuria/polydipsia and tremor. Thus, adverse event discontinuation was seen in 15.6% of patients taking lithium and 3.6% of patients taking divalproex, so that the NNH for adverse event discontinuation with lithium compared with divalproex was 9. The rate of polyuria/polydipsia was significantly higher with lithium (34.4%) than with divalproex (1.6%), and the NNH for polyuria/polydipsia with lithium compared with divalproex was 3. Tremor was significantly more common with lithium (28.1%) than with divalproex (3.6%), so that the NNH for tremor with lithium compared with divalproex was 5 (Calabrese et al. 2005b). Limitations of this study, such as the small sample size and the relatively conservative divalproex dosing, may have contributed to the inability to demonstrate a statistically significant efficacy advantage of divalproex over lithium.

In view of the limitations of lithium monotherapy in patients with rapid-cycling bipolar disorder, combination therapy may be worth considering. Reports suggest that combining lithium with carbamazepine (Denicoff et al. 1997; Di Costanzo and Schifano 1991) or with divalproex (Sharma et al. 1993) may yield benefits in rapid-cycling bipolar disorder. For example, in a 1-year-per-phase, ran-

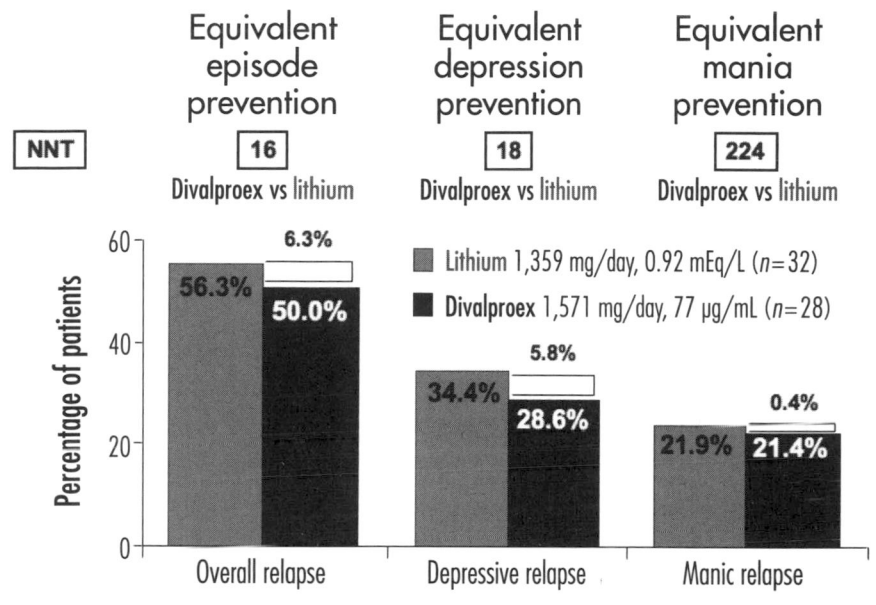

FIGURE 9–4. Overview of 20-month lithium monotherapy versus divalproex monotherapy in rapid-cycling bipolar disorder, numbers needed to treat (NNT), and relapse rates.

Lithium monotherapy (gray bars) compared with divalproex monotherapy (black bars) after manic or hypomanic episodes yielded similar prevention of overall, depressive, and manic episodes. Patients were stabilized on open lithium plus divalproex for 4 weeks before randomization. The relapse criterion was intervention for a mood episode. All lithium versus divalproex differences were nonsignificant. For both treatments, depressive relapses were numerically more common than manic relapses.

Source. Data from Calabrese et al. 2005b.

domized, double-blind, crossover trial, patients with a prior history of rapid cycling had a significantly higher response rate with lithium combined with carbamazepine (56.3%, 9/16) than with lithium monotherapy (28.0%, 7/25, NNT=4) or with carbamazepine monotherapy (19.0%, 4/21, NNT=3) (Figure 9–5, right) (Denicoff et al. 1997). However, as noted above, open lithium plus divalproex combination therapy only yielded adequate efficacy and tolerability in 24% (60/254) of patients with rapid-cycling bipolar disorder (Calabrese et al. 2005b). Hence, additional randomized controlled combination therapy trials are needed in patients with rapid-cycling bipolar disorder. Given the substantial depressive burden in this illness subtype, assessment of combinations of lamotrigine with lithium and/or divalproex is warranted (Calabrese et al. 2005b).

In summary, lithium appears to have less efficacy in rapid-cycling than in non-rapid-cycling bipolar disorder, consistent with its less robust prevention of depression than of mania. This phenomenon may also occur with carbamazepine and lamotrigine, and perhaps to a lesser extent with divalproex. As noted in Chapter 13, "Mood Stabilizers and Antipsychotics," adverse effects with lithium may be challenging, but conservative dosing can enhance tolerability. Clinicians and patients may deem lithium to have inferior tolerability as compared with lamotrigine and divalproex but superior tolerability as compared with antipsychotics.

Divalproex

Divalproex compared with lithium has different mechanisms of action and therapeutic and adverse effects, and therefore has been suggested to be an important treatment option in the management of rapid-cycling bipolar disorder. In the early 1990s, a series of uncontrolled reports described the use of open divalproex monotherapy and combination therapy in patients with rapid-cycling bipolar disorder (Calabrese and Delucchi 1990; Calabrese et al. 1992, 1993).

In 101 patients with rapid-cycling bipolar disorder, divalproex (43%, 43/101 monotherapy; 57%, 58/101 combination therapy) yielded substantial acute and prophylactic relief of manic and mixed symptoms but much more modest relief of depressive symptoms. Predictors of good antimanic response included decreasing or stable episode frequencies and nonpsychotic mania. Predictors of good antidepressant response included nonpsychotic mania worsening over the years of the illness and absence of borderline personality disorder comorbidity (Calabrese et al. 1993). These data along with other observations were subsequently cited as evidence that depression (often treatment-resistant) was the hallmark of rapid-cycling bipolar disorder (Calabrese et al. 2001).

In an analysis of a small, uncontrolled report (Schaff et al. 1993), Tondo et al. (2003) found that the rate of partial prophylactic response (Clinical Global Impression—Improvement Scale) to divalproex (as monotherapy or combination therapy) was similar in patients with rapid-cycling bipolar disorder and patients with non-rapid-cycling bipolar disorder (92%, 24/26 vs. 87%, 32/37, NNT=18) (Figure 9–3, second graph from left) and exceeded that seen with other mood stabilizers in different studies. Such observations, as well as other controlled (Swann et al. 1999) and uncontrolled (Lepkifker et al. 1995) reports, raised the possibility that divalproex may be effective in rapid-cycling bipolar disorder, and thus might prove superior to lithium in treating this illness subtype.

However, as noted above in the section on lithium, in a recent 20-month, randomized, double-blind, controlled trial in patients with rapid-cycling bipolar disorder, divalproex compared with lithium yielded similar efficacy (Figure 9–4) but somewhat better tolerability (Calabrese et al. 2005b). Limitations of the study, such as small sample size (60 patients in the randomized phase) and relatively conservative divalproex dosing (mean dosage 1,571 mg/day, mean serum level 77 µg/mL), may have contributed to the inability to demonstrate a statistically significant efficacy advantage of divalproex over lithium. The findings of the study were consistent with the view that rapid cycling was similarly resistant to both lithium and divalproex.

In view of the limitations of monotherapy in patients with rapid-cycling bipolar disorder, combination therapy may be worth considering. Case reports and case series suggest that divalproex combined with lithium (Sharma et al. 1993), carbamazepine (Ketter et al. 1992), or lamotrigine (Becker et al. 2004; da Rocha et al. 2007; Woo et al. 2007) may yield benefits in rapid-cycling bipolar disorder. However, as noted above, in the open stabilization phase of a controlled trial, lithium plus divalproex combination therapy yielded only adequate efficacy and tolerability in 24% (60/254) of patients with rapid-cycling bipolar disorder (Calabrese et al. 2005b). Thus, additional randomized controlled combination therapy trials are needed in patients with rapid-cycling bipolar disorder. Indeed, Calabrese et al. (2005b) suggested that assessment of combinations of lamotrigine with divalproex and/or lithium is warranted.

In summary, although divalproex was initially considered potentially more effective than lithium as a treatment option for rapid-cycling bipolar disorder, a small randomized controlled trial failed to confirm this hypothesis. Adverse effects with divalproex may be challenging, but conservative dosing can enhance tolerability. Clinicians and patients may deem divalproex to have inferior tolerability compared with lamotrigine but superior tolerability compared with lithium and antipsychotics.

Carbamazepine

Compared with lithium, carbamazepine, like divalproex, has different mechanisms of action and therapeutic and adverse effects, and thus has been suggested to be an alternative in the management of rapid-cycling bipolar disorder. In the 1980s and early 1990s, a series of reports described the use of carbamazepine monotherapy and combination therapy in patients with rapid-cycling bipolar disorder. Early observations suggesting that carbamazepine might prove superior to lithium in patients with rapid-cycling bipolar disorder were followed by reports indicating that carbamazepine was less effective in patients with rapid-cycling bipolar disorder than in those with non-rapid-cycling bipolar disorder, and had comparable efficacy to lithium in both rapid-cycling and non-rapid-cycling patients.

In Tondo et al.'s (2003) meta-analysis of three studies (Denicoff et al. 1997; Fujiwara et al. 1998; Okuma 1993), the rate of *partial* prophylactic response (improvement) to carbamazepine (as monotherapy or combination therapy) was found to be lower in rapid-cycling patients than in non-rapid-cycling patients (45%, 73/133 vs. 67%, 21/63, NNH=5) (Figure 9–3, third graph from left). Similarly, in a meta-analysis of three studies (Joyce 1988; Okuma 1993; Wehr et al. 1988), Tondo et al. (2003) found that the rate of *full* prophylactic response (complete mood episode prevention) to carbamazepine (as monotherapy or combination therapy) was lower in patients with rapid-cycling bipolar disorder than in those with non-rapid-cycling bipolar disorder (16%, 33/202 vs. 36%, 150/415, NNH=6, not illustrated). Across studies, in both rapid-cycling and non-rapid-cycling patients, carbamazepine and lithium had similar efficacy to one another.

In view of the limitations of monotherapy in patients with rapid-cycling bipolar disorder, combination therapy may be worth considering. Reports suggest that combining carbamazepine with lithium (Denicoff et al. 1997; Di Costanzo and Schifano 1991) or divalproex (Ketter et al. 1992) may yield benefits in rapid-cycling bipolar disorder.

In a 1-year-per-phase, randomized, double-blind, crossover trial, Denicoff et al. (1997) assessed carbamazepine monotherapy (mean serum level 7.67 µg/mL), lithium monotherapy (mean serum level 0.84 mEq/L), and combined carbamazepine (mean serum level 7.69 µg/mL) plus lithium (mean serum level 0.84 mEq/L). Patients were randomized to one drug the first year, the other drug the second year, and the combination the third year. The sample included 63.5% (33/52) patients with bipolar I disorder and 36.5% (19/52) patients with bipolar II disorder. Most patients (60.8%, 31/51) had a lifetime history of rapid cycling. The Clinical Global Impression (CGI) response rate (moderate to marked response) for combination therapy compared with carbamazepine monotherapy and lithium monotherapy was similar in the entire sample (55.2%, 31.4%, and 33.3%, respectively) and in patients without a lifetime history of rapid cycling (53.8%, 53.8%, and 41.2%, respectively) (Figure 9–5, left). However, patients with a lifetime history of rapid cycling had a significantly higher CGI response rate with carbamazepine combined with lithium (56.3%, 9/16) compared with carbamazepine monotherapy (19.0%, 4/21, NNT=3) and lithium monotherapy (28.0%, 7/25, NNT=4) (Figure 9–5, right).

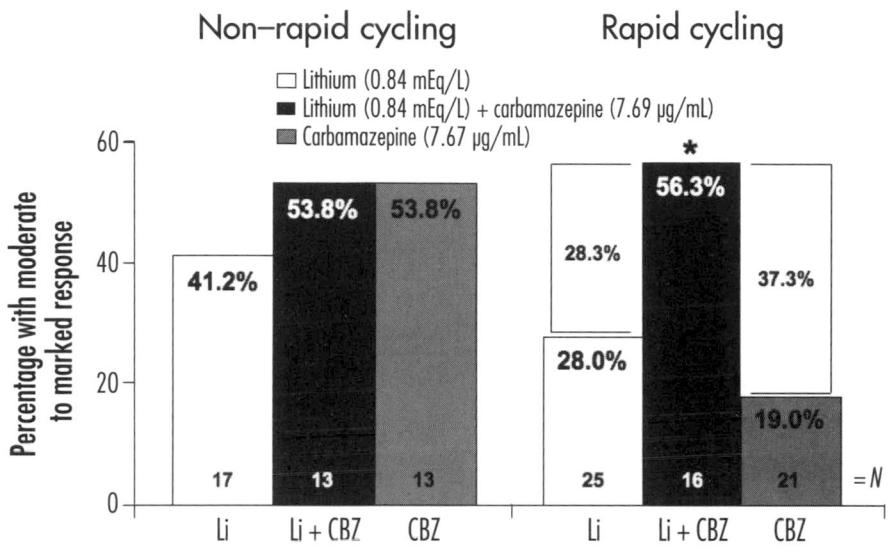

FIGURE 9–5.   Responses of patients with rapid-cycling and non-rapid-cycling bipolar disorder to 1-year-per-phase, randomized, double-blind crossover trial of lithium monotherapy (white bars), carbamazepine monotherapy (gray bars), and carbamazepine plus lithium combination therapy (black bars).

Combination therapy was superior to monotherapy in rapid-cycling but not non-rapid-cycling patients. CBZ=carbamazepine; Li=lithium. *$P<0.05$ compared with Li and CBZ.

Source.   Data from Denicoff et al. 1997.

Early discontinuation rates for combination therapy, carbamazepine monotherapy, and lithium monotherapy for inefficacy were 24.1% (7/29), 37.1% (13/35), and 31.0% (13/42), respectively, and for adverse effects were 0.0% (0/29), 28.6% (10/35), and 4.8% (2/42), respectively. Nine of the 10 carbamazepine adverse effect discontinuations were due to rash. In 30 patients evaluable in both phases, mean weight at the end of the carbamazepine monotherapy phase was modestly but significantly lower than at the end of the lithium monotherapy phase (182.0 lb vs. 185.4 lb).

Carbamazepine drug interactions may limit the utility of combination therapy with agents with hepatic metabolism, as discussed in Chapter 13 of this volume.

In summary, carbamazepine is an alternative treatment option for patients with rapid-cycling bipolar disorder. Adverse effects and drug interactions with carbamazepine may be challenging, but selected patients may experience adequate tolerability compared with mood stabilizers such as lithium and divalproex, or compared with antipsychotics.

Lamotrigine

Lamotrigine has distinctive mechanisms of action and therapeutic and adverse effects compared with other agents used in the treatment of bipolar disorders. Lamotrigine's generally very good tolerability and ability to prevent depressive symptoms suggest that this agent may prove to be an important treatment option for the management of rapid-cycling bipolar disorder.

In a two-study (Calabrese et al. 2000; Walden et al. 2000) meta-analysis, the rate of *full* prophylactic response (complete mood episode prevention) to lamotrigine monotherapy was 40% (40/100) in patients with rapid-cycling bipolar disorder, which was similar to that with divalproex and greater than that with lithium or carbamazepine in other studies (Tondo et al. 2003). However, in a meta-analysis of two studies (Bowden et al. 1999; Walden et al. 2000), the rate of *partial* prophylactic response (improvement) to lamotrigine (as monotherapy or combination therapy) tended to be lower in patients with rapid-cycling bipolar disorder than in patients with non-rapid-cycling bipolar disorder (48%, 23/48 vs. 68%, 23/34, NNH=6) and similar to that seen with lithium and carbamazepine (Tondo et al. 2003) (Figure 9–3, second graph from right).

Results from an early 48-week, open, uncontrolled study suggested that lamotrigine yielded benefits as adjunctive therapy (*n*=60) and monotherapy (*n*=15) in 41 rapid-cycling and 34 non-rapid-cycling bipolar disorder patients with current syndromal mood episodes (Bowden et al. 1999). Mean final lamotrigine dosages were lower in patients with rapid-cycling bipolar disorder (273 mg/day monotherapy, 141 mg/day adjunctive therapy) than in those with non-rapid-cycling bipolar disorder (375 mg/day monotherapy, 193 mg/day adjunctive therapy). Lamotrigine yielded significant improvement from baseline to last visit in both depressive and mood elevation symptoms in both rapid-cycling and non-rapid-cycling patients. For patients with baseline acute major depressive episodes, relief of depression was similar in the two groups. In contrast, among patients with baseline acute manic, mixed, or hypomanic episodes, rapid cyclers compared with non–rapid cyclers had less relief of manic symptoms (particularly if they were severe at baseline). Adverse effect discontinuation rates were similar in rapid cyclers (17.1%, 7/41) and non–rapid cyclers (20.6%, 7/21). Three rapid cyclers and 4 non–rapid cyclers discontinued because of rash, with one of the latter requiring hospitalization for serious rash. Otherwise, lamotrigine was generally adequately tolerated, with dizziness, headache, and benign rash being the most common adverse effects.

A 6-week, randomized, double-blind, placebo-controlled, crossover study found that lamotrigine (mean dosage 274 mg/day) monotherapy but not gabapentin (mean dosage 3,987 mg/day) monotherapy was superior to placebo for overall response in treatment-resistant patients with mood disorder (primarily rapid-cycling bipolar disorder) (Frye et al. 2000). The sample included primarily bipolar disorder patients (80.6%, 25/31, 11 bipolar I and 14 bipolar II) with rapid cycling (74.2%, 23/31), but also included a few patients with non-rapid-cycling bipolar disorder (6.5%, 2/31) or unipolar major depressive disorder (19.3%, 6/31). CGI overall response rates with lamotrigine, gabapentin, and placebo were 51.6%, 25.8%, and 22.6%, respectively, with lamotrigine but not gabapentin being superior to placebo, yielding NNTs for overall response compared with placebo of 4 and 31, respectively (Figure 9–6, left). Lamotrigine, but not gabapentin, also tended to be superior to placebo with respect to CGI antidepressant response rates (Figure 9–6, center) but not CGI antimanic response rates (Figure 9–6, right).

One patient taking lamotrigine developed toxic epidermal necrolysis that required hospitalization but resolved fully. This may have been related to relatively rapid lamotrigine dosage escalation reflective of early epilepsy trials, and more rapid than that subsequently recommended in the U.S. prescribing information dosing recommendations. Otherwise, lamotrigine and gabapentin were generally well tolerated. The most common other adverse effects with lamotrigine were diarrhea (in 6%), headache (in 3%), ataxia (in 3%), and benign rash (in 3%), and with gabapentin were headache (in 13%), fatigue (in 10%), diplopia (in 10%), ataxia (in 10%), and diarrhea (in 6%). Mean weight change with lamotrigine, gabapentin, and placebo was −0.96 kg, +1.83 kg, and −0.40 kg, respectively, with gabapentin compared with lamotrigine yielding a significant increase in mean weight. Limitations of the study included the small sample size and crossover design.

A multicenter, randomized, double-blind, placebo-controlled trial indicated that lamotrigine monotherapy (mean dosage 288 mg/day) may have efficacy in rapid-cycling bipolar II disorder (Calabrese et al. 2000). In the open lead-in phase, lamotrigine was added and was titrated to clinical effect, and stabilized patients were tapered off other psychotropics. More than half of the patients (56.2%, 182/324) were transitioned to lamotrigine monotherapy with stable mood for 2 weeks, and thus randomized to lamotrigine monotherapy versus placebo for the 26-week randomized controlled phase. In this phase, the

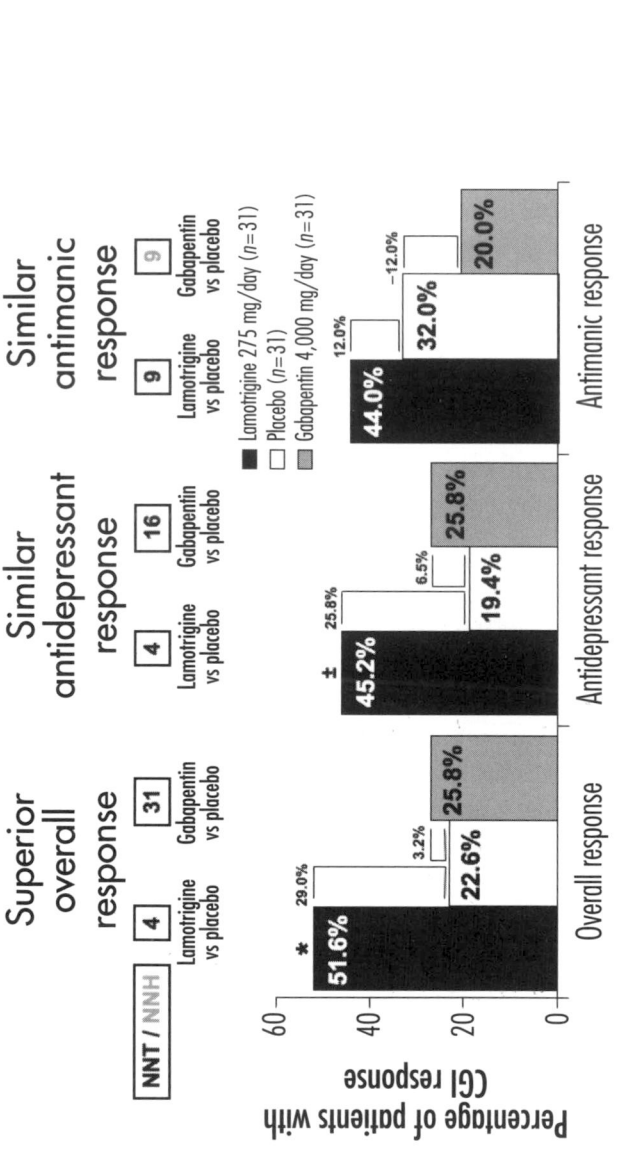

FIGURE 9–6. **Overview of 6-week double-blind lamotrigine monotherapy versus gabapentin monotherapy versus placebo in treatment-resistant mood disorders, numbers needed to treat (NNT), numbers needed to harm (NNH), and response rates.**

The sample consisted primarily of patients with rapid-cycling bipolar disorder (74.2%, 23/31). Clinical Global Impression (CGI) response rates with lamotrigine (black bars) but not gabapentin (gray bars) compared with placebo (white bars) were superior for overall response and tended to be superior for antidepressant (but not antimanic) response. ± P<0.1, *P<0.05 versus placebo.

Source.   Data from Frye et al. 2000.

adverse event discontinuation rate was 10.8% (35/324), and the most common adverse effects were headache, infection, influenza, nausea, dream abnormality, dizziness, and benign rash. Thus, 7.7% (25/324) of patients had benign rash, with no patient in either this phase or the subsequent randomized phase having serious rash.

In the randomized controlled phase, lamotrigine monotherapy was numerically superior to placebo on the primary outcome measure of time to additional pharmacotherapy for emerging symptoms, but the difference was not statistically significant. However, lamotrigine monotherapy was significantly superior to placebo on several secondary outcomes, such as time to any premature discontinuation, percentage of patients stable without relapse for 6 months, and changes in the Global Assessment of Functioning scale and CGI—Severity (CGI-S) scale. Thus, the percentage of patients without relapse for 6 months with lamotrigine compared with placebo was significantly higher in the entire sample (41.1% vs. 26.4%, NNT=7) (Figure 9–7, left) and in patients with bipolar II disorder (45.8% vs. 17.9%, NNT=4) (Figure 9–7, right) but not in patients with bipolar I disorder (38.2% vs. 30.0%, NNT=13) (Figure 9–7, center). Among all patients requiring additional pharmacotherapy for emerging symptoms, depression was four times as common as mood elevation (80% vs. 20%). These data, along with other observations, were subsequently cited as evidence that depression (often treatment-resistant) was the hallmark of rapid-cycling bipolar disorder (Calabrese et al. 2001). Additional analyses using detailed life-chart data indicated that lamotrigine compared with placebo was 1.8 times more likely to achieve euthymia at least once every week and yielded a mean of 0.7 more days per week euthymic (Goldberg et al. 2008a).

In the randomized controlled phase, lamotrigine was generally well tolerated, with an adverse event discontinuation rate of 2.2% (2/92) compared to 2.3% (2/88) with placebo. The most common adverse effects were headache, nausea, infection, pain, and accidental injury. Benign rash was seen in 3.3% (3/92) with lamotrigine and 2.2% (3/88) with placebo. Weight change in completers was +1.1 kg with lamotrigine and −0.3 kg with placebo.

In view of the limitations of monotherapy in patients with rapid-cycling bipolar disorder, combination therapy may be worth considering. Reports suggest that combining lamotrigine with divalproex (Becker et al. 2004; da Rocha et al. 2007; Woo et al. 2007) may yield benefits in patients with rapid-cycling bipolar disorder. Lamotrigine is the target rather than the instigator of clinically significant drug interactions; for example, divalproex doubles and carbamazepine halves serum lamotrigine concentrations, as discussed in detail in Chap-

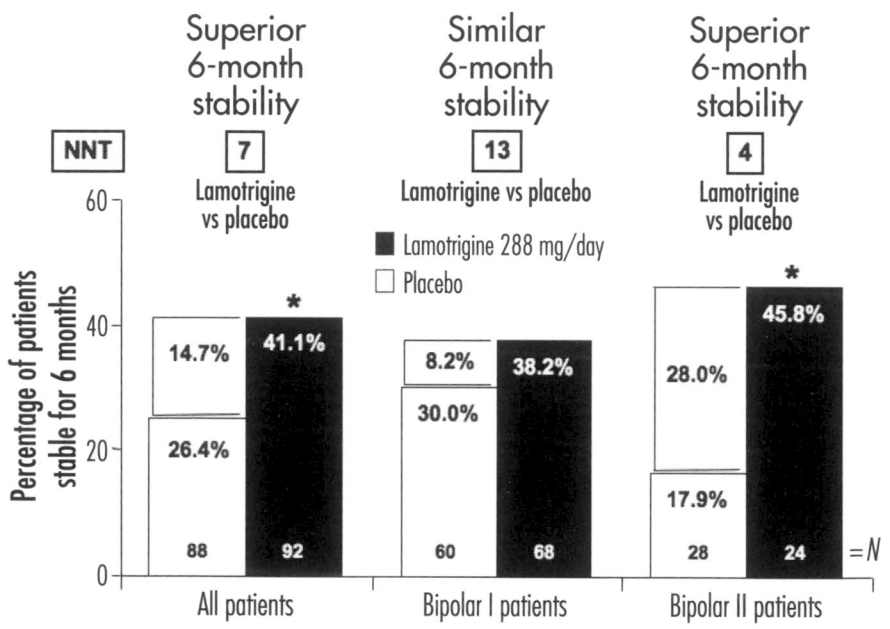

FIGURE 9–7.　Overview of 26-week double-blind study of lamotrigine monotherapy versus placebo in patients with rapid-cycling bipolar disorder after mood episodes or euthymia, numbers needed to treat (NNT), and response rates.

Patients were stabilized on open lamotrigine for 2 weeks before randomization. The stability criterion was stable without relapse for 6 months. Lamotrigine monotherapy (black bars) was superior to placebo (white bars) overall and in patients with bipolar II disorder, but not in patients with bipolar I disorder. *P<0.05 versus placebo.

Source.　Data from Calabrese et al. 2000.

ter 13 of this volume. Nevertheless, lamotrigine's generally good tolerability and ability to prevent depressive episodes suggest that it may be a worthwhile component in combination therapy for rapid-cycling bipolar disorder.

In summary, lamotrigine is a promising medication for the management of rapid-cycling bipolar disorder. Clinicians and patients may deem lamotrigine to have superior tolerability compared with other mood stabilizers, as well as compared with antipsychotics, and thus consider it an attractive treatment option.

Second-Generation Antipsychotics

Second-generation antipsychotics are commonly used in acute mania and are increasingly used for acute bipolar depression and maintenance treatment. Among these agents, olanzapine and aripiprazole have maintenance monotherapy indications, and quetiapine has an adjunctive (added to lithium or divalproex) maintenance indication. Quetiapine may have balanced bimodal antimanic and antidepressant effects, whereas other agents in this class appear to have more robust antimanic than antidepressant effects.

Olanzapine

Olanzapine was the initial second-generation antipsychotic to receive indications for acute mania, bipolar depression (in combination with fluoxetine), and bipolar maintenance. Post hoc secondary analyses of the registration studies for these indications suggested variable utility in patients with rapid-cycling bipolar disorder.

Preliminary assessment of relationships between olanzapine therapeutic effects and rapid cycling was obtained utilizing pooled data from two 3- and 4-week randomized, double-blind, placebo-controlled olanzapine acute mania trials (total $N=254$) (Tohen et al. 1999, 2000), and an up to 1 year extension ($N=113$) of open olanzapine that also permitted open adjunctive fluoxetine and/or lithium (Sanger et al. 2001). Patients with rapid-cycling bipolar disorder compared with those with non-rapid-cycling bipolar disorder appeared to have better acute outcomes (perhaps related to more quickly cycling out of the index manic episode) (Vieta et al. 2004). The Young Mania Rating Scale (YMRS) response ($\geq50\%$ decrease) rate during treatment of acute mania was significantly higher in all 90 patients with rapid-cycling bipolar disorder compared with all 164 patients with non-rapid-cycling bipolar disorder (63.5% vs. 49.1%, $P=0.03$, NNT=7) (Figure 9–8, gray bars); tended to be higher in 44 rapid-cycling compared with 81 non-rapid-cycling patients taking olanzapine (76.7% vs. 60.5%, $P<0.07$, NNT=7) (Figure 9–8, black bars); and was nonsignificantly higher in 46 rapid-cycling compared with 83 non-rapid-cycling patients taking placebo (50.0% vs. 37.5%, $P=0.18$, NNT=8) (Figure 9–8, white bars). The YMRS response rate with olanzapine was greater than with placebo in both rapid-cycling patients (76.7% vs. 50.0%, $P=0.01$, NNT=4) (Figure 9–8, left) and non-rapid-cycling patients (60.5%% vs. 37.5%, $P=0.004$, NNT=5) (Figure 9–8, right).

However, rapid-cycling patients compared with non-rapid-cycling patients had poorer longer-term outcomes (perhaps related to more quickly cycling into a subsequent major depressive episode) (Vieta et al. 2004). During the 12-month

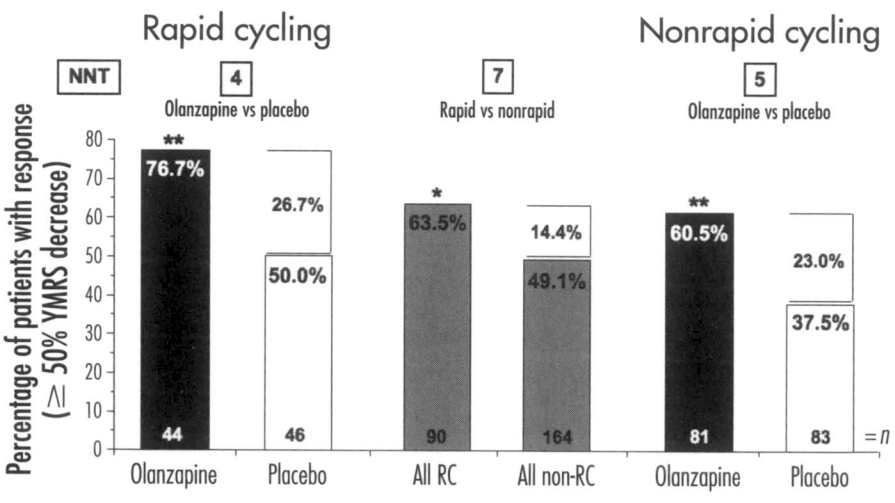

FIGURE 9–8. Overview of 3- and 4-week double-blind olanzapine versus placebo trials in patients with acute mania with and without rapid cycling, numbers needed to treat (NNT), and response rates.

The Young Mania Rating Scale (YMRS) response (≥50% decrease) rate with olanzapine (black bars) was greater than with placebo (white bars) in both rapid cyclers (*left*) and non–rapid cyclers (*right*), as well as in all rapid cyclers (RC) compared with all non–rapid cyclers (Non-RC) (gray bars). *P<0.05, all rapid cyclers versus all non–rapid cyclers; **P<0.01, olanzapine versus placebo.

Source.   Data from Vieta et al. 2004.

open olanzapine extension phase, rapid-cycling patients compared with non-rapid-cycling patients had a significantly lower percentage of visits with symptomatic remission (YMRS≤7, Hamilton Rating Scale for Depression [Ham-D]≤7, CGI≤2, 34.6% vs. 52.5%, P=0.006, NNH=6), as well as significantly higher rates of depressive recurrence (53.8% vs. 14.9%, P<0.001, NNH= 3) (Figure 9–9, left), hospitalization (38.5% vs. 16.2%, P=0.01, NNH=5) (Figure 9–9, center), and suicide attempts (22.2% vs. 7.0%, P=0.03, NNH=7) (Figure 9–9, right). In this phase, rapid-cycling patients compared with non-rapid-cycling patients also had a higher rate of adjunctive fluoxetine use (25.6% vs. 5.4%, P=0.005) but a lower rate of adjunctive lithium use (0.0% vs. 21.6%, P=0.001).

Additional preliminary assessment of relationships between olanzapine therapeutic effects and rapid cycling may be obtained utilizing data from the 8-week, randomized, double-blind, placebo-controlled olanzapine plus fluoxetine acute bipolar I depression registration study (Tohen et al. 2003b). In this study, among depressed rapid cyclers, the olanzapine plus fluoxetine combina-

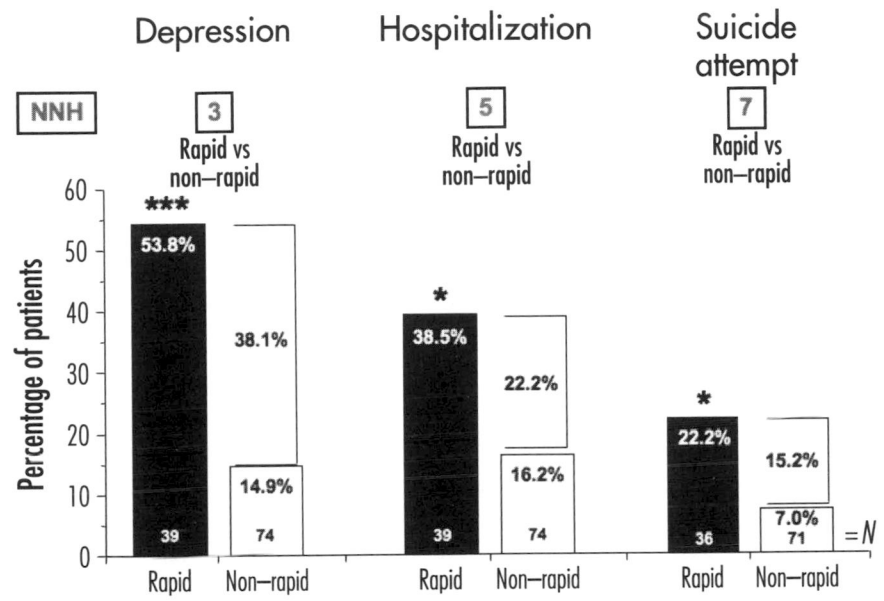

FIGURE 9–9.   More depressive recurrence, hospitalization, and suicide attempts in rapid cyclers compared with non–rapid cyclers during 12-month open olanzapine extension therapy, numbers needed to harm (NNH), recurrence rates, and adverse effect rates.

Rapid cyclers (black bars) compared with non–rapid cyclers (white bars) had significantly higher rates of depressive recurrence (*left*), hospitalization (*center*), and suicide attempts (*right*). Mean olanzapine dosage was 12.4 mg/day. Mean duration was 28 weeks. *$P<0.05$, ***$P<0.001$, rapid versus non–rapid cycling.

Source.   Data from Vieta et al. 2004.

tion (but not olanzapine monotherapy) was more effective than placebo for acute bipolar depression (Keck et al. 2003a).

Thus, among depressed rapid cyclers with bipolar I disorder, the Montgomery-Åsberg Depression Rating Scale (MADRS) response ($\geq$50% decrease) rate in 35 patients taking the olanzapine plus fluoxetine combination was significantly higher than in 129 patients taking placebo (77.8% vs. 39.4%), yielding an NNT of 3 (Figure 9–10, left) (Keck et al. 2003a). In contrast, the MADRS response rate in 132 patients taking olanzapine monotherapy (35.7%) was statistically similar to that in patients taking placebo. The olanzapine plus fluoxetine combination was generally fairly well tolerated, yielding an adverse event discontinuation rate statistically similar to placebo (5.4% and 2.9%, respectively,

NNH=40, Figure 9–10, center). However, olanzapine monotherapy compared with placebo yielded a significantly higher adverse event discontinuation rate (11.4% vs. 2.9%, NNH=12, Figure 9–10, center). Treatment-emergent affective switch rates were low and statistically similar across treatments (Figure 9–10, right). The olanzapine plus fluoxetine combination (but not olanzapine) compared with placebo also yielded significantly greater improvement in quality of life, as evidenced by scores on several 36-item Short Form Health Survey domains (general health, mental health, and social functioning) and the Quality of Life in Depression total score (Shi et al. 2003).

In a 12-month, multicenter, randomized, double-blind, placebo-controlled trial of olanzapine in patients after manic or mixed episodes, almost half (49.6%, 179/361) of patients had rapid-cycling bipolar disorder (Tohen et al. 2006). Olanzapine compared with placebo yielded a significantly longer time to symptomatic relapse in patients with as well as without rapid cycling, but more detailed analyses regarding the polarity of relapse in rapid-cycling patients were not provided. In contrast, a 12-month, multicenter, randomized, double-blind trial comparing olanzapine and lithium in patients after manic or mixed episodes excluded patients with histories of resistance to olanzapine or lithium and thus included only 3% (13/431) with rapid cycling, and hence was not informative regarding relationships between rapid cycling and olanzapine or lithium responses (Tohen et al. 2005).

A post hoc analysis of pooled data included 779 patients from the olanzapine-versus-placebo (Tohen et al. 2006) and olanzapine-versus-lithium (Tohen et al. 2005) maintenance studies. Considering all treatments collectively, earlier relapse was related to rapid-cycling course, as well as mixed index episode, having more than one mood episode in the prior year, onset age≤20 years, having a first-degree relative with bipolar disorder, female gender, and not being hospitalized for bipolar disorder in the prior year (Tohen et al. 2004a). However, history of rapid cycling and mixed index episode were the strongest predictors of earlier relapse. An important limitation of this study was that all treatments were considered collectively rather than individually.

A 44-week, multicenter, randomized, double-blind extension of a 3-week comparison of olanzapine monotherapy and divalproex monotherapy in the treatment of acute manic and mixed episodes (Tohen et al. 2002a) yielded 47-week olanzapine-versus-divalproex information (Tohen et al. 2003a). These data were subsequently analyzed to assess olanzapine and divalproex longer-term efficacy in the 57.6% (144/250) of patients with rapid-cycling bipolar disorder and the 42.4% (106/250) of patients with non-rapid-cycling bipolar

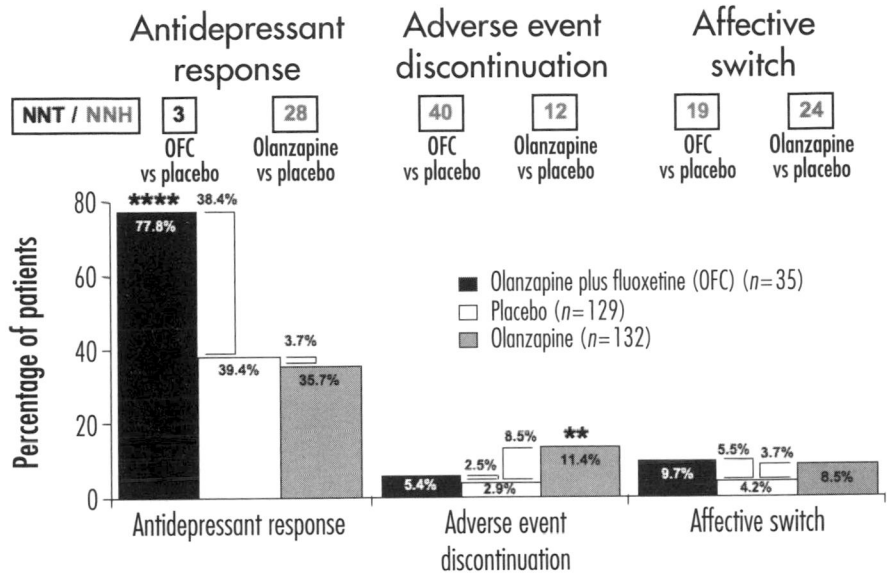

FIGURE 9–10. Overview of 8-week double-blind olanzapine plus fluoxetine versus olanzapine monotherapy versus placebo in acute bipolar I depression in rapid cyclers, numbers needed to treat (NNT), numbers needed to harm (NNH), response rates, and adverse effect rates.

The olanzapine plus fluoxetine combination (OFC; black bars) but not olanzapine monotherapy (gray bars) compared with placebo (white bars) yielded a significantly greater Montgomery-Åsberg Depression Rating Scale (MADRS) response (≥50% decrease) rate (*left*). Olanzapine (but not olanzapine plus fluoxetine) compared with placebo yielded a higher adverse effect discontinuation rate (*center*). Treatment-emergent affective switch rates were low and statistically similar across treatments (*right*). **P<0.01, ****P<0.0001, versus placebo.

Source. Data from Keck et al. 2003a.

disorder (Suppes et al. 2005). Overall, rapid-cycling compared with non-rapid-cycling patients had poorer mania but similar depression outcomes. Among rapid cyclers, olanzapine and divalproex were similarly effective. Changes in YMRS (but not Ham-D) total scores were influenced by a significant three-way cycle frequency × medication × time interaction. YMRS improvement with olanzapine compared with divalproex among rapid-cycling patients was statistically similar, but among non-rapid-cycling patients was significantly greater across the trial and at most time points. YMRS improvement with olanzapine was numerically poorer in rapid-cycling patients than in non-rapid-cycling patients throughout the trial, with differences being statistically significant at weeks 11,

15, and 39. In contrast, YMRS improvement with divalproex was significantly better in rapid cyclers compared with non–rapid cyclers during the first 2 weeks but comparable thereafter.

An 18-month, multicenter, randomized, double-blind extension of a 6-week comparison of adjunctive olanzapine (added to lithium or divalproex) versus adjunctive placebo in the treatment of acute manic and mixed episodes (Tohen et al. 2002b) yielded 18-month adjunctive olanzapine versus adjunctive placebo information (Tohen et al. 2004b). In this study 41.4% (41/99) of patients had rapid cycling, and 58.6% (58/99) did not, and no significant interaction occurred between treatment outcomes and presence or absence of a history of rapid cycling. Suboptimal statistical power related to sample size was a limitation of this study.

In summary, olanzapine is a treatment option for rapid-cycling bipolar disorder that appears to have more robust antimanic compared with antidepressant effects. Patients with rapid cycling compared with those without may have better acute mania outcomes with olanzapine (perhaps because of more quickly cycling out of the index manic episode) but poorer subsequent longer-term outcomes (perhaps because of more quickly cycling into a subsequent major depressive episode). Adverse effects with olanzapine may be challenging, and clinicians and patients may deem this agent to have inferior tolerability compared with mood stabilizers such as lamotrigine and divalproex, as well as some other antipsychotics such as aripiprazole and quetiapine.

Quetiapine

Quetiapine is the only medication with monotherapy indications for both mania and bipolar depression. Quetiapine also has an adjunctive (added to lithium or divalproex) indication for the longer-term treatment of bipolar I disorder, preventing both mania and depression. The latter effect of quetiapine was independent of any specific subgroup, such as assigned mood stabilizer, sex, age, race, most recent bipolar episode, or rapid-cycling course. This broad spectrum of efficacy that includes attenuating both manic and depressive symptoms suggests that quetiapine may have the potential to be useful in rapid-cycling bipolar disorder. However, the post hoc rapid-cycling subgroup analysis of the longer-term adjunctive quetiapine registration studies is not yet available. Also, even preliminary controlled acute mania data were limited, because the multicenter, randomized, controlled immediate-release quetiapine monotherapy (Bowden et al. 2005; McIntyre et al. 2005) and adjunctive therapy (Yatham et al. 2004) acute mania studies excluded patients with rapid cycling. Thus, data regarding quetiapine treatment of rapid-cycling bipolar disorder remained limited to small, uncontrolled, 4-month (Vieta et al. 2002b) and 12-month (Goldberg et al. 2008b) studies, as well as a post hoc analysis of the subset of rapid cyclers in an 8-week, multicenter, randomized controlled acute bipolar depression study (Vieta et al. 2007).

In a 4-month uncontrolled study in 14 patients with rapid-cycling bipolar disorder in various mood states, open adjunctive quetiapine yielded significant baseline to end-point decreases in mania but not depression ratings (Vieta et al. 2002b). Mean quetiapine dosages were significantly higher in patients presenting with mania (720 mg/day) than in patients with depression (183 mg/day). The most common side effect, sedation, was seen in 43% (6/14) of patients.

A small, 12-month, uncontrolled study suggested that open quetiapine may have some efficacy in rapid-cycling bipolar disorder, but the relatively high (68%) discontinuation rate underscored the challenge of managing such patients (Goldberg et al. 2008b). Open, flexibly dosed quetiapine (mean maximal dosage 197 mg/day) as adjunctive therapy ($n=22$) or monotherapy ($n=19$) was assessed in 41 patients with rapid-cycling bipolar disorder (33 bipolar I disorder, 7 bipolar II disorder, 1 not otherwise specified) who entered in various mood states. Quetiapine yielded significant decreases in both mania (YMRS) and depression (Ham-D) ratings. Response (at least 50% improvement) rates with quetiapine were 41% (11/27) for mania, 29% (4/14) for depression, and 37% (15/41) overall. However, 68% of patients discontinued early, including 37% because of inefficacy/mood episode and 12% because of adverse effects/intolerance. Adverse effects included sedation (in 64%), dry mouth (in 24%), weight gain (in 17%), and cognitive impairment, constipation, and dizziness (in 15% each). Mean weight decreased from baseline to end point by 1.65 lb, but this difference was not statistically significant.

A post hoc analysis of data from one of the acute bipolar depression registration studies (Calabrese et al. 2005a) assessed efficacy of quetiapine 300 mg/day and 600 mg/day compared with placebo in 108 patients with rapid-cycling bipolar disorder (Vieta et al. 2007). Although the findings were encouraging, the brief (8-week) duration of the study made interpretation of efficacy in rapid-cycling bipolar disorder challenging. On the primary outcome measure, both dosages of quetiapine compared with placebo yielded greater MADRS decreases from baseline to end point in both 108 rapid cyclers and 402 non–rapid cyclers, as well as subgroups of 67 rapid cyclers with bipolar I disorder, 41 rapid cyclers with bipolar II disorder, and 45 non–rapid cyclers with bipolar I disorder, but not in 127 non–rapid cyclers with bipolar I disorder. The latter subgroup had an attenuated quetiapine effect as well as an increased placebo effect.

Among rapid cyclers, the findings were similar across patients with bipolar I disorder and patients with bipolar II disorder, and across quetiapine dosages (aside from more adverse effects with the higher dosage). Thus, we discuss pooled data for the two quetiapine dosages and the two bipolar subtypes. Among rapid cyclers, quetiapine compared with placebo yielded a significantly higher MADRS response ($\geq$50% MADRS decrease) rate (65.8% vs. 28.6%, $P<$ 0.001, NNT=3) (Figure 9–11, left). Quetiapine was generally adequately tolerated, with only a nonsignificantly higher rate of adverse event discontinuation (18.8% vs. 8.6%, P=0.17, NNH=10); the most common adverse effects were dry mouth, sedation, dizziness, constipation, fatigue, and somnolence. Quetiapine compared with placebo yielded a significantly higher rate of sedation (30.0% vs. 14.9%, NNH= 7, $P<$0.02) (Figure 9–11, center) but only a statistically insignificant greater rate of clinically significant ($\geq$7%) weight gain (11.6% vs. 3.3%, P=0.16, NNH=13) (Figure 9–11, right) and extrapyramidal symptoms (6.3% vs. 0.0%, P=0.17, NNH=16). Mean weight change from baseline to end point was +1.9 kg with quetiapine and −0.2 kg with placebo. Treatment-emergent affective switch rates were similarly low with quetiapine (5.5%) and placebo (2.9%), yielding an NNH for quetiapine versus placebo of 39.

In summary, the broad spectrum of efficacy of quetiapine, which includes attenuating both manic and depressive symptoms, suggests that this agent may have the potential to be useful in rapid-cycling bipolar disorder and that randomized controlled studies in this population are indicated. Adverse effects with this agent may be challenging, and clinicians and patients may deem this agent to have inferior tolerability compared not only to mood stabilizers such as lithium, lamotrigine, and divalproex, but also to some other antipsychotics such as aripiprazole.

Risperidone

Prior to 2008, very limited data were available regarding the utility of risperidone in rapid-cycling bipolar disorder. Even preliminary controlled acute mania data were limited, because most multicenter, randomized, controlled risperidone monotherapy (Hirschfeld et al. 2004; Khanna et al. 2005) and adjunctive therapy (Sachs et al. 2002; Yatham et al. 2003) acute mania studies did not report the prevalence of rapid cycling in their samples or the drug's efficacy in patients with rapid cycling. One multicenter, randomized, controlled risperi-

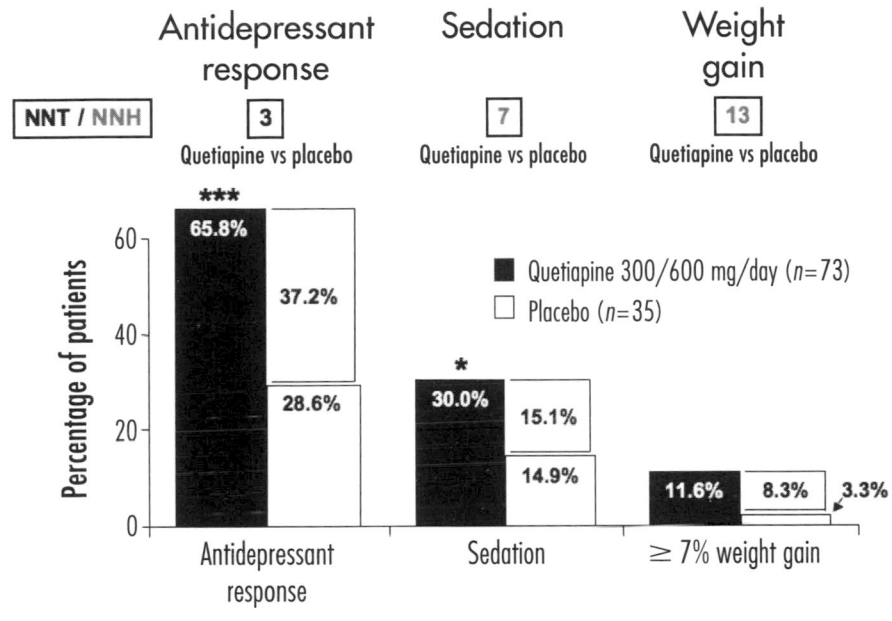

FIGURE 9–11. Overview of 8-week, double-blind quetiapine monotherapy versus placebo in acute bipolar depression in rapid cyclers, numbers needed to treat (NNT), numbers needed to harm (NNH), response rates, and adverse effect rates.

Quetiapine monotherapy (black bars) compared with placebo (white bars) yielded a significantly greater Montgomery-Åsberg Depression Rating Scale (MADRS) response (≥50% decrease) rate (*left*), and sedation rate (*center*), but the increase in clinically significant (≥7%) weight gain rate fell short of statistical significance. *P<0.05, ***P<0.001 quetiapine versus placebo.

Source. Data from Vieta et al. 2007.

done adjunctive therapy acute mania study excluded patients with rapid cycling (Smulevich et al. 2005).

A 6-month, uncontrolled study assessed open, primarily adjunctive (in 9/ 10 cases added to mood stabilizers and/or benzodiazepines) risperidone (mean dosage 3.2 mg/day) in 10 patients with rapid-cycling bipolar disorder (8 with bipolar I disorder, 2 with bipolar II disorder) in various mood states (including 5 with psychotic features and 5 with mixed features) (Vieta et al. 1998). Risperidone yielded significant baseline to end point decreases in mean YMRS (56.4%, from 14.0 to 6.1) and Ham-D (34.3%, from 17.5 to 11.5) scores, as well as episode frequency (63.6%, from 0.92 to 0.33 per month), and was generally well tolerated, with only one adverse effect discontinuation (due to agitation).

However, in 2008, a randomized controlled study suggested that risperidone long-acting injectable (RLAI) added to treatment as usual (TAU) may prevent relapse (particularly manic relapse) in a type of rapid cycling called frequently relapsing bipolar disorder (patients with four or more mood episodes requiring treatment in the prior year) (MacFadden et al. 2008). During a 16-week, open stabilization phase, RLAI (25–50 mg intramuscularly every 2 weeks) plus TAU yielded remission (YMRS≤10, MADRS≤10, CGI–Bipolar Disorder–Severity ≤3) for 4 weeks in 50.5% (139/275) of patients, who thus entered a subsequent 52-week randomized, double-blind, placebo-controlled maintenance trial with RLAI (25–50 mg intramuscularly) plus TAU versus placebo plus TAU. At the beginning of the randomized phase, for 95.7% (133/139) of patients, TAU included taking at least one psychotropic medication, and in this phase 72 patients taking RLAI (mean dosage 2.1 mg/day, 29.7 mg every 2 weeks) plus TAU compared with 67 patients taking placebo plus TAU had significantly lower rates of relapse into any mood episode (22.2% vs. 47.8%, $P<0.003$, NNT=4) (Figure 9–12, left) and relapse into mania (9.7% vs. 26.9%, $P<0.02$, NNT=6) (Figure 9–12, right) but not relapse into depression (12.5% vs. 20.9%, $P=0.25$, NNT=12) (Figure 9–12, center).

Both RLAI plus TAU and placebo plus TAU were generally well tolerated, with similar low adverse event discontinuation rates (4.2% vs. 1.5%, $P=0.62$, NNH=38). The most common adverse events with RLAI plus TAU compared with placebo plus TAU included tremor (23.6% vs. 16.4%, $P=0.40$, NNH=14), muscle rigidity (11.1% vs. 6.0%, $P=0.55$, NNH=20), weight gain (6.9% vs. 1.5%, $P=0.21$, NNH=18), and hypokinesia (6.9% vs. 0.0%, $P=0.059$, NNH=15). In the randomized phase, mean weight change was +0.7 kg with RLAI plus TAU versus −1.8 kg with placebo plus TAU ($P=0.002$), and mean prolactin change was +12.2 ng/mL with RLAI plus TAU versus −19.2 ng/mL with placebo plus TAU ($P<0.001$).

In summary, one multicenter randomized controlled trial suggested that the long-acting injectable formulation of risperidone may help prevent manic relapses in patients with rapid-cycling bipolar disorder who have required frequent medical interventions. However, extrapyramidal symptoms, hyperprolactinemia, and weight gain may limit the utility of risperidone.

Aripiprazole

Aripiprazole has indications for both acute mania and bipolar maintenance therapy. Limited data from post hoc secondary analyses of the registration studies

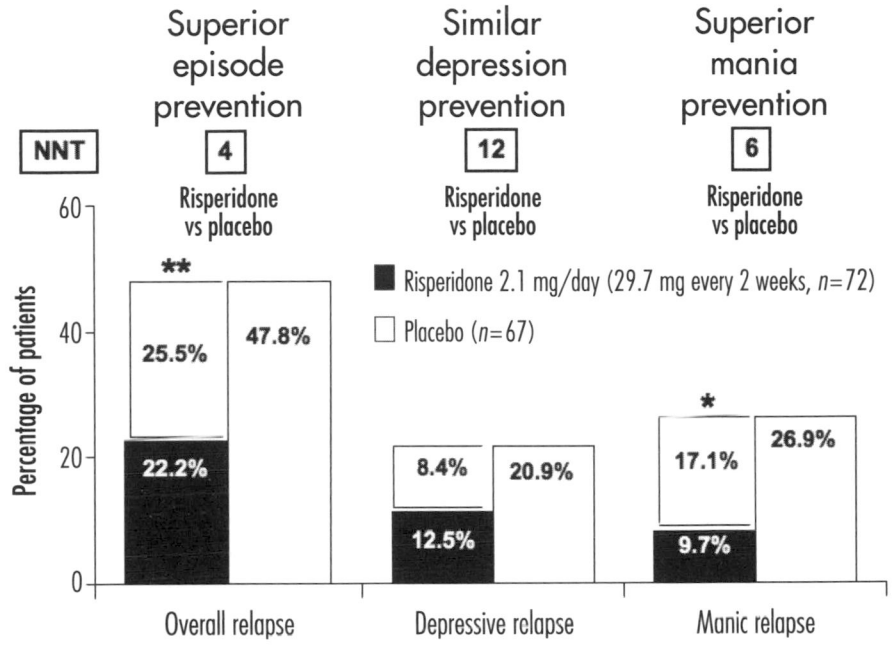

FIGURE 9–12.   Overview of 56-week, double-blind adjunctive risperi-done long-acting injectable (RLAI) versus adjunctive placebo in patients with rapid-cycling bipolar disorder, numbers needed to treat (NNT), and relapse rates.

Adjunctive RLAI (black bars) compared with adjunctive placebo (white bars) yielded a significantly lower recurrence of overall episodes (*left*) and manic episodes (*right*) but not depressive episodes (*center*). Patients were stabilized on RLAI plus treatment as usual for 4 weeks prior to randomization. With RLAI, recurrences of depression were numerically higher than recurrences of mood elevation. *$P<0.05$, **$P<0.01$ adjunctive risperidone versus adjunctive placebo.

Source.   Data from MacFadden et al. 2008.

for these indications suggested potential utility in patients with rapid-cycling bipolar disorder.

Preliminary assessment of relationships between aripiprazole therapeutic effects and rapid cycling was obtained utilizing pooled data from two 3-week randomized, double-blind, placebo-controlled aripiprazole acute mania trials (total $N=516$) (Suppes et al. 2008). Aripiprazole appeared to yield somewhat more robust antimanic effects in patients with rapid cycling compared with patients without rapid cycling, although this finding could have been confounded by quicker cycling out of the index manic episode in the patients with rapid cycling. Aripiprazole significantly reduced mean YMRS total scores at end point compared with placebo in patients with rapid-cycling (-10.9 vs. -5.0, $P<0.01$) and non-rapid-cycling (-10.7 vs. -5.7, $P<0.01$) illness. The YMRS response rate with aripiprazole was greater than with placebo in both rapid cyclers (50.0% vs. 19.6%, $P<0.01$, NNT=4) (Figure 9–13, left) and non–rapid cyclers (45.9%% vs. 27.1%%, $P=0.004$, NNT=6) (Figure 9–13, right).

Preliminary assessment of relationships between aripiprazole therapeutic effects and rapid cycling is not available from the two 8-week randomized, double-blind, placebo-controlled aripiprazole acute bipolar depression trials (Thase et al. 2008). In these trials, aripiprazole was no better than placebo, and the percentage of patients with rapid cycling and results in individuals with rapid cycling were not reported.

In a 26-week, multicenter, randomized, double-blind, placebo-controlled aripiprazole maintenance registration trial in patients after manic or mixed episodes, 17.5% (28/160) of patients had rapid cycling (Keck et al. 2006a). Aripiprazole (mean dosage 25.3 mg/day) compared with placebo yielded a significantly longer time to relapse in patients with rapid cycling (as well as without rapid cycling), but more detailed analyses regarding the polarity of relapse in rapid-cycling patients were not provided (Muzina et al. 2008). Rates of inefficacy discontinuation (a proxy for relapse) tended to be lower with aripiprazole compared with placebo (14.3%, 2/14 vs. 50.0%, 7/14, $P=0.10$, NNT=3). In rapid cyclers, baseline to end point mean YMRS scores increased 3.0 with aripiprazole and 6.6 with placebo ($P=0.21$), and mean MADRS scores increased 8.3 with aripiprazole and 11.5 with placebo ($P=0.52$). The most commonly reported adverse effects with aripiprazole were anxiety ($n=4$) and depression ($n=3$), and one aripiprazole-treated patient discontinued because of an adverse effect (akathisia). There were no significant between-group differences in mean changes in weight or metabolic parameters. Mean weight change at week 26 was -3.8 kg with aripiprazole and $+0.3$ kg with placebo. The small sample size limits the interpretation of these findings.

In summary, aripiprazole appears to provide more robust acute and prophylactic antimanic, rather than antidepressant, effects in bipolar disorder patients in general, and limited data suggest that aripiprazole may have potential in the treatment of the mood elevation component of rapid-cycling bipolar disorder. Adverse effects with aripiprazole may be challenging, and clinicians and patients may deem this agent to have inferior tolerability as compared with mood stabilizers such as lamotrigine and divalproex but superior tolerability as compared with olanzapine or quetiapine.

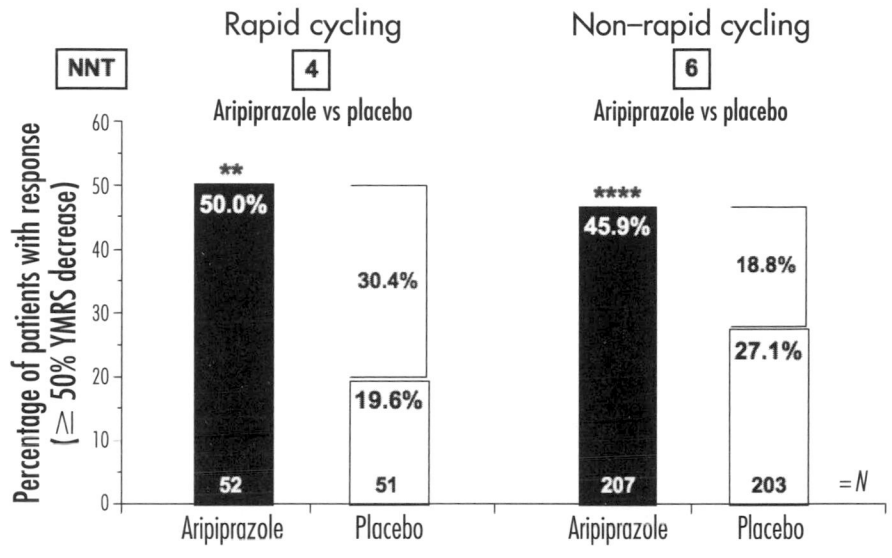

FIGURE 9–13. Overview of 3-week double-blind aripiprazole versus placebo trials in acute mania with and without rapid cycling, numbers needed to treat (NNT), and response rates.

The Young Mania Rating Scale (YMRS) response (≥50% decrease) rate with aripiprazole (black bars) was greater than with placebo (white bars) in both rapid cyclers (*left*) and in non–rapid cyclers (*right*). **P<0.01, ****P<0.0001 aripiprazole versus placebo.

Source. Data from Suppes et al. 2008.

Ziprasidone

Very limited data are available regarding the utility of ziprasidone in rapid-cycling bipolar disorder. Even preliminary data are limited, because the multicenter, randomized, controlled ziprasidone monotherapy acute mania studies do not report the prevalence of rapid cycling in their samples or the acute antimanic efficacy of the drug in patients with rapid cycling (Keck et al. 2003b; Potkin et al. 2005).

A single case report suggested that in a treatment-resistant obese patient with a mixed episode and a history of rapid cycling, ziprasidone titrated to 240 mg/day yielded acute improvement in depression more than in mood elevation, which at 3-month follow-up persisted and was accompanied by a 16-lb weight loss (Mech 2008).

In summary, controlled trials are necessary to assess the utility of ziprasidone in the treatment of rapid-cycling bipolar disorders. Although initiation may be complex and some patients may experience akathisia, the relative lack of problems with weight gain and metabolic complications suggests that controlled trials are warranted.

Clozapine

Clozapine, although not approved for the treatment of bipolar disorder, is approved for treatment-resistant schizophrenia and for decreasing suicidal behavior in schizophrenia. As noted in other chapters in this volume, limited evidence suggests that clozapine may have utility in treatment-resistant bipolar disorders, with perhaps more robust antimanic than antidepressant effects.

There is an absence of controlled trials of clozapine in rapid-cycling bipolar disorder. Several early, small (two- to four-patient) case series suggested that clozapine as monotherapy or adjunctive therapy with dosages ranging between 150 mg/day and 400 mg/day might have utility in patients with treatment-resistant rapid-cycling bipolar disorder with or without psychotic features (Calabrese et al. 1991; Frye et al. 1996; Suppes et al. 1992, 1994).

However, later larger case series suggested that clozapine was less effective in patients with rapid-cycling bipolar disorder than in those with non-rapid cycling bipolar disorder. In a 13-week, open acute mania trial in patients with treatment-resistant bipolar I disorder and schizoaffective disorder, bipolar type, clozapine monotherapy yielded less improvement in patients with than without rapid cycling (Calabrese et al. 1996). This study included 11 patients (7 bipolar and 4 schizoaffective) with rapid cycling and 14 patients (3 bipolar and 11 schizoaffective) without rapid cycling. The mean maximum clozapine dosage was similar in patients with and without rapid-cycling bipolar disorder (498 mg/day vs. 491 mg/day). Patients with rapid cycling had less baseline to end-point improvement in mean Brief Psychiatric Rating Scale (BPRS) scores but similar improvement in mean YMRS scores compared with patients without rapid cycling.

Similarly, in a 1-year, open trial in patients with treatment-resistant bipolar I disorder and schizoaffective disorder, bipolar type, clozapine added to TAU yielded less improvement in patients with rapid cycling than in those without rapid cycling (Suppes et al. 2004). This study included 15 patients (13 bipolar and 2 schizoaffective) with rapid cycling and 13 patients (7 bipolar and 6 schizoaffective) without rapid cycling. The mean clozapine dosage was nonsignificantly lower in patients with rapid cycling than in those without rapid cycling (238 mg/day vs. 329 mg/day). Rapid cyclers demonstrated a marked first-month 14.8-point improvement in mean BPRS score, which was followed by gradual worsening by 0.1 points per month for the remaining 11 months. Non–rapid cyclers demonstrated a more modest first-month 5.0-point improvement in mean BPRS score, which was followed by gradual improvement by 1.3 points per month for the remaining 11 months. Thus, over the entire trial, patients with rapid cycling had significantly less improvement than patients without rapid cycling.

In summary, in view of the challenging adverse effect profile of this agent, clozapine is usually held in reserve for patients with treatment-resistant illness. Controlled trials of clozapine in patients with rapid-cycling bipolar disorder are needed to inform clinical practice.

Effectiveness Studies of the Treatment of Rapid-Cycling Bipolar Disorder

The STEP-BD (Schneck et al. 2008) and the Stanley Foundation Bipolar Network (SFBN; Kupka et al. 2005) have published studies of the naturalistic treatment of patients with rapid-cycling bipolar disorder. In the STEP-BD study (Schneck et al. 2008), among 1,191 patients followed for 1 year while receiving naturalistic treatment using model practice procedures, the rate of prospective rapid cycling (4.9%) was substantially lower than the rate of retrospectively reported rapid cycling for the prior year (29.9%). Although polarity of mood symptoms in the prospective year was not the focus of this report, it appeared consistent among patients with rapid-cycling bipolar disorder compared with patients with non-rapid-cycling bipolar disorder struggling with more depression, based on percentages of patients treated with antidepressants (82.8%, 48/58 vs. 59.3%, 672/1,133, $P<0.0002$).

In the SFBN study (Kupka et al. 2005), among 539 patients with 1 year of daily life-chart data, the rate of prospective rapid cycling (38.2%) was similar to the rate of retrospectively reported rapid cycling for the prior year (40.6%). In this study, among patients with prospective rapid cycling receiving naturalistic treatment according to current standards or in more formal pharmacotherapy protocols, depression was the most pervasive mood state, accounting for 39.5% of the time, whereas mood elevation or ultradian cycling accounted for 27.1% of the time.

Treatment-Resistant Depression as the Hallmark of Rapid-Cycling Bipolar Disorder

The above sections demonstrate that although mood stabilizers and second-generation antipsychotics may have some efficacy in patients with rapid-cycling bipolar disorder, their utility in controlling (especially depressive) symptoms is limited. Indeed, in a 2001 review of rapid-cycling bipolar disorder, Calabrese and associates identified depression (often treatment-resistant) as the hallmark of rapid-cycling bipolar disorder (Calabrese et al. 2001), citing data from controlled and uncontrolled studies of lithium monotherapy (Dunner et al. 1976), divalproex monotherapy and adjunctive therapy (Calabrese et al. 1993), lamotrigine monotherapy (Calabrese et al. 2000), and lithium plus divalproex (Calabrese et al. 2001). Subsequent clinical trials of lithium monotherapy (Calabrese et al. 2005b) (Figure 9–4), divalproex monotherapy (Calabrese et al. 2005b) (Figure 9–4), RLAI adjunctive therapy (MacFadden et al. 2008) (Figure 9–12), and naturalistic treatment (Coryell et al. 2003; Kupka et al. 2005; Schneck et al. 2008) have been consistent with the view that treatment-resistant depression is a crucial unmet need in the management of rapid-cycling bipolar disorder (Table 9–2).

Other Adjunctive Treatments

Treatment resistance or intolerance is sufficiently common in patients with rapid-cycling bipolar disorders that even the above-mentioned armamentarium is insufficient to meet clinical needs. In this section, we describe adjunctive treatments with even more limited evidence of efficacy than the previously mentioned treatments. These treatments include antidepressants, supraphysiological L-thyroxine [T_4], psychotherapy, and other novel interventions such as other anticonvulsants (gabapentin, topiramate, levetiracetam, tiagabine), nimodipine, nutriceuticals (omega-3 fatty acids, choline, melatonin, chromium), electroconvulsive therapy [ECT], sleep deprivation, light therapy, and vagus nerve stimulation [VNS]).

Adjunctive Antidepressants

As noted, effective treatment of depression constitutes a crucial unmet need for patients with rapid-cycling bipolar disorder. Thus, it is understandable that adjunctive antidepressants are commonly administered to such patients. Indeed, in the STEP-BP, the rate of antidepressant usage for patients receiving naturalistic treatment using model practice procedures was higher in patients with prospective rapid cycling (82.8%, 48/58) than in those without (59.3%, 672/1133) (Schneck et al. 2008).

However, for almost three decades, concerns have been raised that antidepressants (particularly tricyclics and monoamine oxidase inhibitors) can yield cycle acceleration (at least two more syndromal episodes with antidepressant

TABLE 9–2. **Treatment-resistant depression: the hallmark of rapid-cycling bipolar disorder**

Depression compared with mood elevation is more resistant to

Lithium ($n=6$; Dunner et al. 1976) ($n=32$; Calabrese et al. 2005b)

Divalproex ($n=101$, $n=28$) (Calabrese et al. 2005b; Calabrese et al. 1993)

Lamotrigine ($n=182$) (Calabrese et al. 2000)

Lithium plus divalproex ($n=215$, $n=56$) (Calabrese et al. 2001)

Risperidone long-acting injectable ($n=139$) (MacFadden et al. 2008)

Naturalistic treatment (CDS, $n=89$; Coryell et al. 2003) (SFBN, $n=206$; Kupka et al. 2005) (STEP-BD, $n=58$; Schneck et al. 2008)

Note. CDS=Collaborative Depression Study; SFBN=Stanley Foundation Bipolar Network; STEP-BD=Systematic Treatment Enhancement Program for Bipolar Disorder.

Source. Adapted and updated from Calabrese et al. 2001.

treatment compared with a similar duration immediately prior to antidepressant treatment) and hence rapid cycling in patients with bipolar disorders (Wehr and Goodwin 1979). Unfortunately, the evidence is limited, consisting of a few uncontrolled or small controlled studies.

For example, in an early, uncontrolled, retrospective study, among 115 patients who developed continuous cycling, prior antidepressant treatment was common, and a common feature of the transformation was the first switch from depression into hypomania, and in rapid cyclers the lithium response rate increased from 16% to 78% with antidepressant discontinuation (Kukopulos et al. 1980).

Also, two small ($n=5$ and $n=51$), prospective, double-blind, placebo-controlled, but not randomized (i.e., subjects used as their own controls) trials found that tricyclics plus lithium compared with lithium monotherapy yielded decreased cycle length (time from onset of mood elevation to time of next onset of mood elevation) (Wehr et al. 1979, 1988).

In an uncontrolled retrospective study, 25.7% (9/35) of patients with treatment-refractory bipolar disorder had a history of heterocyclic antidepressant–induced cycle acceleration (Altshuler et al. 1995). The rate of heterocyclic antidepressant–induced cycle acceleration was higher in patients with a history of antidepressant-induced mood elevation (46.2%, 6/13) than in those without (13.6%, 3/22, $P<0.03$).

Uncontrolled naturalistic/retrospective studies of newer antidepressants have reported rates of cycle acceleration varying from 0.0% (0/37) with bupropion and 7.9% (6/69) with selective serotonin reuptake inhibitors (Joffe et al.

2002) to 22.9% (8/35) with unspecified antidepressants (Ghaemi et al. 2000) and 25.6% (10/39) with various antidepressants (primarily selective serotonin reuptake inhibitors and bupropion) (Ghaemi et al. 2004).

In contrast, other data suggest that associations between antidepressant use and rapid cycling are primarily related to the frequent occurrence of depression in patients with such an illness course. In a large (n=919), longitudinal (1- to 5-year follow-up), but uncontrolled study, the onset of rapid cycling in 45 patients appeared more related to index major depressive episodes than to antidepressant exposure (Coryell et al. 1992). In a subsequent report by the same group, in a large (n=345), longitudinal (mean 13.7-year follow-up), but uncontrolled trial, in 89 patients with rapid cycling, antidepressants were no more often present in the weeks preceding switches from depression to mood elevation than in other weeks when depression was present, and decreased use of antidepressants was not associated with cessation of rapid cycling (Coryell et al. 2003). Indeed, depressive morbidity was particularly evident when lithium was administered without antidepressants. Also, other investigators have, on the basis of retrospective data, questioned the putative relationship between antidepressants and cycle acceleration (Angst 1985; Lewis and Winokur 1982).

Finally, a recent post hoc analysis of a small (43 subjects, including 27 rapid cyclers), 12-week, randomized, open study in depressed patients with bipolar II disorder suggested that venlafaxine monotherapy compared with lithium monotherapy yielded superior antidepressant effects with no increase in treatment-emergent affective switching, and these findings were similar in patients with and without rapid cycling (Amsterdam and Shults 2008). These data are at variance with controlled data that suggest that venlafaxine yields increased treatment-emergent affective switch more often than other antidepressants in patients with bipolar disorder (Post et al. 2006; Vieta et al. 2002a).

In summary, the use of adjunctive antidepressants in the treatment of rapid-cycling bipolar disorder remains controversial. Although these agents are commonly used, considerable expert opinion recommends limiting exposure. The controversy over their use persists in part because of the variable findings in uncontrolled and small controlled studies, and the lack of large, randomized controlled trials to address the use of antidepressants in rapid cycling. Variable findings may be related to subgroup differences. For example, one retrospective study suggested that in women (but not in men) with bipolar disorder, antidepressant use prior to the first manic or hypomanic episode increased the risk of a rapid-cycling course (Yildiz and Sachs 2003). Thus, among 71 female (but not 58 male) patients with bipolar disorder, the lifetime prevalence of rapid cycling was higher in those with antidepressant use prior to the first manic or hypomanic episode than in those without (77% vs. 41%).

Adjunctive Supraphysiological T₄

Hypothyroidism has been suggested to be associated with rapid-cycling bipolar disorder (Cowdry et al. 1983; Kusalic 1992). However, in a recent review of studies assessing this relationship, only two studies were positive (Cowdry et al. 1983; Kusalic 1992) and five were negative (Bartalena et al. 1990; Joffe et al. 1988; Maj et al. 1994; Post et al. 1997; Wehr et al. 1988), and a meta-analysis of these seven studies was negative (Kupka et al. 2003). The nature of such a putative association remains to be established because rapid cycling might increase the risk of hypothyroidism, particularly in the presence of lithium (Cho et al. 1979), or hypothyroidism might increase the risk of rapid cycling (Bauer et al. 1990).

As reviewed by Kupka (2006), three small uncontrolled open case series suggested that, commonly, adjunctive supraphysiological T_4 (maximum dosages 325–500 μg/day) yielded response in 59% (16/27), partial response in 22% (6/27), and nonresponse in 19% (5/27) of primarily (81%, 22/27) female patients with rapid-cycling bipolar disorder (Afflelou et al. 1997; Bauer and Whybrow 1990; Stancer and Persad 1982). Additional information regarding the use of supraphysiological T_4 is presented in Chapter 7, "Management of Acute Major Depressive Episodes in Bipolar Disorders."

Adjunctive Psychotherapy

In view of the efficacy and tolerability limitations of pharmacotherapy, adjunctive psychosocial interventions are worth considering for rapid-cycling bipolar disorder. Unfortunately, limited data are available regarding such use of psychotherapy. Adjunctive cognitive-behavioral therapy (CBT) adapted for patients with rapid-cycling bipolar disorder has been suggested (Reilly Harrington and Knauz 2005). This intervention entails 20 individual 50-minute weekly sessions administered over 5 months, followed by a booster session 4 weeks later, and comprises four flexible modules covering 1) adherence, 2) managing mood shifts, 3) cognitive restructuring of depressive/manic thoughts, and 4) CBT skills for managing comorbid (e.g., anxiety) disorders. A recent uncontrolled pilot study assessed the effectiveness of CBT in 10 bipolar I disorder patients with rapid cycling (Reilly Harrington et al. 2007). Patients with acute manic or mixed episodes, psychosis, alcohol or substance dependence, or confounding medical conditions were excluded. Six of 10 (60%) patients completed this regimen, with three patients discontinuing because of time demands. Among completers, from baseline to posttreatment, mean MADRS, YMRS, and Beck Anxiety Inventory scores decreased, but the difference was only statistically significant for MADRS scores. The authors suggested that CBT may help to relieve depressive symptoms, which are considered to be the hallmark of rapid-cycling bipolar disorder. The discontinuation of three of 10 patients due to time constraints indicates the need for careful patient selection for this treatment. Indeed, as discussed in Chapter 15, "Adjunctive Psychosocial Interventions in the Management of Bipolar Disorders," CBT efficacy may be limited in patients with severe and recurrent bipolar disorders (Scott et al. 2006).

Other Novel Interventions

Other novel treatments, most often used as adjuncts, may have efficacy in the treatment of rapid-cycling bipolar disorders. These treatments include other anticonvulsants (gabapentin, topiramate, levetiracetam, tiagabine), nimodipine, nutriceuticals (omega-3 fatty acids, choline, melatonin, chromium), ECT, sleep deprivation, light therapy, and VNS. Unfortunately, data regarding the utility of these agents in rapid-cycling bipolar disorders are limited.

In view of the utility of divalproex, lamotrigine, and carbamazepine in treating bipolar disorders, researchers have been interested in exploring the potential of other anticonvulsants, such as gabapentin, topiramate, levetiracetam, and tiagabine, in treating patients with rapid-cycling bipolar disorders. Limited data from uncontrolled, open case series suggest that adjunctive gabapentin may benefit some patients with rapid-cycling bipolar disorders (Altshuler et al. 1999; Wang et al. 2000; Young et al. 1999). However, as noted above in the section on lamotrigine, a 6-week, randomized, double-blind, placebo-controlled, crossover study found that lamotrigine (mean dosage 274 mg/day) monotherapy, but not gabapentin (mean dosage 3,987 mg/day) monotherapy, was superior to placebo for overall response in 31 inpatients with treatment-resistant (primarily rapid-cycling bipolar) mood disorder (Frye et al. 2000). Moreover, gabapentin has been reported to exacerbate rapid cycling in occasional patients (Schaffer and Schaffer 1997).

Also, limited uncontrolled, open treatment, case report (Chen et al. 2005) and case series (Kusumakar et al. 1999; Marcotte 1998) data suggest that adjunctive topiramate may benefit some patients with rapid-cycling bipolar disorder. In a chart review, primarily adjunctive topiramate (mean dosage approximately 200 mg/day, mean duration 16 weeks) yielded moderate to marked improvement in 52% (23/44) of outpatients with treatment-resistant rapid-cycling bipolar disorders (Marcotte 1998). Similarly, in a 16-week study, adjunctive open topiramate (mean maximum dosage 105 mg/day) yielded clinically significant improvement in 56% (15/27) of women with treatment-resistant rapid-cycling bipolar disorder (Kusumakar et al. 1999).

Similarly, limited uncontrolled, open treatment, case report and case series data suggest that adjunctive levetiracetam (Braunig and Kruger 2003; Kaufman 2004; Post et al. 2005) and adjunctive tiagabine (Schaffer et al. 2002) may benefit some patients with rapid-cycling bipolar disorder. For example, in one report, 57% (4/7) of outpatients with treatment-resistant rapid-cycling bipolar disorder were much or very much improved with adjunctive tiagabine (mean dosage in responders 4.9 mg/day, mean duration 9.7 weeks) (Schaffer et al. 2002). As noted in Chapter 6, "Management of Acute Manic and Mixed Episodes in Bipolar Disorders," reports of tolerability problems suggest that considerable caution should be exercised in using tiagabine to treat patients with bipolar disorders (Grunze et al. 1999; Suppes et al. 2002).

In view of the importance of calcium to intracellular signaling, and because limited evidence supports the utility of the calcium channel antagonist verapamil in bipolar disorders, nimodipine, another such agent with greater lipid solubility (and hence better central nervous system penetration) as well as some anticonvulsant effects, has been assessed in rapid-cycling bipolar disorders. Limited case report (Davanzo et al. 1999; Goodnick 1995; McDermut et al. 1995) and case series (Manna 1991; Pazzaglia et al. 1993, 1998) data suggest that nimodipine as monotherapy or as adjunctive therapy may offer benefit in some patients with rapid-cycling bipolar disorder.

In a 6-month, open, uncontrolled, crossover study, the combination of nimodipine (90 mg/day) plus lithium, compared with both nimodipine monotherapy and lithium monotherapy, yielded better outcome in 75% (9/12) of patients with rapid-cycling bipolar disorder (Manna 1991). In an uncontrolled, double-blind study, in inpatients with treatment-resistant primarily bipolar disorder (33%, 4/12 bipolar I; 58%, 7/12 bipolar II; 9%, 1/12 unipolar; 92%, 11/12 with rapid, ultra-rapid, or ultradian cycling), nimodipine monotherapy (mean dosage 413 mg/day, mean duration 8.2 weeks) yielded marked improvement in 25% (3/12) and partial improvement in 17% (2/12) of patients (Pazzaglia et al. 1993). In a subsequent uncontrolled, double-blind expansion of the original cohort, 30% (7/23) of inpatients with treatment-resistant bipolar disorder (commonly with rapid, ultra-rapid, or ultradian cycling) had moderate to marked improvement with nimodipine monotherapy (Pazzaglia et al. 1998). In addition, 27% (3/11) of bipolar disorder patients resistant to nimodipine monotherapy had moderate to marked improvement when carbamazepine (mean dosage 793 mg/day, mean serum concentration 7.6 µg/mL, mean duration 60 days) was added.

As noted in Chapter 7 of this volume, patients commonly suggest complementary and alternative medicine interventions such as dietary supplements (nutriceuticals). Although generally well tolerated, such interventions appear to have only modest systematic evidence to support their use.

In a 4-month, double-blind, placebo-controlled study in patients with rapid-cycling bipolar disorder, 14 patients taking 9.6 g/day of adjunctive omega-3 fatty acids (6.2 g/day of eicosapentaenoic acid plus 3.4 g/day of docosahexaenoic acid) compared with 16 taking adjunctive placebo (olive oil) had a significantly longer mean duration of remission (Stoll et al. 1999). However, in a randomized, double-blind, placebo-controlled trial in patients with rapid-cycling bipolar disorder, 31 patients taking adjunctive eicosapentaenoic acid (6 g/day) and 28 taking adjunctive placebo had similar mood outcomes (Keck et al. 2006b).

In a small, uncontrolled, open trial, adjunctive choline bitartrate (mean free choline equivalent 4,867 mg/day) yielded improvement in 67% (4/6) of patients with treatment-refractory rapid-cycling bipolar disorder (Stoll et al. 1996). In a small, 12-week, double-blind, placebo-controlled crossover trial, in five women with rapid-cycling bipolar disorder, melatonin 10 mg/day and placebo had similar effects on mood and sleep (Leibenluft et al. 1997). In an uncontrolled, 3-week acute and 2-year continuation, open trial in 30 patients with treatment-resistant rapid-cycling bipolar disorder who were primarily (77%, 23/30) depressed at entry, adjunctive chromium chloride (600–800 µg/day) yielded 30% Ham-D and 39% MADRS acute antidepressant responses (Amann et al. 2007). However, the longer-term results of this study were challenging to interpret, with the mean duration of treatment being 204 days but only 23% of patients completing 1 year (with episodes per year decreasing from 6.0 to 2.6) and only 13% completing 2 years of continuation therapy.

Limited, uncontrolled, open treatment, case report (Berman and Wolpert 1987) and small case series (Koukopoulos et al. 2003) data suggest that acute ECT may provide benefit in some patients with rapid-cycling bipolar disorders. For example, ECT yielded recovery in 26% (11/43) of outpatients with rapid-cycling bipolar disorders (Koukopoulos et al. 2003). However, ECT may fail to offer acute efficacy in patients with the most challenging illness. Thus, ECT failed to yield remission in 100% (24/24) of inpatients with treatment-refractory rapid-cycling bipolar disorders (Wehr et al. 1988). Similarly, limited, uncontrolled, open treatment, case report (Kho 2002) and small case series (Koukopoulos et al. 2003; Vanelle et al. 1994) data suggest that maintenance ECT may yield benefit in some patients with rapid-cycling bipolar disorders. Additional information regarding ECT is provided in Chapter 7 and Chapter 8 of this volume.

Limited, uncontrolled, open treatment, small case series data suggest that acute sleep deprivation may provide benefit in some patients with rapid-cycling bipolar disorders (Gill et al. 1993; Koukopoulos et al. 2003; Papadimitriou et al. 1993). Very limited data suggest that this intervention may be more effective later, rather than earlier, during depressive episodes (Gill et al. 1993). Also, treatment-emergent affective switch may occur (Papadimitriou et al. 1993). Additional information regarding sleep deprivation is provided in Chapter 7 of this volume.

Limited, uncontrolled, open treatment, case report (Eagles 1994) and small case series (Leibenluft et al. 1995) data suggest that acute light therapy and/or light-dark exposure manipulations (Wehr et al. 1998; Wirz-Justice et al. 1999) may provide benefit in some patients with rapid- or ultradian-cycling bipolar disorders. One small study in patients with rapid-cycling bipolar disorder suggested that light therapy administered at midday may be effective but that light therapy administered in the evening may be ineffective and that light therapy administered in the morning may exacerbate cycling (Leibenluft et al. 1995). Additional information regarding light therapy is provided in Chapter 7 of this volume.

The pivotal study of VNS in treatment-resistant depression included primarily patients with unipolar major depressive disorder and a few with bipolar disorder, but specifically excluded patients with rapid-cycling bipolar disorder (Rush et al. 2005). Limited, uncontrolled, open-label, case report (Bajbouj et al. 2006) and case series (Marangell et al. 2008) data suggest that adjunctive VNS may provide benefit in some patients with treatment-resistant rapid-cycling bipolar disorder. In nine primarily depressed outpatients with treatment-resistant rapid-cycling bipolar disorder, VNS yielded improvements of 38.1% in overall illness scores, 37.1% in depression scores, and 40.2% in mood elevation scores (Marangell et al. 2008). The cost and invasiveness of VNS and the relatively modest efficacy raise cost-benefit concerns. Indeed, patients commonly find that their insurance companies deny reimbursement for VNS. Additional information regarding VNS is provided in Chapter 7 and Chapter 8 of this volume.

Combination Therapy

Despite limited controlled data, combination therapy is commonly utilized in patients with rapid-cycling bipolar disorders. As noted in the section on lithium earlier in this chapter, lithium combined with divalproex (Calabrese et al. 2005b) or carbamazepine (Denicoff et al. 1997) may have some utility, but rapid-cycling bipolar disorder (particularly the depressive component) is commonly refractory even to two-drug combination therapy. In view of the common phenomenon of treatment-resistant depression in patients with rapid-cycling bipolar disorders, it appears reasonable to combine agents that "stabilize mood from above" (i.e., have more prominent antimanic effects), such as lithium, divalproex, or carbamazepine, with those that "stabilize mood from below" (i.e., have more prominent antidepressant effects), such as lamotrigine (Ketter and Calabrese 2002); however, controlled studies are needed to assess such approaches. Also, agents with prominent bimodal (antimanic and antidepressant) activity, such as quetiapine, may have utility in combination therapies, but controlled studies are needed to assess such strategies. The only large controlled study of an adjunctive second-generation antipsychotic in rapid-cycling bipolar disorder indicates that long-acting injectable risperidone was efficacious for manic more than for depressive symptoms (MacFadden et al. 2008). Not all medication combinations uniformly offer benefit, and for some patients, certain combinations may yield poorer outcome (e.g., tricyclics combined with lithium have poorer outcome than lithium monotherapy).

Despite very limited efficacy data and some evidence that they may exacerbate illness, adjunctive antidepressants are commonly used in patients with rapid-cycling bipolar disorder. The olanzapine plus fluoxetine combination appears to offer benefit for acute depression in rapid cyclers (Keck et al. 2003a), but longer-term controlled studies are needed to adequately assess the utility of this combination, and olanzapine has longer-term tolerability risks such as metabolic problems. Nevertheless, agents with particularly potent antimanic effects (such as olanzapine) may provide sufficient counterbalance to the destabilizing effects of antidepressants (such as fluoxetine) to permit therapeutic synergy.

Additional adjunctive treatments have been proposed, but controlled trials are needed to establish that these interventions are effective in treating rapid-cycling bipolar disorder. Adjunctive psychotherapy appears to have particular potential in the treatment of rapid-cycling bipolar disorder, based on its utility in treating acute bipolar depression and in the longer-term treatment of bipolar disorder inpatient samples not restricted to rapid cyclers, as discussed in Chapters 7, 8, and 15.

Conclusion

Rapid-cycling bipolar disorders are a common and particularly challenging subset of bipolar disorders. Women and patients with bipolar II disorder appear to be overrepresented among rapid cyclers. Associations of rapid cycling with other illness characteristics, such as early age at onset, history of suicide attempts, anxiety disorders, thyroid disorders, alcohol/substance abuse, and prior antidepressant administration, have been less consistent. Rapid cycling may be either persistent or transient, highlighting the need for effective therapeutics. Treatment-resistant depression appears to be the hallmark of rapid-cycling bipolar disorder.

Limited controlled data are available to inform clinical practice, but mood stabilizers and second-generation antipsychotics (often in combinations) are commonly used. Adjunctive antidepressants are also commonly used, despite concerns that these agents could yield treatment-emergent affective switch and possibly cycle acceleration. We hope that in the coming years, controlled trials will provide new treatment options and resolution of some of the current controversies regarding the longer management of rapid-cycling bipolar disorders.

Case Study: Treatment of Rapid-Cycling Bipolar Disorders

Ms. Gray is a 43-year-old married white homemaker with three children. She has struggled with generalized anxiety disorder, panic disorder with agoraphobia, and hypochondriasis since childhood, and recurrent diagnosed major depressive episodes as well as undiagnosed hypomanic episodes (interpreted as agitated depressions) since her teenage years. She also reported a history of cannabis and alcohol abuse, starting in her late teenage years and ending in her early 20s.

Ms. Gray's syndromal mood episodes have appeared to increase in frequency and severity over the last few years. Thus, over the 12 months prior to presentation, she reported experiencing three syndromal major depressive episodes lasting at least 2 weeks and characterized by pervasive sadness, anhedonia, insomnia, guilty ruminations, decreased self-esteem, distractibility, poor appetite, psychomotor agitation, and suicidal ideation. Careful assessment, including obtaining information from her husband, indicated that over the 12 months prior to presentation, she had experienced at least three syndromal hypomanic episodes lasting at least 4 days and characterized by significant irritability, decreased need for sleep in that 4 hours was sufficient, racing thoughts to the extent that she felt compelled to write them down in order to retain them, distractibility, and psychomotor agitation. Both Ms. Gray and her husband specifically denied that the hypomanic episodes involved euphoria, expansiveness, inflated self-esteem, overtalkativeness, impulsivity, or marked functional impairment, noting that productivity could actually be enhanced. Both Ms. Gray and her husband specifically denied that she had any lifetime history of psychosis, psychiatric hospitalization, suicide attempts, self-mutilation, violence, arrests, or other legal problems.

Ms. Gray's medical history was noncontributory, and her body mass index at presentation was in the high normal range at 24.6 kg/m^2. She reported that her mother had been treated, including being hospitalized, for bipolar disorder and also had problems with substance abuse. Her eldest child had been treated for attention-deficit/hyperactivity disorder and had also struggled with depression and anxiety. She reported significant marital tension regarding the challenge of parenting her eldest child.

Ms. Gray first had mental health treatment in her teenage years, when she received psychotherapy for depression. She first had pharmacotherapy for depression at approximately age 25 years, when she was treated with imipramine, which was discontinued after approximately 5 years because of constipation, tremor, and orthostasis. A brief trial of paroxetine had yielded some improvement in depression but was discontinued because of constipation and weight gain. Escitalopram 10 mg/day for 2 months had yielded weight gain, which improved somewhat with decreasing dosage to 5 mg/day for the 2 months prior to presentation. Because of sedation, benzodiazepines (clonazepam or alprazolam) were used only on an as-needed basis (about once a week for panic or limited symptom anxiety attacks), limiting their utility in controlling anxiety.

Ms. Gray was diagnosed with bipolar II disorder, currently depressed, with rapid-cycling course. It appeared that her hypomanias, which had entailed irritability rather than euphoria or expansiveness, had been interpreted as agitated depressions, resulting in a delay of accurate diagnosis of approximately 25 years from illness onset and first psychotherapy, and of approximately 15 years from first pharmacotherapy.

After a discussion of the risk of serious rash, lamotrigine (added to escitalopram 5 mg/day) was initiated, using the gradual titration described in the prescribing information. After 6 weeks, when the lamotrigine dosage was 100 mg/day, Ms. Gray switched into hypomania, so escitalopram was discontinued and clonazepam was increased from 0.5 mg/day as needed to 0.5 mg twice a day.

Two weeks later (treatment week 8), while taking lamotrigine 150 mg/day and clonazepam 0.5 mg twice a day, Ms. Gray switched back into depression, so the dosage of lamotrigine continued to be increased gradually.

Three weeks later (treatment week 11), while taking lamotrigine 225 mg/day and clonazepam 0.5 mg twice a day, she switched into subsyndromal hypomanic symptoms, so clonazepam was replaced with quetiapine 25 mg/day, and lamotrigine was continued to be increased gradually.

Although Ms. Gray's anxiety was increasingly well controlled, her subsyndromal hypomanic and depressive symptoms continued to alternate. Therefore, lamotrigine and quetiapine were both gradually increased so that by treatment week 18, she was taking lamotrigine 400 mg/day and quetiapine 200 mg/day. At that time, her 12-hour trough serum lamotrigine concentration was 5.1 μg/mL (epilepsy reference range 3–15 μg/mL), so an attempt was made to further gradually increase lamotrigine but was abandoned as dosages over 400 mg/day yielded tremor and ataxia. Similarly, an attempt to further gradually increase quetiapine was abandoned because dosages over 200 mg/day yielded sedation and ataxia.

Thus, by treatment week 26, her medications and clinical status were similar to 8 weeks earlier, and she complained of gradual weight gain over the last 6 months, with her body mass index increasing from high normal range (24.6) to overweight range (26.8). At that point, Ms. Gray commented that her eldest son had been diagnosed with bipolar II disorder and had experienced remarkable improvement with divalproex. Thus, a decision was made to transition her from quetiapine to divalproex, while continuing lamotrigine.

By treatment week 32, her mood had stabilized with her taking divalproex 1,000 mg/day (with a serum valproate concentration of 85 ng/mL), lamotrigine 200 mg/day (lamotrigine dosage had been decreased by 50% because of divalproex's ability to double serum lamotrigine concentrations), and quetiapine 25 mg/day. With diet and exercise, her body mass index had decreased but was still in the overweight range (26.2).

Over the next 6 months, her mood remained stable and anxiety was controlled. Attempts to discontinue quetiapine (to facilitate weight control) had resulted in insomnia and reemergence of anxiety. Similarly, attempts to decrease divalproex had resulted in subsyndromal hypomanic symptoms. However, ongoing efforts with diet and exercise had yielded reduction of her body mass index to the high normal range (24.9).

In summary, Ms. Gray struggled with bipolar II disorder, which had been interpreted as major depressive disorder, resulting in a 25-year delay of accurate diagnosis. Over the few years prior to presentation, her illness had worsened, and she had developed rapid cycling. Careful assessment, including information from a significant other, revealed a diagnosis of bipolar II disorder. Elimination of antidepressants and gradual introduction of first monotherapy and later combination therapy with mood stabilizers and a second-generation antipsychotic ultimately yielded stable mood and control of anxiety, although ongoing efforts with diet and exercise were necessary to yield adequate weight control.

References

Afflelou S, Auriacombe M, Cazenave M, et al: Administration of high-dose levothyroxine in treatment of rapid cycling bipolar disorders: review of the literature and initial therapeutic application apropos of 6 cases [in French]. Encephale 23:209–217, 1997

Altshuler LL, Post RM, Leverich GS, et al: Antidepressant-induced mania and cycle acceleration: a controversy revisited. Am J Psychiatry 152:1130–1138, 1995

Altshuler LL, Keck PE Jr, McElroy SL, et al: Gabapentin in the acute treatment of refractory bipolar disorder. Bipolar Disord 1:61–65, 1999

Amann BL, Mergl R, Vieta E, et al: A 2-year, open-label pilot study of adjunctive chromium in patients with treatment-resistant rapid-cycling bipolar disorder. J Clin Psychopharmacol 27:104–106, 2007

American Psychiatric Association: Diagnostic and Statistical Manual of Mental Disorders, 4th Edition. Washington, DC, American Psychiatric Association, 1994

American Psychiatric Association: Diagnostic and Statistical Manual of Mental Disorders, 4th Edition, Text Revision. Washington, DC, American Psychiatric Association, 2000

Amsterdam JD, Shults J: Comparison of short-term venlafaxine versus lithium monotherapy for bipolar II major depressive episode: a randomized open-label study. J Clin Psychopharmacol 28:171–181, 2008

Angst J: Switch from depression to mania: a record study over decades between 1920 and 1982. Psychopathology 18:140–154, 1985

Avasthi A, Sharma A, Malhotra S, et al: Rapid cycling affective disorder: a descriptive study from North India. J Affect Disord 54:67–73, 1999

Bajbouj M, Danker-Hopfe H, Heuser I, et al: Long-term outcome of vagus nerve stimulation in rapid-cycling bipolar disorder. J Clin Psychiatry 67:837–838, 2006

Baldessarini RJ, Tondo L, Floris G, et al: Effects of rapid cycling on response to lithium maintenance treatment in 360 bipolar I and II disorder patients. J Affect Disord 61:13–22, 2000

Bartalena L, Pellegrini L, Meschi M, et al: Evaluation of thyroid function in patients with rapid-cycling and non-rapid-cycling bipolar disorder. Psychiatry Res 34:13–17, 1990

Bauer MS, Whybrow PC: Rapid cycling bipolar affective disorder, II: treatment of refractory rapid cycling with high-dose levothyroxine: a preliminary study. Arch Gen Psychiatry 47:435–440, 1990

Bauer MS, Whybrow PC, Winokur A: Rapid cycling bipolar affective disorder, I: association with grade I hypothyroidism. Arch Gen Psychiatry 47:427–432, 1990

Bauer MS, Calabrese J, Dunner DL, et al: Multisite data reanalysis of the validity of rapid cycling as a course modifier for bipolar disorder in DSM-IV. Am J Psychiatry 151:506–515, 1994

Becker OV, Rasgon NL, Marsh WK, et al: Lamotrigine therapy in treatment-resistant menstrually related rapid cycling bipolar disorder: a case report. Bipolar Disord 6:435–439, 2004

Berman E, Wolpert EA: Intractable manic-depressive psychosis with rapid cycling in an 18-year-old woman successfully treated with electroconvulsive therapy. J Nerv Ment Dis 175:236–239, 1987

Bowden CL, Calabrese JR, McElroy SL, et al: The efficacy of lamotrigine in rapid cycling and non-rapid cycling patients with bipolar disorder. Biol Psychiatry 45:953–958, 1999

Bowden CL, Grunze H, Mullen J, et al: A randomized, double-blind, placebo-controlled efficacy and safety study of quetiapine or lithium as monotherapy for mania in bipolar disorder. J Clin Psychiatry 66:111–121, 2005

Braunig P, Kruger S: Levetiracetam in the treatment of rapid cycling bipolar disorder. J Psychopharmacol 17:239–241, 2003

Calabrese JR, Delucchi GA: Spectrum of efficacy of valproate in 55 patients with rapid-cycling bipolar disorder. Am J Psychiatry 147:431–434, 1990

Calabrese JR, Meltzer HY, Markovitz PJ: Clozapine prophylaxis in rapid cycling bipolar disorder (letter). J Clin Psychopharmacol 11:396–397, 1991

Calabrese JR, Markovitz PJ, Kimmel SE, et al: Spectrum of efficacy of valproate in 78 rapid-cycling bipolar patients. J Clin Psychopharmacol 12(suppl):53S–56S, 1992

Calabrese JR, Woyshville MJ, Kimmel SE, et al: Predictors of valproate response in bipolar rapid cycling. J Clin Psychopharmacol 13:280–283, 1993

Calabrese JR, Kimmel SE, Woyshville MJ, et al: Clozapine for treatment-refractory mania. Am J Psychiatry 153:759–764, 1996

Calabrese JR, Suppes T, Bowden CL, et al; Lamictal 614 Study Group: A double-blind, placebo-controlled, prophylaxis study of lamotrigine in rapid-cycling bipolar disorder. J Clin Psychiatry 61:841–850, 2000

Calabrese JR, Shelton MD, Bowden CL, et al: Bipolar rapid cycling: focus on depression as its hallmark. J Clin Psychiatry 62 (suppl 14):34–41, 2001

Calabrese JR, Keck PE Jr, Macfadden W, et al: A randomized, double-blind, placebo-controlled trial of quetiapine in the treatment of bipolar I or II depression. Am J Psychiatry 162:1351–1360, 2005a

Calabrese JR, Shelton MD, Rapport DJ, et al: A 20-month, double-blind, maintenance trial of lithium versus divalproex in rapid-cycling bipolar disorder. Am J Psychiatry 162:2152–2161, 2005b

Chen CK, Shiah IS, Yeh CB, et al: Combination treatment of clozapine and topiramate in resistant rapid-cycling bipolar disorder. Clin Neuropharmacol 28:136–138, 2005

Cho JT, Bone S, Dunner DL, et al: The effect of lithium treatment on thyroid function in patients with primary affective disorder. Am J Psychiatry 136:115–116, 1979

Coryell W, Endicott J, Keller M: Rapidly cycling affective disorder: demographics, diagnosis, family history, and course. Arch Gen Psychiatry 49:126–131, 1992

Coryell W, Solomon D, Turvey C, et al: The long-term course of rapid-cycling bipolar disorder. Arch Gen Psychiatry 60:914–920, 2003

Cowdry RW, Wehr TA, Zis AP, et al: Thyroid abnormalities associated with rapid-cycling bipolar illness. Arch Gen Psychiatry 40:414–420, 1983

da Rocha FF, Soares FM, Correa H, et al: Addition of lamotrigine to valproic acid: a successful outcome in a case of rapid-cycling bipolar affective disorder. Prog Neuropsychopharmacol Biol Psychiatry 31:1548–1549, 2007

Davanzo PA, Krah N, Kleiner J, et al: Nimodipine treatment of an adolescent with ultradian cycling bipolar affective illness. J Child Adolesc Psychopharmacol 9:51–61, 1999

Denicoff KD, Smith-Jackson EE, Disney ER, et al: Comparative prophylactic efficacy of lithium, carbamazepine, and the combination in bipolar disorder. J Clin Psychiatry 58:470–478, 1997

Di Costanzo E, Schifano F: Lithium alone or in combination with carbamazepine for the treatment of rapid-cycling bipolar affective disorder. Acta Psychiatr Scand 83:456–459, 1991

Dunner DL, Fieve RR: Clinical factors in lithium carbonate prophylaxis failure. Arch Gen Psychiatry 30:229–233, 1974

Dunner DL, Stallone F, Fieve RR: Lithium carbonate and affective disorders, V: a double-blind study of prophylaxis of depression in bipolar illness. Arch Gen Psychiatry 33:117–120, 1976

Dunner DL, Patrick V, Fieve RR: Rapid cycling manic depressive patients. Compr Psychiatry 18:561–566, 1977

Eagles JM: The relationship between mood and daily hours of sunlight in rapid cycling bipolar illness. Biol Psychiatry 36:422–424, 1994

Frye MA, Altshuler LL, Bitran JA: Clozapine in rapid cycling bipolar disorder. J Clin Psychopharmacol 16:87–90, 1996

Frye MA, Ketter TA, Kimbrell TA, et al: A placebo-controlled study of lamotrigine and gabapentin monotherapy in refractory mood disorders. J Clin Psychopharmacol 20:607–614, 2000

Fujiwara Y, Honda T, Tanaka Y, et al: Comparison of early and late-onset rapid cycling affective disorders: clinical course and response to pharmacotherapy. J Clin Psychopharmacol 18:282–288, 1998

Ghaemi SN, Boiman EE, Goodwin FK: Diagnosing bipolar disorder and the effect of antidepressants: a naturalistic study. J Clin Psychiatry 61:804–808; quiz 809, 2000

Ghaemi SN, Rosenquist KJ, Ko JY, et al: Antidepressant treatment in bipolar versus unipolar depression. Am J Psychiatry 161:163–165, 2004

Gill DS, Ketter TA, Post RM: Antidepressant response to sleep deprivation as a function of time into depressive episode in rapidly cycling bipolar patients. Acta Psychiatr Scand 87:102–109, 1993

Goldberg JF, Bowden CL, Calabrese JR, et al: Six-month prospective life charting of mood symptoms with lamotrigine monotherapy versus placebo in rapid cycling bipolar disorder. Biol Psychiatry 63:125–130, 2008a

Goldberg JF, Kelley ME, Rosenquist KJ, et al: Effectiveness of quetiapine in rapid cycling bipolar disorder: a preliminary study. J Affect Disord 105:305–310, 2008b

Goodnick PJ: Nimodipine treatment of rapid cycling bipolar disorder (letter). J Clin Psychiatry 56:330, 1995

Grunze H, Erfurth A, Marcuse A, et al: Tiagabine appears not to be efficacious in the treatment of acute mania. J Clin Psychiatry 60:759–762, 1999

Hirschfeld RM, Keck PE Jr, Kramer M, et al: Rapid antimanic effect of risperidone monotherapy: a 3-week multicenter, double-blind, placebo-controlled trial. Am J Psychiatry 161:1057–1065, 2004

Joffe RT, Kutcher S, MacDonald C: Thyroid function and bipolar affective disorder. Psychiatry Res 25:117–121, 1988

Joffe RT, MacQueen GM, Marriott M, et al: Induction of mania and cycle acceleration in bipolar disorder: effect of different classes of antidepressant. Acta Psychiatr Scand 105:427–430, 2002

Joyce PR: Carbamazepine in rapid cycling bipolar affective disorder. Int Clin Psychopharmacol 3:123–129, 1988

Kauer-Sant'Anna M, Frey BN, Andreazza AC, et al: Anxiety comorbidity and quality of life in bipolar disorder patients. Can J Psychiatry 52:175–181, 2007

Kaufman KR: Monotherapy treatment of bipolar disorder with levetiracetam. Epilepsy Behav 5:1017–1020, 2004

Keck PE Jr, Corya SA, Andersen SW, et al: Olanzapine/fluoxetine combination use in rapid-cycling bipolar depression (NR476), in 2003 New Research Program and Abstracts, American Psychiatric Association 156th Annual Meeting, San Francisco, CA, May 17–22, 2003a. Washington, DC, American Psychiatric Association, 2003a, p 178

Keck PE Jr, Versiani M, Potkin S, et al: Ziprasidone in the treatment of acute bipolar mania: a three-week, placebo-controlled, double-blind, randomized trial. Am J Psychiatry 160:741–748, 2003b

Keck PE Jr, Calabrese JR, McQuade RD, et al: A randomized, double-blind, placebo-controlled 26-week trial of aripiprazole in recently manic patients with bipolar I disorder. J Clin Psychiatry 67:626–637, 2006a

Keck PE Jr, Mintz J, McElroy SL, et al: Double-blind, randomized, placebo-controlled trials of ethyl-eicosapentanoate in the treatment of bipolar depression and rapid cycling bipolar disorder. Biol Psychiatry 60:1020–1022, 2006b

Ketter TA, Calabrese JR: Stabilization of mood from below versus above baseline in bipolar disorder: a new nomenclature. J Clin Psychiatry 63:146–151, 2002

Ketter TA, Pazzaglia PJ, Post RM: Synergy of carbamazepine and valproic acid in affective illness: case report and review of the literature. J Clin Psychopharmacol 12:276–281, 1992

Khanna S, Vieta E, Lyons B, et al: Risperidone in the treatment of acute mania: double-blind, placebo-controlled study. Br J Psychiatry 187:229–234, 2005

Kho KH: Treatment of rapid cycling bipolar disorder in the acute and maintenance phase with ECT. J ECT 18:159–161, 2002

Koukopoulos A, Reginaldi D, Minnai G, et al: The long term prophylaxis of affective disorders. Adv Biochem Psychopharmacol 49:127–147, 1995

Koukopoulos A, Sani G, Koukopoulos AE, et al: Duration and stability of the rapid-cycling course: a long-term personal follow-up of 109 patients. J Affect Disord 73:75–85, 2003

Kramlinger KG, Post RM: Ultra-rapid and ultradian cycling in bipolar affective illness. Br J Psychiatry 168:314–323, 1996

Kukopulos A, Reginaldi D, Laddomada P, et al: Course of the manic-depressive cycle and changes caused by treatment. Pharmakopsychiatr Neuropsychopharmakol 13:156–167, 1980

Kukopulos A, Caliari B, Tundo A, et al: Rapid cyclers, temperament, and antidepressants. Compr Psychiatry 24:249–258, 1983

Kupka RW: Treatment options for rapid cycling bipolar disorder. Clinical Approaches in Bipolar Disorders 5:22–29, 2006

Kupka RW, Luckenbaugh DA, Post RM, et al: Rapid and non-rapid cycling bipolar disorder: a meta-analysis of clinical studies. J Clin Psychiatry 64:1483–1494, 2003

Kupka RW, Luckenbaugh DA, Post RM, et al: Comparison of rapid-cycling and non-rapid-cycling bipolar disorder based on prospective mood ratings in 539 outpatients. Am J Psychiatry 162:1273–1280, 2005

Kusalic M: Grade II and grade III hypothyroidism in rapid-cycling bipolar patients. Neuropsychobiology 25:177–181, 1992

Kusumakar V, Yatham L, Kutcher S, et al: Preliminary, open-label study of topiramate in rapid cycling bipolar women. Eur Neuropsychopharmacol 50:S357, 1999

Leibenluft E, Turner EH, Feldman-Naim S, et al: Light therapy in patients with rapid cycling bipolar disorder: preliminary results. Psychopharmacol Bull 31:705–710, 1995

Leibenluft E, Feldman-Naim S, Turner EH, et al: Effects of exogenous melatonin administration and withdrawal in five patients with rapid-cycling bipolar disorder. J Clin Psychiatry 58:383–388, 1997

Lepkifker E, Iancu I, Dannon P, et al: Valproic acid in ultra-rapid cycling: a case report. Clin Neuropharmacol 18:72–75, 1995

Lewis JL, Winokur G: The induction of mania: a natural history study with controls. Arch Gen Psychiatry 39:303–306, 1982

MacFadden W, Haskins T, Kujawa M, et al: Adjunctive risperidone long-acting injectable is effective in delaying relapse to a mood episode in patients with frequently relapsing bipolar disorder (abstract 584). Biol Psychiatry 63(suppl):186S, 2008

Maj M, Pirozzi R, Starace F: Previous pattern of course of the illness as a predictor of response to lithium prophylaxis in bipolar patients. J Affect Disord 17:237–241, 1989

Maj M, Magliano L, Pirozzi R, et al: Validity of rapid cycling as a course specifier for bipolar disorder. Am J Psychiatry 151:1015–1019, 1994

Maj M, Pirozzi R, Formicola AM, et al: Reliability and validity of four alternative definitions of rapid-cycling bipolar disorder. Am J Psychiatry 156:1421–1424, 1999

Manna V: Bipolar affective disorders and role of intraneuronal calcium: therapeutic effects of the treatment with lithium salts and/or calcium antagonist in patients with rapid polar inversion [in Italian]. Minerva Med 82:757–763, 1991

Marangell LB, Suppes T, Zboyan HA, et al: A 1-year pilot study of vagus nerve stimulation in treatment-resistant rapid-cycling bipolar disorder. J Clin Psychiatry 69:183–189, 2008

Marcotte D: Use of topiramate, a new anti-epileptic as a mood stabilizer. J Affect Disord 50:245–251, 1998

McDermut W, Pazzaglia P, Huggins T, et al: Use of single case analyses in on-off-on trials in affective illness: a demonstration of the efficacy of nimodipine. Depression 2:259–271, 1995

McIntyre RS, Brecher M, Paulsson B, et al: Quetiapine or haloperidol as monotherapy for bipolar mania: a 12-week, double-blind, randomised, parallel-group, placebo-controlled trial. Eur Neuropsychopharmacol 15:573–585, 2005

McKowen JW, Frye MA, Altshuler LL, et al: Patterns of alcohol consumption in bipolar patients comorbid for alcohol abuse or dependence. Bipolar Disord 7:377–381, 2005

Mech AW: High-dose ziprasidone monotherapy in bipolar I disorder patients with depressed or mixed episodes. J Clin Psychopharmacol 28:240–241, 2008

Muzina DJ, Momah C, Eudicone JM, et al: Aripiprazole monotherapy in patients with rapid-cycling bipolar I disorder: an analysis from a long-term, double-blind, placebo-controlled study. Int J Clin Pract 62:679–687, 2008

Nurnberger J Jr, Guroff JJ, Hamovit J, et al: A family study of rapid-cycling bipolar illness. J Affect Disord 15:87–91, 1988

Okuma T: Effects of carbamazepine and lithium on affective disorders. Neuropsychobiology 27:138–145, 1993

Papadimitriou GN, Christodoulou GN, Katsouyanni K, et al: Therapy and prevention of affective illness by total sleep deprivation. J Affect Disord 27:107–116, 1993

Pazzaglia PJ, Post RM, Ketter TA, et al: Preliminary controlled trial of nimodipine in ultra-rapid cycling affective dysregulation. Psychiatry Res 49:257–272, 1993

Pazzaglia PJ, Post RM, Ketter TA, et al: Nimodipine monotherapy and carbamazepine augmentation in patients with refractory recurrent affective illness. J Clin Psychopharmacol 18:404–413, 1998

Post RM, Rubinow DR, Ballenger JC: Conditioning and sensitisation in the longitudinal course of affective illness. Br J Psychiatry 149:191–201, 1986

Post RM, Roy-Byrne PP, Uhde TW: Graphic representation of the life course of illness in patients with affective disorder. Am J Psychiatry 145:844–848, 1988

Post RM, Kramlinger KG, Joffe RT, et al: Rapid cycling bipolar affective disorder: lack of relation to hypothyroidism. Psychiatry Res 72:1–7, 1997

Post RM, Altshuler LL, Frye MA, et al: Preliminary observations on the effectiveness of levetiracetam in the open adjunctive treatment of refractory bipolar disorder. J Clin Psychiatry 66:370–374, 2005

Post RM, Altshuler LL, Leverich GS, et al: Mood switch in bipolar depression: comparison of adjunctive venlafaxine, bupropion and sertraline. Br J Psychiatry 189:124–131, 2006

Potkin SG, Keck PE Jr, Segal S, et al: Ziprasidone in acute bipolar mania: a 21-day randomized, double-blind, placebo-controlled replication trial. J Clin Psychopharmacol 25:301–310, 2005

Reilly Harrington NA, Knauz RO: Cognitive-behavioral therapy for rapid-cycling bipolar disorder. Cogn Behav Pract 12:66–75, 2005

Reilly Harrington NA, Deckersbach T, Knauz R, et al: Cognitive behavioral therapy for rapid-cycling bipolar disorder: a pilot study. J Psychiatr Pract 13:291–297, 2007

Roy-Byrne P, Post RM, Uhde TW, et al: The longitudinal course of recurrent affective illness: life chart data from research patients at the NIMH. Acta Psychiatr Scand Suppl 317:1–34, 1985

Rush AJ, Marangell LB, Sackeim HA, et al: Vagus nerve stimulation for treatment-resistant depression: a randomized, controlled acute phase trial. Biol Psychiatry 58:347–354, 2005

Sachs GS: Managing Bipolar Affective Disorder. London, UK, Science Press, 2004

Sachs GS, Grossman F, Ghaemi SN, et al: Combination of a mood stabilizer with risperidone or haloperidol for treatment of acute mania: a double-blind, placebo-controlled comparison of efficacy and safety. Am J Psychiatry 159:1146–1154, 2002

Sanger TM, Grundy SL, Gibson PJ, et al: Long-term olanzapine therapy in the treatment of bipolar I disorder: an open-label continuation phase study. J Clin Psychiatry 62:273–281, 2001

Schaff MR, Fawcett J, Zajecka JM: Divalproex sodium in the treatment of refractory affective disorders. J Clin Psychiatry 54:380–384, 1993

Schaffer CB, Schaffer LC: Gabapentin in the treatment of bipolar disorder (letter). Am J Psychiatry 154:291–292, 1997

Schaffer LC, Schaffer CB, Howe J: An open case series on the utility of tiagabine as an augmentation in refractory bipolar outpatients. J Affect Disord 71:259–263, 2002

Schneck CD: Treatment of rapid-cycling bipolar disorder. J Clin Psychiatry 67 (suppl 11):22–27, 2006

Schneck CD, Miklowitz DJ, Calabrese JR, et al: Phenomenology of rapid-cycling bipolar disorder: data from the first 500 participants in the Systematic Treatment Enhancement Program. Am J Psychiatry 161:1902–1908, 2004

Schneck CD, Miklowitz DJ, Miyahara S, et al: The prospective course of rapid-cycling bipolar disorder: findings from the STEP-BD. Am J Psychiatry 165:370–377; quiz 410, 2008

Scott J, Paykel E, Morriss R, et al: Cognitive-behavioural therapy for severe and recurrent bipolar disorders: randomised controlled trial. Br J Psychiatry 188:313–320, 2006

Sharma V, Persad E, Mazmanian D, et al: Treatment of rapid cycling bipolar disorder with combination therapy of valproate and lithium. Can J Psychiatry 38:137–139, 1993

Shi L, Vallarino C, Namjoshi M, et al: Olanzapine/fluoxetine combination and quality of life in rapid-cycling bipolar depression (NR235), in 2003 New Research Program and Abstracts, American Psychiatric Association 156th Annual Meeting, San Francisco, CA, May 17–22, 2003. Washington, DC, American Psychiatric Association, 2003, p 88

Smulevich AB, Khanna S, Eerdekens M, et al: Acute and continuation risperidone monotherapy in bipolar mania: a 3-week placebo-controlled trial followed by a 9-week double-blind trial of risperidone and haloperidol. Eur Neuropsychopharmacol 15:75–84, 2005

Stancer HC, Persad E: Treatment of intractable rapid-cycling manic-depressive disorder with levothyroxine: clinical observations. Arch Gen Psychiatry 39:311–312, 1982

Stoll AL, Sachs GS, Cohen BM, et al: Choline in the treatment of rapid-cycling bipolar disorder: clinical and neurochemical findings in lithium-treated patients. Biol Psychiatry 40:382–388, 1996

Stoll AL, Severus WE, Freeman MP, et al: Omega 3 fatty acids in bipolar disorder: a preliminary double-blind, placebo-controlled trial. Arch Gen Psychiatry 56:407–412, 1999

Suppes T, McElroy SL, Gilbert J, et al: Clozapine in the treatment of dysphoric mania. Biol Psychiatry 32:270–280, 1992

Suppes T, Phillips KA, Judd CR: Clozapine treatment of nonpsychotic rapid cycling bipolar disorder: a report of three cases. Biol Psychiatry 36:338–340, 1994

Suppes T, Chisholm KA, Dhavale D, et al: Tiagabine in treatment refractory bipolar disorder: a clinical case series. Bipolar Disord 4:283–289, 2002

Suppes T, Ozcan ME, Carmody T: Response to clozapine of rapid cycling versus noncycling patients with a history of mania. Bipolar Disord 6:329–332, 2004

Suppes T, Brown E, Schuh LM, et al: Rapid versus non-rapid cycling as a predictor of response to olanzapine and divalproex sodium for bipolar mania and maintenance of remission: post hoc analyses of 47-week data. J Affect Disord 89:69–77, 2005

Suppes T, Eudicone J, McQuade R, et al: Efficacy and safety of aripiprazole in subpopulations with acute manic or mixed episodes of bipolar I disorder. J Affect Disord 107:145–154, 2008

Swann AC, Bowden CL, Calabrese JR, et al: Differential effect of number of previous episodes of affective disorder on response to lithium or divalproex in acute mania. Am J Psychiatry 156:1264–1266, 1999

Thase ME, Jonas A, Khan A, et al: Aripiprazole monotherapy in nonpsychotic bipolar I depression: results of 2 randomized, placebo-controlled studies. J Clin Psychopharmacol 28:13–20, 2008

Tohen M, Sanger TM, McElroy SL, et al: Olanzapine versus placebo in the treatment of acute mania. Olanzapine HGEH Study Group. Am J Psychiatry 156:702–709, 1999

Tohen M, Jacobs TG, Grundy SL, et al: Efficacy of olanzapine in acute bipolar mania: a double-blind, placebo-controlled study. The Olanzapine HGGW Study Group. Arch Gen Psychiatry 57:841–849, 2000

Tohen M, Baker RW, Altshuler LL, et al: Olanzapine versus divalproex in the treatment of acute mania. Am J Psychiatry 159:1011–1017, 2002a

Tohen M, Chengappa KN, Suppes T, et al: Efficacy of olanzapine in combination with valproate or lithium in the treatment of mania in patients partially nonresponsive to valproate or lithium monotherapy. Arch Gen Psychiatry 59:62–69, 2002b

Tohen M, Ketter TA, Zarate CA, et al: Olanzapine versus divalproex sodium for the treatment of acute mania and maintenance of remission: a 47-week study. Am J Psychiatry 160:1263–1271, 2003a

Tohen M, Vieta E, Calabrese J, et al: Efficacy of olanzapine and olanzapine-fluoxetine combination in the treatment of bipolar I depression. Arch Gen Psychiatry 60:1079–1088, 2003b

Tohen MF, Bowden CL, Calabrese JR, et al: Predictors of time to relapse in bipolar I disorder (NR800), in 2004 New Research Program and Abstracts, American Psychiatric Association 157th Annual Meeting, New York, May 1–6, 2004. Washington, DC, American Psychiatric Association, 2004a, p 301

Tohen M, Chengappa KN, Suppes T, et al: Relapse prevention in bipolar I disorder: 18-month comparison of olanzapine plus mood stabiliser v. mood stabiliser alone. Br J Psychiatry 184:337–345, 2004b

Tohen M, Greil W, Calabrese JR, et al: Olanzapine versus lithium in the maintenance treatment of bipolar disorder: a 12-month, randomized, double-blind, controlled clinical trial. Am J Psychiatry 162:1281–1290, 2005

Tohen M, Calabrese JR, Sachs GS, et al: Randomized, placebo-controlled trial of olanzapine as maintenance therapy in patients with bipolar I disorder responding to acute treatment with olanzapine. Am J Psychiatry 163:247–256, 2006

Tondo L, Hennen J, Baldessarini RJ: Rapid-cycling bipolar disorder: effects of long-term treatments. Acta Psychiatr Scand 108:4–14, 2003

Vanelle JM, Loo H, Galinowski A, et al: Maintenance ECT in intractable manic-depressive disorders. Convuls Ther 10:195–205, 1994

Vieta E, Gasto C, Colom F, et al: Treatment of refractory rapid cycling bipolar disorder with risperidone. J Clin Psychopharmacol 18:172–174, 1998

Vieta E, Martinez-Arán A, Goikolea JM, et al: A randomized trial comparing paroxetine and venlafaxine in the treatment of bipolar depressed patients taking mood stabilizers. J Clin Psychiatry 63:508–512, 2002a

Vieta E, Parramon G, Padrell E, et al: Quetiapine in the treatment of rapid cycling bipolar disorder. Bipolar Disord 4:335–340, 2002b

Vieta E, Calabrese JR, Hennen J, et al: Comparison of rapid-cycling and non-rapid-cycling bipolar I manic patients during treatment with olanzapine: analysis of pooled data. J Clin Psychiatry 65:1420–1428, 2004

Vieta E, Calabrese J, Goikolea J, et al: Quetiapine monotherapy in the treatment of patients with bipolar I or II depression and a rapid-cycling disease course: a randomized, double-blind, placebo-controlled study. Bipolar Disord 9:413–425, 2007

Walden J, Schaerer L, Schloesser S, et al: An open longitudinal study of patients with bipolar rapid cycling treated with lithium or lamotrigine for mood stabilization. Bipolar Disord 2:336–339, 2000

Wang PW, Winsberg ME, Santosa CM, et al: Open adjunctive gabapentin effective in bipolar depression (abstract 277). Biol Psychiatry 47(suppl):84S, 2000

Wehr TA, Goodwin FK: Rapid cycling in manic-depressives induced by tricyclic antidepressants. Arch Gen Psychiatry 36:555–559, 1979

Wehr TA, Sack DA, Rosenthal NE, et al: Rapid cycling affective disorder: contributing factors and treatment responses in 51 patients. Am J Psychiatry 145:179–184, 1988

Wehr TA, Turner EH, Shimada JM, et al: Treatment of rapidly cycling bipolar patient by using extended bed rest and darkness to stabilize the timing and duration of sleep. Biol Psychiatry 43:822–828, 1998

Wirz-Justice A, Quinto C, Cajochen C, et al: A rapid-cycling bipolar patient treated with long nights, bedrest, and light. Biol Psychiatry 45:1075–1077, 1999

Woo YS, Chae JH, Jun TY, et al: Lamotrigine added to valproate successfully treated a case of ultra-rapid cycling bipolar disorder. Psychiatry Clin Neurosci 61:130–131, 2007

Wu LH, Dunner DL: Suicide attempts in rapid cycling bipolar disorder patients. J Affect Disord 29:57–61, 1993

Yatham LN, Grossman F, Augustyns I, et al: Mood stabilisers plus risperidone or placebo in the treatment of acute mania: international, double-blind, randomised controlled trial. Br J Psychiatry 182:141–147, 2003

Yatham LN, Paulsson B, Mullen J, et al: Quetiapine versus placebo in combination with lithium or divalproex for the treatment of bipolar mania. J Clin Psychopharmacol 24:599–606, 2004

Yildiz A, Sachs GS: Do antidepressants induce rapid cycling? A gender-specific association. J Clin Psychiatry 64:814–818, 2003

Young LT, Robb JC, Hasey GM, et al: Gabapentin as an adjunctive treatment in bipolar disorder. J Affect Disord 55:73–77, 1999

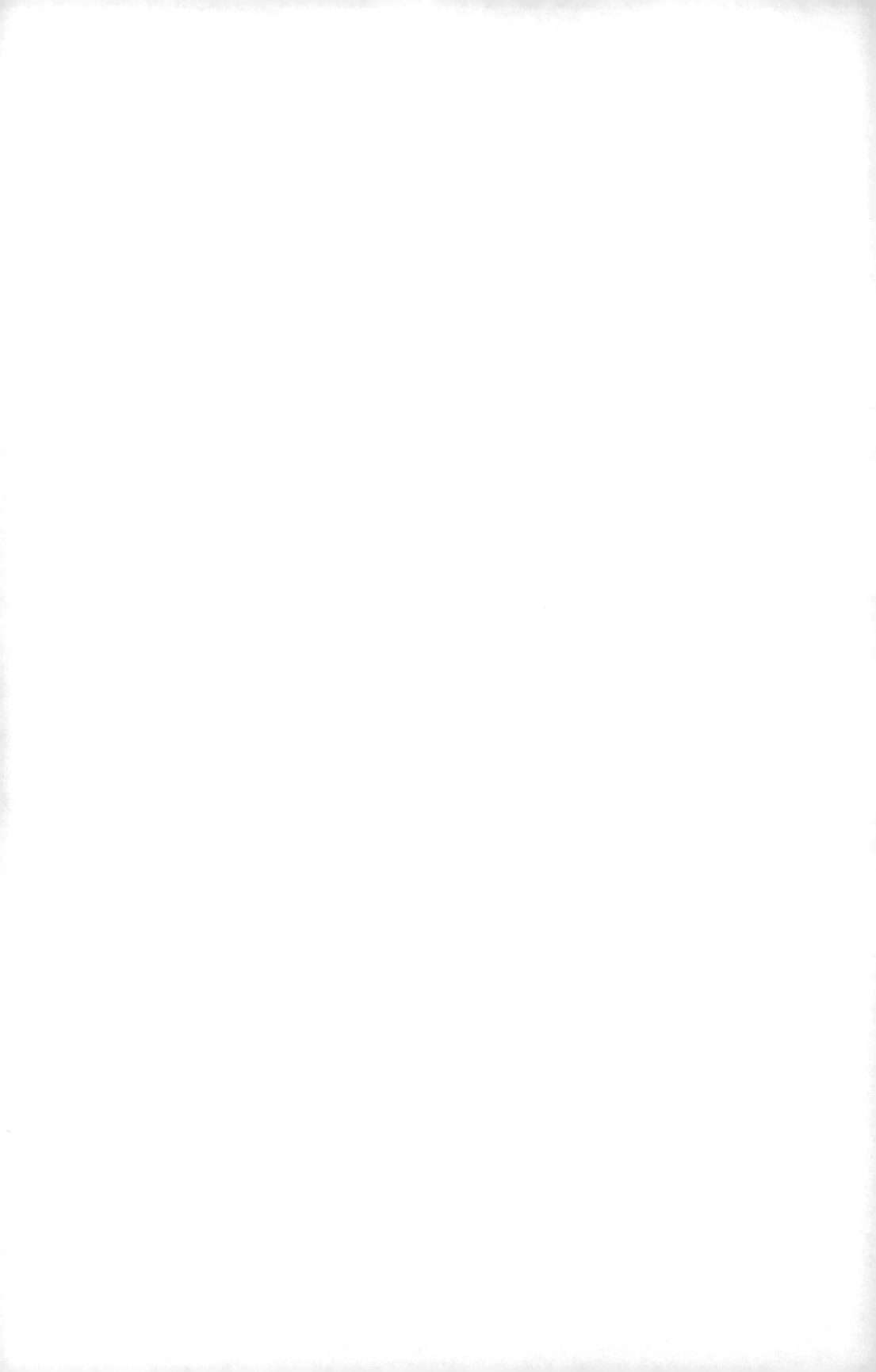

CHAPTER 10

Management of Bipolar Disorders in Children and Adolescents

Kiki D. Chang, M.D.

Manpreet K. Singh, M.D., M.S.

Po W. Wang, M.D.

Meghan Howe, M.S.W.

Although previously thought to begin primarily in late adolescence or early adulthood, bipolar disorder apparently begins before age 18 years in over two-thirds of patients with bipolar disorders (Perlis et al. 2004). Children and adolescents diagnosed with bipolar disorder are particularly at risk for poor psychosocial outcome, with increased risk for suicide attempts, self-injurious behaviors, recurrent syndromal or subsyndromal mood symptoms, co-occurring psychiatric disorders, psychosocial and academic problems, and substance use (McClellan et al. 2007; Singh and Chang 2007). The presentation and developmental course of pediatric bipolar disorder vary with age and pubertal status (Geller and Luby 1997; Geller et al. 2000b, 2000c). Due to these complexities, children and adolescents with bipolar disorder require a multifaceted treatment approach including pharmacotherapy, psychotherapy, and family intervention. Early identification and treatment of pediatric bipolar disorder are essential to prevent or attenuate the chronicity of symptoms and associated complications. Evidence-based treatments that guide clinical decision making for pediatric mood disorders are essential. In this chapter, we provide a summary of the clinical manifestations and controlled therapeutic trials for the treatment of bipolar disorder in children and adolescents, and conclude with some practical suggestions to consider while treating this disorder in pediatric populations.

Bipolar disorders account for an increasingly large percentage of pediatric psychiatry clinic visits and inpatient hospital stays (Youngstrom and Duax 2005). In one tertiary pediatric psychiatry clinic, mania was found in 16% of referrals (Biederman et al. 2005a). In the community, over less than a decade, from 1994–1995 to 2002–2003, outpatient pediatric office visits for bipolar disorders increased an alarming 39-fold, from 25 to 1,003 visits per year per 100,000 population (Moreno et al. 2007). Furthermore, between 1995 and 2000, there was a 90% increase in likelihood of having a bipolar diagnosis among psychiatrically hospitalized children (Harpaz-Rotem et al. 2005). For example, the proportion of male adolescents diagnosed with bipolar disorder from a database of insurance claims was 9.5% in 1995 and 18.9% in 2000. Another group reported that 30% of adolescent inpatients on a psychiatric ward had significant manic symptoms, independent of bipolar diagnosis (Carlson and Youngstrom 2003). Finally, 22% of an incarcerated sample of adolescents in Texas met criteria for bipolar disorder (Pliszka et al. 2000).

This recent dramatic increase in diagnosis of bipolar disorders in the United States has not been reflected internationally (Räsänen et al. 1998; Thomsen et al. 1992; Verhulst et al. 1997). The reasons for this discrepancy with U.S. rates may be multifaceted, including researcher and/or clinician bias against or for the existence of bipolar disorder in children, variable diagnostic interviews used and a lack of trained child psychiatrists internationally (Soutullo et al. 2005). One theory is that the relatively less frequent use of stimulants and antidepressants in pediatric populations in Europe may account for less "creation" of bipolar disorder in children (Reichart and Nolen 2004), but this phenomenon has not been well studied. In therapy, decreasing the use of antidepressants in children and adolescents might decrease the "creation" of bipolar disorder, but the potential costs of such an approach need to be considered. Since the U.S. Food and Drug Administration (FDA) stipulated that the prescribing information of all antidepressants include a boxed warning of the risk of increased suicidality in children and adolescents, the resulting decreased use of antidepressants has been accompanied by an increase in the suicide rate in this population (Gibbons et al.

2007). A similar finding was noted in the Netherlands (Gibbons et al. 2007). More international research in pediatric mood disorders in general and pediatric bipolar disorder in particular is clearly needed to address these important issues.

Clinical Characteristics

Children and adolescents with bipolar disorder may present with severe mood swings, hypersexuality, irritability, distractibility, decreased need for sleep, impulsivity, and racing thoughts. A child or adolescent who has at least one episode of mania is diagnosed with bipolar I disorder according to the *Diagnostic and Statistical Manual of Mental Disorders,* 4th Edition, Text Revision (DSM-IV-TR; American Psychiatric Association 2000). With one or more episodes of major depression and at least one episode of hypomania, the child or adolescent is diagnosed with bipolar II disorder. The DSM-IV-TR criteria for manic and hypomanic episodes are identical for adults, adolescents, and children, and are provided in Chapter 2, "DSM-IV-TR Diagnosis of Bipolar Disorders." Curiously, the DSM-IV-TR criteria for major depressive episodes in children and adolescents not only require the presence of either sadness or anhedonia (as in adults) but also allow the mood to be irritable, creating overlap with the criteria for mood elevation episodes. Cyclothymia is a disorder of at least a 1-year duration, during which a child or adolescent 1) experiences periods of hypomanic and depressive symptoms that do not meet criteria for mania or major depression and 2) is not without symptoms for more than 2 months at a time. Bipolar disorder not otherwise specified is a diagnostic category frequently used in children and adolescents because their mood episodes might not meet full DSM-IV-TR criteria for duration of symptoms or because they might have recurrent hypomanic episodes without depression.

DSM-IV-TR does not provide codes for family history of illnesses. In contrast, the *International Classification of Diseases,* 10th Edition (ICD-10; World Health Organization 1992), has such codes, including codes for having a family history of mental and behavioral disorders such as bipolar disorder. Hopefully, the next DSM revision will provide clinicians with a way to report the important phenomenon of having a relative (particularly a parent) with bipolar disorder.

Evaluation and Differential Diagnosis

Currently, children and adolescents are diagnosed using the same DSM-IV-TR criteria for bipolar disorder that are used to diagnose adults. This convention might change in the next DSM revision, similar to the change in depression criteria in DSM-IV-TR, which now allow children to have irritability as the main mood symptom. Allowing for developmentally relevant symptom presentations will help make diagnoses more valid and relevant across the age span.

Pediatric bipolar disorder is defined as a mood disorder in which children experience significant periods of irritability or euphoria, usually with periods of depression as well. These periods can be distinct or overlapping; frequently, they present together in mixed manic states similar to those reported in adults. During these mood disturbances, children with bipolar disorder also must meet DSM-IV-TR criteria. Examples of DSM-IV-TR criteria for mania in children and adolescents are provided in Table 10–1.

Diagnosing pediatric bipolar disorder requires differentiating it from attention-deficit/hyperactivity disorder (ADHD); oppositional defiant disorder; conduct disorder; anxiety disorders, including posttraumatic stress disorder (PTSD); substance use disorders; and pervasive developmental disorders. However, pediatric bipolar disorder commonly presents with co-occurring disruptive behaviors, attention deficits, and pervasive developmental, anxiety, and substance use disorders. Therefore, the assessment of a child or adolescent for bipolar disorder should include identifying age-specific clinical manifestations of bipolar disorder. For example, children and adolescents with ADHD without bipolar disorder do not have grandiosity, elation, euphoria, extreme irritability, hypersexuality, feelings of guilt or worthlessness, or suicidal ideation. With careful delineation of specific symptoms, these disorders can be separated. Fristad et al. (1992) used the Mania Rating Scale, which was developed for adults, to evaluate a group of prepubertal children with either mania or ADHD. These investigators found this scale to be useful in differentiating manic children from hyperactive children, with the manic children reporting elevated mood, increased motor activity/energy, decreased need for sleep, increased irritability, pressured speech, flight of ideas, disruptive behavior, thought disorders, and a lack of insight.

Children and adolescents with conduct disorder and without a mood disorder typically do not feel remorseful for their predatory actions. Like children and adolescents with mood disorders, those with PTSD might also present with mood lability and difficulty with sleep and concentration. However, the presence of nightmares, startle and avoidance behaviors, flashbacks, and severe anxiety with a history of trauma suggests PTSD as a primary diagnosis. Although the hypersexuality associated with bipolar disorder might be confused with PTSD, less than 1% of children with bipolar disorder with hypersexual behav-

TABLE 10–1. Examples of DSM-IV-TR criteria for mood elevation in children and adolescents

Elevated or expansive mood: Being much happier than situation warrants; inappropriate "goofiness" and silliness; having no insight about inappropriateness of moods.

Irritability: Becoming very belligerent, highly irritable with frequent, intense, and prolonged temper tantrums or "affective storms"; being extremely oppositional, belligerent, short, curt, or hostile, risking misdiagnosis of oppositional defiant or conduct disorder.

Inflated self-esteem or grandiosity: Thinking one has "superpowers" or "can beat up anyone in the world" or "can teach the class better than any of the teachers," despite failing in school. These self-beliefs are more excessive than developmentally appropriate (e.g., feeling like one has superpowers at age 12).

Decreased need for sleep: In a 10-year-old, not being able to fall asleep before 1 A.M. or 2 A.M. and sleeping only 5–7 hours a night without tiring. Amount of sleep is less than typical for one's age.

More talkative than usual: Repeatedly blurting out answers during class; talking "a mile a minute" with friends; very rapid and pressured speech, to the point of being continuous, and at times unintelligible or difficult to follow.

Flight of ideas or racing thoughts: Having "too many ideas and can't get them out fast enough"; describing "thinking faster than others" or having a "busy city" in their heads.

Distractibility: Being unable to pay attention in class because thoughts are moving along too quickly or because there is too much going on externally.

Increase in goal-directed activity: Extreme restlessness and shifting from activity to activity rapidly, without necessarily completing them; taking on elaborate projects or business schemes and working excessively on them in an age-inappropriate manner.

Excessive involvement in pleasurable activities that have a high potential for painful consequences: Being hypersexual and inappropriately touching dolls, peers, or adults in attempts to engage them in "sex"; reckless daredevil tricks on bicycles or jumping off roofs; for adolescents, promiscuous sexual behavior, binge drinking, drug abuse, or excessive shopping.

---

iors have been sexually abused (Geller et al. 2000a). Additionally, although substance use and mood disorders commonly co-occur, it is important to assess for substance-induced mood disorders. Tracking mood symptoms during periods of abstinence, recording the duration and severity of mood symptoms, and performing drug screens might be helpful in determining the relationship between mood symptoms and substance use.

Medical illnesses can cause mood disturbances and need to be investigated prior to assuming a primary psychiatric etiology. For example, symptoms of thyroid disease, infectious mononucleosis, systemic lupus, temporal lobe epilepsy, Wilson's disease, or anemia may mimic those of bipolar disorder. Additionally, medications such as antidepressants, psychostimulants, corticosteroids, antimalarial agents, and thyroxine may induce mania and should be considered in the diagnostic evaluation.

In summary, diagnosis of pediatric bipolar disorder can be complex and challenging. Table 10–2 provides diagnostic guidelines for pediatric bipolar disorder, based on the work of McClellan and associates (2007).

Treatment

Individuals with bipolar disorder often require a comprehensive treatment plan to address a complex array of symptoms and associated morbidities. A multimodal treatment approach combining pharmacological agents and psychosocial interventions is suggested, with the goals of improving symptoms, providing psychoeducation about bipolar disorder, and promoting treatment adherence for relapse prevention and attenuation of long-term complications from the illness (Madaan and Chang 2007). Clinicians should advocate prevention, early intervention, and biopsychosocial treatments that promote the healthy growth and development of all children affected by bipolar disorder, in any cultural context.

Prevention and Early Intervention

Pediatric bipolar disorder is being increasingly diagnosed and recognized as a chronic mood disorder associated with a significant deterioration in quality of life for patients and their families. Recent research indicates that the following may predict a worse outcome: a younger age at onset; lower socioeconomic status; a strong family history of bipolar disorder; and clinical features including the presence of mixed episodes, psychotic symptoms, rapid cycling, co-occurring substance use, and neurocognitive deficits (Post and Kowatch 2006). Optimal clinical suspicion, an early diagnosis, and adequate management of this chronic mood disorder may lessen its impact on the quality of life of children and their families. Some even argue that early intervention may prevent the evolution of this disorder to bipolar disorder in children and adolescents and its associated morbidities (Chang et al. 2006a; Lewinsohn et al. 2003).

Pediatric offspring of parents with bipolar disorder have a substantially increased risk of developing bipolar disorders themselves. Effective early intervention strategies for individuals with such familial risk might delay the pro-

TABLE 10–2. **Diagnostic guidelines for pediatric bipolar disorder**

Challenge	Recommendations
Screening	Inquire about distinct, spontaneous changes in mood, associated with sleep disturbance, and psychomotor activation.
	Inquire about past personal and family histories of mood disorders.
	Inquire about past exposure to antidepressants and psychostimulants.
	Assess symptoms in the context of family, peer, and school interactions.
Assessment	Use DSM-IV-TR criteria to make a diagnosis of mania or hypomania in children and adolescents:
	• Bipolar I disorder: The individual has had at least one episode of mania.
	• Bipolar II disorder: The individual has had one or more episodes of major depression and at least one episode of hypomania.
	• Cyclothymia: The individual has had at least a 1-year duration of hypomanic and depressive symptoms that do not meet criteria for mania or major depression, and has not been symptom-free for more than 2 months at a time.
	• Bipolar disorder not otherwise specified: The individual has had manic symptoms that last <4 days or chronic manic-like symptoms associated with significant functional impairment.
	Assess for suicidality, co-occurring substance use and other disorders, psychosocial stressors, and medical problems.
Differential diagnosis	Consider age-specific manifestations of bipolar disorder to distinguish diagnosis from other conditions that commonly co-occur (e.g., attention-deficit/hyperactivity disorder, oppositional defiant disorder, conduct disorder, anxiety disorders including posttraumatic stress disorder, substance use disorders, and pervasive developmental disorders).
	Use caution when applying a diagnosis of bipolar disorder in preschool children; the diagnostic validity of bipolar disorder in young children has yet to be established.
Comorbidity	High rates of suicide attempts, completed suicides, substance use, and school failure can occur in patients with pediatric bipolar disorder.
	Cognitive, speech, and language disorders and other developmental concerns should be addressed if indicated.

Source. Adapted from McClellan et al. 2007.

gression of already manifesting mood disorders (Chang et al. 2006a). Such mood disorders may include depressive disorders (Geller et al. 1994; Strober and Carlson 1982) or subthreshold bipolar disorder, also referred to as a spectrum of milder bipolar disorders (Birmaher et al. 2006), which may precede or elevate the risk for developing bipolar I disorder. Individuals at high risk for developing bipolar disorder may also be exposed to antidepressants or psychostimulants, which while attempting to treat mood, behavioral, and attentional symptoms may precipitate, exacerbate (Baumer et al. 2006), or accelerate the onset of mania (Soutullo et al. 2002). Strategies designed to identify high-risk symptom complexes and prevent the full development of bipolar disorder might result in avoidance of inappropriate interventions that may precipitate mania.

Unfortunately, the burden of bipolar disorder illness is not matched by sufficient data from randomized intervention studies to facilitate the practice of evidence-based medicine in this population (Post and Kowatch 2006). However, a few intervention studies have demonstrated some benefits of intervening early. Pharmacological studies in children and adolescents with non–bipolar I mood disorders and a familial risk for bipolar disorder (Chang et al. 2003; Findling et al. 2007a; Geller et al. 1998b; Saxena et al. 2006) aim to intervene using medications that may have neuroprotective properties. In these studies, "familial risk" was defined as having a first-degree relative (parent or sibling) with bipolar I disorder (DelBello et al. 2007a) or a parent with either bipolar I or bipolar II disorder (Chang et al. 2003; Findling et al. 2007a; Saxena et al. 2006). Chang et al. (2003) found open-label divalproex monotherapy to be efficacious in 78% of their sample of 24 children and adolescents (ages 6–18 years) who had a current or past diagnosis of major depressive disorder, dysthymia, cyclothymia, or ADHD and were offspring of parents with bipolar disorder. This same group found that 71% of their subjects responded to divalproex, with a significant decrease in scores on the Overt Aggression Scale and the Young Mania Rating Scale (YMRS) (Saxena et al. 2006). In contrast, Findling et al. (2007a) found divalproex to be no more effective than placebo in cyclothymia or bipolar disorder not otherwise specified in children and adolescents with a bipolar parent, using time to treatment discontinuation for any reason and treatment due to a mood event as primary outcome measures. DelBello and colleagues used the Clinical Global Impression—Improvement Scale and the Childhood Depression Rating Scale—Revised in addition to the YMRS to demonstrate the effectiveness and tolerability of quetiapine for adolescents with mood symptoms and a first-degree relative with bipolar I disorder (DelBello et al. 2007a). Although these studies vary methodologically, they are important because effective treatment could improve long-term outcomes for children and adolescents at familial risk (DelBello and Kowatch 2006). However, acute improvement in mood symptoms does not necessarily mean prevention or delay of fully developed bipolar disorder. Therefore, additional long-term pharmacological and psychotherapeutic studies in these high-risk populations are needed.

Pharmacological Interventions

Several case reports, open-label trials, and chart reviews have described the effectiveness of various pharmacological agents for children and adolescents who have already developed bipolar disorder. However, few double-blind, placebo-controlled studies in this population have been published. Nevertheless, the FDA has recently approved two second-generation antipsychotics—risperidone as monotherapy, and aripiprazole as monotherapy or adjunctive to lithium or valproate—for acute manic and mixed episodes in children and adolescents ages 10–17 years. Also recently, the American Academy of Child and Adolescent Psychiatry published guidelines for the treatment of pediatric bipolar disorder, endorsing lithium, divalproex, and second-generation antipsychotics as optimal first-line agents (McClellan et al. 2007). In addition, these guidelines recommend that clinicians initiate medications that are already FDA approved for the treatment of bipolar disorder in adults. These recommendations mirror those of an expert panel of child psychiatrists published 2 years earlier (Kowatch et al. 2005).

Lithium

Lithium was the first medication approved by the FDA for mania in adolescents ages 12 years and older, although no large, multicenter, double-blind, placebo-controlled studies of lithium have been done in adolescents with mania. Results of a placebo-controlled study in youth with bipolar disorder indicated that lithium was effective for decreasing comorbid substance abuse (Geller et al. 1998a), but this study did not specifically evaluate symptoms of mania. In another study, after initiating youth with bipolar disorder on therapeutic serum levels of lithium for 4 weeks and then randomly assigning responders to placebo or continued lithium treatment, Kafantaris et al. (2004) found no statistically significant differences in mania ratings between the groups after 2 weeks. This controlled discontinuation study had a sufficient sample ($N=40$) to detect a 40% difference between the randomized groups and showed high rates of manic relapse in both the ongoing lithium therapy and the placebo groups, suggesting that lithium may not be efficacious beyond an acute stabilization period.

Adverse effects reported with lithium include thyroid dysfunction, weight gain, nausea, polydipsia and polyuria, acne, and tremor. Because lithium has a narrow therapeutic index, blood level monitoring is required, to attenuate the risk of toxicity. In prepubertal children (ages 6–12 years), lithium 30 mg/kg/day (three divided doses) would result in a theoretical therapeutic concentration of 0.6–1.2 mmol/L (Weller et al. 1986). However, it is not clear if children share the same therapeutic range as adults. In a magnetic resonance spectroscopy study, children were found to have lower brain/serum concentration ratios than did adults, indicating that children might need higher serum concentrations to maintain therapeutic lithium levels in the brain (Moore et al. 2002). Recommendations are that baseline complete blood counts, creatinine, pregnancy status, thyroid function panels, serum urea nitrogen, urinalysis, and serum calcium be checked prior to initiating lithium and be monitored every 3–6 months.

Divalproex

Anticonvulsant therapies demonstrated possible efficacy in open-label studies of pediatric mania. Divalproex appeared efficacious in open-label studies in juvenile bipolar disorder (Findling et al. 2005; Kowatch et al. 2000). However, a recently completed large placebo-controlled study of extended-release divalproex (divalproex ER) for pediatric mania was negative (Wagner 2009). The YMRS response rates were 24% and 23% for divalproex ER and placebo, respectively. The most common adverse events were headache and vomiting. Given the potential efficacy data in open studies, it is not clear whether this was a failed study or whether the extended-release preparation acts differently than immediate-release divalproex for pediatric acute mania. For example, in the large divalproex ER pediatric mania trial, the mean final serum valproate level was only 79.9 μg/mL, despite recommendations of 80–120 μg/mL to treat acute mania (Madaan et al. 2007). However, as described in Chapter 6, "Management of Acute Manic and Mixed Episodes in Bipolar Disorders," extended-release divalproex was approved by the FDA as monotherapy for acute manic and mixed episodes in adults, based on a positive multicenter, randomized, double-blind, placebo-controlled trial (Bowden et al. 2006).

Optimal serum levels of divalproex, like those of lithium, remain to be determined for pediatric bipolar disorder but are generally recommended in the range of 80–120 μg/mL (Chang et al. 2003; Kowatch and DelBello 2006). Side effects commonly associated with divalproex include polycystic ovary syndrome, weight gain, sedation, hepatotoxicity, thrombocytopenia, and tremor. Patients taking divalproex should receive baseline liver function tests and complete blood counts, be checked for pregnancy status, and have their divalproex levels measured, with follow-up occurring no less often than every 6 months (McClellan et al. 2007). In 2008, the FDA released an alert regarding increased risk of suicidality (suicidal behavior or ideation) in patients with epilepsy or psychiatric disorders for 11 anticonvulsants (including divalproex, carbamazepine, and lamotrigine). In the FDA's analysis, anticonvulsants compared with placebo yielded approximately twice the risk of suicidality (0.43% vs. 0.22%). The relative risk for suicidality was higher in the patients with epilepsy than in those with psychiatric disorders.

Carbamazepine

Case reports have suggested benefit with carbamazepine in pediatric bipolar disorder either as monotherapy (Woolston 1999) or as an adjunct to lithium (Kowatch et al. 2003) and in adolescents with bipolar disorder who do not respond to lithium (Hsu 1986). One open trial reported a 38% response rate in children with bipolar disorder receiving carbamazepine monotherapy (Kowatch et al. 2000). Therapeutic serum carbamazepine concentrations, extrapolated from the epilepsy literature, range from 4 to 12 µg/mL. Important considerations are that carbamazepine can decrease lamotrigine and divalproex levels, whereas divalproex can increase carbamazepine epoxide levels (Bourgeois 2000; Reimers et al. 2005). Carbamazepine can cause sedation, dizziness, ataxia, and blurred vision, and has less commonly been associated with Stevens-Johnson syndrome, hyponatremia, aplastic anemia, and agranulocytosis. Good clinical practice involves taking baseline complete blood counts and educating the subject regarding the possibilities of hematological and dermatological events and the need to carefully monitor for rash, fever, sore throat, and easy bruising.

Lamotrigine

Based on multicenter, randomized, double-blind, placebo-controlled studies, lamotrigine has been approved for maintenance treatment in adults (Goodwin et al. 2004) and, although not approved, may have modest efficacy in acute bipolar depression in adults (Calabrese et al. 2008; Geddes et al. 2009). In contrast, lamotrigine lacked efficacy for acute mania in adults (Bowden et al. 2000). Because such trials are lacking in children and adolescents, lamotrigine lacks FDA approval for the treatment of pediatric bipolar disorder. However, an 8-week open-label study of lamotrigine as adjunctive or monotherapy in adolescents with bipolar depression demonstrated an 84% response rate in the primary outcome measure of improved Clinical Global Impression—Improvement Scale scores, and a 58% remission rate as determined by low depression and overall bipolar illness severity scores (Chang et al. 2006b). Placebo-controlled studies of lamotrigine for bipolar depression and maintenance in pediatric populations are necessary.

Although controlled efficacy data are lacking for pediatric bipolar disorder, safety and tolerability information from controlled trials of lamotrigine in pediatric epilepsy may be informative, because lamotrigine is approved for the treatment of epilepsy in patients ages 2 years and older. Lamotrigine is generally well tolerated but can yield common benign and rare serious rashes (including Stevens-Johnson syndrome and toxic epidermal necrolysis). Risk factors for rash include age less than 16 years, overly rapid initiation, and concurrent valproate (which doubles serum lamotrigine concentrations). Among 1,983 pediatric epilepsy patients ages 16 years and younger, adjunctive lamotrigine yielded serious rash in 0.3% (3 per 1,000) and one rash-related death. Gradual introduction of lamotrigine is necessary to attenuate the risk of rash. In pediatric epilepsy patients ages 2–12 years not taking the enzyme inhibitor valproate or enzyme inducers such as carbamazepine, lamotrigine is started at 0.3 mg/kg/day (rounded down to the nearest whole tablet) in one or two divided doses for weeks 1 and 2, increased to 0.6 mg/kg/day (rounded down to the nearest whole tablet) in two divided doses for weeks 3 and 4, and thereafter increased every 1–2 weeks by 0.6 mg/kg/day (rounded down to the nearest whole tablet), with usual maintenance dosages of 4.5–7.5 mg/kg/day, and a maximum of 300 mg/day in two divided doses. These dosages are halved in patients concurrently receiving valproate and doubled in patients concurrently receiving carbamazepine or other enzyme inducers. In pediatric epilepsy patients over age 12 years, lamotrigine is introduced in a fashion similar to that in adults, as described in Chapter 13, "Mood Stabilizers and Antipsychotics." (Other lamotrigine adverse effects as well as drug interactions are described in Chapter 13.) In adult bipolar disorder patients, lamotrigine may be administered once daily, in contrast to the two divided doses per day recommended in epilepsy patients. Thus, pediatric bipolar disorder patients commonly take lamotrigine in a single daily dose. Lamotrigine-related rashes tend to occur during the first 3 months of treatment. Benign rash may be seen in 10% of patients, but because any rash is potentially serious, rashes require discontinuation of lamotrigine, unless they are clearly not drug related.

Second-Generation Antipsychotics

Multicenter, randomized, double-blind, placebo-controlled studies have demonstrated the efficacy of the second-generation antipsychotics risperidone, aripiprazole, olanzapine, quetiapine, and ziprasidone as monotherapy in pediatric acute mania. Indeed, risperidone and aripiprazole have been approved for the treatment of acute manic and mixed episodes in children and adolescents ages 10–17 years. For risperidone, aripiprazole, olanzapine, quetiapine, and ziprasidone, compared with placebo, the number needed to treat (NNT) for response ranged between 4 and 5 (Figure 10–1), similar to the pattern seen in adult acute mania studies.

This evidence base is augmented by open-label trials and retrospective chart reviews suggesting the effectiveness of second-generation antipsychotics in pediatric bipolar disorder. The incidence of extrapyramidal symptoms or neuroleptic malignant syndrome is lower with second-generation antipsychotics than with first-generation antipsychotics, but these conditions may still occur with second-generation agents and should be monitored. Patients need to be carefully monitored because these medications can cause significant weight gain in youth and subsequent metabolic problems such as an increased risk of developing type II (non-insulin-dependent) diabetes mellitus and metabolic syndrome (Correll and Carlson 2006).

Risperidone was the initial second-generation antipsychotic to receive FDA approval as monotherapy for the treatment of acute manic and mixed episodes in children and adolescents ages 10–17 years (*Physicians' Desk Reference* 2008). In a 3-week, multicenter, randomized, double-blind, placebo-controlled trial, risperidone 0.5–2.5 mg/day (mean modal dosage 1.9 mg/day) and risperidone 3–6 mg/day (mean modal dosage 4.7 mg/day) yielded greater YMRS decreases than did placebo. Response rates were 59% in the low-dose risperidone group, 63% in the high-dose group, and 28% in the placebo group. Thus, the combined (low-dose and high-dose) risperidone group had a response rate of 61%, which, compared to 28% with placebo, yielded an NNT for response of 3 for risperidone compared with placebo (Figure 10–1, far left). The most common adverse effects with risperidone were somnolence, headache, and fatigue. Somnolence was seen in 49.5% of patients taking risperidone and 19.0% of patients taking placebo (NNH=4). Extrapyramidal symptoms were seen in 25% of the risperidone 3–6 mg/day group (vs. 5% of the placebo group, NNH=5), but in only 8% of the risperidone 0.5–2.5 mg/day group (NNH=34). Weight gain was 1.9 kg with risperidone 0.5–2.5 mg/day, 1.4 kg with risperidone 3–6 mg/day, and 0.7 kg with placebo. Clinically significant (≥7%) weight gain was seen in

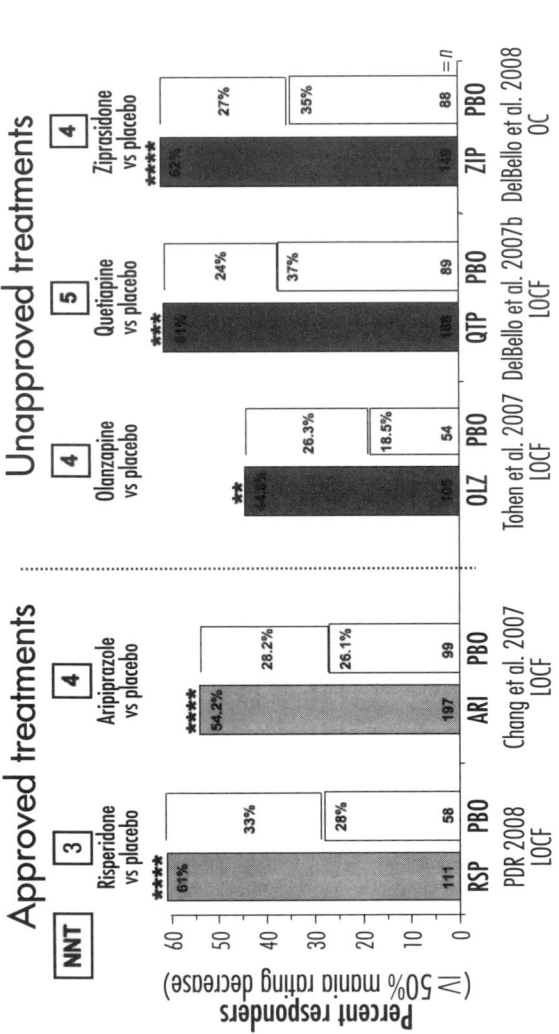

FIGURE 10–1. Overview of second-generation antipsychotic acute mania studies in children and adolescents, numbers needed to treat (NNT), and response rates.

Five second-generation antipsychotics have been effective in multicenter, randomized, double-blind, placebo-controlled pediatric acute mania studies, with single-digit NNTs comparable to those seen in adult studies. The age range was 10–17 years in all studies except the olanzapine study, which had a range of 13–17 years. Response rates are based on last observation carried forward (LOCF) analyses, except that the ziprasidone study is based on less stringent observed cases (OC) analysis. ARI=aripiprazole; OLZ=olanzapine; PBO=placebo; QTP=quetiapine; RSP=risperidone; ZIP=ziprasidone.
$**P<0.01$, $***P<0.001$, $****P<0.0001$ versus placebo.

Source.   Data from Chang et al. 2007; DelBello et al. 2007b, 2008; *Physicians' Desk Reference*

11.9% of patients taking risperidone and 5.3% of patients taking placebo (NNH = 16). Prolactin-related adverse events were seen in 4.5% of patients taking risperidone and 1.7% of patients taking placebo (NNH = 36). Adverse event discontinuations with risperidone included 5% due to somnolence, 3% due to nausea, 2% due to abdominal pain, and 2% due to vomiting.

In children and adolescents ages 10–17 years with acute manic or mixed episodes, risperidone should be started at 0.5 mg/day and increased daily by 0.5–1 mg/day, with a target dosage of 2.5 mg/day (*Physicians' Desk Reference* 2008). The FDA recommends 2.5 mg/day as the target because no evidence has indicated that dosages above 2.5 mg/day are more effective. Based on other open studies and our own clinical experience, children and adolescents with bipolar disorder may benefit from taking two or three divided doses a day. Open-label risperidone studies also have suggested possible efficacy for pediatric bipolar disorder (Biederman et al. 2005c, 2005d). Because risperidone is commonly associated with weight gain and hyperprolactinemia, physicians should consider monitoring weight every 3 months and prolactin levels prior to treatment and every 6 months thereafter.

Aripiprazole, a partial dopamine agonist, has also received FDA approval as monotherapy and, by inference from adult studies, adjunctive therapy (added to lithium or valproate) for the treatment of acute manic and mixed episodes as well as, by inference adult studies, for the maintenance monotherapy treatment of manic and mixed episodes in children and adolescents ages 10–17 years (*Physicians' Desk Reference* 2008). In a 4-week multicenter, randomized, double-blind, placebo-controlled trial in adolescents ages 10–17 years with acute manic or mixed episodes, the response (at least 50% decrease in YMRS) rates in 98 subjects receiving aripiprazole 10 mg/day (44.8%) and 99 subjects receiving aripiprazole 30 mg/day (63.6%) were higher than in 99 subjects receiving placebo (26.1%) (Chang et al. 2007). Thus, the pooled aripiprazole YMRS response rate was 54.2%, which, compared with placebo (26.1%), yielded an NNT for YMRS response of 4 (Figure 10–1, second set of bars from left). On the primary outcome measure (decrease in YMRS), aripiprazole was superior to placebo at week 1 and thereafter. Common adverse effects with aripiprazole were somnolence, extrapyramidal disorder, fatigue, nausea, akathisia, blurred vision, salivary hypersecretion, and dizziness. Rates of somnolence, extrapyramidal disorder, akathisia, salivary hypersecretion, and clinically significant (≥7%) weight gain appeared to increase with aripiprazole dosage. Adverse event discontinuation rates were 7% with aripiprazole and 2% with placebo.

In children and adolescents ages 10–17 years with acute manic or mixed episodes, aripirazole should be started at 2 mg/day, increased to 5 mg/day after 2 days, and increased to the target dosage of 10 mg/day after 2 additional days (*Physicians' Desk Reference* 2008). Subsequent dosage increases should be administered in 5-mg/day increments.

Limited additional uncontrolled data support the efficacy of aripiprazole in pediatric bipolar disorder (Barzman et al. 2004; Biederman et al. 2005b). As in adult populations, the most common side effects of aripiprazole reported in retrospective studies of youth with bipolar disorder were sedation, akathisia, and gastrointestinal disturbances.

In a 3-week, multicenter, randomized, double-blind, placebo-controlled trial in adolescents ages 13–17 years with acute manic or mixed episodes, olanzapine (mean modal dosage 10.7 mg/day) yielded a YMRS response rate that was higher than that with placebo (44.8% vs. 18.5%, NNT=4) (Tohen et al. 2007) (Figure 10–1, middle). On the primary outcome measure (decrease in YMRS), olanzapine was superior to placebo at week 1 and thereafter. However, olanzapine compared with placebo yielded a greater increase in mean weight (3.7 kg vs. 0.3 kg); a higher incidence of clinically significant (≥7% increase) weight gain (41.9% vs. 1.9%, NNH=3); and greater increases in prolactin, fasting glucose, fasting total cholesterol, uric acid, and the hepatic enzymes aspartate transaminase and alanine transaminase. Adverse event discontinuation rates were 2.8% (3/107) with olanzapine and 1.9% (1/54) with placebo. In this trial, olanzapine was started at 2.5 or 5 mg/day and could be increased by 2.5 or 5 mg/day to as high as 20 mg/day. Olanzapine has not been approved by the FDA for the treatment of acute manic and mixed episodes in adolescents.

In a 3-week, multicenter, randomized, double-blind, placebo-controlled trial in children and adolescents ages 10–17 years with acute manic episodes, the YMRS response rates with quetiapine 400 mg/day (64%) and quetiapine 600 mg/day (58%) were higher than with placebo (37%) (DelBello et al. 2007b). Thus, the pooled quetiapine YMRS response rate was 61%, which, compared with placebo (37%), yielded an NNT for YMRS response of 5 (Figure 10–1, second from right). Common adverse effects with quetiapine were somnolence (placebo, 10.0%; 400 mg, 28.4%; 600 mg, 31.6%), sedation (placebo, 4.4%; 400 mg, 23.2%; 600 mg, 25.5%), dizziness (placebo, 2.2%; 400 mg, 18.9%; 600 mg, 17.3%), and headache (placebo, 15.6%; 400 mg, 15.8%; 600 mg, 13.3%). Mean weight gain was 0.4 kg for the placebo group and 1.7 kg for both quetiapine groups. The rates of clinically significant (≥7%) weight gain were 0% with placebo, 14.5% with quetiapine 400 mg/day, and 9.9% with quetiapine 600 mg/

day. Thus, the pooled quetiapine ≥7% weight gain rate was 12.2%, which, compared with placebo (0%), yielded a NNH of 9 for ≥7% weight gain. In this trial, quetiapine was started at 50 mg at bedtime on day 1, increased to 400 mg/day in divided doses by day 5, and increased to 600 mg/day in divided doses by day 7. Quetiapine has not been approved by the FDA for the treatment of acute manic episodes in children and adolescents.

In addition, results from two small controlled studies suggest that quetiapine is a useful medication for the treatment of adolescent mania. In a double-blind, placebo-controlled adjunctive study in children and adolescents with bipolar disorder, DelBello et al. (2002) reported that combined divalproex and quetiapine reduced manic symptoms significantly more than did combined divalproex and placebo. In another double-blind study, DelBello et al. (2006) found that adolescent patients with bipolar disorder receiving quetiapine monotherapy had faster resolution of their manic symptoms and higher rates of remission than did those treated with divalproex monotherapy, and quetiapine was well tolerated. Quetiapine is associated with sedation and orthostatic hypotension, presumably secondary to its affinity for histamine and alpha-adrenergic receptors, respectively. Weight gain in children taking quetiapine appears to be slightly less than that for children taking olanzapine or risperidone (Correll 2007).

In a 4-week, multicenter, randomized, double-blind, placebo-controlled trial in children and adolescents ages 10–17 years with acute manic or mixed episodes, ziprasidone (80–160 mg/day) compared with placebo yielded a greater mean YMRS decrease (DelBello et al. 2008). Response rates using a less stringent observed cases analysis were 62% for the ziprasidone group and 35% for the placebo group, yielding an NNT for response for ziprasidone compared with placebo of 4 (Figure 10–1, far right). The most common adverse effects with ziprasidone were sedation (33%), somnolence (25%), headache (21%), nausea (13%), fatigue (13%), and dizziness (11%). Mean weight change was −0.6 kg and −0.2 kg for the ziprasidone and placebo groups, respectively. Clinically significant (≥7%) weight gain rates were 7% with ziprasidone and 4% with placebo. There were no significant changes in mean body mass index, lipids, liver enzymes, or glucose levels. One ziprasidone-treated subject had a QT prolongation to more than 460 milliseconds. Ziprasidone has not been approved by the FDA for the treatment of acute manic and mixed episodes in children and adolescents.

The prototypical second-generation antipsychotic clozapine lacks randomized controlled trials to support its use in pediatric bipolar disorder. The data regarding the safety and efficacy of clozapine for pediatric bipolar disorder are limited to a few case series (Kowatch et al. 1995; Masi et al. 2002). Clozapine is not considered a first-line agent, because of the lack of evidence of its efficacy, as well as its risk of agranulocytosis, which necessitates frequent blood draws for monitoring. Thus, clozapine is usually reserved for treatment-resistant patients. Clozapine has a particularly challenging adverse effect profile; the U.S. prescribing information includes boxed warnings regarding the risks of 1) agranulocytosis; 2) seizures; 3) myocarditis; 4) other adverse cardiovascular and respiratory effects; and 5) increased mortality (primarily cardiovascular or infectious) in elderly patients with dementia-related psychosis (a second-generation antipsychotic class warning). More frequently reported common side effects in younger populations include sialorrhea, constipation, orthostatic hypotension, weight gain, and sedation. Also, because clozapine is metabolized primarily by the cytochrome P450 1A2, tobacco smoking can cause an induction of clozapine (and similarly olanzapine) metabolism.

When a child or adolescent starts taking a second-generation antipsychotic, the clinician should obtain a personal and family history of obesity, diabetes, dyslipidemia, and cardiovascular disease (Correll and Carlson 2006). Furthermore, the clinician should monitor blood pressure and fasting lipids and glucose beginning at the initial appointment, 3 months after the initial appointment, and then annually. A body mass index should be calculated every 3 months. If a relative weight gain of 5% compared with baseline weight occurs during the first 3 months of treatment, consideration should be given to discontinuing or switching to another agent. The clinician should also discuss lifestyle and dietary measures with patients and their families, and refer them for nutritional advice if needed (Correll and Carlson 2006). Additionally, oral antihyperglycemics, such as metformin, may also help to reduce the risk of weight gain and metabolic dysfunction in pediatric patients taking second-generation antipsychotics (Klein et al. 2006).

Combination Therapy

Children and adolescents with bipolar disorder usually require combinations of medications to achieve adequate mood stabilization (Kowatch et al. 2003). DelBello et al. (2002) found that patients taking quetiapine and divalproex had higher response rates than those taking divalproex alone. Similarly, Pavuluri et al. (2004b) performed an open-label prospective trial evaluating the effectiveness of risperidone in combination with either divalproex or lithium, and reported an improvement in both groups, with almost identical response rates. When psychotic symptoms are present in conjunction with pediatric mania, combination therapy is an optimal choice. For example, Kafantaris et al. (2001) observed lower relapse rates in adolescents with acute psychotic mania who were treated with a second-generation antipsychotic medication in combination with lithium for at least 4 weeks than in those treated with lithium monotherapy.

Newer Anticonvulsants

Unlike valproate, carbamazepine, and lamotrigine, other anticonvulsants lack an evidence base to support their utility in bipolar disorders. Indeed, as described in Chapter 6 of this volume, for some of these agents, multicenter, randomized, double-blind, placebo-controlled trials have failed to demonstrate efficacy in adults. Randomized controlled trials in adults found adjunctive gabapentin to be no better than adjunctive placebo in outpatients with acute mania (Pande et al. 2000) and found gabapentin monotherapy to be no better than placebo in treatment-resistant mood disorder (mainly rapid-cycling bipolar disorder) in-patients (Frye et al. 2000). However, in adults, gabapentin appeared effective in several comorbid conditions commonly seen in patients with bipolar disorders, such as social phobia, panic disorder, and pain syndromes. Similarly, randomized controlled trials have failed to demonstrate efficacy for topiramate in adults (Kushner et al. 2006) and adolescents (DelBello et al. 2005). However, in adults, topiramate appeared effective in several comorbid conditions commonly seen in patients with bipolar disorders, such as obesity, binge-eating disorder, olanzapine-associated weight gain, bulimia, alcohol abuse, essential tremor, chronic low back pain, and borderline personality disorder, as well as in preventing migraine headaches. Oxcarbazepine, a congener of carbamazepine, may differ from other newer anticonvulsants in that, like carbamazepine and valproate, it may have efficacy in acute mania, but this has not been supported by adequately powered randomized controlled trials in adult or pediatric patients with bipolar disorder (Wagner et al. 2006).

Treating Comorbid Disorders

Children and adolescents with bipolar disorder commonly present with co-occurring anxiety disorders, ADHD, oppositional defiant disorder, and conduct disorder (Pavuluri et al. 2005). Furthermore, bipolar disorder in adolescents is a significant risk factor for a substance abuse disorder independent of conduct disorder (Wilens et al. 2004). However, few studies have been reported to inform the treatment of co-occurring disorders in youth with bipolar disorder.

Up to 40% of adolescents with bipolar disorder have a co-occurring substance use disorder. In a small controlled study, Geller et al. (1998a) demonstrated a greater decrease in positive urine toxicology screens in adolescents who were treated with lithium than in those who received placebo (46% vs. 8%). However, the effect of lithium on mood symptoms was not evaluated. Further treatment studies are needed to assess both mood symptoms and substance abuse in youth with comorbid bipolar disorder and substance abuse.

Co-occurring anxiety disorders can be challenging to treat in patients with bipolar disorder because the use of antidepressants such as selective serotonin reuptake inhibitors (SSRIs) may lead to destabilization of mood symptoms (Baumer et al. 2006; DelBello and Kowatch 2006). If a co-occurring anxiety disorder is treated with an SSRI, the child should be carefully monitored for the development of manic or hypomanic symptoms. To avoid mood destabilization, alternative pharmacological and nonpharmacological interventions for the treatment of co-occurring anxiety should be considered. Gabapentin is similar in structure to γ-aminobutyric acid (GABA) and, in contrast to SSRIs, it modulates sodium channels and increases the release of GABA from the glia. Although adjunctive and monotherapy double-blind, placebo-controlled trials showed gabapentin to be no more effective than placebo for the treatment of mania in adults, gabapentin may be helpful in divided doses for anxiety in children and adolescents with bipolar disorder while not destabilizing their mood symptoms (DelBello and Kowatch 2006).

Similar to antidepressants, stimulants and atomoxetine may also adversely affect mood symptoms in children and adolescents with bipolar disorder; therefore, a second-generation antipsychotic or an antimanic mood stabilizer should be used prior to starting these medications for comorbid ADHD (Biederman et al. 1999). In a randomized, placebo-controlled trial, Scheffer et al. (2005) found that 40 children and adolescents with co-occurring bipolar disorder and ADHD were safely and effectively treated with low-dose mixed amphetamine salts after their mood symptoms were stabilized with divalproex. Similarly, another group found that methylphenidate added to divalproex was more effective than placebo added to divalproex in euthymic children and adolescents with bipolar disorder and ADHD (Findling et al. 2007b). Nonetheless, children with bipolar disorder taking psychostimulants should be carefully monitored for mood destabilization.

Disruptive behavior disorders often co-occur with bipolar disorder in children and adolescents. Both divalproex and quetiapine were found to significantly reduce aggression in adolescents with comorbid bipolar disorder and disruptive behavior disorders (inclusive of oppositional defiant and conduct disorders) in a post hoc analysis of a prospective controlled study of adolescents with mania (Barzman et al. 2006). In a secondary analysis of a controlled study, Biederman et al. (2006) reported that risperidone compared with placebo was effective in decreasing manic and depressive symptomatology in children with co-occurring disruptive behavioral disorders and subaverage intelligence at 2, 4, and 6 weeks after treatment initiation. Although no controlled studies of topiramate monotherapy for comorbid bipolar and disruptive behavioral disorders have been reported, adjunctive topiramate may be helpful for these co-occurring disorders (Barzman and DelBello 2006). Randomized controlled studies are needed for co-occurring disorders in pediatric bipolar disorder.

Adjunctive Psychosocial Interventions

As discussed in Chapter 15, "Adjunctive Psychosocial Interventions in the Management of Bipolar Disorders," emerging evidence supports the use of adjunctive psychosocial interventions in adults with bipolar disorders. Similarly, data are beginning to emerge to support the use of such interventions in pediatric bipolar disorder. Psychosocial interventions may include individual, psychoeducational, and family psychotherapies; intervening to improve social and family dysfunction, or academic and occupational dysfunction; and providing community consultation and strategies for relapse prevention. Few of these psychosocial interventions have been systematically studied in pediatric bipolar disorder, and despite advances in pharmacological interventions, problems related to mood symptom relapse, medication nonadherence, and poor outcome continue to emerge (Geller et al. 2004).

The course and onset of bipolar disorder are influenced by both genetic and environmental factors. For example, Geller et al. (2000a) found that low maternal-child warmth, high maternal-child tension, and high paternal-child tension were significantly greater in families of children with bipolar disorder as compared with control groups of children without a family history of mood disorders. Negative life events, sleep problems, and social dysfunction have also been associated with poor outcome for adults with bipolar disorder (Johnson and McMurrich 2006). For these reasons, psychosocial interventions to target challenges that may be inadequately treated by pharmacotherapy alone may add benefit and lead to improved outcomes.

As discussed in detail in Chapter 15 of this volume, adjunctive psychoeducation, bipolar-specific cognitive-behavioral therapy (CBT), family therapy, and interpersonal and social rhythm therapy (see also Chapters 7, "Management of Acute Major Depressive Episodes in Bipolar Disorders," and 8, "Longer-Term Management of Bipolar Disorders") may significantly improve the overall well-being, treatment adherence, and functioning of adults with bipolar disorder (Miklowitz 2006). In the last 10 years, cumulative research has also supported the use of adjunctive psychosocial interventions in pediatric bipolar disorder (Chang et al. 2006a; Kowatch and DelBello 2006). Current guidelines recommend that all patients with pediatric bipolar disorder receive a combination of both medication and psychotherapy (Kowatch et al. 2005).

Understanding the impact of the environment on the developing brain of the child is often challenging. Burns et al. (1999) suggested including family and a manualized intervention to clarify environmental influences, whereas other researchers have proposed a psychoeducational component and the inclusion of CBT to intervene on environmental factors (Lofthouse and Fristad 2004). Psychoeducation aims to teach patients and their families about bipolar disorder and its course, prognosis, and treatment. The goal of CBT is to modify automatic thoughts and behaviors to positively influence emotions and outcomes. Psychoeducation and CBT can be used in individual or group therapeutic settings (Miklowitz 2006).

Researchers have recently begun to study the effectiveness of adjunctive psychosocial interventions for children and adolescents with bipolar disorder. Treatments currently being developed and assessed include adjunctive multifamily psychoeducation groups (MFPG; Fristad et al. 2003), family-focused treatment for adolescents (FFT-A; Miklowitz et al. 2004), and child- and family-focused cognitive-behavioral therapy (CFF-CBT; Pavuluri et al. 2004a). These have all shown preliminary success in decreasing symptom severity and preventing relapse in children with bipolar disorder.

MFPG has been found to be effective for adult-onset bipolar disorder, childhood unipolar depression, anger management in children, and childhood bipolar disorder (Fristad et al. 2003). Adjunctive to pharmacotherapy, MFPG implements a biopsychosocial theoretical approach to working with children with bipolar disorder and their families. For a period of 8 weeks, weekly 90-minute group sessions include psychoeducation on mood disorders, symptoms, medication, medication treatment adherence, problem-solving skills, coping mechanisms, and self-preservation skills using cognitive-behavioral techniques. Additional recreational activity is implemented to foster social skills in the children. In a 6-week randomized controlled trial in 35 children ages 7–12 years with bipolar disorder, parents reported an improved relationship with their children and increased knowledge of mood disorders. Additionally, children perceived an increase in social support from baseline (Fristad et al. 2003).

FFT-A uses a focused psychoeducational approach in conjunction with pharmacotherapy, similar to MFPG. Miklowitz et al. (2004) modified the successful adult version of family-focused treatment (Miklowitz et al. 2000) to address the unique developmental concerns and clinical presentations of adolescents with bipolar disorder; 20 adolescents with bipolar disorder who had experienced an exacerbation of manic, depressed, or mixed symptoms within the previous 3 months received FFT-A in 21 sessions. In addition to the introductory and final wrap-up sessions, 9 sessions were devoted to psychoeducation, 5 to enhancing communication skills, and 5 to learning problem-solving skills. The open FFT-A intervention in combination with standard pharmacotherapy was associated with decreased depression and mania symptoms and behavioral problems over the course of 1 year. A larger controlled study randomly assigned 58 adolescents with bipolar disorder to receive either FFT-A or enhanced care (EC), which consisted of three family psychoeducational sessions. While there were no significant effects on manic symptoms, patients in FFT-A recovered from their baseline depressive symptoms faster than patients in EC and spent fewer weeks in depressive episodes over 2 years (Miklowitz et al. 2008).

Finally, CFF-CBT adds contact with school personnel to combined psycho-education, CBT, and family involvement. CFF-CBT, which uses 12 individual parent and child sessions over a 12-week period, was developed for children with bipolar disorder ages 8–12 years (Pavuluri et al. 2004a). CFF-CBT has demonstrated decreases in bipolar disorder symptom severity and increases in overall well-being in an open study of 34 children with bipolar disorder (Pavuluri et al. 2004a).

Children with bipolar disorder may require special accommodations in school to facilitate healthy academic and social development. Frequent mood swings and adverse effects from medications used to treat bipolar disorder can affect a child's attendance, concentration, motivation, and energy level in school. Moreover, children with bipolar disorder may suffer from neurocognitive deficits even when their mood is euthymic. In a neuropsychological evaluation, impairments in attention, executive functioning, working memory, and verbal learning were found in 28 unmedicated and 28 medicated subjects with bipolar disorder, regardless of illness state, compared with 28 demographically matched healthy controls (Pavuluri et al. 2006b). The cognitive deficits found in this study suggested traitlike characteristics of bipolar disorder, with significant involvement of working and verbal memory functions (Pavuluri et al. 2006b).

The neuropsychological data on co-occurring bipolar disorder and ADHD have been mixed. One study of 28 subjects with bipolar disorder alone versus 27 subjects with bipolar disorder plus ADHD found no difference between these two groups in neuropsychological function or academic difficulties (Pavuluri et al. 2006a). In another study, Rucklidge (2006) compared 12 subjects with bipolar disorder only, 12 subjects with bipolar disorder plus ADHD, 30 subjects with ADHD only, and 41 healthy controls, and found the ADHD-only and combined groups to be most impaired in the domains of processing and naming speed, working memory, and response inhibition. Working memory was the only domain in which the bipolar disorder–only and the healthy control groups differed (Rucklidge 2006).

Regardless of the sample diagnostic variability of these studies, they all demonstrate that a proper educational setting is integral to the therapeutic plan for children with bipolar disorder. Parents and clinicians may collaborate with school personnel to determine the appropriate educational plan for the child with bipolar disorder, taking into consideration accommodations for transitions to new teachers and new schools, return to school from vacations and absences, and any change in medication, which can all result in increased symptomatology and declining school performance. A determination should be made about whether an individualized education program (IEP) is needed and whether input from the clinician on the IEP team would be useful in developing an appropriate academic curriculum for the child.

In summary, psychosocial interventions have demonstrated efficacy in augmenting pharmacological treatment of pediatric bipolar disorder. Moreover, such interventions have been manualized to provide a framework for individual treatment, they have been developed with a child's developmental status in mind, and participation of family members has been encouraged. Additional research is necessary to provide evidence for the long-term benefits of these modalities and to inform future interventions designed to meet the individual needs of the child and family.

Conclusion

The recognition and treatment of pediatric bipolar disorder remain major challenges for clinicians. Despite recent advances in the field, investigations of safety and efficacy of pharmacological interventions, longitudinal outcomes with treatment, and the underlying neurobiological mechanisms of mood disorders remain in their infancy, and additional studies are necessary to further advance the understanding of bipolar disorders in children and adolescents. Recent clinical practice parameters (McClellan et al. 2007) have suggested a systematic approach to the diagnostic challenges associated with evaluating children with mood and associated symptoms (Table 10–2). A multimodal treatment approach, combining psychopharmacological and psychosocial interventions, is indicated (Table 10–3). Furthermore, of equal importance is ensuring that the child's educational setting is appropriate, both for educational and therapeutic purposes. Children and adolescents and their families and teachers need to be educated about mood disorders, the importance of treatment adherence, and the need for regular monitoring of response to treatment and side effects. Patients and/or their parents should be instructed to keep a daily record of the level of depressive and manic symptoms ("mood charting"), which may help monitor symptom presence and recurrence (Denicoff et al. 1997). Careful titration of pharmacotherapy should parallel careful monitoring for treatment response and adverse effects, and unnecessary polypharmacy should be avoided. Attainment of the goal of preventing symptom chronicity and associated complications of pediatric mood disorders may be facilitated with early identification and early implementation of a comprehensive treatment approach.

Case Study: Management of Children and Adolescents With Bipolar Disorders

Charlie is a 15-year-old boy with bipolar I disorder, ADHD, and anxiety disorder not otherwise specified, who presents with ultradian cycling; daily predominant depressive symptoms; and, beginning in the evening and lasting until sleep, mood elevation symptoms of euphoria, irritability, racing thoughts, and increased energy and goal-directed activity.

Charlie's mother has bipolar II disorder, with onset at age 18 years with an initial depressive episode. In addition, he has a maternal aunt with bipolar I disorder and a paternal great-grandmother with possible psychotic depression or schizophrenia.

As an infant and toddler, Charlie was energetic and difficult to soothe. In preschool, he had difficulty attending to tasks and was unable to ever sit quietly. He was perceived as "moody and intense" by his parents. In first grade, at age 5 years, Charlie was seen by a pediatrician, who diagnosed ADHD and prescribed methylphenidate, with some benefit. Charlie took various forms of methylphenidate until age 11 years, when it was discontinued because of attenuation of perceived benefit and concerns that his mood was worsening. Thus, between ages 8 and 11, Charlie had increasing frequent and severe problems with episodic irritability, exploding in anger with his parents or siblings several times each week. He also struggled with symptoms of generalized anxiety disorder, worrying at night about robbers and experiencing some fears regarding separation from his parents.

TABLE 10–3. Multimodal prevention, early intervention, and treatment in pediatric bipolar disorder

Treatment modality	Recommendations	Level of evidence to support recommendations
Prevention and early intervention	To prevent onset and progression of illness, consider: Careful assessment of risk factors for the development of mania and early intervention – family history of mood disorders and psychosis – depressive or bipolar spectrum disorders – exposure to psychostimulants and antidepressants Predictors of poor outcome – younger age at onset, lower socioeconomic status, strong family history of bipolar disorder, mixed episodes, psychotic symptoms, rapid cycling, co-occurring substance use, and neurocognitive deficits (Post and Kowatch 2006).	Open-label trials with divalproex (Chang et al. 2003) and quetiapine (DelBello et al. 2007a) have shown improvement in non–bipolar I mood symptomatology in children with a parent or sibling with bipolar disorder.

TABLE 10–3. Multimodal prevention, early intervention, and treatment in pediatric bipolar disorder (continued)

Treatment modality	Recommendations	Level of evidence to support recommendations
Pharmacotherapy		
U.S. Food and Drug Administration (FDA)–approved agents for adults Lithium Divalproex Carbamazepine Second-generation antipsychotics Aripiprazole Olanzapine Risperidone Quetiapine Ziprasidone Other anticonvulsants Lamotrigine (maintenance)	Consider the following factors when choosing a medication: – Evidence for efficacy – Phase of illness (mania, depression, mixed) – Presence of psychosis or rapid cycling – Safety and side-effect profile – History of prior medication response – Patient and family preferences Use FDA-approved agents for bipolar disorder first. Monitor symptoms, side effects, and labs at baseline and follow-up. Avoid unnecessary polypharmacy and discontinue any agents that have not demonstrated benefit. Ongoing and possibly lifelong medication for relapse prevention may be necessary.	Case reports, open-label trials, and chart reviews have predominated over controlled trials to describe effectiveness of medications in pediatric bipolar disorder. Standard recommendations to start with lithium, divalproex, and/or second-generation antipsychotics for mood stabilization are based on adult randomized controlled trials and emerging controlled pediatric acute mania trials. Lithium is an FDA-approved mood stabilizer for acute mania and maintenance for children age 12 years and older. Lithium is beneficial for comorbid substance use disorders (Geller et al. 1998a). Also, one controlled discontinuation study showed high rates of manic relapse in adolescents in both ongoing lithium and placebo groups (Kafantaris et al. 2004). Risperidone is FDA approved for the treatment of acute manic or mixed episodes as monotherapy in pediatric patients age 10–17 years (Figure 10–1, left). Aripiprazole is FDA approved for the treatment of acute manic or mixed episodes as monotherapy or adjunctive to lithium or valproate, as well as for the monotherapy maintenance treatment of manic or mixed episodes in pediatric patients ages 10–17 years (Figure 10–1, second from left).

TABLE 10–3. Multimodal prevention, early intervention, and treatment in pediatric bipolar disorder (*continued*)

Treatment modality	Recommendations	Level of evidence to support recommendations
Pharmacotherapy (*continued*)		Emerging data suggest efficacy for olanzapine, quetiapine, and ziprasidone in pediatric acute mania (Figure 10–1, right). Other controlled trials have commonly been limited by small sample size and diagnostic variability.
		Divalproex in combination with lithium or quetiapine may decrease relapse or reduce manic symptoms compared with divalproex alone (DelBello et al. 2002); otherwise efficacy data are inconsistent across trials.
		Carbamazepine in pediatric bipolar disorder is supported by very limited data.
		Quetiapine monotherapy has shown faster symptom resolution and higher rates of remission than divalproex monotherapy (DelBello et al. 2006).
Psychosocial therapies Individual Family School Work	Combine pharmacotherapy with psychosocial interventions, because the latter are useful for medication-refractory patients with functional, academic, and developmental impairments and provide education and support, promote treatment adherence, prevent relapse, and address preexisting and co-occurring behavioral and substance use disorders.	Controlled data are emerging for the efficacy of family-focused therapy for adolescents (Miklowitz et al. 2004), child- and family-focused cognitive-behavioral therapy (Pavuluri et al. 2004a), functional family therapy adapted from adult therapeutic models (Miklowitz et al. 2004), and psychoeducational approaches (Fristad et al. 2003). Dialectical behavioral therapy may be useful for youths with mood and behavioral dysregulation (McClellan et al. 2007).

At age 13 years, at the beginning of seventh grade, he had a syndromal major depressive episode, manifested by extreme irritability and dysphoria, insomnia, anhedonia, guilt, and passive suicidal ideation. At this point, he was no longer taking stimulants and he began taking sertraline 50 mg/day. Over the next 2 weeks, Charlie experienced surges of irritability and euphoria, slept only 4–5 hours each night, and was even more agitated and explosive. After assessment by a child psychiatrist, sertraline was discontinued and divalproex was started and titrated to 750 mg twice a day. After 2 weeks, affective symptoms resolved. After 3 months, because of weight gain, divalproex was replaced with lithium 600 mg twice a day.

However, the next spring Charlie experienced a syndromal manic episode. During this time, he slept 3–4 hours/night, reported racing thoughts, had pressured speech, and had grandiose ideas of trapping animals in his backyard and selling them online. He stayed up late at night on the Internet working on this plan, and was also hypersexual, surfing Internet pornography sites. Aripiprazole 5 mg/day was added and then titrated up to 20 mg/day. After 3 weeks, he was close to euthymic, but continued to have difficulties in school, with school refusal and not turning in homework. Neuropsychological testing revealed impaired processing speed and significant difficulties with attention, distractibility, and forgetfulness. At age 14 years, early in eighth grade, OROS-methylphenidate 18 mg/day was added to his aripiprazole and divalproex, resulting in fairly good relief of cognitive symptoms. However, because he had significant appetite suppression and some continuing irritability, he was switched from OROS-methylphenidate to atomoxetine 100 mg/day, which resulted in continued relief of cognitive symptoms.

Now presenting at age 15 years in the spring of eighth grade with significant symptoms of depression, Charlie was found to have practically no friends and poor self-esteem, and he was 35 lb overweight. Lamotrigine was added to aripiprazole, lithium, and atomoxetine, and gradually titrated up to 100 mg twice a day, resulting in some relief of depression, but he continued to have residual periods of dysphoria and generally few social interactions. He joined a psychotherapy group and attended a summer camp for adolescents with bipolar disorder and increased his social network. He began an exercise regimen, including running and training for races, lost 30 lb, and was able to decrease dosages of some of his medications. He was successfully maintained over the following year on lithium 450 mg twice a day, lamotrigine 100 mg twice a day, aripiprazole 5 mg/day, and atomoxetine 70 mg/day. He was enrolled in a private school for students with learning disabilities and continued individual and group therapy. Of note, his mother also maintained relative stability during the year, and several sessions of family therapy aided in improving communication and decreasing stress in the home environment.

References

American Psychiatric Association: Diagnostic and Statistical Manual of Mental Disorders, 4th Edition, Text Revision. Washington, DC, American Psychiatric Association, 2000

Barzman DH, DelBello MP: Topiramate for co-occurring bipolar disorder and disruptive behavior disorders. Am J Psychiatry 163:1451–1452, 2006

Barzman DH, DelBello MP, Kowatch RA, et al: The effectiveness and tolerability of aripiprazole for pediatric bipolar disorders: a retrospective chart review. J Child Adolesc Psychopharmacol 14:593–600, 2004

Barzman DH, DelBello MP, Adler CM, et al: The efficacy and tolerability of quetiapine versus divalproex for the treatment of impulsivity and reactive aggression in adolescents with co-occurring bipolar disorder and disruptive behavior disorder(s). J Child Adolesc Psychopharmacol 16:665–670, 2006

Baumer FM, Howe M, Gallelli K, et al: A pilot study of antidepressant-induced mania in pediatric bipolar disorder: characteristics, risk factors, and the serotonin transporter gene. Biol Psychiatry 60:1005–1012, 2006

Biederman J, Mick E, Prince J, et al: Systematic chart review of the pharmacologic treatment of comorbid attention deficit hyperactivity disorder in youth with bipolar disorder. J Child Adolesc Psychopharmacol 9:247–256, 1999

Biederman J, Faraone SV, Wozniak J, et al: Clinical correlates of bipolar disorder in a large, referred sample of children and adolescents. J Psychiatr Res 39:611–622, 2005a

Biederman J, McDonnell MA, Wozniak J, et al: Aripiprazole in the treatment of pediatric bipolar disorder: a systematic chart review. CNS Spectr 10:141–148, 2005b

Biederman J, Mick E, Hammerness P, et al: Open-label, 8-week trial of olanzapine and risperidone for the treatment of bipolar disorder in preschool-age children. Biol Psychiatry 58:589–594, 2005c

Biederman J, Mick E, Wozniak J, et al: An open-label trial of risperidone in children and adolescents with bipolar disorder. J Child Adolesc Psychopharmacol 15:311–317, 2005d

Biederman J, Mick E, Faraone SV, et al: Risperidone for the treatment of affective symptoms in children with disruptive behavior disorder: a post hoc analysis of data from a 6-week, multicenter, randomized, double-blind, parallel-arm study. Clin Ther 28:794–800, 2006

Birmaher B, Axelson D, Strober M, et al: Clinical course of children and adolescents with bipolar spectrum disorders. Arch Gen Psychiatry 63:175–183, 2006

Bourgeois BF: Pharmacokinetic properties of current antiepileptic drugs: what improvements are needed? Neurology 55 (suppl 3):S11–S16, 2000

Bowden C, Calabrese J, Ascher J, et al: Spectrum of efficacy of lamotrigine in bipolar disorder: overview of double-blind placebo-controlled studies. Paper presented at the annual meeting of the American College of Neuropsychopharmacology, San Juan, Puerto Rico, December 2000

Bowden CL, Swann AC, Calabrese JR, et al: A randomized, placebo-controlled, multicenter study of divalproex sodium extended release in the treatment of acute mania. J Clin Psychiatry 67:1501–1510, 2006

Burns BJ, Hoagwood K, Mrazek PJ: Effective treatment for mental disorders in children and adolescents. Clin Child Fam Psychol Rev 2:199–254, 1999

Calabrese JR, Huffman RF, White RL, et al: Lamotrigine in the acute treatment of bipolar depression: results of five double-blind, placebo-controlled clinical trials. Bipolar Disord 10:323–333, 2008

Carlson GA, Youngstrom EA: Clinical implications of pervasive manic symptoms in children. Biol Psychiatry 53:1050–1058, 2003

Chang KD, Dienes K, Blasey C, et al: Divalproex monotherapy in the treatment of bipolar offspring with mood and behavioral disorders and at least mild affective symptoms. J Clin Psychiatry 64:936–942, 2003

Chang K, Howe M, Gallelli K, et al: Prevention of pediatric bipolar disorder: integration of neurobiological and psychosocial processes. Ann NY Acad Sci 1094:235–247, 2006a

Chang K, Saxena K, Howe M: An open-label study of lamotrigine adjunct or monotherapy for the treatment of adolescents with bipolar depression. J Am Acad Child Adolesc Psychiatry 45:298–304, 2006b

Chang K, Nyilas M, Aurang C, et al: Efficacy of aripiprazole in children (10–17 years old) with mania. Paper presented at the annual meeting of the American Academy of Child and Adolescent Psychiatry, Boston, MA, October 2007

Correll CU: Weight gain and metabolic effects of mood stabilizers and antipsychotics in pediatric bipolar disorder: a systematic review and pooled analysis of short-term trials. J Am Acad Child Adolesc Psychiatry 46:687–700, 2007

Correll CU, Carlson HE: Endocrine and metabolic adverse effects of psychotropic medications in children and adolescents. J Am Acad Child Adolesc Psychiatry 45:771–791, 2006

DelBello MP, Kowatch RA: Pharmacological interventions for bipolar youth: developmental considerations. Dev Psychopathol 18:1231–1246, 2006

DelBello MP, Schwiers ML, Rosenberg HL, et al: A double-blind, randomized, placebo-controlled study of quetiapine as adjunctive treatment for adolescent mania. J Am Acad Child Adolesc Psychiatry 41:1216–1223, 2002

DelBello MP, Findling RL, Kushner S, et al: A pilot controlled trial of topiramate for mania in children and adolescents with bipolar disorder. J Am Acad Child Adolesc Psychiatry 44:539–547, 2005

DelBello MP, Kowatch RA, Adler CM, et al: A double-blind randomized pilot study comparing quetiapine and divalproex for adolescent mania. J Am Acad Child Adolesc Psychiatry 45:305–313, 2006

DelBello MP, Adler CM, Whitsel RM, et al: A 12-week single-blind trial of quetiapine for the treatment of mood symptoms in adolescents at high risk for developing bipolar I disorder. J Clin Psychiatry 68:789–795, 2007a

DelBello MP, Findling RL, Earley WR, et al: Efficacy of quetiapine in children and adolescents with bipolar mania: a 3-week, double-blind, randomized, placebo-controlled trial. Paper presented at the annual meeting of the American College of Neuropsychopharmacology, Boca Raton, FL, December 2007b

DelBello M, Findling RL, Wang PP, et al: Safety and efficacy of ziprasidone in pediatric bipolar disorder (abstract 892). Biol Psychiatry 63(suppl):283S, 2008

Denicoff KD, Smith-Jackson EE, Disney ER, et al: Preliminary evidence of the reliability and validity of the prospective life-chart methodology (LCM-p). J Psychiatr Res 31:593–603, 1997

Findling RL, McNamara NK, Youngstrom EA, et al: Double-blind 18-month trial of lithium versus divalproex maintenance treatment in pediatric bipolar disorder. J Am Acad Child Adolesc Psychiatry 44:409–417, 2005

Findling RL, Frazier TW, Youngstrom EA, et al: Double-blind, placebo-controlled trial of divalproex monotherapy in the treatment of symptomatic youth at high risk for developing bipolar disorder. J Clin Psychiatry 68:781–788, 2007a

Findling RL, Short EJ, McNamara NK, et al: Methylphenidate in the treatment of children and adolescents with bipolar disorder and attention-deficit/hyperactivity disorder. J Am Acad Child Adolesc Psychiatry 46:1445–1453, 2007b

Fristad MA, Weller EB, Weller RA: The Mania Rating Scale: can it be used in children? A preliminary report. J Am Acad Child Adolesc Psychiatry 31:252–257, 1992

Fristad MA, Goldberg-Arnold JS, Gavazzi SM: Multi-family psychoeducation groups in the treatment of children with mood disorders. J Marital Fam Ther 29:491–504, 2003

Frye MA, Ketter TA, Kimbrell TA, et al: A placebo-controlled study of lamotrigine and gabapentin monotherapy in refractory mood disorders. J Clin Psychopharmacol 20:607–614, 2000

Geddes JR, Calabrese JR, Goodwin GM: Lamotrigine for treatment of bipolar depression: independent meta-analysis and meta-regression of individual patient data from five randomised trials. Br J Psychiatry 194:4–9, 2009

Geller B, Luby J: Child and adolescent bipolar disorder: a review of the past 10 years. J Am Acad Child Adolesc Psychiatry 36:1168–1176, 1997

Geller B, Fox LW, Clark KA: Rate and predictors of prepubertal bipolarity during follow-up of 6- to 12-year-old depressed children. J Am Acad Child Adolesc Psychiatry 33:461–468, 1994

Geller B, Cooper TB, Sun K, et al: Double-blind and placebo-controlled study of lithium for adolescent bipolar disorders with secondary substance dependency. J Am Acad Child Adolesc Psychiatry 37:171–178, 1998a

Geller B, Cooper TB, Zimerman B, et al: Lithium for prepubertal depressed children with family history predictors of future bipolarity: a double-blind, placebo-controlled study. J Affect Disord 51:165–175, 1998b

Geller B, Bolhofner K, Craney JL, et al: Psychosocial functioning in a prepubertal and early adolescent bipolar disorder phenotype. J Am Acad Child Adolesc Psychiatry 39:1543–1548, 2000a

Geller B, Zimerman B, Williams M, et al: Diagnostic characteristics of 93 cases of a prepubertal and early adolescent bipolar disorder phenotype by gender, puberty and comorbid attention deficit hyperactivity disorder. J Child Adolesc Psychopharmacol 10:157–164, 2000b

Geller B, Zimerman B, Williams M, et al: Six-month stability and outcome of a prepubertal and early adolescent bipolar disorder phenotype. J Child Adolesc Psychopharmacol 10:165–173, 2000c

Geller B, Tillman R, Craney JL, et al: Four-year prospective outcome and natural history of mania in children with a prepubertal and early adolescent bipolar disorder phenotype. Arch Gen Psychiatry 61:459–467, 2004

Gibbons RD, Brown CH, Hur K, et al: Early evidence on the effects of regulators' suicidality warnings on SSRI prescriptions and suicide in children and adolescents. Am J Psychiatry 164:1356–1363, 2007

Goodwin GM, Bowden CL, Calabrese JR, et al: A pooled analysis of 2 placebo-controlled 18-month trials of lamotrigine and lithium maintenance in bipolar I disorder. J Clin Psychiatry 65:432–441, 2004

Harpaz-Rotem I, Leslie DL, Martin A, et al: Changes in child and adolescent inpatient psychiatric admission diagnoses between 1995 and 2000. Soc Psychiatry Psychiatr Epidemiol 40:642–647, 2005

Hsu LK: Lithium-resistant adolescent mania. J Am Acad Child Psychiatry 25:280–283, 1986

Johnson SL, McMurrich S: Life events and juvenile bipolar disorder: conceptual issues and early findings. Dev Psychopathol 18:1169–1179, 2006

Kafantaris V, Coletti DJ, Dicker R, et al: Adjunctive antipsychotic treatment of adolescents with bipolar psychosis. J Am Acad Child Adolesc Psychiatry 40:1448–1456, 2001

Kafantaris V, Coletti DJ, Dicker R, et al: Lithium treatment of acute mania in adolescents: a placebo-controlled discontinuation study. J Am Acad Child Adolesc Psychiatry 43:984–993, 2004

Klein DJ, Cottingham EM, Sorter M, et al: A randomized, double-blind, placebo-controlled trial of metformin treatment of weight gain associated with initiation of atypical antipsychotic therapy in children and adolescents. Am J Psychiatry 163:2072–2079, 2006

Kowatch RA, DelBello MP: Pediatric bipolar disorder: emerging diagnostic and treatment approaches. Child Adolesc Psychiatr Clin N Am 15:73–108, 2006

Kowatch RA, Suppes T, Gilfillan SK: Clozapine treatment of children and adolescents with bipolar disorder and schizophrenia: a clinical case series. J Child Adolesc Psychopharmacol 5:241–253, 1995

Kowatch RA, Suppes T, Carmody TJ, et al: Effect size of lithium, divalproex sodium, and carbamazepine in children and adolescents with bipolar disorder. J Am Acad Child Adolesc Psychiatry 39:713–720, 2000

Kowatch RA, Sethuraman G, Hume JH, et al: Combination pharmacotherapy in children and adolescents with bipolar disorder. Biol Psychiatry 53:978–984, 2003

Kowatch RA, Fristad M, Birmaher B, et al: Treatment guidelines for children and adolescents with bipolar disorder. J Am Acad Child Adolesc Psychiatry 44:213–235, 2005

Kushner SF, Khan A, Lane R, et al: Topiramate monotherapy in the management of acute mania: results of four double-blind placebo-controlled trials. Bipolar Disord 8:15–27, 2006

Lewinsohn PM, Seeley JR, Klein DN: Bipolar disorders during adolescence. Acta Psychiatr Scand Suppl 418:47–50, 2003

Lofthouse N, Fristad MA: Psychosocial interventions for children with early onset bipolar spectrum disorder. Clin Child Fam Psychol Rev 7:71–88, 2004

Madaan V, Chang KD: Pharmacotherapeutic strategies for pediatric bipolar disorder. Expert Opin Pharmacother 8:1801–1819, 2007

Masi G, Mucci M, Millepiedi S: Clozapine in adolescent inpatients with acute mania. J Child Adolesc Psychopharmacol 12:93–99, 2002

McClellan J, Kowatch R, Findling RL: Practice parameter for the assessment and treatment of children and adolescents with bipolar disorder. J Am Acad Child Adolesc Psychiatry 46:107–125, 2007

Miklowitz DJ: An update on the role of psychotherapy in the management of bipolar disorder. Curr Psychiatry Rep 8:498–503, 2006

Miklowitz DJ, Simoneau TL, George EL, et al: Family focused treatment of bipolar disorder: 1-year effects of a psychoeducational program in conjunction with pharmacotherapy. Biol Psychiatry 48:582–592, 2000

Miklowitz DJ, George EL, Axelson DA, et al: Family focused treatment for adolescents with bipolar disorder. J Affect Disord 82 (suppl 1):S113–S128, 2004

Miklowitz DJ, Axelson DA, Birmaher B, et al: Family-focused treatment for adolescents with bipolar disorder: results of a 2-year randomized trial. Arch Gen Psychiatry 65:1053–1061, 2008

Moore CM, Demopulos CM, Henry ME, et al: Brain-to-serum lithium ratio and age: in vivo magnetic resonance spectroscopy study. Am J Psychiatry 159:1240–1242, 2002

Moreno C, Laje G, Blanco C, et al: National trends in the outpatient diagnosis and treatment of bipolar disorder in youth. Arch Gen Psychiatry 64:1032–1039, 2007

Pande AC, Crockatt J, Janney CA, et al; Gabapentin Bipolar Disorder Study Group: Gabapentin in bipolar disorder: a placebo-controlled trial of adjunctive therapy. Bipolar Disord 2:249–255, 2000

Pavuluri MN, Graczyk PA, Henry DB, et al: Child- and family-focused cognitive-behavioral therapy for pediatric bipolar disorder: development and preliminary results. J Am Acad Child Adolesc Psychiatry 43:528–537, 2004a

Pavuluri MN, Henry DB, Carbray JA, et al: Open-label prospective trial of risperidone in combination with lithium or divalproex sodium in pediatric mania. J Affect Disord 82 (suppl 1):S103–S111, 2004b

Pavuluri MN, Birmaher B, Naylor MW: Pediatric bipolar disorder: a review of the past 10 years. J Am Acad Child Adolesc Psychiatry 44:846–871, 2005

Pavuluri MN, O'Connor MM, Harral EM, et al: Impact of neurocognitive function on academic difficulties in pediatric bipolar disorder: a clinical translation. Biol Psychiatry 60:951–956, 2006a

Pavuluri MN, Schenkel LS, Aryal S, et al: Neurocognitive function in unmedicated manic and medicated euthymic pediatric bipolar patients. Am J Psychiatry 163:286–293, 2006b

Perlis RH, Miyahara S, Marangell LB, et al: Long-term implications of early onset in bipolar disorder: data from the first 1000 participants in the Systematic Treatment Enhancement Program for Bipolar Disorder (STEP-BD). Biol Psychiatry 55:875–881, 2004

Physicians' Desk Reference, 62nd Edition. Montvale, NJ, Thomson Healthcare, 2008

Pliszka SR, Sherman JO, Barrow MV, et al: Affective disorder in juvenile offenders: a preliminary study. Am J Psychiatry 157:130–132, 2000

Post RM, Kowatch RA: The health care crisis of childhood-onset bipolar illness: some recommendations for its amelioration. J Clin Psychiatry 67:115–125, 2006

Räsänen P, Tiihonen J, Hakko H: The incidence and onset-age of hospitalized bipolar affective disorder in Finland. J Affect Disord 48:63–68, 1998

Reichart CG, Nolen WA: Earlier onset of bipolar disorder in children by antidepressants or stimulants? An hypothesis. J Affect Disord 78:81–84, 2004

Reimers A, Skogvoll E, Sund JK, et al: Drug interactions between lamotrigine and psychoactive drugs: evidence from a therapeutic drug monitoring service. J Clin Psychopharmacol 25:342–348, 2005

Rucklidge JJ: Impact of ADHD on the neurocognitive functioning of adolescents with bipolar disorder. Biol Psychiatry 60:921–928, 2006

Saxena K, Howe M, Simeonova D, et al: Divalproex sodium reduces overall aggression in youth at high risk for bipolar disorder. J Child Adolesc Psychopharmacol 16:252–259, 2006

Scheffer RE, Kowatch RA, Carmody T, et al: Randomized, placebo-controlled trial of mixed amphetamine salts for symptoms of comorbid ADHD in pediatric bipolar disorder after mood stabilization with divalproex sodium. Am J Psychiatry 162:58–64, 2005

Singh MK, Chang K: The impact of bipolar disorder on selected areas of pediatric development: a research update. Pediatric Health 1:199–215, 2007

Soutullo CA, DelBello MP, Ochsner JE, et al: Severity of bipolarity in hospitalized manic adolescents with history of stimulant or antidepressant treatment. J Affect Disord 70:323–327, 2002

Soutullo CA, Chang KD, Diez-Suarez A, et al: Bipolar disorder in children and adolescents: international perspective on epidemiology and phenomenology. Bipolar Disord 7:497–506, 2005

Strober M, Carlson G: Predictors of bipolar illness in adolescents with major depression: a follow-up investigation. Adolesc Psychiatry 10:299–319, 1982

Thomsen PH, Moller LL, Dehlholm B, et al: Manic-depressive psychosis in children younger than 15 years: a register-based investigation of 39 cases in Denmark. Acta Psychiatr Scand 85:401–406, 1992

Tohen M, Kryzhanovskaya L, Carlson G, et al: Olanzapine versus placebo in the treatment of adolescents with bipolar mania. Am J Psychiatry 164:1547–1556, 2007

Verhulst FC, van der Ende J, Rietbergen A: Ten-year time trends of psychopathology in Dutch children and adolescents: no evidence for strong trends. Acta Psychiatr Scand 96:7–13, 1997

Wagner KD, Kowatch RA, Emslie GJ, et al: A double-blind, randomized, placebo-controlled trial of oxcarbazepine in the treatment of bipolar disorder in children and adolescents. Am J Psychiatry 163:1179–1186, 2006

Wagner KD, Redden L, Kowatch RA, et al: A double-blind, randomized, placebo-controlled trial of divalproex extended-release in the treatment of bipolar disorder in children and adolescents. J Am Acad Child Adolesc Psychiatry 48:519–532, 2009

Weller EB, Weller RA, Fristad MA: Lithium dosage guide for prepubertal children: a preliminary report. J Am Acad Child Psychiatry 25:92–95, 1986

Wilens TE, Biederman J, Kwon A, et al: Risk of substance use disorders in adolescents with bipolar disorder. J Am Acad Child Adolesc Psychiatry 43:1380–1386, 2004

Woolston JL: Case study: carbamazepine treatment of juvenile-onset bipolar disorder. J Am Acad Child Adolesc Psychiatry 38:335–338, 1999

World Health Organization: The ICD-10 Classification of Mental and Behavioural Disorders: Clinical Descriptions and Diagnostic Guidelines. Geneva, World Health Organization, 1992

Youngstrom EA, Duax J: Evidence-based assessment of pediatric bipolar disorder, part I: base rate and family history. J Am Acad Child Adolesc Psychiatry 44:712–717, 2005

CHAPTER 11

Management of Bipolar Disorders in Women

Laurel N. Zappert, Psy.D.

Natalie L. Rasgon, M.D., Ph.D.

Clinically significant gender differences are commonly encountered in the management of medical disorders in general and psychiatric disorders in particular. For example, the prevalence of unipolar major depressive disorder is twice as high in women as in men. Although the prevalence of bipolar disorders is equal between genders, presentations and treatment responses in men and women may differ, and diverse special considerations need to be taken into account when treating female patients with bipolar disorders (Burt and Rasgon 2004).

In this chapter, we review data relevant to best clinical practice in the management of women with bipolar disorders. Topics include the reasons women may be more likely to develop severe forms of the illness, such as rapid cycling; the relationship between the phases of female reproductive life (e.g., menarche, menstrual cycle, pregnancy, menopause) and the course of bipolar disorders; the effects of medications on metabolic and reproductive function in women; and the effects of medication in pregnant and breast-feeding women with bipolar disorders.

Clinical Characteristics: Gender Differences

Although bipolar disorders affect similar numbers of males and females, research has suggested significant gender differences in symptom presentation. For example, bipolar II subtype and rapid-cycling course are overrepresented in women (Tondo and Baldessarini 1998). Many studies have noted gender differences in the clinical course of bipolar disorders, with women tending to suffer more frequently than men from depressive (Angst 1978; Perugi et al. 1990), mixed (McElroy et al. 1995; Taylor and Abrams 1981), and dysphoric hypomanic (Suppes et al. 2005) episodes, and from rapid cycling (Berk and Dodd 2004). While depressed, women also may experience atypical features more often than men (Benazzi 1999).

Research on the etiology and course of seasonal affective disorder and rapid-cycling mood disorders suggests that reproductive hormones may contribute significantly to the course of affective illness during different menstrual cycle phases (Rubinow and Schmidt 2006). In addition, an increased vulnerability for mood episodes in women with bipolar disorders has been reported in relation to the premenstrual period, the postpartum period, and the menopausal transition (Blehar et al. 1998; Marsh et al. 2008).

The number and type of manic episodes also appear to be related to gender. The first affective episode appears more likely to be a major depressive episode in females but a manic episode in males. In women, the predominance of major depressive episodes over manic episodes may be even greater than in men (Roy-Byrne et al. 1985). Rapid cycling (Robb et al. 1998; Tondo and Baldessarini 1998) and mixed mania (Arnold et al. 2000; Kessing 2004; Robb et al. 1998) also occur with greater frequency in women, and both are associated with a poorer prognosis (Keller et al. 1986). A study by Rasgon et al. (2005b) determined that compared with men, women were more likely not only to be depressed but also to have cyclical changes in mood. Women with bipolar disorders are also more likely to experience later onset of mania, impaired physical health, and pain disorders (Robb et al. 1998).

Notable between- and within-group gender differences also occur with regard to comorbidity of alcoholism and bipolar disorders. Specifically, in patients with bipolar disorders, fewer women than men have a lifetime history of alcoholism (29.1% vs. 49.1%). However, women with bipolar disorders are at greater risk for alcoholism compared with the general female population than are men with bipolar disorders in comparison to the general male population (odds ratios 7.4 vs. 2.8) (Frye et al. 2003).

Differences in treatment response may also be attributed to the differences in the clinical presentation between women and men. Although Viguera et al. (2000b) found no gender differences in response to lithium in their review of 17 studies, Freeman and McElroy (1999) noted that mixed states (which respond more poorly to lithium) occurred more frequently in women than in men. Women may also be more likely to receive antidepressant treatment, because depressive symptoms are very much the predominant presentation in women with bipolar disorders. Therefore, some of the risk for rapid cycling in women may reflect greater exposure to the mood-destabilizing effects of antidepressants (Tondo and Baldessarini 1998). Leibenluft suggested that compared with men, women may also be at higher risk for antidepressant-induced hypomania or mania (Leibenluft 1997). It is therefore of particular importance to optimize use of mood stabilizers and only use antidepressants with substantial caution, because antidepressants may be a factor in the development of mania and cycle acceleration in women (Leibenluft 1997).

For treating rapid-cycling bipolar disorder, lithium has only modest efficacy (Dunner and Fieve 1974). Early reports suggested that valproate, carbamazepine, and clozapine were useful for patients with rapid-cycling bipolar disorder (Calabrese et al. 2001). Although both valproate and carbamazepine have been cited as being effective in treating rapid cycling, these medications often require adjunctive agents, including lithium, lamotrigine, and antidepressants (Cruz et al. 2008), although antidepressants may destabilize mood (Ghaemi 2008). One study found that even the combination of open lithium and valproate yielded only modest benefit in rapid cycling (Calabrese et al. 2005).

Some reports have demonstrated lamotrigine's efficacy in depression prophylaxis (Goodwin et al. 2004) and to a more limited extent in acute bipolar depression (Calabrese et al. 1999, 2008). In addition, initial evidence supports lamotrigine's efficacy in treating rapid-cycling bipolar disorder (Becker et al. 2004; Calabrese et al. 2000; Goldberg et al. 2008). Despite encouraging early open reports, later controlled trials suggested that gabapentin and topiramate are not effective as primary therapies in bipolar disorders but may be useful adjuncts for mood or comorbid symptoms.

Although more systematic clinical trials are needed to clarify this issue, some anticonvulsant mood stabilizers may be appropriate for use in female patients. Some of these medications, compared with lithium, may be more effective in treating mixed symptoms (e.g., divalproex or carbamazepine) and depressive symptoms or rapid cycling (e.g., lamotrigine) without increasing the risk of escalation to hypomania or mania. Chapter 9 in this volume discusses the management of rapid-cycling bipolar disorders in detail.

Differential Diagnosis and Evaluation

When an evaluation for bipolar disorders is being conducted, other psychiatric disorders to be considered include major depressive disorder, a condition that is approximately twice as prevalent in women as in men. For women, dysphoric states with prominent irritability may be difficult to distinguish from manic, mixed, or dysphoric hypomanic episodes. As a result, this distinction requires a careful clinical evaluation of the presence of manic or hypomanic symptoms. In addition, bipolar disorder is associated with anxiety disorders, conditions that are also approximately twice as prevalent in women as in men. Alcohol and other substance use disorders, conditions more prevalent in men than in women, co-occur with bipolar disorder in many individuals, and individuals with earlier onset of bipolar I disorder are more likely to have a history of current alcohol or other substance abuse. Individuals with bipolar disorder and concomitant alcohol or other substance use have an increased number of hospitalizations and a poorer course of illness.

In addition to other psychiatric disorders, medical disorders that should be considered include thyroid disorder and other endocrinopathies that may have differential prevalences and presentations in women compared with men. As described in Chapter 12, "Management of Bipolar Disorders in Older Adults," if the age at onset for a first manic episode is over 40 years, the symptoms may more likely be due to a general medical condition or substance use than to primary bipolar disorders.

Careful attention to menstrual history is crucial for the optimal management of bipolar disorders in women. Thus, it is important to assess baseline menstrual history and related questions (Table 11–1) and reproductive cycle history, and repeat menstrual history and related questions yearly, and if clinically significant weight gain ($\geq 7\%$) or new onset of menstrual abnormalities or hirsutism occurs.

Treatment

In treating bipolar I disorder, it is best to follow evidence-based pharmacotherapy as described elsewhere in this volume. Patients should be given the lowest effective dosages of drugs, to minimize side effects. Monotherapy is the preferred treatment regimen unless more than one agent is absolutely needed. Be-

TABLE 11–1. Menstrual history and related questions

- How often do you menstruate a year?
- How long is your cycle?
- Do you have any irregular bleeding, including spotting?
- Is there pain when you menstruate, and how much pain?
- Do you have any black hair growth on your abdomen, breasts, face, or back?
- Have you noticed recent weight gain?
- Have you noticed your hairline receding or hair loss?

fore proceeding to the continuation phase of treatment, the clinician needs to be certain that the patient is stable and has shown acute response (clinically significant improvement) or, better still, remission (virtual absence of mood symptoms), recognizing that improvement can be slow and that some medications may take 4–6 weeks to achieve steady state in the patient's blood. When treating women of childbearing age, the clinician needs to discuss the possibility of pregnancy before treating with psychotropic medications, because of the risk of adverse effects to the fetus.

Another consideration when treating women is the effects of certain medications on metabolic and reproductive functioning. Although lithium, certain anticonvulsants (valproate, carbamazepine, lamotrigine), and second-generation antipsychotics (olanzapine, risperidone, quetiapine, ziprasidone, and aripiprazole) have demonstrated acute and/or prophylactic efficacy in bipolar disorders, these medications may alter metabolic and endocrine function, as described in other chapters in this volume. Treatment decisions must therefore include careful consideration of the interactions between medications and metabolic and reproductive endocrine function.

Metabolic Consequences of Bipolar Disorder and Treatment

People with bipolar disorders and other serious mental illnesses are at elevated risk for developing metabolic disorders (Garcia-Portilla et al. 2008; van Winkel et al. 2008). Other physiological alterations have been observed, including dysregulation of the hypothalamic-pituitary-adrenal axis, a common finding in patients with bipolar disorders, yielding hypercortisolemia, which is associated with a high risk for metabolic syndrome (Rasgon et al. 2005a). In a study of women with bipolar disorders taking antimanic medications, Rasgon et al. (2005a) found a significant positive correlation of body mass index with insulin resistance and free testosterone levels, which was independent of medication used. Because of these associations, patients treated for bipolar disorders should be monitored closely for weight gain and, if feasible, treated with agents that are not associated with weight gain.

Bipolar Disorder and Obesity

Fagiolini et al. (2003) evaluated the relationship of obesity to demographic and clinical characteristics, in addition to treatment outcome, in 175 patients with bipolar I disorder. Of the subjects who were treated for an acute affective episode and followed through a period of maintenance treatment, 35.4% met criteria for obesity. Overall, the obese patients had fewer years of education, had more previous depressive and manic episodes, had higher baseline Hamilton Rating Scale for Depression scores, and required more time in acute treatment to stabilize mood. Furthermore, the number of patients experiencing a depressive recurrence was significantly higher in the obese than in the nonobese group, suggesting that obesity is correlated with a poorer outcome in patients with bipolar disorders.

Metabolic Syndrome

The management of female patients with bipolar disorders may often be complicated by concern about weight gain and other metabolic effects of psychotropic drugs, as well as preexisting obesity and metabolic problems. Obesity and diabetes are both strongly associated with metabolic syndrome, a set of co-occurring abnormalities that include insulin resistance, impaired glucose tolerance, abdominal obesity, disturbances of lipid metabolism, hypertension, microalbuminuria, and prothrombotic and proinflammatory states (Grundy et al. 2004). The health implications of metabolic syndrome are striking, including a three- to fivefold increase in cardiovascular disease mortality (Alexander et al. 2003; Bonora et al. 2004; Lakka et al. 2002) and a sixfold increase in risk for developing type 2 diabetes (Laaksonen et al. 2002). Therefore, health care providers need to take into account a medication's weight gain and metabolic profiles when making a decision about treatment.

Weight Changes With Central Nervous System Drugs

Weight gain is a common adverse effect of pharmacotherapy for bipolar disorders, with a predominant increase in central adiposity (Vestergaard et al. 1988). Increased rates of impaired glucose tolerance and diabetes have been correlated with antipsychotic and antidepressant use (Müller-Oerlinghausen et al. 1978; Paykel et al. 1973). Weight increases have also been observed in patients receiving acute and maintenance treatment with the mood stabilizers lithium (Bowden et al. 2000, 2006; Sachs et al. 2006) and divalproex (Bowden et al. 2000) and with the second-generation antipsychotics olanzapine (Tohen et al. 2006), clozapine (Leppig et al. 1989), risperidone (Vieta et al. 2001), and quetiapine (Adler et al. 2007) (Table 11–2). Carbamazepine (Ketter et al. 2004) and aripiprazole (Keck et al. 2006) appear less likely to cause weight gain. Chronic high-dose gabapentin has also been associated with weight gain (DeToledo et al. 1997). Interestingly, divalproex is associated with a lower mean weight gain than olanzapine. Possibly because of its binding to peroxisome proliferator-activated receptor alpha (PPARα), valproate may yield beneficial lipid changes (as seen with fibrates) (Horie and Suga 1985) and increased weight but improved metabolism (as with thiazolidinediones) (Lampen et al. 2001).

Medications that are considered weight neutral include lamotrigine (Bowden et al. 2006; Sachs et al. 2006), oxcarbazepine (Reinstein et al. 2003), and ziprasidone (Warrington et al. 2007). In contrast, medications that have been found to decrease weight include bupropion (Anderson et al. 2002), topiramate (Kushner et al. 2006), and zonisamide (Gadde et al. 2003; Wang et al. 2008).

Managing Weight Gain

Patients should be advised of the risk of weight gain with medications, counseled to use diet and exercise to avoid gaining weight, and carefully monitored for weight gain to facilitate early intervention. The risk of weight gain needs to be considered when choosing agents, especially agents that may be used in longer-term treatment. If weight gain is detected, options that need to be considered include additional efforts with diet and exercise, minimizing dosages of

TABLE 11–2. Weight change with central nervous system drugs

Increase	Neutral	Decrease
Clozapine ↑↑↑	Ziprasidone	Topiramate ↓↓
Olanzapine ↑↑↑	Oxcarbazepine	Zonisamide ↓↓
Divalproex ↑↑	Lamotrigine	Bupropion ↓
Lithium ↑↑		
Risperidone ↑		
Quetiapine ↑		
Carbamazepine ↑		
Aripiprazole ↑		
Gabapentin ↑		

medications with dosage-related weight gain, and switching to medication(s) with lower likelihood for causing weight gain. In some instances, none of these options will prove feasible, in which case the use of adjunctive agents to permit weight loss may need to be considered.

Topiramate (50–200 mg/day) may yield weight loss and may maintain weight loss (Astrup et al. 2004). However, topiramate has potential adverse effects, including cognitive impairment, which can compound the impairment associated with the mood state and that related to the concomitant use of other medications, such as lithium. Cognitive impairment associated with topiramate use may be minimized by slow titration (by increments of 25 mg/day every 1 or 2 weeks) and taking topiramate in a single dose at bedtime.

Sustained-release bupropion (300–450 mg/day) has an anorectic effect, which is more robust at 450 mg/day in some obese individuals. For instance, obese subjects with depressive symptoms, but not major depressive disorder, lost an average of 4.6% of baseline weight during treatment with 300–400 mg/day of sustained-release bupropion, compared with a 1.8% loss among placebo recipients (Jain et al. 2002). As it may be activating, bupropion is dosed early in the day.

Zonisamide, 400–600 mg/day, has also been shown to decrease weight. In a study by Gadde et al. (2003), 57% of the treatment group lost more than 5% of body weight, compared with 10% of the placebo group. In another controlled trial, zonisamide yielded more weight loss than placebo in obese patients with binge-eating disorder (McElroy et al. 2006). In an open study, zonisamide yielded weight loss in obese, medicated patients with euthymic bipolar disorder (Wang et al. 2008). However, central nervous system and gastrointestinal adverse effects may limit zonisamide's utility. Because of adverse effects and a long half-life, zonisamide needs to be gradually titrated (e.g., starting with 100 mg/day and increasing every 2 weeks by 100 mg/day). A single bedtime dose may yield better tolerability.

Finally, sibutramine, a serotonin-norepinephrine reuptake inhibitor, has been approved by the U.S. Food and Drug Administration for weight loss since 1997. Some data suggest that sibutramine reduces triglyceride levels and increases high-density lipoprotein cholesterol levels in obese patients with dyslipidemia. In a placebo-controlled trial, adjunctive sibutramine yielded weight loss in patients with schizophrenia or schizoaffective disorder who were taking olanzapine (Henderson et al. 2005). In a randomized trial in overweight or obese bipolar disorder patients with psychotropic-associated weight gain, adjunctive sibutramine and topiramate had comparable weight loss effects, but both were associated with similarly high discontinuation rates (McElroy et al. 2007). Because sibutramine can cause hypertension, blood pressure needs to be monitored. Sibutramine is commonly started at 10 mg/day and increased to 15 mg/day after 4 weeks.

Medication Effects on Reproductive Function

Mood stabilizers, anticonvulsants, and some antipsychotics may influence serum levels of reproductive hormones and consequently impact reproductive function. In women, the investigation of the effects of these medications on reproductive endocrine function is especially crucial. Although most second-generation antipsychotics generally have modest effects on prolactin, risperidone and first-generation antipsychotics can yield clinically significant prolactin elevation, resulting in galactorrhea, menstrual irregularities, and problems with sexual desire and function.

Knowledge is limited of anticonvulsants' effects on the reproductive endocrine function of women with bipolar disorders. However, a few studies have been published that specifically address medication effects on reproductive endocrine function in women with bipolar disorders (Joffe et al. 2006b; Rasgon et al. 2000). In addition, several reports have addressed this topic in women with epilepsy. Specifically, studies have suggested an association between anticonvulsants used in treating epilepsy and reproductive abnormalities in both girls and women ranging from menstrual dysfunction to polycystic ovary syndrome (PCOS). Vainionpää et al. (1999) reported valproate-induced hyperandrogenism during pubertal maturation in 41 girls with epilepsy, ages 8–18 years, and found that the mean serum testosterone concentrations of prepubertal, pubertal, and postpubertal female adolescents taking valproate were significantly higher than those in age-matched control groups. Additionally, the postpubertal female adolescents taking valproate were more often obese than the controls. These consequences and their clinical implications have stimulated further investigation of the effect of anticonvulsants on female reproductive function.

Polycystic Ovary Syndrome in Women With Bipolar Disorder

PCOS is a serious endocrine disorder, characterized by ovulatory dysfunction and hyperandrogenism, that is thought to have a higher prevalence in women with bipolar disorders. Limited data suggest that the risk of bipolar disorder may be increased in women with PCOS (Klipstein and Goldberg 2006). Various theories have been offered to explain the higher prevalence of PCOS and other reproductive disorders in bipolar disorders, including the effects of the disease itself and of anticonvulsant drugs. In particular, valproate may directly cause PCOS or indirectly lead to the disorder by causing weight gain that triggers insulin resistance, increased testosterone levels, and other reproductive abnormalities.

As listed in Table 11–3, clinical manifestations of PCOS include hirsutism, seborrhea, acne, alopecia, menstrual irregularities, obesity, and infertility (Dunaif et al. 1989). Anovulation resulting from PCOS may manifest clinically as amenorrhea or irregular menses and ultimately may result in infertility. Although PCOS does not by definition require the presence of polycystic ovaries, these are very common in PCOS.

A definitive association between reproductive endocrine function and treatment of bipolar disorders, however, has not been established (O'Donovan et al. 2002). Emerging data are providing more information on the prevalence of PCOS in women with bipolar disorder receiving mood stabilizers. Data from the Systematic Treatment Enhancement Program for Bipolar Disorder (STEP-BD) study suggest that valproate use in adult females may carry a modest risk of PCOS, because nine of 86 women (10.5%) taking valproate developed PCOS (Joffe et al. 2006b). Of the 230 women who were evaluated, 2 (1.4%) of 144 women taking lithium or a nonvalproate anticonvulsant (e.g., lamotrigine, topiramate, gabapentin, carbamazepine, oxcarbazepine) and 9 (10.5%) of 86 women taking valproate developed oligomenorrhea with hyperandrogenism. In addition, in the valproate-treated women who developed oligomenorrhea, it always developed within 12 months of starting valproate.

In a follow-up study of the valproate-treated women who developed new-onset menstrual cycle irregularities and hyperandrogenism, Joffe et al. (2006a) attempted to determine whether discontinuation of valproate resulted in a reversal of PCOS features. Of the seven women who developed PCOS associated with valproate use, three of four women who discontinued valproate achieved remission from PCOS reproductive features, whereas PCOS persisted in all three women who continued valproate use. Overall, improved reproductive features of PCOS were seen in most valproate discontinuers, including a trend for lower serum testosterone ($P=0.06$), despite static body weight, indicating that menstrual cycle–related mood changes can be reversed after valproate cessation. Larger controlled trials are needed to further examine the effects of valproate cessation on female reproductive function.

Rasgon et al. (2005a) examined reproductive function and prevalence of PCOS in women, ages 18–45 years, who were taking antimanic medications to treat bipolar disorders. Fifty-two of the 80 female participants (65%) reported current menstrual abnormalities, and 40 of 80 (50%) subjects reported one or

TABLE 11–3.   Clinical signs of polycystic ovary syndrome

- Hirsutism
- Seborrhea
- Acne
- Alopecia

- Menstrual irregularities
- Obesity
- Infertility

more menstrual abnormalities that preceded the diagnosis of bipolar disorders. Of the 15 (38%) who reported developing menstrual abnormalities after starting treatment for bipolar disorders, 14 developed abnormalities after beginning valproate treatment ($P=0.04$). In addition, three of the 50 women (6%) taking valproate and none of the 22 taking other antimanic medications met criteria for PCOS.

Rasgon et al. (2005c) conducted a separate longitudinal study as a follow-up to findings from several cross-sectional studies that reported high rates of menstrual abnormalities in women with bipolar disorders, which in some cases were associated with valproate use (Rasgon 2003; Rasgon et al. 2000, 2002, 2003a, 2003b, 2005b). Reproductive endocrine and metabolic function was evaluated in 25 women, ages 18–45, treated for bipolar disorders over a 2-year time period while controlling for valproate use (Rasgon et al. 2005c). At study commencement, 10 subjects were currently receiving valproate as a mood-stabilizing agent. Of the remaining subjects, six were receiving lithium and five were receiving second-generation antipsychotics. Forty percent of all subjects reported oligomenorrhea before starting medication, whereas 41.7% reported current oligomenorrhea. However, rates of oligomenorrhea and clinical hyperandrogenism did not differ by medication use. Additionally, 80% of women had a high homeostatic model assessment of insulin resistance at baseline, while all other measures were normal. All subjects exhibited a significant decrease in luteal phase progesterone and increase in free testosterone concentrations over time, and valproate use was associated with an increase over time in total testosterone.

Overall, the findings from these studies suggest that valproate may be associated with new-onset oligomenorrhea and hyperandrogenism, which are characteristic of PCOS. Weight gain associated with use of valproate may be responsible for these neuroendocrine effects; however, the evidence regarding the possible impact of weight on neuroendocrine dysfunction in bipolar disorder is inconclusive. Further controlled studies are needed to investigate the effects of these medications on reproductive function.

Hormonal Contraceptives and Treatment of Bipolar Disorder

When initiating therapy for bipolar disorders, the clinician needs to consider that some medications may alter the efficacy of hormonal contraceptives (Burt and Rasgon 2004). Mood stabilizers such as carbamazepine and to a lesser extent oxcarbazepine and topiramate (for the latter, especially above 200 mg/day) may affect the metabolism of hormonal contraceptives, presumably by inducing hepatic cytochrome P450 3A4 activity and thus decreasing levels of hormonal contraceptives (Crawford 2002).

Likewise, hormonal contraceptives may alter the efficacy of other medications. Sabers et al. (2001) presented a case series of seven women with epilepsy who received hormonal contraceptives while being treated with lamotrigine to determine the effect of hormonal contraceptives on lamotrigine plasma levels. Overall, hormonal contraceptives reduced lamotrigine plasma levels by 41%–64%, with a mean decrease in plasma lamotrigine levels of 49%. The authors concluded that women with epilepsy who are treated with both lamotrigine and hormonal contraceptives should have their lamotrigine plasma levels monitored closely and their lamotrigine dosage adjusted as necessary. No drug interactions with hormonal contraceptives have been reported to date with valproate, lithium, gabapentin, or the second-generation antipsychotics (*Physicians' Desk Reference* 2008).

The potential mood-stabilizing effects of hormonal contraceptives in women are worthy of examination. In the previously mentioned study of mood changes across the menstrual cycle, women taking hormonal contraceptives did not have significant mood changes, whereas those not taking hormonal contraceptives did have significant mood changes (Rasgon et al. 2003a). This finding is consistent with several studies that have reported the mood-stabilizing effects of exogenous gonadal steroids in women with treatment-resistant bipolar disorder (Chouinard et al. 1987; Hatotani et al. 1979; Price and Giannini 1985). Similar effects in women with PCOS have been observed, as hormonal contraceptive treatment has been associated with decreased rates of depression (Pearlstein and Steiner 2000). In addition, hormonal contraceptives may ameliorate perimenstrual mood changes in women with premenstrual syndrome (Patten and Lamarre 1992). However, in healthy women, exogenous gonadal steroids, such as those used for hormonal contraception or hormonal replacement, can affect mood negatively (Price and DiMarzio 1986). Thus, some women with bipolar disorders, as well as some women with PCOS and premenstrual syndrome, may represent subpopulations in which hormonal contraceptives may have mood-stabilizing effects. Taken together, these studies of the effects of hormonal contraceptives on those patients with endocrine and mood disorders may represent a link between reproductive endocrine dysfunction and affective illness. Because the effects of hormonal contraceptives are heterogeneous, clinicians need to ascertain whether the mood effects of hormonal contraceptives for a particular patient are positive, negative, or neutral.

Treatment During Pregnancy

In pregnant patients with bipolar disorders, the potential for the development of fetal or neonatal adverse effects should be considered when assessing the use of medications (Burt and Rasgon 2004). Potential side effects include intrauterine death, perinatal toxicity, teratogenicity, growth retardation, and neurobehavioral toxicity (Holmes et al. 2001). Other considerations include special treatment issues associated with pregnancy (e.g., the need for dosage adjustments) and risk of recurrence and exacerbation of mood episodes. Substantial risk for relapse has been found to exist during the pregnancy period following discontinuation of mood-stabilizing medication (Viguera et al. 2002). Viguera and associates found similar rates of recurrence during the first 40 weeks after lithium discontinuation for women who were pregnant (52%) and those not pregnant (58%); however, relapse rates had been much lower for both groups in the year before lithium was discontinued (21%) (Viguera et al. 2000a).

As previously discussed, information remains limited regarding the risk of recurrence of bipolar disorders in pregnant women after discontinuation of lithium or other mood stabilizers. Although teratogenic effects of lithium (Ebstein's anomaly in 0.1%) (Cohen et al. 1994), valproate (neural tube defects and other major malformations in as many as 10%) (Koren et al. 2006), and carbamazepine (spina bifida in 3%, craniofacial defects in 11%, fingernail hypoplasia in 26%, and developmental delay in 20%) (Jones et al. 1989; Rosa 1991) are fairly well documented, the same cannot be said for most second-generation antipsychotics and other anticonvulsants, many of which have emerged more recently (see Table 11–4). Recent data indicate that the malformation risk with valproate is greater than had previously been appreciated, but the malformation risk with lamotrigine may be comparable to that with no anticonvulsant exposure and lower than that with valproate (Cunnington and Tennis 2005). A preliminary study demonstrated no increased risk of teratogenicity in 23 cases during which olanzapine was used antenatally (Goldstein et al. 2000).

Teratogenic effects in pregnancy have not been demonstrated with use of verapamil. In an uncontrolled naturalistic study of 37 women with bipolar disorders, Wisner et al. (2002) found that verapamil was effective for acute treatment

TABLE 11–4.　Evaluations of bipolar treatment during pregnancy

Medication	Treatment concerns and *recommendations*
Lithium	Greatest concerns: higher rate of cardiovascular abnormalities and lithium toxicity, in addition to Epstein's anomaly in 0.1%. *Monitor lithium levels during delivery.*
Valproate	Human teratogen: neural tube defects and other malformations (risk as high as 10%), possible neurocognitive adverse effects, and complications at delivery. *Switch patient's medication before conception; supplement with folate.*
Carbamazepine	Low birth weight and human teratogen: spina bifida in 3%, craniofacial defects in 11%, fingernail hypoplasia in 26%, and developmental delay in 20%. *Avoid use during pregnancy if possible; supplement with vitamin K and folate.*
Lamotrigine	Normal rates of defects overall, but modest increase in occurence of cleft lip and/or palate; rash, hepatotoxicity, and fetal metabolism of drug. *Currently cleared for use during pregnancy.*
First-generation antipsychotic	No increased rate of malformation; some short-lived withdrawal and extrapyramidal symptoms in infants. *May want to switch patient to antipsychotic if deemed effective.*
Second-generation antipsychotic	Limited data. Olanzapine associated with weight gain, insulin resistance, gestational diabetes, and preeclampsia. *Monitor patient's weight, glucose, and blood pressure.*
Calcium channel blockers	Efficacy in bipolar disorder treatment unproven, but data show no drug-related reproductive adverse effects. *Consider use, but beware of potential efficacy limitations.*
Benzodiazepines	Potential increased risk for cleft lip and/or palate, possible developmental delay. Withdrawal symptoms observed. *Neonatal toxicity should be monitored. High-potency compounds may be preferable.*
Electroconvulsive therapy (ECT)	Few side effects and risks. *Fetal cardiac monitoring should be used to detect arrhythmias. ECT parameters should be adjusted according to hormone levels.* Additional concerns regarding anesthesiology during pregnancy. *Consider use in very acute and/or severe mood disturbance.*

of mania and for prevention of bipolar recurrence when used as a maintenance medication. However, a small, uncontrolled trial of verapamil in acute mania was negative (Janicak et al. 1998), and more adequately powered controlled studies are necessary to ascertain the efficacy of verapamil before it can be considered effective (Leibenluft 2000).

Although limited data suggest that lithium discontinuation during pregnancy carries relapse rates similar to discontinuation at other times, further studies are needed to assess the effect of discontinuation of medication and resulting acute psychiatric illness on fetal development (Viguera et al. 2002). However, the following recommendations are helpful if the pregnant patient is to be treated with mood stabilizers.

- Pharmacotherapy
  - Pharmacotherapy during pregnancy should be avoided if clinically possible (Iqbal et al. 2001), especially during the first trimester. This, however, may not be possible for women with bipolar disorders, who have historically demonstrated rapid relapse upon discontinuation of mood stabilizers. Discontinuation of medications in women with histories of suicidal depression or psychotic manias should be approached with particular caution.
  - During pregnancy, monotherapy is preferred, and the woman should be treated with the minimal effective dosage of medication that sustains psychiatric stability (Iqbal et al. 2001). Partial treatment carries the risks of both teratogenesis and maternal psychiatric decompensation (Llewellyn et al. 1998).
  - Dosing changes related to hemodynamic changes, reduced absorption, liver metabolism changes, and decreased protein binding may be required during pregnancy. Dosage requirements may rise during pregnancy, in part because of the increased extracellular fluid volume. Following delivery, prepregnancy dosages should be reinstated, unless acute postpartum destabilization occurs.

- Psychotherapy
  - Psychotherapy may be a useful adjunctive treatment. In an uncontrolled small study of 13 pregnant depressed women utilizing a modified version of interpersonal psychotherapy, all subjects appeared to respond with full remission of depressive symptoms (Spinelli 1997). Although interpersonal psychotherapy has been endorsed as a treatment for major de-

pression with postpartum onset (O'Hara et al. 2000), no reports have been published on the efficacy of psychotherapy in the management of bipolar disorders during pregnancy.

- Women with bipolar disorders should be encouraged to seek support from family and friends for infant care, optimize sleep, and minimize other responsibilities. Support from the partner has been of significant benefit for women experiencing postpartum depression (Rapkin et al. 2002).

- Prenatal Counseling
  - At least 3 months before pregnancy, prenatal counseling should be instituted, and patients should be suitably educated about the known possible risks of taking medications during pregnancy, the genetic risk of transmission of bipolar disorder to offspring, and the risks to the mother and the unborn child of antenatal bipolar decompensation (Iqbal et al. 2001).

- Folate Supplementation
  - Folate supplementation 3 months before conception and continuing into the first trimester of pregnancy may reduce the risk of neural tube defects (Iqbal et al. 2001). Whereas folate supplementation of 0.4 mg/day is recommended for all women of childbearing age to prevent spina bifida and other neural tube defects, dosages of 4 mg/day are recommended for high-risk women who have previously delivered infants with neural tube defects. Although no formal guidelines are available for folic acid supplementation in women taking valproate and carbamazepine, these women are at increased risk for having babies with neural tube defects. Therefore, women with bipolar disorders who are taking these medications should take 4 mg/day of folate when they are actively attempting pregnancy and during the first 3 months of pregnancy ("Use of Psychoactive Medication" 2000).

- Electroconvulsive Therapy
  - Although electroconvulsive therapy is not a standard first-line treatment for bipolar disorders, this treatment modality may be an important alternative to medication during pregnancy, especially in cases of suicidal or homicidal ideation (infanticide) or psychotic decompensation. Llewellyn et al. (1998) found no indication of teratogenesis associated

with electroconvulsive therapy, and the treatment is relatively safe during pregnancy if special precautions are taken to reduce potential risks (Miller 1994).

- Postpartum Management
  - In women who have psychotic decompensation during the postpartum period, treatment should be aggressive, because of the risks to both mother and infant. Early treatment allows the mother to recover and proceed with mother-infant attachment. Because of the particular danger of infanticide, contact between a psychotic mother and infant needs to be regulated and supervised carefully. Hospitalization is often required, especially if the mother appears dangerous to herself or her infant (Rapkin et al. 2002).
  - Recommended treatments for postpartum psychosis include mood stabilizers (e.g., lithium); neuroleptics (high-potency antipsychotics such as haloperidol are preferred over low-potency antipsychotics and are often required for severe psychosis); olanzapine, risperidone, and quetiapine; and electroconvulsive therapy (for those patients who do not respond to pharmacotherapy or whose symptoms threaten to escalate) (Rapkin et al. 2002).

Treatment During Breast-feeding

A substantial risk of relapse, ranging from 20% to 82%, is associated with the postpartum period, and the decision about treatment for prophylaxis is generally decided on the basis of the patient's ability to avoid major mood episodes without medication (Viguera et al. 2002). Studies examining the effectiveness of lithium to attenuate high postpartum risk for recurrence of bipolar disorder have found lithium treatment resulted in a two- to fivefold decrease in postpartum recurrences of bipolar disorder. Specifically, among subjects who remained stable over the first 40 weeks after lithium discontinuation, postpartum recurrences were 2.9 times more frequent than recurrences in nonpregnant women during weeks 41–64 (70% vs. 24%) (Viguera et al. 2000a). For patients with bipolar disorders who chose to breast-feed, continuing antenatal psychotropic treatment into the postpartum period and/or commencing prophylaxis after delivery may also pose very real problems. Many of the medications currently used to treat bipolar disorders lack sufficient data regarding use during breast-feeding. Although breast-feeding has many advantages for maternal-infant bonding and infant health, breast-feeding commonly entails sleep deprivation, which can undermine psychiatric stability in patients with bipolar disorders. In addition, many medications are secreted in breast milk during lactation, posing other treatment dilemmas. Llewellyn et al. (1998) recommended close monitoring of the infant and a low threshold for cessation or suspension of breast-feeding during use of medication. In addition, because breast-feeding does not always prevent conception, patients should receive education about birth control options (Newport et al. 2002).

Conclusion and Practical Suggestions

Of patients with bipolar disorders, women are significantly more likely than men to present with depression, mixed episodes, and rapid cycling, all of which appear to be less responsive to lithium treatment. Because women with bipolar disorders are more likely than men to be treated with antidepressants and to develop rapid cycling and antidepressant-induced mania and hypomania, treating women entails optimal mood stabilization and considerable caution with antidepressants. Although it is an option for treatment, valproate has substantial safety and tolerability limitations in women of reproductive potential. Other treatment alternatives for women with bipolar disorders include the newer anticonvulsant lamotrigine; controlled studies have demonstrated the efficacy of this agent in treating depressive symptoms and rapid cycling, with little evidence of manic switching. To date, reports are lacking on whether other newer anticonvulsants have utility in treating female patients with bipolar disorders and whether these medications will produce fewer side effects (on mood and neuroendocrine function) in women. Although newer anticonvulsants in general do not appear as effective as monotherapy for mania, some of these medications may emerge as useful adjuncts in female patients for mood or comorbid symptoms. However, care must be taken regarding the potential of some such agents to interfere with oral contraception.

During pregnancy, lithium, valproate, and carbamazepine entail teratogenic risk. Recent data indicate that the malformation risk with valproate is greater than had previously been appreciated, but the malformation risk with lamotrigine may be comparable to that with no anticonvulsant exposure and lower than that with valproate. Research has not yet established whether the newer anticonvulsants or second-generation antipsychotics are safe or effective in this regard. At present, of the antimanic mood stabilizers (lithium, carbamazepine, and valproate), lithium may carry a somewhat lower risk of birth defects. However, if the decision is made to treat a woman during pregnancy, it may be most prudent to treat with an agent of proven utility in an individual patient rather than another agent with less putative teratogenicity but unproven utility in that person.

For women who are breast-feeding, lithium is contraindicated, and more data are needed to evaluate the safety of valproate, carbamazepine, lamotrigine, and newer anticonvulsants and second-generation antipsychotics for exposed breast-fed babies.

The influence of the menstrual cycle, pregnancy, postpartum period, and menopause on the course of bipolar illness requires investigation. Considerably more research is needed to elucidate distinctive symptom presentations and the course of bipolar disorders in female patients. Also, the development of treatment guidelines and modalities better suited to the needs of the female bipolar population are needed to optimize the management of bipolar disorder in women.

Case Study: Management of Bipolar Disorders in Women

Ms. White, a 43-year-old, married, white woman, presented with treatment-resistant bipolar II disorder with rapid-cycling course, and a history of monthly mood swings since age 13 years (Becker et al. 2004).

The patient reported worsening of her cyclic mood changes about 4 years prior, and thus started charting her mood changes across the menstrual cycle at that time. She recorded monthly depressive symptoms with an average duration of 2 weeks beginning with the onset of menses, followed by a switch to elevated mood at the time of ovulation that lasted throughout the luteal phase. She documented a total of five syndromal depressions and five syndromal hypomanias within the past year. Medications at the time of evaluation included divalproex 500 mg/day (serum valproate 21 µg/mL) with dosage limited by sedation, venlafaxine 225 mg/day, and levothyroxine 175 µg/day (serum thyrotropin 1.9 µIU/mL).

Ms. White denied any history of suicide attempts, psychotic symptoms, or antidepressant-induced hypomania. She admitted to a history of binge weekend drinking and amphetamine and marijuana use in her teenage years, but denied current drug or alcohol abuse. Prior medication trials included lithium, which yielded fatigue and incoordination; bupropion, which increased irritability; fluoxetine, which yielded mild attenuation of depression; and sertraline, which provided no benefit. Venlafaxine attenuated intensity of depression but caused cycle acceleration. Hormonal contraceptives provided no benefit. Her past medical history was remarkable for thyroidectomy at the age of 15 for hyperthyroidism, followed by chronic replacement therapy with levothyroxine 175 µg/day. The subject was never pregnant.

Because she reported cycle acceleration with venlafaxine, this medication was tapered gradually as lamotrigine was started at 5 mg/day. The daily dosage of lamotrigine was initially increased by 5 mg each week until a dosage of 55 mg/

day was attained, and then accelerated to weekly increments of 10–15 mg/day until a dosage of 300 mg was attained. The patient continued taking divalproex 500 mg/day and levothyroxine 175 μg/day. Computerized daily self-reported mood ratings were obtained from the patient, starting when venlafaxine was discontinued and lamotrigine was started. For a 6-month period, the subject recorded mood, menstrual data, psychiatric medication, and life events daily. The patient also used urine ovulation test kits and basal body temperature charting to track her menstrual cycle.

Upon discontinuation of venlafaxine, the patient initially experienced a longer and more severe than average depression. As lamotrigine was titrated gradually over the next 6 months, the patient's mood cycle amplitude gradually attenuated. She experienced a notable decrease in the severity and duration of depressive symptoms specifically during the follicular phase of the menstrual cycle. Response to lamotrigine was noted at a dosage of 105 mg/day. Remission with lamotrigine was seen at 290 mg/day. Her blood lamotrigine concentration at a dosage of 300 mg/day was 9.3 μg/mL (reference range 4.0–18.0 μg/mL).

The patient experienced a period of recovery for the first time in decades, and this sustained wellness lasted 14 months. Lamotrigine was gradually increased to 525 mg/day to relieve subsyndromal cyclic mood symptoms that were still entrained to her menstrual cycle. An attempt to discontinue divalproex led to depression, so divalproex 500 mg/day was restarted, and lamotrigine was further titrated to as high as 600 mg/day, yielding a blood lamotrigine concentration of 11.6 μg/mL. This yielded a second period of recovery for 11 months.

In summary, in this middle-aged woman with bipolar II disorder with rapid cycling entrained to her menstrual cycle, the foundation of her psychotropic therapy proved to be lamotrigine 300–600 mg/day plus divalproex 500 mg/day, a regimen that was well tolerated and ultimately led to two periods of recovery lasting 14 and 11 months. Thus, her rate of mood episodes decreased approximately 20-fold, from 10 per year in the year prior to this regimen to 0.48 per year (one in 25 months). One concern is that with menopause in the future, she may be at risk for mood destabilization.

References

Adler CM, Fleck DE, Brecher M, et al: Safety and tolerability of quetiapine in the treatment of acute mania in bipolar disorder. J Affect Disord 100 (suppl 1):S15–S22, 2007

Alexander CM, Landsman PB, Teutsch SM, et al: NCEP-defined metabolic syndrome, diabetes, and prevalence of coronary heart disease among NHANES III participants age 50 years and older. Diabetes 52:1210–1214, 2003

Anderson JW, Greenway FL, Fujioka K, et al: Bupropion SR enhances weight loss: a 48-week double-blind, placebo-controlled trial. Obes Res 10:633–641, 2002

Angst J: The course of affective disorders, II: typology of bipolar manic-depressive illness. Arch Psychiatr Nervenkr 226:65–73, 1978

Arnold LM, McElroy SL, Keck PE Jr: The role of gender in mixed mania. Compr Psychiatry 41:83–87, 2000

Astrup A, Caterson I, Zelissen P, et al: Topiramate: long-term maintenance of weight loss induced by a low-calorie diet in obese subjects. Obes Res 12:1658–1669, 2004

Becker OV, Rasgon NL, Marsh WK, et al: Lamotrigine therapy in treatment-resistant menstrually related rapid cycling bipolar disorder: a case report. Bipolar Disord 6:435–439, 2004

Benazzi F: Gender differences in bipolar II and unipolar depressed outpatients: a 557-case study. Ann Clin Psychiatry 11:55–59, 1999

Berk M, Dodd S: Review: rapid cycling bipolar disorder associated with female gender and bipolar type II subgroup (comment). Evid Based Ment Health 7:91, 2004

Blehar MC, DePaulo JR Jr, Gershon ES, et al: Women with bipolar disorder: findings from the NIMH Genetics Initiative sample. Psychopharmacol Bull 34:239–243, 1998

Bonora E, Targher G, Formentini G, et al: The metabolic syndrome is an independent predictor of cardiovascular disease in type 2 diabetic subjects: prospective data from the Verona Diabetes Complications Study. Diabet Med 21:52–58, 2004

Bowden CL, Calabrese JR, McElroy SL, et al: A randomized, placebo-controlled 12-month trial of divalproex and lithium in treatment of outpatients with bipolar I disorder. Divalproex Maintenance Study Group. Arch Gen Psychiatry 57:481–489, 2000

Bowden CL, Calabrese JR, Ketter TA, et al: Impact of lamotrigine and lithium on weight in obese and nonobese patients with bipolar I disorder. Am J Psychiatry 163:1199–1201, 2006

Burt VK, Rasgon N: Special considerations in treating bipolar disorder in women. Bipolar Disord 6:2–13, 2004

Calabrese JR, Bowden CL, Sachs GS, et al: A double-blind placebo-controlled study of lamotrigine monotherapy in outpatients with bipolar I depression. Lamictal 602 Study Group. J Clin Psychiatry 60:79–88, 1999

Calabrese JR, Suppes T, Bowden CL, et al: A double-blind, placebo-controlled, prophylaxis study of lamotrigine in rapid-cycling bipolar disorder. Lamictal 614 Study Group. J Clin Psychiatry 61:841–850, 2000

Calabrese JR, Shelton MD, Rapport DJ, et al: Current research on rapid cycling bipolar disorder and its treatment. J Affect Disord 67:241–255, 2001

Calabrese JR, Keck PE Jr, Macfadden W, et al: A randomized, double-blind, placebo-controlled trial of quetiapine in the treatment of bipolar I or II depression. Am J Psychiatry 162:1351–1360, 2005

Calabrese JR, Huffman RF, White RL, et al: Lamotrigine in the acute treatment of bipolar depression: results of five double-blind, placebo-controlled clinical trials. Bipolar Disord 10:323–333, 2008

Chouinard G, Steinberg S, Steiner W: Estrogen-progesterone combination: another mood stabilizer? (letter) Am J Psychiatry 144:826, 1987

Cohen LS, Friedman JM, Jefferson JW, et al: A reevaluation of risk of in utero exposure to lithium. JAMA 271:146–150, 1994

Crawford P: Interactions between antiepileptic drugs and hormonal contraception. CNS Drugs 16:263–272, 2002

Cruz N, Vieta E, Comes M, et al: Rapid-cycling bipolar I disorder: course and treatment outcome of a large sample across Europe. J Psychiatr Res 42:1068–1075, 2008

Cunnington M, Tennis P: Lamotrigine and the risk of malformations in pregnancy. Neurology 64:955–960, 2005

DeToledo JC, Toledo C, DeCerce J, et al: Changes in body weight with chronic, high-dose gabapentin therapy. Ther Drug Monit 19:394–396, 1997

Dunaif A, Segal KR, Futterweit W, et al: Profound peripheral insulin resistance, independent of obesity, in polycystic ovary syndrome. Diabetes 38:1165–1174, 1989

Dunner DL, Fieve RR: Clinical factors in lithium carbonate prophylaxis failure. Arch Gen Psychiatry 30:229–233, 1974

Fagiolini A, Kupfer DJ, Houck PR, et al: Obesity as a correlate of outcome in patients with bipolar I disorder. Am J Psychiatry 160:112–117, 2003

Freeman MP, McElroy SL: Clinical picture and etiologic models of mixed states. Psychiatr Clin North Am 22:535–546, vii, 1999

Frye MA, Altshuler LL, McElroy SL, et al: Gender differences in prevalence, risk, and clinical correlates of alcoholism comorbidity in bipolar disorder. Am J Psychiatry 160:883–889, 2003

Gadde KM, Franciscy DM, Wagner HR 2nd, et al: Zonisamide for weight loss in obese adults: a randomized controlled trial. JAMA 289:1820–1825, 2003

Garcia-Portilla MP, Saiz PA, Benabarre A, et al: The prevalence of metabolic syndrome in patients with bipolar disorder. J Affect Disord 106:197–201, 2008

Ghaemi SN: Treatment of rapid-cycling bipolar disorder: are antidepressants mood destabilizers? Am J Psychiatry 165:300–302, 2008

Goldberg JF, Bowden CL, Calabrese JR, et al: Six-month prospective life charting of mood symptoms with lamotrigine monotherapy versus placebo in rapid cycling bipolar disorder. Biol Psychiatry 63:125–130, 2008

Goldstein DJ, Corbin LA, Fung MC: Olanzapine-exposed pregnancies and lactation: early experience. J Clin Psychopharmacol 20:399–403, 2000

Goodwin GM, Bowden CL, Calabrese JR, et al: A pooled analysis of two placebo-controlled 18-month trials of lamotrigine and lithium maintenance in bipolar I disorder. J Clin Psychiatry 65:432–441, 2004

Grundy SM, Brewer HB Jr, Cleeman JI, et al: Definition of metabolic syndrome: report of the National Heart, Lung, and Blood Institute/American Heart Association conference on scientific issues related to definition. Circulation 109:433–438, 2004

Hatotani N, Nomura J, Inoue K, et al: Psychoendocrine model of depression. Psycho-neuroendocrinology 4:155–172, 1979

Henderson DC, Copeland PM, Daley TB, et al: A double-blind, placebo-controlled trial of sibutramine for olanzapine-associated weight gain. Am J Psychiatry 162:954–962, 2005

Holmes LB, Harvey EA, Coull BA, et al: The teratogenicity of anticonvulsant drugs. N Engl J Med 344:1132–1138, 2001

Horie S, Suga T: Enhancement of peroxisomal beta–oxidation in the liver of rats and mice treated with valproic acid. Biochem Pharmacol 34:1357–1362, 1985

Iqbal MM, Gundlapalli SP, Ryan WG, et al: Effects of antimanic mood-stabilizing drugs on fetuses, neonates, and nursing infants. South Med J 94:304–322, 2001

Jain AK, Kaplan RA, Gadde KM, et al: Bupropion SR vs. placebo for weight loss in obese patients with depressive symptoms. Obes Res 10:1049–1056, 2002

Janicak PG, Sharma RP, Pandey G, et al: Verapamil for the treatment of acute mania: a double-blind, placebo-controlled trial. Am J Psychiatry 155:972–973, 1998

Joffe H, Cohen LS, Suppes T, et al: Longitudinal follow-up of reproductive and meta-bolic features of valproate-associated polycystic ovarian syndrome features: a pre-liminary report. Biol Psychiatry 60:1378–1381, 2006a

Joffe H, Cohen LS, Suppes T, et al: Valproate is associated with new-onset oligoamen-orrhea with hyperandrogenism in women with bipolar disorder. Biol Psychiatry 59:1078–1086, 2006b

Jones KL, Lacro RV, Johnson KA, et al: Pattern of malformations in the children of women treated with carbamazepine during pregnancy. N Engl J Med 320:1661–1666, 1989

Keck PE Jr, Calabrese JR, McQuade RD, et al: A randomized, double-blind, placebo-controlled 26-week trial of aripiprazole in recently manic patients with bipolar I disorder. J Clin Psychiatry 67:626–637, 2006

Keller MB, Lavori PW, Coryell W, et al: Differential outcome of pure manic, mixed/cycling, and pure depressive episodes in patients with bipolar illness. JAMA 255:3138–3142, 1986

Kessing LV: Gender differences in the phenomenology of bipolar disorder. Bipolar Dis-ord 6:421–425, 2004

Ketter TA, Kalali AH, Weisler RH: A 6-month, multicenter, open-label evaluation of beaded, extended-release carbamazepine capsule monotherapy in bipolar disorder patients with manic or mixed episodes. J Clin Psychiatry 65:668–673, 2004

Klipstein KG, Goldberg JF: Screening for bipolar disorder in women with polycystic ovary syndrome: a pilot study. J Affect Disord 91:205–209, 2006

Koren G, Nava-Ocampo AA, Moretti ME, et al: Major malformations with valproic acid. Can Fam Physician 52:441–442, 444, 447, 2006

Kushner SF, Khan A, Lane R, et al: Topiramate monotherapy in the management of acute mania: results of four double-blind placebo-controlled trials. Bipolar Disord 8:15–27, 2006

Laaksonen DE, Lakka HM, Niskanen LK, et al: Metabolic syndrome and development of diabetes mellitus: application and validation of recently suggested definitions of the metabolic syndrome in a prospective cohort study. Am J Epidemiol 156:1070–1077, 2002

Lakka HM, Laaksonen DE, Lakka TA, et al: The metabolic syndrome and total and cardiovascular disease mortality in middle-aged men. JAMA 288:2709–2716, 2002

Lampen A, Carlberg C, Nau H: Peroxisome proliferator–activated receptor delta is a specific sensor for teratogenic valproic acid derivatives. Eur J Pharmacol 431:25–33, 2001

Leibenluft E: Issues in the treatment of women with bipolar illness. J Clin Psychiatry 58 (suppl 15):5–11, 1997

Leibenluft E: Women and bipolar disorder: an update. Bull Menninger Clin 64:5–17, 2000

Leppig M, Bosch B, Naber D, et al: Clozapine in the treatment of 121 out-patients. Psychopharmacology (Berl) 99(suppl):S77–S79, 1989

Llewellyn A, Stowe ZN, Strader JR Jr: The use of lithium and management of women with bipolar disorder during pregnancy and lactation. J Clin Psychiatry 59 (suppl 6):57–64; discussion 65, 1998

Marsh WK, Templeton A, Ketter TA, et al: Increased frequency of depressive episodes during the menopausal transition in women with bipolar disorder: preliminary report. J Psychiatr Res 42:247–251, 2008

McElroy SL, Strakowski SM, Keck PE Jr, et al: Differences and similarities in mixed and pure mania. Compr Psychiatry 36:187–194, 1995

McElroy SL, Kotwal R, Guerdjikova AI, et al: Zonisamide in the treatment of binge eating disorder with obesity: a randomized controlled trial. J Clin Psychiatry 67:1897–1906, 2006

McElroy SL, Frye MA, Altshuler LL, et al: A 24-week, randomized, controlled trial of adjunctive sibutramine versus topiramate in the treatment of weight gain in overweight or obese patients with bipolar disorders. Bipolar Disord 94:426–434, 2007

Miller LJ: Use of electroconvulsive therapy during pregnancy. Hosp Community Psychiatry 45:444–450, 1994

Müller-Oerlinghausen B, Passoth PM, Poser W, et al: Effect of long-term treatment with neuroleptics or lithium salts on carbohydrate metabolism [in German]. Arzneimittelforschung 28:1522–1524, 1978

Newport DJ, Hostetter A, Arnold A, et al: The treatment of postpartum depression: minimizing infant exposures. J Clin Psychiatry 63 (suppl 7):31–44, 2002

O'Donovan C, Kusumakar V, Graves GR, et al: Menstrual abnormalities and polycystic ovary syndrome in women taking valproate for bipolar mood disorder. J Clin Psychiatry 63:322–330, 2002

O'Hara MW, Stuart S, Gorman LL, et al: Efficacy of interpersonal psychotherapy for postpartum depression. Arch Gen Psychiatry 57:1039–1045, 2000

Patten SB, Lamarre CJ: Can drug-induced depressions be identified by their clinical features? Can J Psychiatry 37:213–215, 1992

Paykel ES, Mueller PS, De la Vergne PM: Amitriptyline, weight gain and carbohydrate craving: a side effect. Br J Psychiatry 123:501–507, 1973

Pearlstein T, Steiner M: Non-antidepressant treatment of premenstrual syndrome. J Clin Psychiatry 61 (suppl 12):22–27, 2000

Perugi G, Musetti L, Simonini E, et al: Gender-mediated clinical features of depressive illness: the importance of temperamental differences. Br J Psychiatry 157:835–841, 1990

Physicians' Desk Reference, 62nd Edition. Montvale, NJ, Thomson Healthcare, 2008

Price WA, DiMarzio L: Premenstrual tension syndrome in rapid-cycling bipolar affective disorder. J Clin Psychiatry 47:415–417, 1986

Price WA, Giannini AJ: Antidepressant effects of estrogen (letter). J Clin Psychiatry 46:506, 1985

Rapkin AJ, Mikacich JA, Moatakef-Imani B, et al: The clinical nature and formal diagnosis of premenstrual, postpartum, and perimenopausal affective disorders. Curr Psychiatry Rep 4:419–428, 2002

Rasgon NL: Anatomic, functional, and clinical studies of neuroendocrine function in bipolar disorder. Advanced Studies in Medicine 3 (suppl 8A):S726–S732, 2003

Rasgon NL, Altshuler LL, Gudeman D, et al: Medication status and polycystic ovary syndrome in women with bipolar disorder: a preliminary report. J Clin Psychiatry 61:173–178, 2000

Rasgon NL, Carter MS, Elman S, et al: Common treatment of polycystic ovarian syndrome and major depressive disorder: case report and review. Curr Drug Targets Immune Endocr Metabol Disord 2:97–102, 2002

Rasgon N, Bauer M, Glenn T, et al: Menstrual cycle related mood changes in women with bipolar disorder. Bipolar Disord 5:48–52, 2003a

Rasgon NL, Rao RC, Hwang S, et al: Depression in women with polycystic ovary syndrome: clinical and biochemical correlates. J Affect Disord 74:299–304, 2003b

Rasgon NL, Altshuler LL, Fairbanks L, et al: Reproductive function and risk for PCOS in women treated for bipolar disorder. Bipolar Disord 7:246–259, 2005a

Rasgon N, Bauer M, Grof P, et al: Sex-specific self-reported mood changes by patients with bipolar disorder. J Psychiatr Res 39:77–83, 2005b

Rasgon NL, Reynolds MF, Elman S, et al: Longitudinal evaluation of reproductive function in women treated for bipolar disorder. J Affect Disord 89:217–225, 2005c

Reinstein MJ, Sonnenberg JG, Hedberg TG, et al: Oxcarbazepine versus divalproex sodium for the continuing treatment of mania. Clin Drug Investig 23:671–677, 2003

Robb JC, Young LT, Cooke RG, et al: Gender differences in patients with bipolar disorder influence outcome in the Medical Outcomes Survey (SF-20) subscale scores. J Affect Disord 49:189–193, 1998

Rosa FW: Spina bifida in infants of women treated with carbamazepine during pregnancy. N Engl J Med 324:674–677, 1991

Roy-Byrne P, Post RM, Uhde TW, et al: The longitudinal course of recurrent affective illness: life chart data from research patients at the NIMH. Acta Psychiatr Scand Suppl 317:1–34, 1985

Rubinow DR, Schmidt PJ: Gonadal steroid regulation of mood: the lessons of premenstrual syndrome. Front Neuroendocrinol 27:210–216, 2006

Sabers A, Buchholt JM, Uldall P, et al: Lamotrigine plasma levels reduced by oral contraceptives. Epilepsy Res 47:151–154, 2001

Sachs G, Bowden C, Calabrese JR, et al: Effects of lamotrigine and lithium on body weight during maintenance treatment of bipolar I disorder. Bipolar Disord 8:175–181, 2006

Spinelli MG: Interpersonal psychotherapy for depressed antepartum women: a pilot study. Am J Psychiatry 154:1028–1030, 1997

Suppes T, Mintz J, McElroy SL, et al: Mixed hypomania in 908 patients with bipolar disorder evaluated prospectively in the Stanley Foundation Bipolar Treatment Network: a sex-specific phenomenon. Arch Gen Psychiatry 62:1089–1096, 2005

Taylor MA, Abrams R: Gender differences in bipolar affective disorder. J Affect Disord 3:261–271, 1981

Tohen M, Calabrese JR, Sachs GS, et al: Randomized, placebo-controlled trial of olanzapine as maintenance therapy in patients with bipolar I disorder responding to acute treatment with olanzapine. Am J Psychiatry 163:247–256, 2006

Tondo L, Baldessarini RJ: Rapid cycling in women and men with bipolar manic-depressive disorders. Am J Psychiatry 155:1434–1436, 1998

Use of psychoactive medication during pregnancy and possible effects on the fetus and newborn. Committee on Drugs. American Academy of Pediatrics. Pediatrics 105:880–887, 2000

Vainionpää LK, Rättyä J, Knip M, et al: Valproate-induced hyperandrogenism during pubertal maturation in girls with epilepsy. Ann Neurol 45:444–450, 1999

van Winkel R, De Hert M, Van Eyck D, et al: Prevalence of diabetes and the metabolic syndrome in a sample of patients with bipolar disorder. Bipolar Disord 10:342–348, 2008

Vestergaard P, Poulstrup I, Schou M: Prospective studies on a lithium cohort, 3: tremor, weight gain, diarrhea, psychological complaints. Acta Psychiatr Scand 78:434–441, 1988

Vieta E, Goikolea JM, Corbella B, et al: Risperidone safety and efficacy in the treatment of bipolar and schizoaffective disorders: results from a 6-month, multicenter, open study. J Clin Psychiatry 62:818–825, 2001

Viguera AC, Nonacs R, Cohen LS, et al: Risk of recurrence of bipolar disorder in pregnant and nonpregnant women after discontinuing lithium maintenance. Am J Psychiatry 157:179–184, 2000a

Viguera AC, Tondo L, Baldessarini RJ: Sex differences in response to lithium treatment. Am J Psychiatry 157:1509–1511, 2000b

Viguera AC, Cohen LS, Baldessarini RJ, et al: Managing bipolar disorder during pregnancy: weighing the risks and benefits. Can J Psychiatry 47:426–436, 2002

Wang PW, Yang YS, Chandler RA, et al: Adjunctive zonisamide for weight loss in euthymic bipolar disorder patients: a pilot study. J Psychiatr Res 42:451–457, 2008

Warrington L, Lombardo I, Loebel A, et al: Ziprasidone for the treatment of acute manic or mixed episodes associated with bipolar disorder. CNS Drugs 21:835–849, 2007

Wisner KL, Peindl KS, Perel JM, et al: Verapamil treatment for women with bipolar disorder. Biol Psychiatry 51:745–752, 2002

Management of Bipolar Disorders in Older Adults

John O. Brooks III, Ph.D., M.D.

Barbara R. Sommer, M.D.

Terence A. Ketter, M.D.

Older adults, particularly the oldest-old, constitute the fastest-growing age subgroup in the U.S. population and face substantial unmet needs. Bipolar disorders are associated with significant health care challenges for older adults, including disability, functional decline, diminished quality of life, increased mortality from comorbid medical conditions or suicide, demands on caregivers, and increased service utilization (Charney et al. 2003). Mental health care access is inadequate for most older adults and is further limited by a lack of information regarding the treatment of bipolar disorders in older adults. For example, no large-scale, multicenter studies of therapeutic agents have yet been published and no U.S. Food and Drug Administration (FDA) treatments have been approved specifically for older adults with bipolar disorders.

Pharmacological interventions in older adults are challenging because of comorbid conditions, altered metabolism, and potential drug interactions. In this chapter, we review the state of current knowledge of the management of bipolar disorders in older adults. We review unique aspects of the clinical presentation and treatment of older adults with bipolar disorders to clarify special diagnostic considerations and to aid in optimizing therapeutic outcomes.

Epidemiology

Approximately 0.1% of Americans age 65 years or older have bipolar I disorder, and a similar percentage of older adults have bipolar II disorder (Weissman et al. 1988), a figure that is three- to 10-fold lower than for adults ages 30–44 years with the disorder. Despite the low prevalence of bipolar disorders in older adults in community samples, bipolar disorder in older adults represents a substantial public health challenge. For example, bipolar disorder appears to account for similar proportions (approximately 10%) of psychiatric hospitalizations of older and younger patients (Depp and Jeste 2004). Moreover, bipolar disorder accounts for approximately 5% of older adult outpatient visits and nursing home beds, as well as 15% of older adult psychiatric emergency room visits (Depp and Jeste 2004). Older veterans with bipolar disorder are greater users of health services than their younger counterparts (Sajatovic et al. 2004). Furthermore, older patients with bipolar disorder appear more likely to have cognitive disorders and are more likely to need conservatorship and case management services (Depp et al. 2005).

Clinical Characteristics

Clinical Presentation

Overall, bipolar disorder has a unimodal age-at-onset distribution, peaking in the late teens to early 20s, with only approximately 10% of patients having an onset after age 50 years (Yassa et al. 1988) and 5% after age 60 (Goodwin and Jamison 2007). In samples of older adults with bipolar disorders, the mean age at onset was 48 years, and the average duration of affective illness was 20 years (Depp and Jeste 2004). Older patients with bipolar disorders are more often female, and although mania may be less intense, individuals in this age group have more index depressive (rather than manic) episodes and longer hospitalizations than do younger adults (Depp and Jeste 2004). Evidence indicates that older adults with bipolar disorders use substances slightly less often than younger adults with bipolar disorders (7.0% vs. 8.3% current prevalence) (Depp et al. 2005). However, among older patients with bipolar disorders and dementia, comorbid alcohol abuse or dependence is associated with a greater risk of inpatient hospitalization (Brooks et al. 2006).

Late-onset bipolar disorder is often associated with comorbid neurological disease and may be accompanied by vascular disease and psychotic features. Late-onset bipolar disorder is commonly not associated with family psychiatric history and stressful life events, consistent with the hypothesis that organic, genetic, and psychosocial factors play differing roles depending on the age at onset of bipolar disorder (Ahearn et al. 1998; Hays et al. 1998; Krishnan 2002; Wylie et al. 1999).

Major Depressive Episodes

Depression in older individuals may represent a primary psychiatric disorder or be symptomatic of medical abnormalities. Therefore, it is important to perform a complete medical evaluation to assess the etiology of affective symptoms in this population. Depressive episodes can be associated with *pseudodementia*, the distractibility and poor concentration of an apparent presentation of dementia (e.g., memory loss, decreased executive function, cognitive slowing), which is actually a reflection of depressive symptoms (Lantz and Buchalter 2001). Pseudodementia can be distinguished from dementia by the more acute onset of cognitive decline over weeks or months rather than over years. Classically, the pseudodementia patient complains of both short- and long-term memory deficits, whereas the patient with dementia will at first have short-term memory deficits. The concept of pseudodementia has been complicated by the more recent literature that demonstrates depression as a risk factor for dementia (Jorm 2000). Older patients with depression and cognitive complaints need close monitoring for sustained cognitive decline over time.

Hypomanic or Manic Episodes

In older adults, clinicians may have difficulty differentiating between hypomanic or manic episodes and neuropsychiatric disorders. Mania can be primary in the sense that it results from bipolar disorder, or it may be secondary and reflect one or more nonpsychiatric conditions (Brooks and Hoblyn 2005). In considering a diagnosis of mania or hypomania in an older adult, the clinician should try to find out whether the patient has a past history of bipolar disorder. In any case, it is important to attempt to rule out secondary mania (some causes of which are listed in Table 12–1). However, even patients with primary bipolar disorder may experience affective exacerbations related to medical problems, such as the development of depressive episodes from lithium-induced hypothyroidism. The acute symptomatic treatment of secondary mania, with mood stabilizers, antipsychotics, and/or less commonly benzodiazepines, is

TABLE 12–1.　Possible causes of secondary mania in older adults

Neurological diseases

Cerebral tumor (particularly temporal, orbitofrontal, or thalamic)	Multiple sclerosis
	Seizure disorder
Cerebrovascular disease	Traumatic brain injury
Delirium	
Dementia	

Endocrine diseases

Addison's disease
Cushing's syndrome
Hyperthyroidism
Hypothyroidism

Infectious diseases

HIV/AIDS
Tertiary syphilis

Nonpsychotropic medications

Anticholinergics (e.g., diphenhydramine)	Metrizamide
Baclofen	Phenytoin
Bromides	Procainamide
Captopril	Steroids
Dopamine agonists (e.g., L-dopa)	Thyroxine
Hydralazine	Yohimbine

Psychotropic medications/somatic therapies

Antidepressants	Phototherapy
Electroconvulsive therapy	Stimulants

Substances

Alcohol	Illicit stimulants
Cocaine	

similar to the treatment of primary mania, but needs to be undertaken with particular caution with respect to dosage titration and tolerability, and accompanied by aggressive medical interventions to address the underlying medical illnesses.

Euthymic Phase

Evaluating patients during the euthymic, or minimally symptomatic, phase may be the best way to assess the effect of bipolar disorder on cognition. Although little research has been reported in this area, older adults with bipolar disorders appear to exhibit deficits in memory, attention, and executive function (Brooks et al. 2007; Gildengers et al. 2004, 2007; Hoblyn et al. 2007). Cognitive dysfunction during euthymia affects quality of life in many ways. For example, the ability to perform activities of daily living and adherence to medication regimens may be negatively affected. Currently, with no controlled studies of pharmacological interventions for cognitive enhancement in bipolar disorder, efforts are targeted toward avoiding relapse. On occasion, clinicians may determine that cognitive symptoms during euthymia are sufficiently concerning that they necessitate empirical treatment with agents indicated for dementia (Gildengers et al. 2008). In such instances, the clinician needs to monitor carefully for drug interactions and medical and psychiatric adverse effects in patients who are already receiving pharmacotherapy for bipolar disorder.

Differential Diagnosis and Evaluation

Presentations in older adults with bipolar disorders are often complex, involving mixed, psychotic, and secondary symptoms that overlap those of unipolar major depressive disorder, dementia, delirium, neurological disorders, substance abuse, and general medical conditions. Older adults with mania, especially late-onset mania, require careful assessment for medical contributors, particularly neurological and cerebrovascular disease.

Some patients with unipolar major depressive disorder progress to bipolar disorder, with the development of manic or hypomanic episodes in late life. The latency period from first major depressive episode to first episode of mood elevation is commonly a decade, and may be as long as 25 years (Snowdon 1991). Although euphoric presentations of mood elevation episodes may be relatively straightforward, the prominent depressive symptoms in dysphoric mania and mixed episodes may resemble agitated depression. Mixed episodes may have psychotic features and prominent cognitive symptoms, raising the possibility of late-onset nonaffective psychotic disorder, psychosis related to dementia, or even delirium (Weintraub and Lippmann 2001).

As noted earlier, mood disorders secondary to medical problems or their treatments are not unusual in older patients (Brooks and Hoblyn 2005; Krauthammer and Klerman 1978). The range of medical, neurological, and medication- or substance-related causes of secondary mania highlights the need for thoughtful and thorough assessments in older patients with mania, especially those with first-episode mania. Table 12–1, adapted from several medical texts, is a compendium of some of the many causes of secondary mania.

Treatment Overview

Before considering psychopharmacological intervention in an older adult with bipolar disorder, the clinician should obtain a complete medical and psychiatric history, physical examination, and baseline laboratories as indicated, and then carefully consider the impact of comorbid medical conditions and other medications. Older adults require careful monitoring of medical conditions and other medications throughout the course of treatment.

Despite the impact of bipolar disorder in older patients, there is a relative dearth of research specifically about older patients or even secondary analyses governed by age. This lack of research is unfortunate not only because of the physiological differences between older and younger adults, but also because of the fact that older adults commonly have experienced a longer time course with bipolar disorder and hence have different treatment needs and responses.

In view of the absence of evidence specific to older adults, medications with proven efficacy and tolerability in mixed-age populations with bipolar disorders have highest priority. In addition, some information can be inferred from controlled data on the treatment of acute agitation and psychosis in older adults. Thus, in Table 12–2, we provide a summary of principles to guide pharmacotherapy of bipolar disorders in older adults.

Medication dosing regimens in older adults can differ substantially from those used in younger adults. Older adult patients may be characterized as "frail" (i.e., those having substantive medical or neurological comorbidity) or "nonfrail" (i.e., those without substantive medical or neurological comorbidity). In frail older adults, the initial target dosage should be very low (e.g., 25%–50% of young adult full dosage) because of markedly increased risks of adverse effects. In older adults as in younger adults, dosages during acute depression and maintenance may be as much as 50% lower than during acute mania. In view of the increased risk of adverse effects and drug interactions in older adults, the clinician needs to carefully explore the dosage range of individual agents before prescribing combinations. This approach leads to the dosage titration and final dosage guidelines in Table 12–3, which are broadly in agreement with clinical observations and expert-suggested dosages in older adults with bipolar disorders.

In the following sections, medications are discussed in terms of their potential benefits and precautions in older patients. The limited data regarding pharmacotherapy in older adults with bipolar disorders are supplemented with uncontrolled and controlled data regarding treatment of older adults with epilepsy, psychosis, and dementia with agitation.

TABLE 12–2.   **Principles of pharmacotherapy of bipolar disorder in older adults**

1.   Start with careful diagnostic evaluation, including complete medical and psychiatric history, physical examination, mental status examination (including cognition), and baseline laboratories as indicated.

2.   Provide ongoing careful psychiatric, medical, and cognitive clinical monitoring and laboratory monitoring.

3.   Give highest priority to psychotropic medications with proven efficacy and tolerability in mixed-aged populations with bipolar disorder.

4.   Select psychotropic medication, taking into account concurrent medical conditions and nonpsychotropic medications.

5.   Start psychotropic medications (one at a time) at low dosages (e.g., 10%–50% of young adult full dosage) and gradually increase dosages (e.g., in increments of 5%–10% of young adult full dosage every 4–7 days) as necessary and tolerated.

6.   Initially target dosages to 25%–50% of young adult full dosage in frail older adults (i.e., those with substantive medical or neurological comorbidity) and to 50% of young adult dosage in nonfrail older adults (i.e., those without substantive medical or neurological comorbidity).

7.   Consider higher subsequent dosages, up to 75% of young adult full dosage, as necessary and tolerated in some patients (e.g., nonfrail older adults with acute mania).

8.   Prescribe dosages that are as much as 50% lower during acute depression and maintenance than during acute mania.

9.   Carefully explore dosage range of individual agents before prescribing combinations.

Additional information regarding mood stabilizers and antipsychotics is provided in Chapter 13 of this volume, "Mood Stabilizers and Antipsychotics." Additional information regarding other medications is provided in Chapter 14, "Antidepressants, Anxiolytics/Hypnotics, and Other Medications."

Mood Stabilizers

The mood stabilizers lithium, valproate, carbamazepine, and lamotrigine are considered fundamental treatments for both younger and older patients with bipolar disorders. Although lithium is used almost exclusively in mood disorders, valproate, carbamazepine, and lamotrigine are also approved for the treatment of epilepsy. In addition, valproate is approved for prevention of migraine headaches, and carbamazepine is approved for the treatment of trigeminal neuralgia.

TABLE 12–3.　Dosing guideline schema for older adults with bipolar disorders

Medication	Starting dosage (mg/day)	Dosage increment[a] (mg/day)	Initial target (mg/day and/or level)
Mood stabilizers			
Lithium	150[b]	150	Dosage varies with renal clearance (0.3–0.6 mEq/L)
Valproate	250[b]	125–250	250–1,000 (30–60 μg/mL)
Carbamazepine	100[b]	100	400–800[c] (3–6 μg/mL)
Lamotrigine	12.5–25[b]	12.5–25	50–100
Second-generation antipsychotics			
Olanzapine	1.25–2.5	1.25–2.5	2.5–10
Risperidone	0.25–0.5[b]	0.25–0.5	0.5–2[c]
Quetiapine	25–50[b]	25–50	200–400[c]
Ziprasidone	20	20	40–80[d]
Aripiprazole	2–5	2–5	2–15[c]
Clozapine	6.25–25[b]	6.25–25	112.5–225[c]

Note.　Except for lamotrigine, dosages are for acute agitation/mania; for bipolar depression and maintenance, dosages may be up to 50% lower. Dosages are guidelines only—concurrent medications (e.g., carbamazepine-related enzyme induction, valproate-related enzyme inhibition), medical comorbidity, and genetic variation in metabolism will affect dosing in individual patients.
[a]Increase every 4–7 days, except lamotrigine (12.5–25 mg/day for 2 weeks, 25–50 mg/day for 2 weeks, then increasing weekly by 12.5–25 mg/day).
[b]In divided dosages.
[c]Frail older adults may only tolerate even lower dosages (i.e., carbamazepine 100–300 mg/day, risperidone 0.5–1.5 mg/day, quetiapine 50–200 mg/day, aripiprazole 2–10 mg/day, clozapine 25–100 mg/day).
[d]Low doses may yield akathisia, while high doses may yield sedation.

Lithium

Historically, lithium was considered the treatment of choice for both younger and older patients with bipolar disorders.

In the 1990s, there was a marked migration from lithium to valproate in the management of older adults with bipolar disorders. Concerns have been raised that this change was not based on demonstrations of superior efficacy and tolerability for valproate in randomized controlled trials (Shulman et al. 2003). However, there are limited uncontrolled retrospective (Chen et al. 1999; Hewick et al. 1977; Himmelhoch et al. 1980; Sanderson 1998; Stone 1989; Van der Velde 1970) and prospective (Abou-Saleh and Coppen 1983; Murray et al. 1983; Sajatovic et al. 2005; Schaffer and Garvey 1984; Schneider and Wilcox 1998) data suggesting the efficacy of lithium in older adults with bipolar disorders. In a post hoc analysis of older adults in mixed-age, maintenance registration studies, lithium (mean dosage 750 mg/day) delayed mood elevation episodes, while lamotrigine (mean dosage 240 mg/day) delayed overall and depressive episodes (Sajatovic et al. 2005).

The U.S. prescribing information for lithium includes a boxed warning regarding the risk of lithium toxicity that can occur at dosages yielding close to therapeutic levels. Lithium is almost exclusively eliminated unchanged in the urine. Thus, lithium's adverse effect profile can be challenging in older adults because of their decreased renal capacity and circulation (Goodwin 2003; Sproule et al. 2000). Use of lower doses and sustained-release formulations and weighting the dosage toward bedtime may help limit adverse effects. However, polyuria and polydipsia may occur in approximately one-third of older adults who are taking lithium (Hewick et al. 1977). Another consideration is lithium-related nocturia, which contributes to increased risk of nocturnal falls and sleep disturbance.

Hypothyroidism, another side effect of lithium, may have a more deleterious course in older adults than in younger adults, although it can be corrected with levothyroxine. As many as one-third of older adults taking lithium may require concomitant thyroid hormone therapy (Head and Dening 1998). Other side effects of lithium in older adults may include tremor, renal impairment, weight gain, ataxia, increased fasting blood glucose, and cognitive dysfunction (Stoudemire et al. 1998). Hand tremor associated with lithium tends to increase with age (Murray et al. 1983). Older adult patients taking lithium appear to be at increased risk for adverse cardiac effects such as arrhythmias (Roose et al. 1979a, 1979b).

Because of decreased renal clearance, the half-life of lithium in older adults may be approximately twice that observed in younger patients (Chapron 1988; Hardy et al. 1987). Thus, consultation with a nephrologist may be helpful when considering whether to continue lithium in an individual. Some case series have suggested that older patients show positive clinical response to lower plasma lithium levels (0.5–0.8 mEq/L) than are commonly used in younger populations (e.g., 0.8–1.2 mEq/L) (Schaffer and Garvey 1984; Shulman et al. 1987), although other data suggest that levels of at least 0.8 mEq/L are needed for optimal responses (Chen et al. 1999). Importantly, lithium toxicity in older adults with bipolar disorders can occur at serum levels that are therapeutic in younger patients (Sproule et al. 2000). Consequently, it may be advisable to reduce lithium dosages 25%–50% in older adults (Sproule et al. 2000) and to carefully monitor patients' clinical status and serum lithium concentrations.

After baseline medical status, electrolytes, renal and thyroid function, and electrocardiograms are assessed in older adult patients, the prudent approach is to start lithium at 150 mg/day and, as necessary and tolerated, increase by 150 mg/day every 4–7 days, carefully monitoring clinical status and serum lithium concentrations. The initial target dosages are commonly between 450 and 900 mg/day, and initial target serum concentrations are commonly between 0.3 and 0.6 mEq/L (Table 12–3).

Older patients are more likely to be taking other medications or to have other conditions that can have significant interactions with lithium. For example, nonsteroidal anti-inflammatory agents such as ibuprofen, thiazide diuretics, angiotensin-converting enzyme inhibitors, sodium-restricted diets, and dehydration may significantly increase serum lithium levels; theophylline may decrease lithium levels (Sproule et al. 2000). Older patients appear susceptible to additive neurotoxicity (delirium, tremor, and cerebellar dysfunction) when combining lithium with first-generation antipsychotic medications, even when low dosages of the latter agents are used (Miller et al. 1986).

In view of lithium's safety and tolerability limitations in older adults, clinicians often prefer to utilize other treatment options such as valproate for acute mania and mania prevention, or lamotrigine for acute depression and depression prevention. Some providers contend that the migration away from lithium may have been excessive, leaving this option relatively underutilized.

Valproate

Valproate, typically in the divalproex formulation, is used increasingly in older patients with bipolar disorders. This increasing usage appears to be related to efficacy and tolerability limitations of lithium that may be particularly significant in older patients.

Limited case report and case series data suggest that valproate is safe and effective in the treatment of mania in older adults (Chen et al. 1999; Goldberg et al. 2000; Kando et al. 1996; McFarland et al. 1990; Mordecai et al. 1999; Niedermier and Nasrallah 1998; Noaghiul et al. 1998; Puryear et al. 1995; Risinger et al. 1994; Sanderson 1998; Schneider and Wilcox 1998; Sharma et al. 1993). In such reports, final mean valproate dosages were approximately 750–1,500 mg/day, with final mean valproate serum concentrations of 50–75 µg/mL. In view of the risk of adverse effects, even more conservative initial dosing may be necessary (Table 12–3). Medically frail older adults with bipolar disorder may only tolerate the low valproate serum concentrations (40–60 µg/mL) used in older adults with epilepsy or dementia.

The U.S. prescribing information for valproate includes boxed warnings regarding the risks of hepatotoxicity, teratogenicity, and pancreatitis. However, the risks of hepatotoxicity and pancreatitis appear to decrease with age. Common dose-related adverse effects with valproate include gastrointestinal (nausea, vomiting, dyspepsia, diarrhea), hepatic (transaminase elevations), central nervous system (tremor, sedation, dizziness), and metabolic (weight gain, osteoporosis) events, as well as hair loss. In mid-2008, the FDA released an alert regarding increased risk of suicidality (suicidal behavior or ideation) in patients with epilepsy or psychiatric disorders for 11 anticonvulsants, including valproate, carbamazepine, and lamotrigine. In the FDA's analysis, anticonvulsants compared with placebo yielded approximately twice the risk of suicidality (0.43% vs. 0.22%). The relative risk for suicidality was higher in the patients with epilepsy than in the patients with psychiatric disorders.

In older adults, the effects of valproate on cognition tend to be mild for many patients (Gallassi et al. 1990; Gillham et al. 1990), although occasional individuals may experience difficulties. Although previous research is somewhat controversial in this regard, results indicate that valproate may be associated with mild memory or attention deficits. However, encephalopathy, on occasion with elevated ammonia levels, and parkinsonian symptoms, on occasion with cognitive decline, appear to be uncommon adverse effects, seen primarily in older patients with neurological disorders. Nonetheless, valproate in older adult patients (as in younger patients) appears to be generally better tolerated than lithium (Conney and Kaston 1999). Interestingly, despite valproate's generally milder cognitive side effects profile, lithium and valproate appear to yield similar rates of delirium (Shulman et al. 2005).

Valproate is extensively metabolized and can cause hepatotoxicity, so particular caution is needed in older patients with decreased hepatic function. Indeed, hepatic insufficiency may decrease valproate clearance by as much as 50%, requiring dosage adjustment or, in cases of hepatotoxicity, discontinuation. The half-life of valproate can almost double in older adults because of decreased elimination (Bryson et al. 1983).

An important issue that affects valproate dosage and use in older adults is the fact that valproic acid is highly protein bound in the blood and the remaining free valproate is metabolized. Thus, factors that affect the protein binding of valproate affect the level of free valproate, which may be a primary determinant of adverse effects in some older adults (Fenn et al. 2006). Unbound valproate is of concern because its clearance is reduced by up to 40% in older adults (Perucca et al. 1984); clearance can be further reduced because of renal insufficiency (Stephen 2003). As the fraction of free valproate increases, the measure of total valproate becomes more misleading. Thus, when the total valproate level is used to guide dosing strategies, the dosage may be too high in older adults. Although the optimal therapeutic levels of valproate in older adults with bipolar disorders are not clearly established, a range of 40–90 µg/mL may be reasonable (Chen et al. 1999).

Thus, in older adults, after baseline medical status, complete blood count with platelets, and hepatic function have been assessed, the prudent approach is to start valproate at 250 mg/day and, as necessary and tolerated, increase by 125–250 mg/day every 4–7 days, carefully monitoring clinical status and serum valproate concentrations. The initial targeted dosage is 250–1,000 mg/day, and the initial target serum concentrations are commonly 30–60 µg/mL (Table 12–3).

Valproate inhibits hepatic enzymes, increasing blood concentrations of other drugs, including lamotrigine; carbamazepine epoxide; amitriptyline; nortriptyline; anticonvulsants such as ethosuximide, phenobarbital, and phenytoin; and other agents such as zidovudine. Several medications that may be commonly used in older adults can interfere with the protein binding of valproate. For example, aspirin can decrease the protein-bound portion of valproate and inhibit valproate metabolism (Abbott et al. 1986). Valproate can displace warfarin and lead to greater unbound fractions (Panjehshahin et al. 1991). Older patients should be more closely monitored if they are taking both valproate and warfarin.

Despite the limited data regarding the efficacy of valproate in older adults with bipolar disorders, contemporary clinicians focusing on acute mania and prevention of mania tend to choose this treatment option over lithium in view of valproate's more favorable tolerability profile, and over carbamazepine in view of valproate's more favorable tolerability and drug interaction profiles. In contrast, clinicians focusing on acute depression and prevention of depression may tend to choose lamotrigine over valproate in view of lamotrigine's more favorable efficacy (for the depressive component of bipolar disorder) and tolerability profiles.

Carbamazepine

Carbamazepine is occasionally used in both younger and older patients with bipolar disorders. However, carbamazepine's adverse effect and drug interaction profiles limit its utility, particularly in older adults, who are more vulnerable to these problems. Very limited case report and case series data are available regarding the use of carbamazepine in older adult patients with bipolar disorders (Cullen et al. 1991; Kellner and Neher 1991; Sanderson 1998; Schneier and Kahn 1990).

The U.S. prescribing information for carbamazepine includes boxed warnings regarding the risks of aplastic anemia (16/million patient-years), agranulocytosis (48/million patient-years), and serious dermatological reactions and the HLA-B*1502 allele. In older adults taking carbamazepine, concern has been raised that rashes may be associated with blood dyscrasias (Cates and Powers 1998). In 2008, the FDA released an alert regarding an increased risk of suicidality in patients with epilepsy or psychiatric disorders for carbamazepine as well as 10 other anticonvulsants.

Carbamazepine's most common dose-related adverse effects involve the central nervous system (diplopia, blurred vision, fatigue, sedation, dizziness, ataxia) or gastrointestinal system (nausea, vomiting). Because carbamazepine is metabolized by the liver and can yield hepatotoxicity, particular caution is needed in older patients with hepatic problems, who may require dosage adjustment or, in cases of hepatotoxicity, discontinuation. The metabolic rate of carbamazepine in older adults is more than 20% lower than in younger adults (Battino et al. 2003). Gradual initiation, conservative initial target serum levels (e.g., 3–6 μg/mL), use of sustained-release formulations, and weighting the dosage toward bedtime may help to limit these adverse effects.

Older patients are also more sensitive to carbamazepine-induced hyponatremia, which may present as confusion (Cullen et al. 1991). Older adult patients may also be at increased risk for carbamazepine-related cardiac conduction delay (Kasarskis et al. 1992), as well as gastrointestinal problems, hepatotoxicity, and rash (Cullen et al. 1991). Although data regarding the neurocognitive effects of carbamazepine in older adults are limited, some studies of younger adults have suggested motor speed slowing (Duncan et al. 1990; Gillham et al. 1990).

Thus, in older adults, after baseline medical status, complete blood count, hepatic function, serum electrolytes, and electrocardiograms have been assessed, the prudent approach is to start carbamazepine at 100 mg/day and, as necessary and tolerated, increase the dosage by 100 mg/day every 4–7 days, carefully monitoring clinical status and serum carbamazepine concentrations. Initial target dosages are commonly 400–800 mg/day, and initial target serum concentrations are commonly 3–6 µg/mL (Table 12–3), although frail older adults may only tolerate 100–300 mg/day.

Carbamazepine decreases blood concentrations of multiple other psychotropic medications (compromising their efficacy unless a dosage adjustment is made), including the mood stabilizers valproate and lamotrigine; the antipsychotics haloperidol, clozapine, olanzapine, risperidone, quetiapine, ziprasidone, and aripiprazole; the antidepressants citalopram, escitalopram, mirtazapine, mianserin, sertraline, bupropion, amitriptyline, nortriptyline, imipramine, desipramine, doxepin, and clomipramine; and the benzodiazepines clonazepam, alprazolam, and midazolam (Ketter et al. 1991a, 1991b). Valproate interacts with carbamazepine in two important additional ways. First, valproate displaces carbamazepine from serum proteins and increases the free carbamazepine fraction. Second, valproate inhibits metabolism of the active carbamazepine epoxide metabolite, which can result in toxicity developing at parent drug therapeutic levels. Combination of clozapine with carbamazepine is not recommended in view of the hypothetical possibility of synergistic bone marrow suppression. Although carbamazepine and lithium lack kinetic interactions, this combination may give rise to additive neurotoxicity.

Carbamazepine decreases blood concentrations of multiple other medications, including anticonvulsants such as topiramate, tiagabine, oxcarbazepine, levetiracetam, and zonisamide; dihydropyridine calcium channel blockers such as nimodipine and felodipine; methylxanthines such as theophylline and aminophylline; antibiotics such as doxycycline; antivirals such as protease inhibitors; neuromuscular blockers such as pancuronium, vecuronium, and doxacurium; analgesics such as methadone; immunosuppressants such as sirolimus and tacrolimus; and the anticoagulant warfarin. Such interactions can compromise the effectiveness of these other medications, unless a dosage adjustment is made.

Also, multiple other medications inhibit carbamazepine metabolism, yielding increased serum carbamazepine concentrations and intoxication (unless a dosage adjustment is made). These medications include antidepressants such as fluoxetine, fluvoxamine, and nefazodone; nondihydropyridine calcium channel blockers such as verapamil and diltiazem; isoniazid; azole antifungals such as ketoconazole; macrolide antibiotics such as erythromycin and clarithromycin; protease inhibitors such as ritonavir and nelfinavir; hypolipidemics such as gemfibrozil and nicotinamide; and the carbonic anhydrase inhibitor acetazolamide. The risk of hyponatremia is increased if a patient is taking sodium-wasting diuretics.

Taken together, carbamazepine's adverse effect and drug interaction profiles are challenging enough in older adults that clinicians often prefer other treatment options, such as valproate or lithium for mood elevation symptoms or lamotrigine for depressive symptoms.

Lamotrigine

Lamotrigine, approved by the FDA for bipolar disorder maintenance treatment in 2003, has become the most frequently prescribed mood stabilizer, overtaking lithium, valproate, and carbamazepine. This increase in usage has been in part related to lamotrigine's generally excellent tolerability, efficacy for the depressive component of bipolar disorder, and relatively limited drug interactions, assets of particular value in older adults.

Limited case report data in older adults suggest that lamotrigine may help delay relapse or recurrence of bipolar depression (Robillard and Conn 2002). In a post hoc analysis, controlled data suggested that lamotrigine maintenance delayed overall and depressive episodes and was well tolerated in older adults with bipolar I disorder (Sajatovic et al. 2005).

The U.S. prescribing information for lamotrigine includes a boxed warning regarding the risk of serious rashes requiring hospitalization. Stevens-Johnson syndrome occurred in 0.8% of adult patients with epilepsy receiving adjunctive therapy and in 0.08% and 0.13% of adult patients with mood disorder receiving monotherapy and adjunctive therapy, respectively. The risk of rash may be higher when lamotrigine is coadministered with valproate, when the recommended initial lamotrigine dosage is exceeded, or when the recommended rate of lamotrigine dosage escalation is exceeded. Benign rash may be seen in 10% of patients, but because any rash is potentially serious, rashes require discontinuation of lamotrigine, unless they are clearly not drug related. Nearly all cases of life-threatening rashes have occurred within 2–8 weeks of starting lamotrigine. Other warnings in the prescribing information include the risks of hypersensitivity reactions (with fever and lymphadenopathy, but not necessarily rash); acute multiorgan failure (fatalities observed in about 1 in 1,800 adult patients with epilepsy, but not in patients with bipolar disorders); blood dyscrasia; and possibly withdrawal seizures in patients with bipolar disorders, so that unless safety concerns demand abrupt discontinuation, lamotrigine should be tapered over 2 weeks.

Lamotrigine can also cause adverse effects of the central nervous system (headache, somnolence, insomnia, dizziness, tremor) and gastrointestinal system (nausea, diarrhea). In most instances, these problems attenuate or resolve with time or lamotrigine dosage adjustment, but occasional patients may require lamotrigine discontinuation. Unlike other mood stabilizers, lamotrigine has not been associated with weight gain. In general, lamotrigine appears to be very well tolerated in older adults (Bowden et al. 2004; Brodie et al. 1999).

Lamotrigine dosage is initially titrated *very slowly* to decrease the risk of rash. When lamotrigine is added to valproate (which doubles lamotrigine levels), lamotrigine dosages are halved. When lamotrigine is added to carbamazepine (which halves lamotrigine levels), lamotrigine dosages are doubled.

Overall, even though there are limited data regarding the efficacy of lamotrigine in older adults with bipolar disorders, its favorable adverse effect and drug interaction profiles may lead contemporary clinicians to choose this treatment option over valproate, lithium, or carbamazepine for patients with prominent depressive symptoms. However, given lamotrigine's lack of acute and relatively modest prophylactic antimanic effects, other agents may be necessary in patients with prominent mood elevation symptoms.

Antipsychotics

In the past, first-generation antipsychotics were often prescribed for acute symptoms of bipolar disorder, such as psychosis associated with mania or depression, but adverse events such as emotional blunting and neurological side effects limited their use. As large-scale studies have demonstrated the efficacy of second-generation antipsychotic drugs in the acute and maintenance treatment of bipolar disorder, their use has expanded.

Although second-generation antipsychotic drugs are associated with fewer severe neurological effects, they have substantive other adverse effects. Thus, all (i.e., both first-generation and second-generation) antipsychotics carry class warnings for neuroleptic malignant syndrome and tardive dyskinesia. The U.S. prescribing information for both first-generation and second-generation antipsychotics includes a boxed warning that these agents may increase mortality in older adults with dementia-related psychosis. The increased mortality appears to be due primarily to cardiac and infectious processes, already the most common causes of death in this population. Some second-generation agents (olanzapine, risperidone, and aripiprazole) also have been associated with increased risk of cerebrovascular accidents in older adults with dementia. Some agents (e.g., clozapine, olanzapine, risperidone, quetiapine) are associated with sedation, weight gain, and metabolic adverse effects, whereas others (e.g., aripiprazole, ziprasidone) are associated with akathisia in all age groups. As with other medications, dosages of antipsychotics in older compared with younger patients are commonly 25%–50% lower to limit adverse effects.

First-Generation Antipsychotics

Limited data are available on the use of first-generation antipsychotics in older adults with bipolar disorders (Chen et al. 1999; Stone 1989) or with psychotic disorders (Barak et al. 2002; Cowley and Glen 1979; Howanitz et al. 1999; Jeste et al. 1999b; Kennedy et al. 2003; Weisbard et al. 1997).

Tardive dyskinesia with first-generation antipsychotics is of concern because its incidence appears much higher in older adults (26%, 52%, and 60%, after 1, 2, and 3 years, respectively) (Jeste et al. 1995) than in younger adults (5%/year) (Kane et al. 1988b). Higher-potency antipsychotics (e.g., haloperidol, fluphenazine) have a higher incidence of extrapyramidal symptoms, which in turn may increase agitation. In addition, older patients experience extrapyramidal symptoms more frequently than do younger patients (Lanctot et al. 1998). Furthermore, evidence indicates that first-generation antipsychotics (particularly higher-potency agents) may exacerbate the depressive component of bipolar disorder (Ahlfors et al. 1981; Sachs and Thase 2000).

Lower-potency medications such as chlorpromazine and thioridazine have anticholinergic side effects that can yield memory impairment, confusion, and, in severe cases, delirium. Sedation and orthostatic hypotension are more common among low-potency than high-potency first-generation antipsychotics, further limiting the use of low-potency agents in older adults.

Cardiac arrhythmia may play a role in the choice of antipsychotic medication. Thioridazine, for example, has been associated with abnormal QT intervals and ventricular arrhythmias in patients of all ages (Timell 2000). Although pimozide, droperidol, and haloperidol have been associated with *torsades de pointes* and sudden death, the greatest risk may be with thioridazine (Glassman and Bigger 2001). However, for all antipsychotics, preexisting cardiac conduction abnormalities increase the risk of QT abnormalities, making a baseline electrocardiogram essential before initiating treatment (Glassman and Bigger

2001). Indeed, in a recent epidemiological study, current use of first- and second-generation antipsychotics was associated with dose-related increases in rates of sudden cardiac death (1.99 and 2.26, respectively) (Ray et al. 2009).

Interestingly, evidence regarding the effects of first-generation antipsychotics on cognitive function in older adults is equivocal. In two studies of older patients with dementia, no change was found in overall cognitive status associated with the use of first-generation antipsychotics after 4–6 weeks (Burton et al. 1992) or 1 year (Woerner et al. 1995). However, another study (McShane et al. 1997) found that the rate of cognitive decline in patients with dementia treated with first-generation antipsychotics was twice that of patients who were not— even after adjusting for aggression, diurnal rhythm disturbances, and delusions. Thus, the combination of dementia and first-generation antipsychotics may accelerate dementia-related cognitive decline.

Carbamazepine may decrease serum concentrations of first-generation antipsychotics. In view of potential additive sedative effects, caution is necessary when combining them with sedating agents such as benzodiazepines. Case reports suggest that occasional patients receiving lithium combined with antipsychotics, particularly first-generation antipsychotics, can experience an encephalopathic syndrome that is difficult to distinguish from neuroleptic malignant syndrome.

Second-Generation Antipsychotics

Second-generation antipsychotics have surpassed first-generation antipsychotics in the treatment of older adults (Jeste et al. 1999c), and the growing consensus is that second-generation antipsychotics are the drugs of choice (Gareri et al. 2006), based not only on enhanced safety and tolerability but also on greater efficacy in treatment of mood disorders and negative symptoms of psychosis. Whereas second-generation antipsychotics are often thought of as treatments for acute mania (olanzapine, risperidone, quetiapine, ziprasidone, and aripiprazole all have indications), both quetiapine and the combination of olanzapine and fluoxetine are indicated for bipolar depression. Three of these agents (olanzapine and aripiprazole as monotherapy, and quetiapine as adjunctive therapy) have indications for maintenance treatment, and some authors have suggested that the other second-generation antipsychotics may ultimately prove to have utility not only in acute mania but also in bipolar depression (Jarema 2007). However, aripiprazole and ziprasidone monotherapy were no better than placebo in controlled acute bipolar depression trials. Nevertheless, emerging data suggest that at least some of these agents may be useful as adjuncts to antidepressants in the treatment of unipolar major depressive disorders.

Limited data are available on the use of second-generation antipsychotics in older adults with bipolar disorders (Gareri et al. 2006; Madhusoodanan et al. 1995; Sajatovic et al. 2008; Shulman et al. 1997).

A crucial safety concern with second-generation antipsychotics is the increase in mortality of older adult dementia patients using these drugs. In 2005, the FDA noted that in 17 controlled trials involving 5,106 older adults with dementia and behavioral disorders, olanzapine, risperidone, quetiapine, and aripiprazole yielded an approximately 1.7-fold increase in mortality (an increase from 2.6% to 4.5% with 10 weeks of exposure), primarily because of cardiovascular-related events (e.g., heart failure, sudden death) or infections (mostly pneumonia) (U.S. Food and Drug Administration 2005). Because this increase was seen with second-generation antipsychotic medications in three different chemical classes, the FDA stipulated a boxed warning in the prescribing information for all second-generation antipsychotics, which included clozapine and ziprasidone. As noted above, in 2008, a similar warning was applied to first-generation antipsychotics. The prescribing information for olanzapine, risperidone, and aripiprazole warns of increased cerebrovascular adverse events, including stroke in older adults with dementia-related psychosis, likely presenting a risk similar to that of first-generation antipsychotics (Herrmann et al. 2004).

The FDA has stipulated that the prescribing information for all second-generation antipsychotics include a warning of the risks of hyperglycemia and diabetes mellitus. However, the report of a recent consensus development conference on antipsychotics and obesity, diabetes, and hyperlipidemia emphasized differences between second-generation antipsychotics, with clozapine and olanzapine being the most implicated, risperidone and quetiapine being less implicated, and ziprasidone and aripiprazole being the least implicated (*Physicians' Desk Reference* 2008).

Second-generation antipsychotics appear to have complex safety and tolerability similarities and differences in older adults. For example, certain anticholinergic and antihistaminic symptoms, such as dry mouth, blurred vision, constipation, and urinary difficulties, are seen with olanzapine, risperidone, and quetiapine at roughly twice the rate seen with placebo (Kennedy et al. 2001). However, blurred vision and urinary disturbances were infrequent with olanzapine and quetiapine (Kennedy et al. 2001). Some second-generation antipsychotics such as ziprasidone have been thought to be associated with QTc interval prolongation, although the degree to which this is clinically relevant remains to be established. In general, patients are at an increased risk of torsades de pointes as a result of QTc prolongation if the QTc interval is greater than 500 milliseconds or if it is 60 milliseconds greater than baseline (Haddad and Anderson 2002).

For the older patient, sedation can be difficult to tolerate, interfering with daily function and increasing the risk of falls and concomitant injuries. Some, but not all, second-generation antipsychotics may cause sedation. Specifically, older second-generation antipsychotics such as olanzapine, risperidone, and quetiapine appear more associated with sedation, weight gain, and metabolic problems, and the newer second-generation antipsychotics such as ziprasidone and aripiprazole appear more frequently associated with akathisia, agitation, and anxiety.

Thus, clinicians considering treating older adults with second-generation antipsychotics are faced with challenging risk-benefit determinations. There are important unmet treatment needs in this population, inadequate evidence regarding the efficacy of these drugs in bipolar disorder, and substantial safety and tolerability concerns arising from therapeutic trials in dementia patients with psychosis and/or agitation. Below, we discuss these agents individually in greater detail.

Olanzapine

There are very limited data regarding the use of olanzapine in older adults with bipolar disorders (Nicolato et al. 2006; Samuels and Fang 2004). Olanzapine's use has been limited by safety and tolerability concerns, including sedation, weight gain, and metabolic problems, as well as risks of increased mortality and cerebrovascular accidents in dementia patients. Other adverse effects include orthostatic hypotension, syncope, seizures, hyperprolactinemia, and benign transaminase elevations (Conley and Meltzer 2000).

In view of these data, if a clinician believes that the potential benefits of using olanzapine outweigh the risks (especially increased mortality, cerebrovascular accidents, weight gain, and metabolic disturbance) for an older adult patient and has very carefully assessed the patient (i.e., baseline medical status, weight, fasting blood total, low-density and high-density lipoprotein and total cholesterol, triglycerides, and glucose), it would be prudent to prescribe olanzapine at 1.25–2.5 mg/day, and, as necessary and tolerated, increase by 1.25–2.5 mg/day every 4–7 days, carefully monitoring clinical status, with initial target doses commonly being between 2.5 and 10 mg/day (Table 12–3).

Carbamazepine decreases serum olanzapine concentrations, whereas fluvoxamine and ciprofloxacin may increase serum olanzapine concentrations. Caution is necessary when combining olanzapine with other sedating agents, such as benzodiazepines, in older adults.

Given the limited data on the efficacy of olanzapine in older adults with bipolar disorders, together with its adverse effect profile, including sedation, weight gain, hypertriglyceridemia, and glucose intolerance, the clinician may want to consider other antipsychotic drugs prior to considering olanzapine in this population.

Risperidone

There are very limited data regarding the use of risperidone in older adults with bipolar disorder (Madhusoodanan et al. 1995). The use of risperidone has been limited by safety and tolerability concerns, including sedation, weight gain, metabolic problems, postural hypotension, extrapyramidal symptoms, and increased mortality and cerebrovascular accidents in patients with dementia. Although risperidone had a lower risk of tardive dyskinesia than haloperidol in a 9-month prospective trial involving older patients (Jeste et al. 1999a), it exhibits dose-dependent extrapyramidal symptoms (these are lessened with the intramuscular long-acting formulation). There is no evidence that any cardiac risk is different for older adults as compared with younger adults, yet risperidone may be associated with an increase in the QTc interval (Llerena et al. 2004; Yerrabolu et al. 2000).

In view of the above data, clinicians should first weigh the potential benefits against the risks (e.g., weight gain and metabolic disturbance) when deciding whether to treat older adults with risperidone. While the literature on risk for premature death and stroke pertains to patients with dementia, no similar retrospective studies have investigated similar possible effects on older, frail patients with bipolar disorders. Therefore, after carefully discussing these possibilities with the patient and his or her family and carefully evaluating the patient's health (i.e., baseline medical status, weight, fasting blood total, low-density and high-density lipoprotein and total cholesterol, triglycerides, and glucose), it would be prudent to start risperidone at 0.25–0.5 mg/day, increasing the dosage by 0.25–0.5 mg/day every 4–7 days (with initial target doses commonly being between 0.5 and 2 mg/day) as necessary and tolerated, while carefully monitoring clinical status (Table 12–3). Frail older adults may only tolerate even lower doses.

Carbamazepine decreases serum risperidone concentrations, and paroxetine and fluoxetine may increase serum risperidone concentrations. Caution is necessary when combining risperidone with other sedating agents, such as benzodiazepines, in older adults. There are very limited data regarding the efficacy of risperidone in older adults with bipolar disorder. Together with its adverse effect profile that includes sedation, weight gain, metabolic problems, and risk of increased mortality and cerebrovascular accidents in dementia patients, risperidone treatment may prove challenging enough in this population to lead clinicians to first consider other treatment options.

Paliperidone

Paliperidone, an active metabolite of risperidone, has FDA approval for the treatment of schizophrenia (Citrome 2007). However, it has not been approved for the treatment of bipolar disorder, and no studies have been published on paliperidone use in older adults with bipolar disorders, or on the drug's cognitive effects.

Unlike risperidone, paliperidone is cleared primarily unchanged in the urine. Thus, dosage may need to be decreased in patients with renal impairment. Like risperidone, however, paliperidone can cause mild QTc prolongation (Llerena et al. 2004).

Quetiapine

There are very limited data regarding the efficacy of quetiapine in treating older adults with bipolar disorders (Madhusoodanan et al. 2000; Tariot et al. 2000). Quetiapine's use has been limited by safety and tolerability concerns, including sedation, weight gain, metabolic problems, and postural hypotension. As a second-generation antipsychotic, quetiapine also poses an increased risk of mortality in dementia patients. Other warnings in the quetiapine prescribing information include the risk of clinical worsening of depression and suicide risk (an antidepressant class warning). Quetiapine can also cause dry mouth, constipation, increased alanine transaminase, weight gain, dyspepsia, and seizures (Adler et al. 2007).

In view of these data, if a clinician believes that the potential benefits of quetiapine treatment for an older adult outweigh the risks (especially increased mortality, cerebrovascular accidents, weight gain, and metabolic disturbance) and has very carefully assessed the patient's health (i.e., baseline medical status, weight, and fasting blood total, low-density and high-density lipoprotein and total cholesterol, triglycerides, and glucose), it would be prudent to start quetiapine at 25–50 mg/day, increasing by 25–50 mg/day every 4–7 days as necessary and tolerated, carefully monitoring clinical status. Initial target dosages are commonly between 200 and 400 mg/day, although frail older adults may only tolerate 50–200 mg/day (Table 12–3).

Carbamazepine decreases serum quetiapine concentrations, and paroxetine and ketoconazole and erythromycin may increase serum quetiapine concentrations. Because of potential additive sedative effects, caution is necessary when combining quetiapine with other sedating agents, such as benzodiazepines, in older adults. The very limited data regarding the efficacy of quetiapine in older adults with bipolar disorders, together with its adverse effect profile (with safety and tolerability concerns including sedation, weight gain, metabolic problems, and postural hypotension), may suggest consideration of other treatment options.

Ziprasidone

Currently, there are very limited data regarding the use of ziprasidone in older adults with bipolar disorder or schizophrenia (Loebel et al. 2003a, 2003b). Ziprasidone, possibly to a lesser degree than some other second-generation antipsychotics, may cause hyperglycemia, diabetes mellitus, and metabolic abnormalities. Nevertheless, clinical and laboratory monitoring for obesity, diabetes, and hyperlipidemia may be prudent for patients receiving ziprasidone.

Other warnings in the prescribing information include risk of QTc prolongation and sudden death. Although premarketing studies suggested that ziprasidone is associated with cardiac conduction delays, postmarketing experience to date has failed to indicate clinically significant problems with cardiac conduction (Daniel 2003; Harvey and Bowie 2005). Ziprasidone generally is considered safe with respect to adverse cardiac effects (Greenberg and Citrome 2007), yet it is more likely to lead to QTc prolongation than other second-generation antipsychotics (Haddad and Anderson 2002). In younger adults, lower ziprasidone dosages as compared with higher dosages may increase the risk of akathisia (Oral et al. 2006), so that optimal titration of this agent may involve abruptly increasing the dose if akathisia develops at lower doses. Adjunctive lorazepam used in registration acute mania trials decreased the intensity of the akathisia.

Limited studies of ziprasidone in older adults suggest it may be tolerated and effective in some individuals. To date, ziprasidone does not appear to be associated with weight gain, dyslipidemia, or hyperglycemia, which is an important potential advantage for older adults (Greenberg and Citrome 2007).

In view of the above data, if a clinician believes that the potential benefits of ziprasidone treatment outweigh the risks (especially increased mortality, cerebrovascular accidents, weight gain, and metabolic disturbance) for older adults and has very carefully assessed the patient's health (i.e., baseline medical status, weight, fasting blood total, low-density and high-density lipoprotein and total cholesterol, triglycerides, and glucose), it would be prudent to start ziprasidone at 20 mg/day with food, increasing by 20 mg/day every 4–7 days as necessary and tolerated, carefully monitoring clinical status. Initial target doses would be between 40 and 80 mg/day with food (Table 12–3). It is crucial that ziprasidone be taken with food, as this doubles absorption. Doses in bipolar depression or maintenance treatment may need to be as much as 50% lower than in acute mania. Low doses may yield akathisia, while high doses may yield sedation.

Carbamazepine decreases serum ziprasidone concentrations, and ketoconazole may increase serum ziprasidone concentrations, but the clinical significance of these interactions remains to be determined. Caution is necessary when combining ziprasidone with sedating agents, such as benzodiazepines, in older adults. There are very limited data regarding the efficacy of ziprasidone in older adults with bipolar disorders, such that clinicians may consider other treatment options preferable.

Aripiprazole

There are limited data regarding the use of aripiprazole in older adults with bipolar disorders. In a 12-week, open-label, prospective trial in 20 older adults with bipolar I disorder, adjunctive aripiprazole (starting with 5 mg/day and gradually increasing to a mean final dosage of 10.3 mg/day) yielded significant reductions in mean depression and mania scores compared with baseline (Sajatovic et al. 2008). Aripiprazole was overall adequately tolerated, with no adverse effect discontinuations, with restlessness in 15.8% of patients, clinically significant (≥7%) weight gain in 15.8%, and sedation in 10.5%.

A recent open-label study explored the use of aripiprazole as an augmentation to selective serotonin reuptake inhibitors (SSRIs) in depressed older adults (Rutherford et al. 2007). After 6 weeks of augmentation ranging from 5 to 15 mg/day, half of the subjects exhibited a significant improvement in depression. This parallels the experience in younger patients (Berman et al. 2007). The most frequent side effects in older adults were dry mouth (25%), agitation/anxiety (20%), and drowsiness (15%) (Rutherford et al. 2007).

The use of aripiprazole has been limited by safety and tolerability concerns (e.g., akathisia), as well as risks of increased mortality and cerebrovascular accidents in dementia patients. Although weight gain can occur with aripiprazole, it is generally less of a problem than with olanzapine (McQuade et al. 2004). Nevertheless, aripiprazole can cause metabolic problems.

In view of the above data, if a clinician believes the potential benefits outweigh the risks (especially increased mortality, cerebrovascular accidents, weight gain, and metabolic disturbance) for older adults and has very carefully assessed the patient's health (i.e., baseline medical status, weight, and fasting blood total, low-density and high-density lipoprotein and total cholesterol, triglycerides, and glucose), it would be prudent to start aripiprazole at 2–5 mg/day, increasing by 2–5 mg/day every 4–7 days as necessary and tolerated, carefully monitoring clinical status. Initial target doses are commonly between 2 and 15 mg/day, although frail older adults may only tolerate 2–10 mg/day (Table 12–3).

Carbamazepine decreases serum aripiprazole concentrations, and quinidine and ketoconazole increase serum aripiprazole concentrations. Caution is necessary when combining aripiprazole with sedating agents, such as benzodiazepines, in older adults.

As with other second-generation antipsychotics, there are very limited data regarding the efficacy of aripiprazole in older adults with bipolar disorders, and its adverse effect profile (i.e., safety and tolerability concerns, including akathisia, and increased mortality and cerebrovascular accidents in dementia patients) may prove challenging.

Clozapine

Clozapine lacks an indication for bipolar disorder. However, this agent is the only medication with an FDA indication for treatment-resistant schizophrenia and for the prevention of suicidal behaviors in schizophrenia. The absence of a bipolar disorder indication, combined with a particularly challenging adverse effect profile, means that clozapine is held in reserve for patients with treatment-resistant illness.

Limited data are available regarding clozapine's use in older adults with bipolar disorders (Shulman et al. 1997). For example, in three older adults with treatment-resistant bipolar disorder, open clozapine (mean final dosage 80 mg/day, range 25–112.5 mg/day) was effective and adequately tolerated, both acutely and prophylactically (Shulman et al. 1997).

The U.S. prescribing information for clozapine includes boxed warnings regarding the risks of 1) agranulocytosis, 2) seizures, 3) myocarditis, 4) other adverse cardiovascular and respiratory effects, and 5) increased mortality as a second-generation antipsychotic. Whether or not the latter occurs with cloza-pine remains to be established. The most concerning adverse effect of clozapine, agranulocytosis, may occur more frequently in older than in younger patients (Alvir et al. 1993). A frequently underestimated adverse effect with clozapine, magnified in the geriatric population, is severe constipation, which may be life endangering at times, resulting in bowel infarction. Beginning the patient on a high-fiber diet, with standing prescriptions of laxatives, may be indicated prior to prescribing clozapine.

Metabolic adverse effects are particularly common with clozapine and in-clude weight gain, hyperlipidemia, hypertriglyceridemia, and hyperglycemia (Allison et al. 1999; Gaulin et al. 1999). Thus, clinical and (as indicated) labo-ratory monitoring for obesity, diabetes, and hyperlipidemia appear prudent for patients receiving clozapine. Other warnings in the prescribing information in-clude the risk of eosinophilia. Clozapine appears to be the least likely antipsy-chotic to yield extrapyramidal adverse effects.

Somnolence is a common side effect of clozapine and is frequently a reason for discontinuation (Kane et al. 1988a). Seizures, sedation, and confusion are of particular concern in older adults with concurrent neurological illness (Duffy and Kant 1996). Postural hypotension may be particularly problematic in older adults (Chengappa et al. 1995). However, conservative dosing may yield accept-able tolerability, even in patients with neurological disorders (Chengappa et al. 1995; Oberholzer et al. 1992).

In view of the data discussed above, clinicians need to consider whether the potential benefits of clozapine in older adults outweigh the risks (especially agranulocytosis, seizures, myocarditis, other adverse cardiovascular and respi-ratory effects, increased mortality, cerebrovascular accidents, weight gain, con-stipation, and metabolic disturbance). Then, after very careful assessment of baseline medical status, complete blood count with differential, weight, and fasting blood total, low-density and high-density lipoprotein and total choles-terol, triglycerides, and glucose, the prudent approach is to start clozapine at 6.25–25 mg/day and, as necessary and tolerated, increase by 6.25–25 mg/day every 4–7 days, carefully monitoring clinical status. Initial target dosages are commonly 112.5–225 mg/day (Table 12–3), although frail older adults may tol-erate only 25–100 mg/day.

Carbamazepine and tobacco smoking decrease serum clozapine concentra-tions, and fluvoxamine and possibly caffeine (in excess of 400 mg/day) increase serum clozapine concentrations. Caution is necessary when combining cloza-pine with other sedating agents, such as benzodiazepines, in older adults. Clozapine is not recommended in combination with other agents that cause marrow suppression.

In summary, very limited data are available regarding the efficacy of clozapine in older adults with bipolar disorders, and its particularly challenging adverse effect profile may lead clinicians to hold this option in reserve for treatment-resistant cases.

Metabolic Syndrome

As discussed in previous sections of this chapter, some second-generation antipsychotics cause weight gain, hyperglycemia, and dyslipidemia, all of which are symptoms associated with metabolic syndrome (Straker et al. 2005). Some research suggests that the risk of metabolic syndrome is greatest with clozapine and olanzapine, followed by quetiapine and risperidone, and followed in turn by aripiprazole and ziprasidone (Correll et al. 2006). In mixed-age patients taking olanzapine, a weight gain of at least 2 kg in the first 3 weeks predicted substantial weight gain (≥5 kg or ≥7%) by week 30 (Lipkovich et al. 2006). In patients with dementia and behavioral disturbances taking olanzapine, weight gain was greater in those with a body mass index lower than 25 (Lipkovich et al. 2007).

If second-generation antipsychotics are prescribed for short-term treatment of symptoms associated with an affective episode, metabolic issues are of less concern. However, if a patient is to be maintained on a second-generation antipsychotic, the clinician should weigh the individual at the onset of therapy and obtain fasting blood glucose and glycated hemoglobin Hb1Ac. Subsequently, weight can be monitored every 2 months and fasting blood glucose checked every 6 months, or when significant weight gain occurs. In many cases, it may be worthwhile to consider the benefits of adequately treated psychiatric symptoms accompanied by the need for an oral hypoglycemic agent, such as metformin (Wu et al. 2008).

Combination Therapy

Polypharmacy in older adults can be fraught with more challenges than in younger adults. The challenges in older adults may be related to altered drug clearance, comorbid medical illness, concurrent pharmacotherapy, and increased side-effect sensitivity.

Several antipsychotics (e.g., haloperidol, fluphenazine, loxapine, risperidone, aripiprazole) are metabolized to a significant degree by the cytochrome P450 (CYP) enzyme 2D6 isoform. Thus, CYP2D6 inhibitors, such as the antidepressants fluoxetine, paroxetine, duloxetine, and bupropion, may increase serum levels of these antipsychotics, in some instances yielding clinically significant adverse effects. Quetiapine is metabolized to a significant degree by CYP3A4, making it susceptible to induction by carbamazepine, or to inhibition by fluoxetine, fluvoxamine, nefazodone, azole antifungals, and other agents.

Orthostatic hypotension may be a significant adverse event in older adults, particularly if they are taking antihypertensive medications. Thus, when using an antipsychotic that has adrenergic α_1 receptor–blocking characteristics (e.g., any low-potency first-generation antipsychotic, clozapine, olanzapine, and in some instances risperidone), orthostatic hypotension may become a difficult problem, resulting in falls. Patients should be advised to rise slowly from seated or supine positions and may require readjustment of their antihypertensive medication.

The prescription of multiple concurrent second-generation antipsychotics for patients with bipolar disorders is not a standard treatment. Evidence from younger patients with schizophrenia suggests a greater incidence of metabolic syndrome in patients taking more than one second-generation antipsychotic (Correll et al. 2007). Because older adults are more likely to have medical problems such as hypertension, hyperglycemia, and hypertriglyceridemia, clinicians should try to avoid prescribing multiple concurrent second-generation antipsychotics.

Adjunctive Benzodiazepines

Generally, benzodiazepines should be used cautiously in older adults, but in instances of extreme agitation, they may be necessary. The cautions associated with benzodiazepine use by older adults are related to the presence of comorbid medical conditions or drug-drug interactions. In addition, older patients are generally more sensitive than younger patients to central effects of benzodiazepines (Greenblatt et al. 1991a, 1991b), such as disinhibition, ataxia, confusion, and even delirium.

Medical conditions more common in older patients may give rise to specific cautions. For example, patients with chronic obstructive pulmonary disease may be predisposed to respiratory depression, especially when given intramuscular or intravenous benzodiazepines (George 2000; Guilleminault 1990). Patients with end-stage cirrhosis may metabolize certain benzodiazepines more slowly, needing only one-third of the usual dosage of such agents (Sellers 1978).

In addition, benzodiazepines can adversely affect cognition in older adults, which in turn may affect their ability to execute activities of daily living and may lead to diagnostic quandaries (Brooks and Hoblyn 2007). For example, should a patient present to an emergency room, medical personnel may not realize that the patient is taking benzodiazepines and misdiagnose cognitive slowing as a dementia-related process or disinhibition as delirium.

The risks of dependence and physiological tolerance increase with longer-term use of benzodiazepines. If patients with bipolar disorders require long-term medication for anxiety-related symptoms, low dosages of olanzapine, quetiapine, or risperidone may be reasonable alternatives. However, as mentioned above, these medications also have adverse effects associated with them and should be given with caution. The use of cognitive-behavioral psychotherapy should be considered, along with relaxation tapes and other nonpharmacological methods. These techniques may have similar efficacy compared with medications in some situations. SSRIs may be options but can yield treatment-emergent mania.

Additional information regarding benzodiazepines is provided in Chapter 14 of this volume.

Adjunctive Antihistaminergic and Anticholinergic Medications

Antihistaminergic and anticholinergic medications are commonly prescribed as adjunctive medications for patients with bipolar disorders. For example, anticholinergic medications (e.g., benztropine) are often administered with first-generation antipsychotics to lessen extrapyramidal side effects. Antihistamines (e.g., diphenhydramine, hydroxyzine) are often administered as anxiolytics and hypnotics to avoid the use of benzodiazepines. These medications rarely have roles in treating older patients with bipolar disorders because of their anticholinergic load. Older compared with younger adults are more vulnerable to anticholinergic delirium, and both anticholinergic and antihistaminergic medications are associated with cognitive deficits (Brooks and Hoblyn 2007). An extensive literature exists on the overuse of anticholinergic drugs in older adults and their deleterious effects on cognition (Mulsant et al. 2003).

Adjunctive Antidepressants

The role of antidepressants in the management of bipolar disorder is complex and at times controversial. Researchers have suggested that the foundational treatments for bipolar depression are mood stabilizers and that antidepressants are adjuncts that need to be used with caution (Thase and Sachs 2000). However, some evidence indicates that older patients with bipolar disorders who are treated with a mood stabilizer and an antidepressant may be less likely to attempt suicide (Aizenberg et al. 2006). Even though the benefits of antidepressants as adjunctive agents might be unclear, these medications are commonly used to treat depressive episodes. Medications of other classes are effective in treating bipolar depression, although very limited data are available regarding their utility in older adults. For example, quetiapine monotherapy and the olanzapine-fluoxetine combination are effective treatments for acute bipolar depression, whereas lamotrigine is effective in the prophylaxis of bipolar depression (Gao and Calabrese 2005).

Additional information regarding antidepressants is provided in Chapter 14 of this volume.

Other Newer Anticonvulsants

Other newer anticonvulsants (felbamate, gabapentin, levetiracetam, oxcarbazepine, pregabalin, tiagabine, topiramate, zonisamide) do not appear to be generally effective for acute mania in mixed-age populations but may have utility for comorbid conditions (e.g., anxiety or alcohol use disorders or pain syndromes). In view of the absence of evidence of their efficacy in bipolar disorder and because of their potential for adverse effects and drug interactions (Fenn et al. 2006; Sommer et al. 2007), use of these agents in older adults ought to be undertaken with considerable caution.

Electroconvulsive Therapy

Electroconvulsive therapy (ECT) is an important evidence-based treatment option for major depressive episodes. Meta-analyses of randomized controlled trials in mixed-age samples of depressed patients with unipolar or bipolar disorder revealed superior efficacy for 1) real compared with simulated ECT, 2) ECT compared with pharmacotherapy (including tricyclic antidepressants, monoamine oxidase inhibitors, paroxetine, and lithium), and 3) high compared with low electrical stimulus ECT (The UK ECT Review Group 2003). Unfortunately, patients with bipolar disorders in ECT studies are commonly aggregated with patients with major depressive disorder. As discussed in Chapter 6 ("Management of Acute Manic and Mixed Episodes in Bipolar Disorders") of this volume, only limited controlled evidence supports a role for ECT in the treatment of acute mania (Mukherjee et al. 1994).

ECT has been advocated for the treatment of depression in older adults (Kamat et al. 2003), based on limited controlled data in older adults, uncontrolled data in older adults, and imputing findings from mixed-age samples.

Potential adverse effects primarily involve cognitive impairment. Less often, cardiovascular complications, prolonged seizures, prolonged apnea, headaches, muscle soreness, nausea, treatment-emergent mania, and postictal delirium may occur (Kamat et al. 2003). Medical risks that need consideration in older adults consenting to ECT include space-occupying lesions and brain tumors (increased intracranial pressure risk), cerebrovascular disease (hemorrhage, confusion risks), cardiovascular disease (cardiac disease exacerbation risk), diabetes mellitus (hypoglycemia during pre-ECT fasting risk), seizure disorders (prolonged/spontaneous seizure risk), hyperthyroidism (thyroid storm risk), and electrolyte disturbances (hypokalemia—prolonged paralysis risk; hyperkalemia—cardiotoxicity risk; hyponatremia—spontaneous seizure risk) (Kamat et al. 2003). Medications that should be used with caution and that may pose an increased risk during ECT include theophylline (status epilepticus risk), benzodiazepines (increased seizure threshold, decreased cognition), anticonvulsants (increased seizure threshold), lithium (delirium, prolonged seizure risks), diuretics (incontinence, bladder rupture risks), hypoglycemic agents (hypoglycemia during pre-ECT fasting risk), and L-dopa/carbidopa (delirium risk) (Kamat et al. 2003).

Taken together, the very limited data regarding the efficacy of ECT in older adults with bipolar disorders and its adverse effect profile may lead clinicians to hold this option in reserve for treatment-resistant cases. On the other hand, proponents of ECT point out that it may carry a lower risk for complications than some forms of pharmacotherapy among older adults (Kamat et al. 2003). ECT remains the treatment of choice when the acuteness of affective illness compromises the patient's medical stability.

Drug Metabolism in Older Adults

As a group, older adults compared with younger adults have as much as 30% lower hepatic cytochrome P450 enzyme activity (Sotaniemi et al. 1997). In older adults, decreased clearance and associated increased half-lives and serum levels necessitate dosing adjustments and greater care with respect to drug interactions. With important exceptions such as lithium and paliperidone, which rely primarily on renal clearance, most psychotropic medications used in patients with bipolar disorders are metabolized, commonly through the P450 system and/or conjugation reactions. In Chapter 13 of this volume, Table 13–14 provides a classification of many psychotropic medications and their associated enzymes. Potent enzyme inhibitors and inducers can lead to marked increases and decreases in serum drug concentrations, respectively, which may prove particularly problematic in older adults.

Comorbid Medical Conditions

Comorbid medical conditions are common in older adults with bipolar disorders and must be considered when choosing psychotropic medications. One study of older adults with bipolar disorders revealed an average of 2.1 comorbid medical conditions and 1.5 nonpsychiatric medications (Sajatovic et al. 1996). Patients with glaucoma are sensitive to medications with anticholinergic properties (Lachkar and Bouassida 2007) because of the risk of acute angle closure and resultant increased intraocular pressure. Similarly, patients with prostatic hypertrophy may experience increased difficulty with urination when taking anticholinergic agents. Patients with Parkinson's disease may experience dramatic exacerbations of motor symptoms, particularly with higher-potency first-generation antipsychotics, related to the potent dopamine D_2 receptor blockade of these medications and the relative lack of mitigating anticholinergic activity.

Dementia is not uncommon in older adults with bipolar disorders; its prevalence was as high as 3% in a nationwide sample of 37,304 veterans of all ages with bipolar disorders (Brooks et al. 2006). Despite the FDA warnings regarding the use of second-generation antipsychotics for agitation in dementia, as many as 40% of patients with dementia may be taking these drugs (Oborne et al. 2002).

Clinicians treating older adults with psychosis and/or agitation face substantial challenges because no treatments have been approved by the FDA. Although conservatively dosed valproate may be generally well tolerated, data are insufficient to consider this an effective intervention. In view of the crucial unmet need for intervention, a frank discussion with significant others regarding the degree of uncertainty and the potential risks and benefits is indicated in managing older adults with psychosis and/or agitation.

Pulmonary diseases are more common in older patients who smoke than in younger patients. Medications used to treat chronic obstructive pulmonary disease may lead to complications when combined with certain psychopharmacological medications. For example, inhaled medications such as albuterol (a β-adrenergic agonist) may lead to tachycardia, a possible complication in the therapy of a patient with additional cardiac disease who is also taking lithium or first-generation antipsychotics.

Cardiac disease and associated QTc prolongation is more common in older adults, and evidence that some second-generation antipsychotics (most notably ziprasidone) are associated with QTc prolongation is concerning. Of importance, the clinician should remember that the risk of *torsades de pointes* associated with QT prolongation increases when the QTc interval is greater than 500 milliseconds or is 60 milliseconds greater than baseline. In a recent epidemiological study, current use of first- and second-generation antipsychotics was associated with dose-related increases in rates of sudden cardiac death (1.99 and 2.26, respectively) (Ray et al. 2009). Also, sinus node problems are more common in older adults and increase the likelihood of cardiac events when using lithium (Kando et al. 1996).

Psychosocial Interventions in Older Adults

Limited data have been reported regarding the efficacy of such interventions in older adults with bipolar disorders. Thus, clinicians are faced with imputing information regarding the utility of psychosocial interventions from data in mixed-age patients with bipolar disorders (reviewed in detail in Chapter 15, "Adjunctive Psychosocial Interventions in the Management of Bipolar Disorders") or older patients with unipolar major depressive disorder.

Limited data suggest that psychotherapy, particularly cognitive-behavioral therapy (CBT), has utility in depressed older adults. A recent meta-analysis found five randomized controlled trials (153 participants) that suggested that CBT was more effective than a waiting list control condition (Wilson et al. 2008). An expert consensus guideline suggested that the preferred psychotherapy techniques for treating depression in older patients were CBT, supportive psychotherapy, problem-solving psychotherapy, and interpersonal psychotherapy (Alexopoulos et al. 2001).

Integrated psychosocial interventions may offer benefits for patients with bipolar disorders, although few data are available regarding such interventions in older adults. In 441 mixed-age (mean age 44.2 years) patients with bipolar disorders, systematic care management (structured group psychoeducation, monthly telephone monitoring, and feedback to and coordination with a mental health treatment team) provided by nurse care managers yielded lower mean mania ratings over 24 months (Simon et al. 2006). In another randomized controlled trial in 306 mixed-age (mean age 46.6 years) veterans with bipolar disorders, a collaborative model for chronic care (group psychoeducation, nurse care coordinators to improve information flow and access to and continuity of care, and clinician decision support with simplified practice guidelines) reduced weeks in (primarily manic) mood episodes, and improved social role function, mental quality of life, and treatment satisfaction over 36 months (Bauer et al. 2006).

Substantial support already exists for the use of integrated psychosocial interventions for geriatric depression. For example, an expert consensus guideline regarding the management of depression in older adults strongly supported including appropriate psychosocial interventions (e.g., psychoeducation, family counseling, and visiting nurse services) in treatment programs (Alexopoulos et al. 2001).

Taken together, the findings discussed above suggest the potential utility of psychotherapy and psychosocial interventions in older adults with bipolar disorders, and the need for studies of these interventions in this specific population.

Conclusion

Older adults with bipolar disorders present a significant public health challenge. The assessment and treatment of bipolar disorders in this population are complex because of multiple confounding effects, including cognitive changes, medical comorbidities, and drug interactions. Unfortunately, no large, randomized, controlled trials have been reported in this population to provide an evidence base for bipolar disorder therapeutics. Thus, clinicians are faced with deriving evidence from mixed-age populations and inferring safety and tolerability of treatments for older adults with bipolar disorders from the literature on older adults with epilepsy, psychosis, and dementia with agitation. Hopefully, in the future, data from large, randomized controlled trials in older adults with bipolar disorders will provide an evidence base to better inform clinicians treating this population.

Case Study: Management of Older Adults With Bipolar Disorders

Ms. Green, a 78-year-old woman diagnosed with bipolar II disorder with rapid-cycling course, had previously experienced both adverse effects and little effectiveness from medications. Her 50-year history of recurrent severe major depressive episodes required approximately six hospitalizations between ages 36 and 74, and 10 more hospitalizations for ECT of depressive episodes between ages 74 and 78. Ms. Green also had a history of recurrent hypomanic episodes, typically prior to depression, and never accompanied by psychosis, hospitalization, or severe impairment. Lithium was ineffective, valproate yielded a modest increase in euthymic periods but was accompanied by intolerable diarrhea and tremor, and carbamazepine gave rise to confusion. Brief trials of multiple antidepressants were not effective.

Upon her initial presentation, she was taking amlodipine 5 mg/day for hypertension, oxybutynin (a centrally active anticholinergic drug that has been found to decrease cognition in healthy older adults [Katz et al. 1998]) 10 mg/day for stress incontinence, and no psychotropic medication, but was receiving recurrent brief series of ECT, usually comprising two treatments upon the emergence of a depressive episode. She weighed 136 lb, was 5 feet, 4 inches tall (body mass index 23.4), and had normal baseline serum chemistries, including fasting glucose, lipids, and triglycerides.

Olanzapine was started and titrated over 3 months to 7.5 mg/day, which attenuated the frequency and severity of both hypomanic and major depressive episodes, permitting Ms. Green to avoid ECT for several months for the first time in years. Sedation and ataxia precluded olanzapine dosages greater than 7.5 mg/day. Because of persistent affective cycling, lamotrigine was added and titrated over 8 months to 200 mg/day; sedation precluded higher dosages. The combination of lamotrigine and olanzapine was well tolerated.

Ms. Green had a series of breakthrough depressive symptoms that gave rise to a series of trials of antidepressants, all of which either were ineffective or caused adverse effects. For example, fluoxetine, with dosages to 40 mg/day, was ineffective, and agitation precluded higher dosages. Bupropion, at dosages to 300 mg/day, was ineffective, and tremor precluded the administration of higher dosages. When sertraline was added, at a dosage of 75 mg/day, the patient developed a urinary tract infection, more severe depression, and an abrupt deterioration in cognition, which resulted, at age 82, in her first psychiatric hospitalization in 4 years. Evaluation for other medical and neurological contributors was negative, and she responded to treatment of her urinary tract infection as well as a single ECT treatment.

At this point, no further trials of antidepressants were attempted, because of the limited efficacy and tolerability of these agents. Her internist started trimethoprim 100 mg/day to treat recurrent urinary tract infections (apparently correlated with episodic depressive and confusional symptoms). Ms. Green subsequently developed another urinary tract infection accompanied by severe depression and an abrupt deterioration in cognition, resulting in another psychiatric hospitalization, again with a 4-year interval between hospitalizations, at age 86. Cephalexin yielded resolution of the acute urinary tract infection, which was accompanied by resolution of depression and cognitive problems.

In the 3 years since that time, Ms. Green has been maintained on lamotrigine 200 mg/day, olanzapine 7.5–10 mg/day, cephalexin 100 mg/day, and amlodipine 10 mg/day, and has done well psychiatrically and medically. Throughout the course of her treatment, her maximum weight has been 142 lb

(BMI 24.4), and she has continued to have normal fasting glucose, lipids, and triglycerides.

Thus, the foundation of Ms. Green's psychotropic regimen proved to be lamotrigine 200 mg/day plus olanzapine 7.5–10 mg/day, which was well tolerated, and ultimately—combined with effective urinary tract infection prophylaxis—permitted a rate of hospitalization (0.18 incidents per year, 2 in 11 years) that represented a more than 10-fold decrease compared with the 4 years immediately prior (2.5 per year, 10 in 4 years).

References

Abbott FS, Kassam J, Orr JM, et al: The effect of aspirin on valproic acid metabolism. Clin Pharmacol Ther 40:94–100, 1986

Abou-Saleh MT, Coppen A: The prognosis of depression in old age: the case for lithium therapy. Br J Psychiatry 143:527–528, 1983

Adler CM, Fleck DE, Brecher M, et al: Safety and tolerability of quetiapine in the treatment of acute mania in bipolar disorder. J Affect Disord 100 (suppl 1):S15–S22, 2007

Ahearn EP, Steffens DC, Cassidy F, et al: Familial leukoencephalopathy in bipolar disorder. Am J Psychiatry 155:1605–1607, 1998

Ahlfors UG, Baastrup PC, Dencker SJ, et al: Flupenthixol decanoate in recurrent manic-depressive illness: a comparison with lithium. Acta Psychiatr Scand 64:226–237, 1981

Aizenberg D, Olmer A, Barak Y: Suicide attempts amongst elderly bipolar patients. J Affect Disord 91:91–94, 2006

Alexopoulos GS, Katz IR, Reynolds CF 3rd, et al: The expert consensus guideline series: pharmacotherapy of depressive disorders in older patients. Postgrad Med (Spec No Pharmacotherapy):1–86, 2001

Allison DB, Mentore JL, Heo M, et al: Antipsychotic-induced weight gain: a comprehensive research synthesis. Am J Psychiatry 156:1686–1696, 1999

Alvir JM, Lieberman JA, Safferman AZ, et al: Clozapine-induced agranulocytosis: incidence and risk factors in the United States. N Engl J Med 329:162–167, 1993

Barak Y, Shamir E, Zemishlani H, et al: Olanzapine vs. haloperidol in the treatment of elderly chronic schizophrenia patients. Prog Neuropsychopharmacol Biol Psychiatry 26:1199–1202, 2002

Battino D, Croci D, Rossini A, et al: Serum carbamazepine concentrations in elderly patients: a case-matched pharmacokinetic evaluation based on therapeutic drug monitoring data. Epilepsia 44:923–929, 2003

Bauer MS, McBride L, Williford WO, et al: Collaborative care for bipolar disorder, part II: impact on clinical outcome, function, and costs. Psychiatr Serv 57:937–945, 2006

Berman RM, Marcus RN, Swanink R, et al: The efficacy and safety of aripiprazole as adjunctive therapy in major depressive disorder: a multicenter, randomized, double-blind, placebo-controlled study. J Clin Psychiatry 68:843–853, 2007

Bowden CL, Asnis GM, Ginsberg LD, et al: Safety and tolerability of lamotrigine for bipolar disorder. Drug Saf 27:173–184, 2004

Brodie MJ, Overstall PW, Giorgi L: Multicentre, double-blind, randomised comparison between lamotrigine and carbamazepine in elderly patients with newly diagnosed epilepsy. The UK Lamotrigine Elderly Study Group. Epilepsy Res 37:81–87, 1999

Brooks JO 3rd, Hoblyn JC: Secondary mania in older adults. Am J Psychiatry 162:2033–2038, 2005

Brooks JO, Hoblyn JC: Neurocognitive costs and benefits of psychotropic medications in older adults. J Geriatr Psychiatry Neurol 20:199–214, 2007

Brooks JO 3rd, Hoblyn JC, Kraemer HC, et al: Factors associated with psychiatric hospitalization of individuals diagnosed with dementia and comorbid bipolar disorder. J Geriatr Psychiatry Neurol 19:72–77, 2006

Brooks JO, Hoblyn JC, Woodard S, et al: Relations between delayed memory and cerebral metabolism in older euthymic adults with bipolar disorder. Biol Psychiatry 61(8S):114S, 2007

Bryson SM, Verma N, Scott PJ, et al: Pharmacokinetics of valproic acid in young and elderly subjects. Br J Clin Pharmacol 16:104–105, 1983

Burton LC, German PS, Rovner BW, et al: Physical restraint use and cognitive decline among nursing home residents. J Am Geriatr Soc 40:811–816, 1992

Cates M, Powers R: Concomitant rash and blood dyscrasias in geriatric psychiatry patients treated with carbamazepine. Ann Pharmacother 32:884–887, 1998

Chapron DJ: Comment on "Pharmacokinetics of lithium in the elderly." J Clin Psychopharmacol 8:78, 1988

Charney DS, Reynolds CF 3rd, Lewis L, et al: Depression and Bipolar Support Alliance consensus statement on the unmet needs in diagnosis and treatment of mood disorders in late life. Arch Gen Psychiatry 60:664–672, 2003

Chen ST, Altshuler LL, Melnyk KA, et al: Efficacy of lithium vs. valproate in the treatment of mania in the elderly: a retrospective study. J Clin Psychiatry 60:181–186, 1999

Chengappa KN, Baker RW, Kreinbrook SB, et al: Clozapine use in female geriatric patients with psychoses. J Geriatr Psychiatry Neurol 8:12–15, 1995

Citrome L: Paliperidone: quo vadis? Int J Clin Pract 61:653–662, 2007

Conley RR, Meltzer HY: Adverse events related to olanzapine. J Clin Psychiatry 61 (suppl 8):26–29; discussion 30, 2000

Conney J, Kaston B: Pharmacoeconomic and health outcome comparison of lithium and divalproex in a VA geriatric nursing home population: influence of drug-related morbidity on total cost of treatment. Am J Manag Care 5:197–204, 1999

Correll CU, Frederickson AM, Kane JM, et al: Metabolic syndrome and the risk of coronary heart disease in 367 patients treated with second-generation antipsychotic drugs. J Clin Psychiatry 67:575–583, 2006

Correll CU, Frederickson AM, Kane JM, et al: Does antipsychotic polypharmacy increase the risk for metabolic syndrome? Schizophr Res 89:91–100, 2007

Cowley LM, Glen RS: Double-blind study of thioridazine and haloperidol in geriatric patients with a psychosis associated with organic brain syndrome. J Clin Psychiatry 40:411–419, 1979

Cullen M, Mitchell P, Brodaty H, et al: Carbamazepine for treatment-resistant melancholia. J Clin Psychiatry 52:472–476, 1991

Daniel DG: Tolerability of ziprasidone: an expanding perspective. J Clin Psychiatry 64 (suppl 19):40–49, 2003

Depp CA, Jeste DV: Bipolar disorder in older adults: a critical review. Bipolar Disord 6:343–367, 2004

Depp CA, Lindamer LA, Folsom DP, et al: Differences in clinical features and mental health service use in bipolar disorder across the lifespan. Am J Geriatr Psychiatry 13:290–298, 2005

Duffy JD, Kant R: Clinical utility of clozapine in 16 patients with neurological disease. J Neuropsychiatry Clin Neurosci 8:92–96, 1996

Duncan JS, Shorvon SD, Trimble MR: Effects of removal of phenytoin, carbamazepine, and valproate on cognitive function. Epilepsia 31:584–591, 1990

Fenn HH, Sommer BR, Ketter TA, et al: Safety and tolerability of mood-stabilising anticonvulsants in the elderly. Expert Opin Drug Saf 5:401–416, 2006

Gallassi R, Morreale A, Lorusso S, et al: Cognitive effects of valproate. Epilepsy Res 5:160–164, 1990

Gao K, Calabrese JR: Newer treatment studies for bipolar depression. Bipolar Disord 7 (suppl 5):13–23, 2005

Gareri P, De Fazio P, De Fazio S, et al: Adverse effects of atypical antipsychotics in the elderly: a review. Drugs Aging 23:937–956, 2006

Gaulin BD, Markowitz JS, Caley CF, et al: Clozapine-associated elevation in serum triglycerides. Am J Psychiatry 156:1270–1272, 1999

George CF: Perspectives on the management of insomnia in patients with chronic respiratory disorders. Sleep 23 (suppl 1):S31–S35; discussion S36–S38, 2000

Gildengers AG, Butters MA, Seligman K, et al: Cognitive functioning in late-life bipolar disorder. Am J Psychiatry 161:736–738, 2004

Gildengers AG, Butters MA, Chisholm D, et al: Cognitive functioning and instrumental activities of daily living in late-life bipolar disorder. Am J Geriatr Psychiatry 15:174–179, 2007

Gildengers AG, Butters MA, Chisholm D, et al: A 12-week open-label pilot study of donepezil for cognitive functioning and instrumental activities of daily living in late-life bipolar disorder. Int J Geriatr Psychiatry 23:693–698, 2008

Gillham RA, Williams N, Wiedmann KD, et al: Cognitive function in adult epileptic patients established on anticonvulsant monotherapy. Epilepsy Res 7:219–225, 1990

Glassman AH, Bigger JT Jr: Antipsychotic drugs: prolonged QTc interval, torsade de pointes, and sudden death. Am J Psychiatry 158:1774–1782, 2001

Goldberg JF, Sacks MH, Kocsis JH: Low-dose lithium augmentation of divalproex in geriatric mania (letter). J Clin Psychiatry 61:304, 2000

Goodwin FK: Rationale for using lithium in combination with other mood stabilizers in the management of bipolar disorder. J Clin Psychiatry 64 (suppl 5):18–24, 2003

Goodwin FR, Jamison K: Manic-Depressive Illness: Bipolar Disorders and Recurrent Depression, 2nd Edition. New York, Oxford University Press, 2007

Greenberg WM, Citrome L: Ziprasidone for schizophrenia and bipolar disorder: a review of the clinical trials. CNS Drug Rev 13:137–177, 2007

Greenblatt DJ, Harmatz JS, Shader RI: Clinical pharmacokinetics of anxiolytics and hypnotics in the elderly: therapeutic considerations (part I). Clin Pharmacokinet 21:165–177, 1991a

Greenblatt DJ, Harmatz JS, Shader RI: Clinical pharmacokinetics of anxiolytics and hypnotics in the elderly: therapeutic considerations (part II). Clin Pharmacokinet 21:262–273, 1991b

Guilleminault C: Benzodiazepines, breathing, and sleep. Am J Med 88:25S–28S, 1990

Haddad PM, Anderson IM: Antipsychotic-related QTc prolongation, torsade de pointes and sudden death. Drugs 62:1649–1671, 2002

Hardy BG, Shulman KI, Mackenzie SE, et al: Pharmacokinetics of lithium in the elderly. J Clin Psychopharmacol 7:153–158, 1987

Harvey PD, Bowie CR: Ziprasidone: efficacy, tolerability, and emerging data on wide-ranging effectiveness. Expert Opin Pharmacother 6:337–346, 2005

Hays JC, Krishnan KR, George LK, et al: Age of first onset of bipolar disorder: demographic, family history, and psychosocial correlates. Depress Anxiety 7:76–82, 1998

Head L, Dening T: Lithium in the over-65s: who is taking it and who is monitoring it? A survey of older adults on lithium in the Cambridge Mental Health Services catchment area. Int J Geriatr Psychiatry 13:164–171, 1998

Herrmann N, Mamdani M, Lanctot KL: Atypical antipsychotics and risk of cerebrovascular accidents. Am J Psychiatry 161:1113–1115, 2004

Hewick DS, Newbury P, Hopwood S, et al: Age as a factor affecting lithium therapy. Br J Clin Pharmacol 4:201–205, 1977

Himmelhoch JM, Neil JF, May SJ, et al: Age, dementia, dyskinesias, and lithium response. Am J Psychiatry 137:941–945, 1980

Hoblyn JC, Brooks JO, Rosen AC, et al: Cerebral metabolic correlates of attention in older euthymic adults with bipolar disorder. Biol Psychiatry 61(8S):116S, 2007

Howanitz E, Pardo M, Smelson DA, et al: The efficacy and safety of clozapine versus chlorpromazine in geriatric schizophrenia. J Clin Psychiatry 60:41–44, 1999

Jarema M: Atypical antipsychotics in the treatment of mood disorders. Curr Opin Psychiatry 20:23–29, 2007

Jeste DV, Caligiuri MP, Paulsen JS, et al: Risk of tardive dyskinesia in older patients: a prospective longitudinal study of 266 outpatients. Arch Gen Psychiatry 52:756–765, 1995

Jeste DV, Alexopoulos GS, Bartels SJ, et al: Consensus statement on the upcoming crisis in geriatric mental health: research agenda for the next 2 decades. Arch Gen Psychiatry 56:848–853, 1999a

Jeste DV, Lacro JP, Bailey A, et al: Lower incidence of tardive dyskinesia with risperidone compared with haloperidol in older patients. J Am Geriatr Soc 47:716–719, 1999b

Jeste DV, Rockwell E, Harris MJ, et al: Conventional vs. newer antipsychotics in elderly patients. Am J Geriatr Psychiatry 7:70–76, 1999c

Jorm AF: Is depression a risk factor for dementia or cognitive decline? a review. Gerontology 46:219–227, 2000

Kamat SM, Lefevre PJ, Grossberg GT: Electroconvulsive therapy in the elderly. Clin Geriatr Med 19:825–839, 2003

Kando JC, Tohen M, Castillo J, et al: The use of valproate in an elderly population with affective symptoms. J Clin Psychiatry 57:238–240, 1996

Kane J, Honigfeld G, Singer J, et al: Clozapine for the treatment-resistant schizophrenic: a double-blind comparison with chlorpromazine. Arch Gen Psychiatry 45:789–796, 1988a

Kane JM, Woerner M, Lieberman J: Epidemiological aspects of tardive dyskinesia. Encephale 14 (Spec No):191–194, 1988b

Kasarskis EJ, Kuo CS, Berger R, et al: Carbamazepine-induced cardiac dysfunction: characterization of two distinct clinical syndromes. Arch Intern Med 152:186–191, 1992

Katz IR, Sands LP, Bilker W, et al: Identification of medications that cause cognitive impairment in older people: the case of oxybutynin chloride. J Am Geriatr Soc 46:8–13, 1998

Kellner MB, Neher F: A first episode of mania after age 80. Can J Psychiatry 36:607–608, 1991

Kennedy JS, Bymaster FP, Schuh L, et al: A current review of olanzapine's safety in the geriatric patient: from pre-clinical pharmacology to clinical data. Int J Geriatr Psychiatry 16 (suppl 1):S33–S61, 2001

Kennedy JS, Jeste D, Kaiser CJ, et al: Olanzapine vs haloperidol in geriatric schizophrenia: analysis of data from a double-blind controlled trial. Int J Geriatr Psychiatry 18:1013–1020, 2003

Ketter TA, Post RM, Worthington K: Principles of clinically important drug interactions with carbamazepine, part I. J Clin Psychopharmacol 11:198–203, 1991a

Ketter TA, Post RM, Worthington K: Principles of clinically important drug interactions with carbamazepine, part II. J Clin Psychopharmacol 11:306–313, 1991b

Krauthammer C, Klerman GL: Secondary mania: manic syndromes associated with antecedent physical illness or drugs. Arch Gen Psychiatry 35:1333–1339, 1978

Krishnan KR: Biological risk factors in late life depression. Biol Psychiatry 52:185–192, 2002

Lachkar Y, Bouassida W: Drug-induced acute angle closure glaucoma. Curr Opin Ophthalmol 18:129–133, 2007

Lanctot KL, Best TS, Mittmann N, et al: Efficacy and safety of neuroleptics in behavioral disorders associated with dementia. J Clin Psychiatry 59:550–561, 1998

Lantz MS, Buchalter EN: Pseudodementia: cognitive decline caused by untreated depression may be reversed with treatment. Geriatrics 56:42–43, 2001

Lipkovich I, Citrome L, Perlis R, et al: Early predictors of substantial weight gain in bipolar patients treated with olanzapine. J Clin Psychopharmacol 26:316–320, 2006

Lipkovich I, Ahl J, Nichols R, et al: Weight changes during treatment with olanzapine in older adult patients with dementia and behavioral disturbances. J Geriatr Psychiatry Neurol 20:107–114, 2007

Llerena A, Berecz R, Dorado P, et al: QTc interval, CYP2D6 and CYP2C9 genotypes and risperidone plasma concentrations. J Psychopharmacol 18:189–193, 2004

Loebel AD, Mackell J, Leaderer M, et al: Utilization of ziprasidone in elderly nursing facility residents (abstract), in 55th Institute on Psychiatric Services, Boston, MA, October 29–November 1, 2003a

Loebel AD, Siu CO, Romano SJ: Overview of ziprasidone tolerability in patients 55 years of age and older (NR367), in 2003 New Research Program and Abstracts, American Psychiatric Association 156th Annual Meeting, San Francisco, CA, May 17–22, 2003. Washington, DC, American Psychiatric Association, 2003b, pp 137–138

Madhusoodanan S, Brenner R, Araujo L, et al: Efficacy of risperidone treatment for psychoses associated with schizophrenia, schizoaffective disorder, bipolar disorder, or senile dementia in 11 geriatric patients: a case series. J Clin Psychiatry 56:514–518, 1995

Madhusoodanan S, Brenner R, Alcantra A: Clinical experience with quetiapine in elderly patients with psychotic disorders. J Geriatr Psychiatry Neurol 13:28–32, 2000

Marder SR, Meibach RC: Risperidone in the treatment of schizophrenia. Am J Psychiatry 151:825–835, 1994

McFarland BH, Miller MR, Straumfjord AA: Valproate use in the older manic patient. J Clin Psychiatry 51:479–481, 1990

McQuade RD, Stock E, Marcus R, et al: A comparison of weight change during treatment with olanzapine or aripiprazole: results from a randomized, double-blind study. J Clin Psychiatry 65 (suppl 18):47–56, 2004

McShane R, Keene J, Gedling K, et al: Do neuroleptic drugs hasten cognitive decline in dementia? Prospective study with necropsy follow up. BMJ 314:266–270, 1997

Miller F, Menninger J, Whitcup SM: Lithium-neuroleptic neurotoxicity in the elderly bipolar patient. J Clin Psychopharmacol 6:176–178, 1986

Mordecai DJ, Sheikh JI, Glick ID: Divalproex for the treatment of geriatric bipolar disorder. Int J Geriatr Psychiatry 14:494–496, 1999

Mukherjee S, Sackeim HA, Schnur DB: Electroconvulsive therapy of acute manic episodes: a review of 50 years' experience. Am J Psychiatry 151:169–176, 1994

Mulsant BH, Pollock BG, Kirshner M, et al: Serum anticholinergic activity in a community-based sample of older adults: relationship with cognitive performance. Arch Gen Psychiatry 60:198–203, 2003

Murray N, Hopwood S, Balfour DJ, et al: The influence of age on lithium efficacy and side-effects in out-patients. Psychol Med 13:53–60, 1983

Nicolato R, Romano-Silva MA, Correa H, et al: Stuporous catatonia in an elderly bipolar patient: response to olanzapine (letter). Aust N Z J Psychiatry 40:498, 2006

Niedermier JA, Nasrallah HA: Clinical correlates of response to valproate in geriatric inpatients. Ann Clin Psychiatry 10:165–168, 1998

Noaghiul S, Narayan M, Nelson JC: Divalproex treatment of mania in elderly patients. Am J Geriatr Psychiatry 6:257–262, 1998

Oberholzer AF, Hendriksen C, Monsch AU, et al: Safety and effectiveness of low-dose clozapine in psychogeriatric patients: a preliminary study. Int Psychogeriatr 4:187–195, 1992

Oborne CA, Hooper R, Li KC, et al: An indicator of appropriate neuroleptic prescribing in nursing homes. Age Ageing 31:435–439, 2002

Oral ET, Altinbas K, Demirkiran S: Sudden akathisia after a ziprasidone dose reduction (letter). Am J Psychiatry 163:546, 2006

Panjehshahin MR, Bowmer CJ, Yates MS: Effect of valproic acid, its unsaturated metabolites and some structurally related fatty acids on the binding of warfarin and dansylsarcosine to human albumin. Biochem Pharmacol 41:1227–1233, 1991

Perucca E, Grimaldi R, Gatti G, et al: Pharmacokinetics of valproic acid in the elderly. Br J Clin Pharmacol 17:665–669, 1984

Physicians' Desk Reference, 62nd Edition. Montvale, NJ, Thomson Healthcare, 2008

Puryear LJ, Kunik ME, Workman R Jr: Tolerability of divalproex sodium in elderly psychiatric patients with mixed diagnoses. J Geriatr Psychiatry Neurol 8:234–237, 1995

Ray WA, Chung CP, Murray KT, et al: Atypical antipsychotic drugs and the risk of sudden cardiac death. N Engl J Med 360:225–235, 2009

Risinger RC, Risby ED, Risch SC: Safety and efficacy of divalproex sodium in elderly bipolar patients (letter). J Clin Psychiatry 55:215, 1994

Robillard M, Conn DK: Lamotrigine use in geriatric patients with bipolar depression. Can J Psychiatry 47:767–770, 2002

Roose SP, Bone S, Haidorfer C, et al: Lithium treatment in older patients. Am J Psychiatry 136:843–844, 1979a

Roose SP, Nurnberger JI, Dunner DL, et al: Cardiac sinus node dysfunction during lithium treatment. Am J Psychiatry 136:804–806, 1979b

Rutherford B, Sneed J, Miyazaki M, et al: An open trial of aripiprazole augmentation for SSRI non-remitters with late-life depression. Int J Geriatr Psychiatry 22:986–991, 2007

Sachs GS, Thase ME: Bipolar disorder therapeutics: maintenance treatment. Biol Psychiatry 48:573–581, 2000

Sajatovic M, Popli A, Semple W: Health resource utilization over a ten-year period by geriatric veterans with schizophrenia and bipolar disorder. J Geriatr Psychiatry Neurol 15:128–133, 1996

Sajatovic M, Blow FC, Ignacio RV, et al: Age-related modifiers of clinical presentation and health service use among veterans with bipolar disorder. Psychiatr Serv 55:1014–1021, 2004

Sajatovic M, Gyulai L, Calabrese JR, et al: Maintenance treatment outcomes in older patients with bipolar I disorder. Am J Geriatr Psychiatry 13:305–311, 2005

Sajatovic M, Coconcea N, Ignacio RV, et al: Aripiprazole therapy in 20 older adults with bipolar disorder: a 12-week, open-label trial. J Clin Psychiatry 69:41–46, 2008

Samuels S, Fang M: Olanzapine may cause delirium in geriatric patients. J Clin Psychiatry 65:582–583, 2004

Sanderson DR: Use of mood stabilizers by hospitalized geriatric patients with bipolar disorder. Psychiatr Serv 49:1145–1147, 1998

Schaffer CB, Garvey MJ: Use of lithium in acutely manic elderly patients. Clin Gerontol 3:58–60, 1984

Schneider AL, Wilcox CS: Divalproate augmentation in lithium-resistant rapid cycling mania in four geriatric patients. J Affect Disord 47:201–205, 1998

Schneier HA, Kahn D: Selective response to carbamazepine in a case of organic mood disorders (letter). J Clin Psychiatry 51:485, 1990

Sellers EM: Clinical pharmacology and therapeutics of benzodiazepines. Can Med Assoc J 118:1533–1538, 1978

Sharma V, Persad E, Mazmanian D, et al: Treatment of rapid cycling bipolar disorder with combination therapy of valproate and lithium. Can J Psychiatry 38:137–139, 1993

Shulman KI, Mackenzie S, Hardy B: The clinical use of lithium carbonate in old age: a review. Prog Neuropsychopharmacol Biol Psychiatry 11:159–164, 1987

Shulman KI, Rochon P, Sykora K, et al: Changing prescription patterns for lithium and valproic acid in old age: shifting practice without evidence. BMJ 326:960–961, 2003

Shulman KI, Sykora K, Gill S, et al: Incidence of delirium in older adults newly prescribed lithium or valproate: a population-based cohort study. J Clin Psychiatry 66:424–427, 2005

Shulman RW, Singh A, Shulman KI: Treatment of elderly institutionalized bipolar patients with clozapine. Psychopharmacol Bull 33:113–118, 1997

Simon GE, Ludman EJ, Bauer MS, et al: Long-term effectiveness and cost of a systematic care program for bipolar disorder. Arch Gen Psychiatry 63:500–508, 2006

Snowdon J: A retrospective case-note study of bipolar disorder in old age. Br J Psychiatry 158:485–490, 1991

Sommer BR, Fenn HH, Ketter TA: Safety and efficacy of anticonvulsants in elderly patients with psychiatric disorders: oxcarbazepine, topiramate and gabapentin. Expert Opin Drug Saf 6:133–145, 2007

Sotaniemi EA, Arranto AJ, Pelkonen O, et al: Age and cytochrome P450–linked drug metabolism in humans: an analysis of 226 subjects with equal histopathologic conditions. Clin Pharmacol Ther 61:331–339, 1997

Sproule BA, Hardy BG, Shulman KI: Differential pharmacokinetics of lithium in elderly patients. Drugs Aging 16:165–177, 2000

Stephen LJ: Drug treatment of epilepsy in elderly people: focus on valproic acid. Drugs Aging 20:141–152, 2003

Stone K: Mania in the elderly. Br J Psychiatry 155:220–224, 1989

Stoudemire A, Hill CD, Lewison BJ, et al: Lithium intolerance in a medical-psychiatric population. Gen Hosp Psychiatry 20:85–90, 1998

Straker D, Correll CU, Kramer-Ginsberg E, et al: Cost-effective screening for the metabolic syndrome in patients treated with second-generation antipsychotic medications. Am J Psychiatry 162:1217–1221, 2005

Tariot PN, Salzman C, Yeung PP, et al: Long-term use of quetiapine in elderly patients with psychotic disorders. Clin Ther 22:1068–1084, 2000

Thase ME, Sachs GS: Bipolar depression: pharmacotherapy and related therapeutic strategies. Biol Psychiatry 48:558–572, 2000

Timell AM: Thioridazine: re-evaluating the risk/benefit equation. Ann Clin Psychiatry 12:147–151, 2000

The UK ECT Review Group: Efficacy and safety of electroconvulsive therapy in depressive disorders: a systematic review and meta-analysis. Lancet 361:799–808, 2003

U.S. Food and Drug Administration Center for Drug Evaluation and Research: FDA public health advisory: deaths with antipsychotics in elderly patients with behavioral disturbances. April 11, 2005. Available at: http://www.fda.gov/cder/drug/advisory/antipsychotics.htm. Accessed September 4, 2008.

Van der Velde CD: Effectiveness of lithium carbonate in the treatment of manic-depressive illness. Am J Psychiatry 127:345–351, 1970

Weintraub D, Lippmann S: Delirious mania in the elderly. Int J Geriatr Psychiatry 16:374–377, 2001

Weisbard JJ, Pardo M, Pollack S: Symptom change and extrapyramidal side effects during acute haloperidol treatment in chronic geriatric schizophrenics. Psychopharmacol Bull 33:119–122, 1997

Weissman MM, Leaf PJ, Tischler GL, et al: Affective disorders in five United States communities. Psychol Med 18:141–153, 1988

Wilson KC, Mottram PG, Vassilas CA: Psychotherapeutic treatments for older depressed people. Cochrane Database Syst Rev CD004853, 2008

Woerner MG, Alvir JM, Kane JM, et al: Neuroleptic treatment of elderly patients. Psychopharmacol Bull 31:333–337, 1995

Wu RR, Zhao JP, Jin H, et al: Lifestyle intervention and metformin for treatment of antipsychotic-induced weight gain: a randomized controlled trial. JAMA 299:185–193, 2008

Wylie ME, Mulsant BH, Pollock BG, et al: Age at onset in geriatric bipolar disorder. Effects on clinical presentation and treatment outcomes in an inpatient sample. Am J Geriatr Psychiatry 7:77–83, 1999

Yassa R, Nair NP, Iskandar H: Late-onset bipolar disorder. Psychiatr Clin North Am 11:117–131, 1988

Yerrabolu M, Prabhudesai S, Tawam M, et al: Effect of risperidone on QT interval and QT dispersion in the elderly. Heart Dis 2:10–12, 2000

CHAPTER 13

Mood Stabilizers and Antipsychotics

Pharmacokinetics, Drug Interactions, Adverse Effects, and Administration

Terence A. Ketter, M.D.

Po W. Wang, M.D.

Pharmacotherapy of bipolar disorders is a complex and rapidly evolving field. The development of new treatments has helped refine concepts of illness subtypes and generated important new management options. Although the mood stabilizers lithium, carbamazepine, valproate, and lamotrigine may be argued to be the foundational pharmacotherapies for bipolar disorders, antipsychotics (particularly second-generation agents) have been increasingly used. In addition, antidepressants, anxiolytics/hypnotics, other anticonvulsants, and other medications are commonly combined with mood stabilizers and antipsychotics in clinical settings.

These diverse medications have varying pharmacodynamics, pharmacokinetics, drug-drug interactions, and adverse effects, thus offering not only new therapeutic opportunities but also a variety of new potential pitfalls. Therefore, clinicians are challenged with integrating the complex data regarding efficacy spectra with the pharmacological properties described for mood stabilizers and antipsychotics in this chapter and for antidepressants, anxiolytics, and other medications in Chapter 14 of this volume, in efforts to provide safe, effective, state-of-the-art pharmacotherapy for patients with bipolar disorders. Florida Best Practice Medication Guidelines are provided in Appendix A, and Quick Reference Medication Facts are provided in Appendix B to assist in this endeavor.

Medical Assessment and Monitoring

Baseline evaluation of patients with bipolar disorders includes not only psychosocial assessment but also general medical evaluation, in view of the risk of medical processes that could confound diagnosis or influence management decisions, as well as the risk of adverse effects that may occur with treatment. Assessment commonly includes medical history, physical examination, and laboratory tests such as complete blood count with differential and platelets; renal, hepatic, and thyroid function tests; toxicology and pregnancy tests; and other chemistries and electrocardiograms as clinically indicated (American Psychiatric Association 2002). Such evaluation provides baseline values for parameters that influence decisions regarding choice of medication and intensity of clinical and laboratory monitoring. The specifics of such assessments will vary across agents (Table 13–1) and are discussed in detail in the following sections describing individual medications. The information in Table 13–1 is in broad agreement with recommendations of prescribing information and treatment guidelines.

Medical assessment continues after interventions are initiated. In general, monitoring is more intensive during the first few weeks and months of treatment and less intensive thereafter. Also, monitoring is more intensive in patients with abnormal baseline indices than in those with normal baseline indices. Although schemas such as that shown in Table 13–1 may be a convenient way of organizing complex scheduling information, clinicians should keep in mind that monitoring as clinically indicated is the highest priority (Table 13–2).

In view of the chronic nature of bipolar disorder and the need for maintenance therapy, patients commonly take multiple medications for extended periods of time. In such circumstances, a simplified approach to longer-term medical monitoring may prove useful. Performing annual monitoring at the first visit of each calendar year, as suggested in Figure 13–1, may be one way to ensure that patients receive appropriate scheduled longer-term medical monitoring. However, clinicians should keep in mind that monitoring as clinically indicated is still the highest priority.

Mood Stabilizers

The term *mood stabilizer* is commonly used to refer to medications that are approved for the treatment of bipolar disorder that are not dopamine antagonists; mood stabilizers include lithium and the anticonvulsants valproate, carbamazepine, and lamotrigine. Unfortunately, there is no consensus definition of the term *mood stabilizer,* leading the U.S. Food and Drug Administration (FDA) to avoid using the term and some experts to even suggest abandoning the term. In this volume in general, and in this chapter in particular, *mood stabilizer* is used as defined above, reflecting the common clinical usage of the term.

Mood stabilizers have varying structures, efficacy spectra, pharmacodynamics, pharmacokinetics, drug-drug interactions, and adverse effects, indicating the need to appreciate both the commonalities and differences among these agents. These agents are all available in immediate-release formulations; lithium, valproate, and carbamazepine are available in suspension and extended-release formulations; and valproate is available in an intravenous formulation. Unfortunately, intramuscular and depot formulations have not been feasible, because these agents can cause necrosis when in direct contact with muscle tissue.

Adverse effects of mood stabilizers are commonly intermediate between those of other agents, being somewhat more problematic than with antidepressants and anxiolytics, yet somewhat less problematic than with antipsychotics. However, the complexity of administering mood stabilizers (e.g., because of differential efficacy spectra across illness phases and differential drug interactions) is arguably as challenging as with antipsychotics.

In view of the relative complexity of mood stabilizer therapy, patient education regarding common and serious adverse events is crucial. Information sheets or booklets describing clinical monitoring for problems such as neurotoxicity with lithium, hematological reactions and drug interactions with carbamazepine, hepatic and pancreatic reactions and teratogenicity with valproate, and dermatological reactions with lamotrigine, can aid in prevention and early detection of adverse events to enhance tolerability and safety.

Lithium

Pharmacokinetics and Drug Interactions

Lithium is well absorbed, with a bioavailability close to 100%, is not bound to plasma proteins, and has a moderate volume of distribution of about 1 L/kg and a half-life of about 24 hours (Marcus 1994; Obach et al. 1988; Ward et al. 1994). Sustained-release formulations can decrease peak serum concentrations and

TABLE 13–1. Medical monitoring for mood stabilizers and antipsychotics (in addition to as clinically indicated)

Assessment	Baseline	3 months	6 months	9 months	Yearly	Comments
History						
Rash (LTG, CBZ)	+	+				Each visit for first 3 months
Metabolic, cardiovascular (personal, family) (SGAPs)	+				+	Obesity, diabetes, dyslipidemia, hypertension, cardiovascular disease
Sexual (prolactin-increasing APs)	+	+	+	+	+	Each visit until dose stable, then yearly; prolactin level if indicated by history
Physical examination						
Pulse, blood pressure (SGAPs, medications with cardiovascular effects)	+	+			+	
Weight, height, BMI (Li, VPA, SGAPs)	+	+	+	+	+	BMI monthly for first 3 months when starting SGAPs
Waist circumference (SGAPs)	+				+	
Extrapyramidal (APs)	+	+	+	+	+	Weekly until dose stable, then at each visit
Tardive dyskinesia (APs)	+				+	SGAPs
			+		+	SGAPs, at-risk patients
			+		+	FGAPs
				+	+	FGAPs, at-risk patients
Visual acuity (QTP)	+		+		+	Slit-lamp examination if symptomatic

TABLE 13–1. Medical monitoring for mood stabilizers and antipsychotics (in addition to as clinically indicated) *(continued)*

Assessment	Baseline	3 months	6 months	9 months	Yearly	Comments
Laboratory tests						
Medication levels (Li, VPA, CBZ)	+	+	+		+	
Pregnancy (any medication)	+					
Renal (Li)	+	+	+		+	BUN, creatinine
Urinary (Li)	+	+	+		+	Urinalysis, specific gravity
Thyroid (Li)	+	+	+		+	TSH
Electrolytes (Li, CBZ, VPA)	+	+	+		+	VPA only baseline, yearly
Hematology (VPA, CBZ)	+	+	+		+	CBC, differential, platelets
Hepatic (VPA, CBZ)	+	+	+		+	AST (SGOT), ALT (SGPT), alkaline phosphatase
Metabolic, fasting (SGAPs)	+	+			+	Glucose, triglycerides, cholesterol—HDL, LDL, total (lipids at least every 5 years)
Electrocardiogram (Li, ZIP)	+					Li, if over 40 ZIP, if cardiac risk

Note. ALT (SGPT)=alanine transaminase (serum glutamate pyruvate transaminase); APs=antipsychotics; AST (SGOT)=aspartate transaminase (serum glutamic oxaloacetic transaminase); BMI=body mass index; BUN=blood urea nitrogen; CBC=complete blood count; CBZ=carbamazepine; FGAPs=first-generation antipsychotics; HDL=high-density lipoprotein; LDL=low-density lipoprotein; Li=lithium; LTG= lamotrigine; QTP=quetiapine; SGAPs=second-generation antipsychotics; TSH=thyroid-stimulating hormone; VPA=valproate; ZIP=ziprasidone.

TABLE 13–2.   Examples of clinically indicated laboratory tests

Laboratory tests	Clinical indication
Med levels (Li, VPA, CBZ)	Side effects, inefficacy
Pregnancy (any medication)	Missed menstrual period
Renal (Li)	Polyuria, polydipsia, lithium toxicity
Urinary (Li)	Polyuria, polydipsia, lithium toxicity
Thyroid (Li)	Breakthrough mood symptoms, hyper- or hypothyroidism symptoms
Electrolytes (Li, CBZ, VPA)	Confusion, dehydration.
Hematology (VPA, CBZ)	Fever, bruising, bleeding
Hepatic (VPA, CBZ)	Abdominal complaints, hepatitis symptoms
Metabolic, fasting (SGAPs)	Weight gain≥5 lb
Electrocardiogram (Li, ZIP)	Chest pain, palpitations, syncope

Note.   CBZ=carbamazepine; Li=lithium; SGAPs=second-generation antipsychotics; VPA=valproate; ZIP=ziprasidone.

hence adverse effects related to peak concentrations (Castrogiovanni 2002). Lithium is more than 95% renally excreted unchanged, with a clearance (generally ranging from 10 to 40 mL/min) that is about one-fourth that of creatinine, so that dosage may need to be decreased in patients with decreased renal function. This feature, taken together with evidence suggesting adverse renal effects of lithium, indicates that patients with decreased renal function may not be good candidates for lithium therapy.

Because of its near-exclusive renal excretion unchanged, lithium has renally mediated rather than hepatically mediated pharmacokinetic drug-drug interactions (Amdisen 1982; Finley et al. 1995; Jefferson et al. 1981, 1987). Thus, as described below, certain nonpsychotropic medications with prominent effects on renal function can have clinically significant pharmacokinetic interactions with lithium. Medications with near-exclusive (>95%) renal excretion unchanged (gabapentin, pregabalin) and prominent (50%–95%) renal excretion unchanged (topiramate, levetiracetam) could, in theory, also have clinically significant pharmacokinetic interactions with lithium, but systematic studies are needed to assess if such putative interactions occur. In contrast, most psychotropic and anticonvulsant medications encountered in the management of bipolar disorders have minimal (<5%) renal excretion unchanged (e.g., valproate, carbamazepine, lamotrigine, tiagabine, oxcarbazepine, antipsychotics other than paliperidone) or minor (30%) renal excretion unchanged (e.g., zonisamide) and lack prominent effects on renal function, and are thus not expected to

Annual Medical Monitoring for Bipolar Disorder Patients

Name _____ **Date** ____ / ____

History
Obesity ___ Diabetes ___ Dyslipidemia ___ Hypertension ___ Cardiovascular disease ___
Libido ___ Sexual function ___ Female: Menstrual ___ Galactorrhea (APs) ___
Polyuria/polydipsia (Li, SGAPs) ___ Other _____

Family History (First-Degree Relatives)
Obesity ___ Diabetes ___ Dyslipidemia ___ Hypertension ___ Cardiovascular disease ___
Other _____

Physical Examination
Pulse _____ bpm   Blood pressure _____ / _____ mm Hg
Weight _____ lb   Height _____ inches
Body mass index (703 x weight in lb)/(height in inches)^2 _____ m/kg^2 Waist ____ inches
Extrapyramidal (APs): Tremor ____ Rigid ____ Cogwheel ____ Akathisia ____ TD ____
Visual acuity (quetiapine) _____

Laboratory
Medications: Li _____ mmole/L   VPA _____ µg/mL   CBZ _____ µg/mL
Renal (Li): Blood urea nitrogen _____ mg/dL   Creatinine _____ mg/dL
Urinary (Li): Urinalysis _____   Specific gravity _____
Thyroid (Li): Thyroid-stimulating hormone _____ mIU/mL
Electrolytes (Li, VPA, CBZ): Na ____ K ____ Cl ____ CO$_2$ ____ mmole/L   Ca ____ mg/dL
Complete blood count (VPA, CBZ): WBC _____ K/µL   ANC _____ K/µL   Platelets _____ K/µL
                                     Hb _____ g/dL   Hct _____ %
Hepatic (VPA, CBZ): AST (SGOT) _____ U/L   ALT (SGPT) _____ U/L   Alk phos _____ U/L
Metabolic, fasting (SGAPs): Glucose _____ mg/dL   Triglycerides _____ mg/dL
                               Cholesterol HDL _____ mg/dL   LDL _____ mg/dL   Total ____ mg/dL

FIGURE 13–1.   Annual medical monitoring for bipolar disorder patients.

ALT (SGPT)=alanine aminotransaminase (serum glutamate pyruvate transaminase); ANC=absolute neutrophil count; APs=antipsychotics; AST (SGOT)=aspartate aminotransaminase (serum glutamic oxaloacetic transaminase); CBZ=carbamazepine; Li=lithium; SGAPs= second-generation antipsychotics; TD=tardive dyskinesia; VPA=valproate; WBC=white blood cell count.

generally have clinically significant pharmacokinetic interactions with lith-ium—but again, systematic studies are needed to confirm the lack of such in-teractions.

Based on case reports, concerns have been raised regarding development of an encephalopathic syndrome (weakness, lethargy, fever, tremulousness, confu-sion, extrapyramidal symptoms, leukocytosis, elevated serum enzymes, blood urea nitrogen, and fasting blood sugar) that may overlap with neuroleptic ma-lignant syndrome when lithium is combined with first-generation antipsychot-ics (Addonizio 1985; Cohen and Cohen 1974; Jeffries et al. 1984; Keitner and Rahman 1984; Mann et al. 1983; Miller et al. 1986; Murphy et al. 1989; Nemes et al. 1986; Prakash et al. 1982; Smith and Helms 1982; Spring and Frankel 1981; Yassa 1986). However, systematic efforts to assess such risks in larger numbers of patients (Baastrup et al. 1976; Goldney and Spence 1986; Juhl et al. 1977; Krishna et al. 1978) and clinical trials (Biederman et al. 1979; Sachs et al. 2002; Wilson 1993) have suggested that combining lithium with first-generation antipsy-chotics does not generally yield more than merely additive adverse effects. The absence of compelling consistent evidence of clinically significant pharmaco-kinetic interactions between lithium and first-generation antipsychotics (Aziz-abadi-Farahani et al. 1996; Forsman and Ohman 1977; Ghadirian et al. 1989; Nemes et al. 1986; Pandey et al. 1979; Rivera-Calimlim et al. 1978; Schaffer et al. 1984; Sletten et al. 1966; von Knorring et al. 1982; Werstiuk et al. 1983) suggests that sporadic cases in which problems occur during combination therapy may be due to pharmacodynamic interactions (Goldman 1996).

Case reports also suggest that occasional individuals could develop serious adverse effects such as neuroleptic malignant syndrome when lithium is com-bined with second-generation antipsychotics such as clozapine (Pope et al. 1986), risperidone (Bourgeois and Kahn 2003), olanzapine (Berry et al. 2003), ziprasi-done (Borovicka et al. 2006), and aripiprazole (Ali et al. 2006). However, obser-vational and controlled clinical trials suggest that combining lithium with second-generation antipsychotics such as clozapine (Bender et al. 2004; Kelly et al. 2006; Small et al. 2003), risperidone (Sachs et al. 2002; Yatham et al. 2003), olanzapine (Tohen et al. 2002b), quetiapine (Potkin et al. 2002b; Sachs et al. 2004; Suppes et al. 2009; Vieta et al. 2008b; Yatham et al. 2004), ziprasidone (Weisler et al. 2004b), and aripiprazole (Citrome et al. 2005; Vieta et al. 2008a) does not generally yield more than merely additive adverse effects. Indeed, risperidone (Sachs et al. 2002; Yatham et al. 2003), olanzapine (Tohen et al. 2002b), quetia-pine (Sachs et al. 2004; Yatham et al. 2004), and aripiprazole (Vieta et al. 2008a) have received FDA approval for combination with lithium (or valproate) for the treatment of acute mania. Also, quetiapine has been approved for longer-term treatment in combination with lithium (or divalproex) (Suppes et al. 2009; Vieta et al. 2008b).

As expected, lithium does not appear to generally have clinically significant pharmacokinetic interactions with second-generation antipsychotics. The combination of lithium and second-generation antipsychotics is generally well tolerated. Sporadic instances of serious adverse effects with such combinations could be mediated by pharmacodynamic mechanisms.

Lithium and antidepressants generally lack pharmacokinetic interactions, are commonly administered in combination, and are generally well tolerated in patients with either bipolar disorder or major depressive disorder (Jefferson and Ayd 1983; Nemeroff et al. 2001; Nierenberg et al. 2006; Sachs et al. 2007). However, case reports suggest that some individuals may experience substantive adverse events while taking lithium combined with antidepressants (Adan-Manes et al. 2006; Gabriel et al. 1976; Marchesi et al. 2005; Rogers and Whybrow 1971; Salama and Shafey 1989; Sobanski et al. 1997; Solomon 1979), in most instances presumably related to pharmacodynamic rather than pharmacokinetic mechanisms.

Similarly, in general, lithium and benzodiazepines lack pharmacokinetic interactions. However, occasional patients may experience problematic additive neurotoxicity, presumably related to pharmacodynamic mechanisms (Koczerginski et al. 1989).

Gabapentin (Frye et al. 1998) and topiramate (*Physicians' Desk Reference* 2008) have near-exclusive (>95%) and prominent (50%–70%) renal excretion unchanged, respectively, but do not appear to generally yield clinically significant changes in lithium kinetics. However, case reports have raised the possibility that topiramate causes clinically significant increases in serum lithium concentrations in some individuals (Abraham and Owen 2004; Pinninti and Zelinski 2002). Pregabalin and levetiracetam also have near-exclusive (>95%) and prominent (66%) renal excretion unchanged, respectively, but systematic data are lacking regarding their effects on lithium pharmacokinetic interactions with lithium.

Taken together, the evidence discussed above suggests that for most patients, lithium generally lacks clinically significant pharmacokinetic interactions with psychotropic and anticonvulsant medications encountered in the management of patients with bipolar disorders. However, case reports suggest that occasional patients receiving lithium combined with some of these agents (particularly antipsychotics) can experience serious adverse effects, in most instances presumably related to pharmacodynamic interactions.

In contrast, several agents with prominent renal effects that are commonly used in general medical practice have been clearly implicated in altering lithium pharmacokinetics (Finley et al. 1995; Harvey and Merriman 1994). For example, thiazide diuretics, certain nonsteroidal anti-inflammatory drugs (NSAIDs), angiotensin I converting enzyme inhibitors (ACEIs), and angiotensin II receptor type-1 (AT_1) antagonists can increase lithium reabsorption in the proximal tubule, yielding increased serum lithium concentrations and lithium toxicity (Table 13–3).

Diuretics are commonly prescribed for patients with bipolar disorders, not only for hypertension but also to help attenuate lithium-induced nephrogenic diabetes insipidus (Batlle et al. 1985; des Lauriers et al. 1982; Timmer and Sands 1999). Certain diuretics can induce sodium depletion, resulting in increased proximal tubule sodium and lithium reabsorption. Thus, thiazide diuretics (Crabtree et al. 1991; Himmelhoch et al. 1977; Jefferson and Kalin 1979), but not furosemide (Crabtree et al. 1991; Jefferson and Kalin 1979; Thomsen and Schou 1968) or amiloride (Atherton et al. 1987; Batlle et al. 1985; Bruun et al. 1989), yield clinically significant decreases in lithium excretion. Because of lithium's relatively low therapeutic index, addition of thiazide diuretics can result in clinical lithium toxicity unless a dosage adjustment is made. Amiloride has been suggested to be a particularly attractive option for lithium-induced nephrogenic diabetes insipidus because it has less effect on lithium clearance and does not cause hypokalemia or require sodium restriction (Batlle et al. 1985; Finch et al. 2003; Kosten and Forrest 1986; Timmer and Sands 1999). In contrast, other diuretics such as acetazolamide (Colussi et al. 1989; Thomsen and Schou 1968) and mannitol (Noormohamed and Lant 1995) may increase lithium excretion, potentially yielding clinical inefficacy, if serum lithium concentrations fall below the therapeutic range.

Analgesics are commonly administered to patients with bipolar disorders. Certain NSAIDs inhibit prostaglandin synthesis, decreasing glomerular filtration rate and lithium clearance, thereby potentially yielding lithium toxicity (Monji et al. 2002; Phelan et al. 2003; Ragheb 1990; Stockley 1995; Timmer and Sands 1999). Lithium clearance is decreased with indomethacin (Frolich et al. 1979; Herschberg and Sierles 1983; Ragheb et al. 1980; Reimann et al. 1983), piroxicam (Harrison et al. 1986; Walbridge and Bazire 1985), diclofenac (Reimann and Frolich 1981), naproxen (Ragheb and Powell 1986b), mefenamic acid (Shelley 1987), meloxicam (Turck et al. 2000), and ketoprofen (Singer et al.. 1981), perhaps less consistently so with ibuprofen (Bailey et al. 1989; Kristoff et al. 1986; Ragheb 1987b; Ragheb et al. 1980), and perhaps to a lesser extent with sulindac

TABLE 13–3. **Drug interactions and other factors affecting lithium clearance**

Clearance decreased by	Clearance not changed by	Clearance increased by
Diuretics	*Diuretics*	*Diuretics*
Thiazides	Amiloride	Acetazolamide
	Furosemide	Mannitol
Older NSAIDs	*Analgesics*	
Diclofenac	±ASA (conflicting data)	
±Ibuprofen (less consistent effect)	Acetaminophen	
Indomethacin		
Ketoprofen		
Mefenamic acid		
Meloxicam		
Naproxen (smaller effect with OTC dose)		
Piroxicam		
±Sulindac (conflicting data)		
COX-2 inhibitors		
Celecoxib		
Rofecoxib		
ACEIs		*Methylxanthines*
Captopril		Aminophylline
Enalapril		±Caffeine (conflicting data)
Fosinopril		
Lisinopril		Theophylline
Perindopril		
AT$_1$ antagonists		
Candesartan		
Losartan		
Valsartan		
Physiological/disease states		*Physiological/disease states*
Advanced age		Pregnancy
Dehydration		±Mania (conflicting data)
Renal disease		
Sodium depletion		

Note. ACEIs=angiotensin I converting enzyme inhibitors; ASA=acetylsalicylic acid; AT$_1$ = angiotensin II receptor type-1; COX-2= cyclooxygenase-2; NSAIDs=nonsteroidal anti-inflammatory drugs; OTC=over the counter; ±=variable/inconsistent effect.

(Furnell and Davies 1985; Miller et al. 1989; Ragheb and Powell 1986a, 1986b) (although there are conflicting data [Jones and Stoner 2000]), and not with aspirin (Bikin et al. 1982; Ragheb 1987a; Reimann et al. 1983, 1985) (although there are conflicting data [Bendz and Feinberg 1984]), or with over-the-counter doses of naproxen and acetaminophen (Levin et al. 1998). The newer cyclooxygenase-2 (COX-2) inhibitor NSAIDs celecoxib (Gunja et al. 2002; Phelan et al. 2003; Slordal et al. 2003) and rofecoxib (Lundmark et al. 2002; Phelan et al. 2003; Ratz Bravo et al. 2004) may increase serum lithium concentrations.

Antihypertensives are commonly administered to patients with bipolar disorders. Certain ACEIs and AT_1 antagonists can induce volume depletion and hence decrease glomerular filtration rate and lithium clearance, potentially yielding lithium toxicity (Timmer and Sands 1999). Case reports also suggest that the newer AT_1 antagonists candesartan (Zwanzger et al. 2001), losartan (Blanche et al. 1997), and valsartan (Leung and Remick 2000; Su et al. 2007) can decrease lithium clearance, yielding clinical lithium toxicity.

Methylxanthines such as aminophylline, theophylline, and caffeine are commonly encountered in the management of patients with bipolar disorders. These adenosine antagonists have renal effects that can increase lithium clearance, potentially yielding inefficacy.

Reports of potential interactions between lithium and calcium channel blockers have varied. Neurotoxicity, including nausea, weakness, tremor, ataxia, parkinsonian symptoms, and choreoathetosis, has been reported when combining lithium with verapamil (Helmuth et al. 1989; Price and Giannini 1986; Price and Shalley 1987; Wright and Jarrett 1991), diltiazem (Binder et al. 1991; Valdiserri 1985), and nifedipine (Pinkofsky et al. 1997). Calcium channel blockers are very commonly used, and postmarketing surveillance has failed to provide systematic evidence that problems commonly occur when combining these agents with lithium (Flicker et al. 1988). Taken together, the data suggest the need for some caution when combining lithium and calcium channel blockers, because occasional individuals may have problems.

Different physiological and disease states can have varying effects on lithium clearance. Increasing age is associated with decreased renal clearance and increased sensitivity to adverse effects, yielding the need for (on average approximately 40%–50%) lower lithium dosages and serum concentrations in older adults (Chapron et al. 1982; Greil et al. 1985; Hewick et al. 1977; Shulman et al. 1987; Vestergaard and Schou 1984). Dehydration, renal disease, and sodium depletion also decrease renal lithium clearance, increasing the risk of toxicity (Atherton et al. 1987; Chapron et al. 1982; Norman et al. 1984; Thomsen and

Schou 1968). In contrast, lithium clearance increases during pregnancy (Schou and Weinstein 1980) and may also increase during strenuous exercise (Jefferson et al. 1982). Patients who become manic or hypomanic often have dramatic increases in physical activity, which may yield increased cardiac output and perhaps increased renal lithium filtration and excretion, thereby decreasing serum lithium concentrations at the very time when this medication is needed most in some individuals (Kukopoulos and Reginaldi 1978; Kukopoulos et al. 1985). However, groups of patients with mania as a whole do not appear to have statistically significant mean changes in lithium clearance (Degkwitz et al. 1979; Swann et al. 1990).

Adverse Effects

Common dose-related adverse effects with lithium include renal (polyuria, polydipsia), metabolic (weight gain), central nervous system (sedation, tremor, ataxia, lethargy, decreased coordination, and cognitive problems), gastrointestinal (nausea, vomiting, diarrhea), and dermatological (hair loss, acne) problems, as well as edema (Table 13–4) (Gelenberg 1988). Lithium-induced central nervous system adverse effects can be important reasons for poor adherence (Gitlin et al. 1989). Lithium can compromise memory and information processing speed, even without subjective complaints or awareness of mental slowness (Honig et al. 1999).

TABLE 13–4.   Common and serious adverse effects of mood stabilizers

Lithium	Valproate	Carbamazepine	Lamotrigine
Gastrointestinal	Gastrointestinal	Gastrointestinal	Gastrointestinal
Weight gain	Weight gain	*Rash*	*Rash*
Neurotoxicity	Tremor	Neurotoxicity	Headache
Renal toxicity	*Hepatotoxicity*	Hepatotoxicity	Dizziness
Thyroid toxicity	Thrombocytopenia	Thyroid changes	Pruritus
Hair loss	Hair loss	*Blood dyscrasia*	Dream abnormality
Cardiac toxicity	*Pancreatitis*	Cardiac toxicity	
Acne, psoriasis	Polycystic ovary syndrome	Hyponatremia	
Teratogen	*Teratogen*	Teratogen	Teratogen
	Suicidality	Suicidality	Suicidality

Note.   *Bold italics* indicate those adverse effects that have a boxed warning in the U.S. prescribing information.

The U.S. lithium prescribing information includes a boxed warning regarding the risk of lithium toxicity that can occur at dosages close to therapeutic levels (Bell et al. 1993). Lithium intoxication can present with central nervous system, cardiovascular, renal, and gastrointestinal symptoms (Delva and Hawken 2001; Hansen and Amdisen 1978; Livingstone and Rampes 2006; Timmer and Sands 1999; Vestergaard et al. 1980). In severe cases, lithium intoxication can yield irreversible central nervous system (Verdoux and Bourgeois 1990), cardiac (Terao et al. 1996), or renal problems (Hetmar 1988), and even death (Amdisen et al. 1974). The risk of lithium toxicity is high in patients who have significant renal or cardiovascular disease, severe debilitation, dehydration, or sodium depletion, or who are taking diuretics or angiotensin converting enzyme inhibitors. However, in medically healthy individuals, at dosages of 900 mg/day or less, lithium is usually well tolerated, and even with low serum levels may yield benefit in milder forms of bipolar disorders or when used in combination with other agents.

Other warnings include the risks of renal problems such as nephrogenic diabetes insipidus; morphological changes with glomerular and interstitial fibrosis and nephron atrophy with chronic therapy (as described below); and drug interactions (as described above), such as encephalopathic syndrome with neuroleptics. Patients need to maintain adequate fluid and sodium intake, and caution is indicated when patients have protracted sweating, diarrhea, infection, and fever. Lithium can also yield thyroid problems, as described below.

Many of the adverse effects of taking lithium can be treated through various management options (Table 13–5). Lithium can cause digestive tract disturbances, with the lithium citrate solution having more proximal absorption and thus exacerbating upper (nausea and vomiting) or attenuating lower (diarrhea) gastrointestinal adverse effects. The reverse holds for sustained-release preparations. Administration of divided dosages and with food can help attenuate gastrointestinal adverse effects. Although lithium is often given in divided dosages to decrease peak serum levels and thus minimize adverse effects, dosages can also be weighted toward bedtime, and patients receiving low to moderate dosages may tolerate a single daily dose at bedtime. The latter regimen may aid sleep, attenuate daytime neurotoxicity, and possibly even decrease polyuria (Coppen et al. 1983). Beta-blocking agents can attenuate lithium-induced tremor (Gelenberg and Jefferson 1995; Lapierre 1976).

Lithium has endocrine adverse effects and can yield hypothyroidism in up to one-third of patients, and women and patients with rapid cycling may be at particular risk (Amdisen and Andersen 1982; Bocchetta et al. 2001; Henry 2002;

TABLE 13–5. **Treatment of mood stabilizer adverse effects**

Adverse effect	Management options
General	Decrease, divide, or change time of dose Change mood stabilizer
Gastrointestinal	Give with food Change to extended release if nausea or vomiting Change to suspension or immediate release if diarrhea Provide symptomatic relief with gastrointestinal agents
Weight gain	Give prior warning; diet; exercise Aggressively treat hyperphagic, anergic depression Add topiramate, zonisamide, atomoxetine, or sibutramine
Neurotoxicity	Dose at bedtime Initiate gradually to improve tolerance (with lithium and carbamazepine)
Tremor	Add propranolol, atenolol, pindolol
Hair loss	Add selenium 25–100 µg/day, zinc 10–50 mg/day
Polyuria	Prescribe single daily dose Add amiloride, thiazide, indomethacin
Thyroid	Prescribe thyroid hormone
Hepatic	Discontinue carbamazepine or valproate if hepatic indices >three times upper limit of normal
Rash	Initiate gradually Limit other new antigens during initiation? Seek dermatology consultation regarding risk and management Discontinue carbamazepine or lamotrigine if rash not clearly unrelated to drug
Leukopenia	Add lithium Discontinue carbamazepine if white blood cell count<3,000 or neutrophils<1,000
Hyponatremia	Add lithium, demeclocycline, doxycycline?

Note.   ? = uncertain benfit

Livingstone and Rampes 2006). Moreover, lower serum levothyroxine concentrations appear to be associated with more frequent affective episodes and more depression in patients with mood disorders (Frye et al. 1999). Patients with hypothyroidism (increased thyroid-stimulating hormone [TSH] and decreased free thyroxine) need levothyroxine replacement therapy. However, controversy exists regarding the management of subclinical hypothyroidism (increased TSH and normal free thyroxine). One proposed approach entails 1) instituting levothyroxine if TSH exceeds 10 mU/L, even in the absence of clinical symptoms, because of the risk of progression of thyroid disease, and 2) increasing laboratory monitoring and considering levothyroxine if TSH is between 5 and 10 mU/L (Kleiner et al. 1999). Hyperthyroidism, although far less common, can also occur with lithium therapy (Barclay et al. 1994). Hypercalcemia and hyperparathyroidism can also occur with lithium administration (Bendz et al. 1996; Livingstone and Rampes 2006; Nordenstrom et al. 1994). Thus, if hypercalcemia is detected on electrolyte screening, serum parathyroid hormone needs to be assessed.

As previously noted, lithium has significant interactions with renal function, because lithium clearance is by renal excretion, and lithium can cause common benign as well as rare serious renal adverse effects (Livingstone and Rampes 2006; Vestergaard and Amdisen 1981; Vestergaard et al. 1979). Nephrogenic diabetes insipidus may occur in up to 10% of patients with chronic lithium therapy (Bendz and Aurell 1999). Polyuria and polydipsia (greater than 3 L/24-hour urine volume) can be attenuated by lithium dosage reduction or single daily dose, and by administration of diuretics; however, as noted earlier, care must be taken because such agents can influence lithium clearance. Hence, hydrochlorothiazide 50 mg/day may attenuate polyuria, but using this agent requires decreasing lithium dosage and replacing potassium. Indomethacin has also been considered, but this agent also decreases lithium clearance, and could yield renal problems (Allen et al. 1989). Amiloride 5–10 mg twice a day has been suggested to be a preferable option for lithium-induced nephrogenic diabetes insipidus (Batlle et al. 1985; Finch et al. 2003; Kosten and Forrest 1986; Timmer and Sands 1999). Chronic lithium less commonly yields more long-standing and serious renal complications that are apparently more prevalent in cases with repeated lithium toxicity, advanced age, and concurrent NSAID therapy or chronic medical illness (Bendz 1983; DasGupta and Jefferson 1990; Timmer and Sands 1999). Clinical and laboratory monitoring may help detect problems early, thus allowing interventions to attenuate adverse effects.

Weight gain can occur with lithium therapy (Baptista et al. 1995; Bowden et al. 2000, 2006a; Peselow et al. 1980; Sachs et al. 2006a; Vendsborg et al. 1976) and can be a significant contributor to compliance problems. Weight gain appears to be more of an issue with lithium than with lamotrigine (Sachs et al. 2006a), particularly in patients who are already obese (Bowden et al. 2006a), but less of a problem than with valproate (Bowden et al. 2000) or olanzapine (Tohen et al. 2005). In 12-month maintenance trials, the incidence of weight gain was 13% with lithium, 21% with valproate, and 7% with placebo (Bowden et al. 2000), and 10% with lithium and 30% with olanzapine (Tohen et al. 2005).

Many of the agents used in treating patients with bipolar disorders can yield weight gain, as can residual hyperphagia, hypersomnia, and anergy of bipolar depression, or lithium-induced hypothyroidism. Counseling regarding weight gain early in the maintenance phase of treatment may allow early attention to diet and exercise to attenuate this effect. In some cases, early detection of a rising high normal or modestly elevated TSH can allow crossing over to another mood stabilizer, thus avoiding the need for chronic replacement thyroid hormones, as is necessary in more advanced cases of lithium-induced hypothyroidism. Even in some euthyroid patients, addition of thyroid hormones may offer adjunctive antidepressant effects, increasing energy and activity, and thus attenuating weight gain. Another important approach is to minimize the number of concurrent medications that also yield weight gain, thus avoiding potential synergistic weight increases. Classical prescription weight loss agents and stimulants are most often avoided, because they can destabilize mood and result in abuse or dependence. Adjunctive anticonvulsants, such as topiramate (Bray et al. 2003) and zonisamide (Gadde et al. 2003), and the norepinephrine reuptake inhibitor atomoxetine (McElroy et al. 2007) may allow patients to lose weight without systematically destabilizing mood, provided there is adequate concurrent antimanic therapy.

Acneiform and maculopapular eruptions, psoriasis, and folliculitis can occur with lithium (Chan et al. 2000; Yeung and Chan 2004). In some patients, symptomatic treatment of dermatological adverse effects with topical agents or retinoic acid can yield enough improvement to allow continuation of therapy, whereas in others switching to or adding another mood stabilizer to allow lithium dosage decrease or discontinuation is necessary.

Lithium can have adverse cardiac effects, ranging from benign electrocardiographic T-wave morphological changes to clinically significant sinus node dysfunction or sinoatrial block, and onset or aggravation of ventricular irritability (Mitchell and Mackenzie 1982; Roose et al. 1979; Terao et al. 1996).

Lithium, like the other mood stabilizers, is a teratogen (FDA pregnancy category D) (Gentile 2006), yielding cardiac malformations at a rate of 0.1%–1.0% (Cohen et al. 1994). Ultrasound may allow early detection of such malformations. In patients with milder illness, a medication-free interval during pregnancy may be feasible. Because rapid discontinuation of lithium may yield rebound episodes (Baldessarini et al. 1996), a gradual tapering off of medication is a preferable strategy. Some patients have sufficiently severe illness to merit continuing lithium during pregnancy. Frank counseling and discussion of the risks and benefits of this approach are crucial in the management of such cases. Lithium and other mood stabilizers generally ought to be restarted immediately postpartum in view of the risk of relapse, which may be as high as 60% (Cohen et al. 1995). Because lithium and other mood stabilizers are excreted to varying degrees in breast milk, the most cautious approach is to not breast-feed while taking mood stabilizers. The FDA recommends that the mother discontinue nursing or discontinue taking the drug, depending on the importance of the drug to the mother. However, recent data indicating that lithium concentrations fall 50% from maternal serum to milk, and another 50% from milk to infant serum, yielding adequate tolerability in infants, suggest that recommendations against lithium during breast-feeding may need to be reassessed (Viguera et al. 2007).

Administration

In acute care settings, such as the inpatient treatment of mania, lithium therapy is commonly initiated at 600–1,200 mg/day in two or three divided doses, and increased as necessary and tolerated every 2–4 days by 300 mg/day, with final dosages commonly not exceeding 1,800 mg/day (Table 13–6). Some patients may better tolerate weighting the dosage toward bedtime or even taking the entire daily dosage at bedtime. Euthymic or depressed patients tend to tolerate aggressive initiation less well than manic patients. Thus, in less acute situations, such as the initiation of prophylaxis or adjunctive use, lithium can be started at 300–600 mg/day, and increased as necessary and tolerated by 300 mg/day every 4–7 days. Thus, target dosages are commonly between 900 and 1,800 mg/day, yielding serum levels from 0.6 to 1.2 mEq/L (0.6–1.2 mmol/L), with the higher portion of the range used acutely, and lower dosages used in adjunctive therapy or prophylaxis (Sproule 2002). In acute mania studies of the adjunctive second-generation antipsychotics risperidone, olanzapine, quetiapine, and aripiprazole, target serum lithium concentrations ranged from 0.60 to 1.4 mEq/L, yet mean serum lithium concentrations ranged between 0.70 and 0.76 mEq/L (Sachs et al. 2002; Tohen et al. 2002b; Yatham et al. 2004). Older data suggest that during maintenance treatment, serum lithium concentrations maintained at 0.4–0.6 (median average 0.54) mEq/L compared with 0.8–1.0 (median average 0.83) mEq/L were better tolerated but less effective (Gelenberg et al. 1989). However, in a European lithium-versus-carbamazepine maintenance study, serum trough lithium concentrations were maintained at 0.6–0.8 mEq/L, with a mean of 0.63 mEq/L (Greil et al. 1997). In an American lithium versus carbamazepine maintenance study, serum trough lithium concentrations were maintained at 0.5–1.2 mEq/L, with a mean of 0.84 mEq/L (Denicoff et al. 1997). In a lithium versus valproate versus placebo maintenance study, serum trough lithium concentrations were maintained at 0.8–1.2 mEq/L, with a mean of 1.0 mEq/L at day 30 of randomized treatment (Bowden et al. 2000). In a lithium-versus-lamotrigine versus placebo maintenance study, serum trough lithium concentrations were maintained at 0.8–1.1 mEq/L, with a steady-state mean of 0.8 mEq/L during randomized treatment (Calabrese et al. 2003). In a lithium-versus-olanzapine maintenance study, serum trough lithium concentrations were maintained at 0.6–1.2 mEq/L, with a mean of 0.76 mEq/L during randomized treatment (Tohen et al. 2005).

Clinical and Laboratory Monitoring

Patients taking lithium need to be advised of adverse effects, drug interactions, and the importance of adequate hydration. Clinical assessments with lithium therapy include a baseline physical examination and routinely querying patients regarding central nervous system (sedation, tremor, ataxia), gastrointestinal (nausea, vomiting, diarrhea), metabolic (weight gain), and renal (polyuria, polydipsia) disorders and adverse effects at baseline and during treatment. Laboratory monitoring includes a baseline pregnancy test, an electrocardiogram (in patients over 40 years of age), and renal (blood urea nitrogen, serum creatinine and electrolytes) and thyroid (TSH) indices, with reevaluation of renal and thyroid indices at 3 and 6 months, and then every 6–12 months thereafter, and as clinically indicated (American Psychiatric Association 2002). Serum lithium concentrations are commonly assessed 12 hours after dosing at steady state, which occurs at about 5 days after a dosage change, and then as indicated by inefficacy or adverse effects. More frequent laboratory monitoring is prudent in the medically ill and in patients with abnormal indices.

Valproate (Divalproex)

Pharmacokinetics and Drug Interactions

Valproate is well absorbed, with bioavailability close to 100% (DeVane 2003). It is 80%–90% bound to plasma proteins. This binding is saturable, so that at higher dosages a greater percentage of the drug may be in the free form. Valproate is quite hydrophilic, with a low volume of distribution of about 0.1 L/kg. At higher dosages, the increased free fraction may remain in the blood compartment (rather than escaping into the tissues) and thus be cleared by the liver. This may yield "sublinear" kinetics, so that with higher serum concentrations, greater increases in dosage may be required, to yield the desired increase in serum level (Graves 1995).

TABLE 13–6.   Dosing of mood stabilizers and second-generation antipsychotics

Medication	Start (mg/day or mg/kg/day)[a]	Range (mg/day)	Dosing	Blood levels
Mood stabilizers				
Lithium	600–1,200 acute 300–600 less acute	900–1,800 acute 600–1,200 less acute	div	0.9–1.2 mEq/L acute 0.6–0.9 mEq/L less acute
Valproate	25 mg/kg/day acute 250–500 less acute (?)	2,000–3,000 acute 1,000–2,000 less acute (?)	DR div ER qhs	85–125 µg/mL acute 50–85 µg/mL less acute (?)
Carbamazepine	200–400 acute 100–200 less acute (?)	800–1,600 acute 600–1,200 less acute (?)	div	9–12 µg/mL acute (?) 4–9 µg/mL less acute (?)
Lamotrigine[b]	25×2 wks, 50×2 wks, 100×1 wk, then 200	200–400 (occasionally 500)	qam	3–15 µg/mL epilepsy (?)
Second-generation antipsychotics				
Aripiprazole	15–30 acute 2–5 less acute (?)	15–30 acute 5–10 less acute (?)	qam (qhs if sedating)	
Aripiprazole IM	9.75	15–30	q2h	
Clozapine	25, ↑ 25 qd acute (?) 12.5, ↑ 25 q4d less acute (?)	50–400 acute (?) 25–200 less acute (?)	div/qhs	
Olanzapine	10–15 acute 5 less acute	10–20 acute 5–10 less acute	qhs	
Olanzapine IM	5–10	10–30	q2h–q4h	
Quetiapine	100, ↑ 100 qd acute 50, ↑ 50–100 qd less acute	400–800 acute 300–600 less acute	div/qhs	
Risperidone	2–3 acute 0.25–0.5 less acute (?)	1–6 acute 1–2 less acute (?)	qhs	

TABLE 13–6. Dosing of mood stabilizers and second-generation antipsychotics (*continued*)

Medication	Start (mg/day or mg/kg/day)[a]	Range (mg/day)	Dosing	Blood levels
Second-generation antipsychotics (*continued*)				
Risperidone LAI	25 q2w	25–50 q2w	q2w	
Ziprasidone	80 acute	120–160 acute	div, with food	
	80 less acute (?)	120–160 less acute (?)		
		240–320 in some patients (?)		
Ziprasidone IM (schizophrenia)	10	up to 40	q2h	

Note. div=divided doses recommended, but dose commonly weighted toward bedtime; DR=direct release; ER=extended release; IM=rapid-acting injectable; LAI=long-acting injectable; qam=each morning; qd=once daily; q4d=every 4 days; qhs=daily at bedtime; q2h=every 2 hours; q2w=every 2 weeks; schizophrenia=approved for schizophrenia but not bipolar disorder; XR=extended release; (?)=limited data.
[a]Acute=manic or mixed inpatients; less acute=depressed, euthymic, or hypomanic outpatients.
[b]Halve doses with valproate and double doses with carbamazepine.

In monotherapy, valproate has a half-life of about 12 hours and clearance of about 10 mL/min. When valproate is combined with enzyme inducers, such as carbamazepine, phenytoin, or phenobarbital, valproate's half-life falls 50% to approximately 6 hours and clearance doubles to about 20 mL/min. Valproate is available as valproic acid and as divalproex delayed release, the latter of which has better gastrointestinal tolerability (Zarate et al. 1999). In 2005, the FDA approved an extended-release divalproex formulation (divalproex ER) for the treatment of acute manic and mixed episodes (Bowden et al. 2006b), and this formulation has potentially even better tolerability than the delayed-release divalproex formulation (Smith et al. 2004).

Valproate is extensively metabolized, with less than 3% being excreted unchanged in the urine. Thus, patients with hepatic insufficiency may require lower dosages. Valproate has three principal routes of elimination (Aly and Abdel-Latif 1980; Baillie 1992). Conjugations to inactive glucuronides and other inactive metabolites account for 50% of valproate disposition and appear to be mediated primarily by UGT1A6, UGT1A9, and UGT2B7 (Ethell et al. 2003). In addition, about 40% of valproate undergoes β-oxidation in the mitochondria to several metabolites, including the desaturation product 2-ene-valproate that may contribute to the therapeutic effects of valproate. Preliminary evidence suggests that patients who experience weight gain while taking valproate may have higher levels of 2-ene-valproate, suggesting that dysfunction of the β-oxidation pathway (which metabolizes endogenous lipids) could play a role in this adverse effect (Gidal et al. 1994). About 10% of valproate undergoes cytochrome cytochrome P450 oxidation reactions that appear to be mediated primarily by CYP2C9, CYP2A6, and CYP2B6. P450 oxidation reactions yield a variety of metabolites, including hydroxylation (3-OH-valproate, 4-OH-valproate, 5-OH-valproate) and subsequent ketone (4-oxo-valproate) and dicarboxylic acid (propylsuccinic acid [PSA] and propylglutaric acid [PGA]) products. In addition, the desaturation product, 4-ene-valproate, may be hepatotoxic and teratogenic. Induction of formation of this metabolite by enzyme-inducing anticonvulsants could explain why these problems are a greater concern in certain combination therapies than in valproate monotherapy.

Valproate has a somewhat more favorable therapeutic index than lithium or carbamazepine, with a lower incidence of neurotoxicity being an important advantage. This favorable therapeutic index, along with the existence of three principal metabolic pathways, may account for the fact that clinical drug-drug interactions yielding valproate toxicity appear less prominent than with lithium or carbamazepine.

However, valproate has metabolic interactions with some drugs (Bourgeois 1988) (Table 13–7). Valproate is an inhibitor of hepatic metabolism, including epoxide hydrolase, some glycosyltransferases, and some cytochrome P450 isoforms (Ethell et al. 2003; Svinarov and Pippenger 1995; Wen et al. 2001). In human liver microsomes, valproate inhibits UGT2B7 (Rowland et al. 2006) and CYP2C9 (Wen et al. 2001), but only tends to inhibit CYP2C19, CYP3A4, and CYP2A6 and has minimal effects on CYP1A2, CYP2D6, and CYP2E1.

Thus, valproate can yield increased serum concentrations of carbamazepine-10,11-epoxide by inhibiting epoxide hydrolase (Pisani et al. 1990), and can inhibit glucuronidation of carbamazepine-10,11-trans-diol (Bernus et al. 1997). In addition, carbamazepine induces valproate metabolism, yielding decreased serum valproate concentrations (Jann et al. 1988; Levy et al. 1982). Carbamazepine appears to induce valproate metabolism by increasing clearance via both the conjugation and cytochrome P450 oxidation routes (Levy et al. 1982). Valproate doubles serum lamotrigine concentrations, presumably mediated by inhibition of UGT2B7 (Anderson et al. 1996; Rambeck and Wolf 1993; Rowland et al. 2006), and thus increases the risk of rash with lamotrigine, so that it is particularly important to take care to introduce lamotrigine even more conservatively (halving lamotrigine dosages) in patients who are taking valproate (Faught et al. 1999), as noted below. Lamotrigine may yield only modest (25%), clinically insignificant decreases in valproate levels (Anderson et al. 1996). Valproate and lithium lack clinically significant pharmacokinetic interactions with one another (Granneman et al. 1996).

Valproate does not appear to have clinically significant pharmacokinetic interactions with haloperidol (Hesslinger et al. 1999), risperidone (Spina et al.

TABLE 13–7. Selected valproate metabolic drug interactions

VPA →↑ drug	Drug →↑ VPA	Drug →↓ VPA
Amitriptyline	Aspirin	Carbamazepine
CBZ-E	Felbamate	Carbapenems
Ethosuximide		±Lamotrigine
Lamotrigine		Phenobarbital
Nortriptyline		Phenytoin
Phenobarbital		Rifampin
Phenytoin		
Zidovudine		

Note. CBZ-E=carbamazepine-10,11-epoxide; VPA=valproate; ↑=increased concentrations; ↓=decreased concentrations.

2000a), or aripiprazole (Citrome et al. 2005). Limited data suggest that valproate might decrease clozapine levels (Finley and Warner 1994; Longo and Salzman 1995). Valproate decreased dosage-corrected olanzapine concentrations in four patients (Bergemann et al. 2006), but this potential interaction needs to be confirmed in a larger sample. Valproate may (Aichhorn et al. 2006) or may not (*Physicians' Desk Reference* 2008) increase quetiapine serum concentrations.

Reports vary regarding the effect of valproate on tricyclic antidepressant pharmacokinetics. Valproate may increase serum amitriptyline/nortriptyline (Bertschy et al. 1990; Fu et al. 1994; Wong et al. 1996) and clomipramine (DeToledo et al. 1997) concentrations, but may decrease desipramine (Joseph and Wroblewski 1993) concentrations. Fluoxetine may increase (Cruz-Flores et al. 1995; Lucena et al. 1998; Sovner and Davis 1991) or decrease (Droulers et al. 1997) valproate serum concentrations. In one patient, sertraline increased valproate levels (Berigan and Harazin 1999).

Valproate is commonly administered along with benzodiazepines in patients with bipolar disorders, with merely additive central nervous system adverse effects (e.g., sedation, ataxia). Indeed, contemporary controlled valproate trials routinely permit some adjunctive benzodiazepine (e.g., lorazepam) administration (Bowden et al. 1994, 2000, 2006b; Tohen et al. 2002a; Zajecka et al. 2002). Valproate modestly decreases diazepam (Dhillon and Richens 1982) and lorazepam (Samara et al. 1997) clearance. A pharmacoepidemiological study suggested that valproate and clonazepam only modestly affect one another's metabolism (Yukawa et al. 2003). However, limited data suggest that for at least some patients, caution is indicated when combining valproate with benzodiazepines. Occasional patients might experience serious central nervous system depression when valproate is combined with lorazepam (Lee et al. 2002). Valproate combined with clonazepam may induce absence status in patients with a history of absence status (Watson 1979). A single case report described somnambulism when valproate was combined with zolpidem (Sattar et al. 2003).

Valproate can yield increased serum concentrations of ethosuximide (Mattson and Cramer 1980; Pisani et al. 1984), felbamate (*Physicians' Desk Reference* 2008), phenobarbital (Fernandez de Gatta et al. 1986), and phenytoin (Lai and Huang 1993). Valproate can increase the free fraction of tiagabine (*Physicians' Desk Reference* 2008). Felbamate can yield increased serum valproate concentrations (Wagner et al. 1991), and phenobarbital and phenytoin can yield decreased (Sackellares et al. 1981) serum valproate concentrations.

Aspirin can yield decreased valproate clearance (Abbott et al. 1986), as well as decreased valproate protein binding (Orr et al. 1982). The antimicrobials rifampin (Bachmann and Jauregui 1993) and meropenem (Coves-Orts et al. 2005; Fudio et al. 2006; Nacarkucuk et al. 2004), as well as other carbapenems (e.g., imipenem, doripenem, ertapenem), can yield decreased serum valproate concentrations. Valproate can yield increased serum concentrations of zidovudine (Lertora et al. 1994). In contrast to carbamazepine, valproate does not yield clinically significant decreases in serum concentrations of hormonal contraceptives (Crawford et al. 1986).

Binding interactions can also occur, so that valproate can increase free fractions of diazepam (Calvo et al. 1986; Dhillon and Richens 1982), carbamazepine (Mattson et al. 1982), phenytoin (Lai and Huang 1993), tiagabine (*Physicians' Desk Reference* 2008), tolbutamide (*Physicians' Desk Reference* 2008), and warfarin (Panjehshahin et al. 1991). In contrast, the NSAIDs aspirin (Goulden et al. 1987; Orr et al. 1982; Sandson et al. 2006), diflunisal (Addison et al. 2000a), tolmetin (Dasgupta and Volk 1996), mefenamic acid (Dasgupta and Emerson 1996), fenoprofen (Dasgupta and Emerson 1996), ibuprofen (Dasgupta and Volk 1996), and naproxen (Addison et al. 2000b; Dasgupta and Volk 1996; Grimaldi et al. 1984) can increase the free fraction of valproate.

Adverse Effects

Common, dosage-related adverse effects with valproate include gastrointestinal (nausea, vomiting, dyspepsia, diarrhea), hepatic (transaminase elevations), central nervous system (tremor, sedation, dizziness), and metabolic (weight gain, osteoporosis) problems, as well as hair loss (Dreifuss and Langer 1988). As valproate can cause gastrointestinal disturbances (Schmidt 1984), divalproex ER is preferred because it yields such problems less often than does the divalproex delayed-release formulation (Smith et al. 2004), which in turn appears better tolerated than valproic acid (Zarate et al. 1999). Central nervous system adverse effects may be attenuated by weighting valproate dosage toward bedtime or reducing dosage. Beta-blockers may attenuate valproate-induced tremor. Valproate can cause weight gain, which appears to be more of a problem than with lithium (Bowden et al. 2000) but less of an issue than with olanzapine (Tohen et al. 2003b). For example, the incidence of weight gain was 21% with valproate, 13% with lithium, and 7% with placebo in a 12-month maintenance trial (Bowden et al. 2000), and 18% with valproate and 24% with olanzapine in a 47-week maintenance trial (Tohen et al. 2003b). Valproate-related weight gain can be approached in a fashion similar to that already described for lithium. Limited data suggest that valproate-induced hair loss may be avoided or attenuated by the addition of selenium 25–100 μg/day and zinc 10–50 mg/day, presumably by counteracting valproate-induced depletion of these elements.

The U.S. prescribing information for valproate includes boxed warnings regarding the risks of 1) hepatotoxicity, 2) teratogenicity, and 3) pancreatitis. Hepatic fatalities are of concern in infants receiving valproate along with enzyme-inducing agents, but rates for patients over 10 years of age are about 1 in 609,000 with valproate monotherapy and about 1 in 28,000 when valproate is given with enzyme inducers (Bryant and Dreifuss 1996). Valproate, like carbamazepine, is generally discontinued if hepatic indices rise above three times the upper limit of normal. A general guideline called "Hy's rule" after Hyman Zimmerman recommends discontinuing medications out of a concern regarding hepatotoxicity if the serum alanine aminotransferase level is greater than or equal to three times the upper limit of normal and the serum bilirubin level is greater than or equal to two times the upper limit of normal, as this can entail a mortality risk of 10%–50% for different drugs (Bjornsson 2006). Data suggest that rates of major congenital malformations (spina bifida, heart defects, urogenital defects, and multiple anomalies) with valproate exposure could be higher than rates with carbamazepine or lamotrigine exposure or than rates with no anticonvulsant exposure (Cunnington and Tennis 2005; Morrow et al. 2006; Vajda et al. 2007; Wyszynski et al. 2005). Valproate may also increase the risk of neurodevelopmental or neurocognitive defects (Adab et al. 2001; Gaily et al. 2004). Valproate-induced pancreatitis may occur in as many as 1 in 1,000 patients and is detectable by assessing serum amylase in patients with persistent or severe gastrointestinal problems. Other warnings include the risks of hyperammonemic encephalopathy in patients with urea cycle disorders, somnolence in older adults, and thrombocytopenia. The latter appears to be dosage related, particularly if serum valproate concentrations are above 100 μg/mL (700 μmol/L).

In 2008, the FDA released an alert regarding increased risk of suicidality (suicidal behavior or ideation) in patients with epilepsy or psychiatric disorders for 11 anticonvulsants (including valproate). In the FDA's analysis, anticonvulsants compared with placebo yielded approximately twice the risk of suicidality (0.43% vs. 0.22%). The relative risk for suicidality was higher in the patients with epilepsy than in those with psychiatric disorders.

For over a decade, reports have varied regarding a possible association between valproate therapy and polycystic ovary syndrome in women with epilepsy (Isojarvi et al. 1993; Rasgon 2004). Two studies whose findings were consistent with the possibility of a 6%–10% risk of polycystic ovary syndrome with valproate in women with bipolar disorders (Joffe et al. 2006; Rasgon et al. 2005) have indicated the need for prospective trials to systematically assess this issue.

Valproate, like the other mood stabilizers, is a teratogen (FDA pregnancy category D) (Gentile 2006). As previously noted, data suggest that rates of major congenital malformations with valproate exposure could be higher than rates with carbamazepine or lamotrigine exposure or with no anticonvulsant exposure (Cunnington and Tennis 2005; Morrow et al. 2006; Vajda et al. 2007; Wyszynski et al. 2005). Folate supplementation may attenuate the risk of spina bifida, and ultrasound may allow early detection. In view of these findings, valproate therapy in pregnancy appears to be more problematic than therapy with other mood stabilizers, so careful assessments of the risks and benefits of treatment are particularly crucial for patients who are taking valproate. Although valproate concentrations in breast milk and infant serum are low (less than 10% of maternal serum levels), the FDA recommends considering the discontinuation of nursing by a mother who is taking valproate.

Administration

In acute care settings, such as the inpatient treatment of mania, valproate therapy in the past was commonly initiated at 750–2,000 mg/day and increased, as necessary and tolerated, by 250 mg/day every 1–2 days. In view of its extensive metabolism, patients with hepatic insufficiency may require lower dosages. Over the last decade, studies have described more aggressive valproate initiation in acute mania utilizing divalproex formulations. Thus, with the divalproex delayed-release formulation, initiating at 10 mg/lb (20 mg/kg) or even loading with 30 mg/kg/day for 1 or 2 days, followed by 20 mg/kg/day, appears generally well tolerated in acute mania (Lima et al. 1999; McElroy et al. 1996) (Table 13–6). Because of lower bioavailability, dosages with divalproex ER may need to be 6%–20% higher than with the divalproex direct-release formulation. In a recent acute mania study, divalproex ER was started at 25 mg/kg/day rounded up to the nearest 500 mg, increased by 500 mg on day 3, and intermittently adjusted based on clinical effects targeting serum levels from 85 to 125 µg/mL (600–850 µmol/L) (Bowden et al. 2006b). However, euthymic or depressed patients tend to tolerate aggressive initiation less well than do manic patients. Thus, in less acute situations, such as the initiation of prophylaxis or adjunctive use, valproate is often started at 250–500 mg/day and increased, as necessary and tolerated, by 250 mg/day every 4–7 days. Target dosages in the past have commonly been between 750 and 2,500 mg/day, yielding serum levels from 50 to 125 µg/mL (350–850 µmol/L) (Bowden et al. 1996), with the higher portion of the range used acutely and the lower dosages used in adjunctive therapy or prophylaxis. Divalproex ER (Bowden et al. 2006b), and, in some cases, all or the majority of the divalproex delayed-release formulation (Winsberg et al. 2001), can be given in a single dose at bedtime. In a recent meta-analysis of controlled acute mania studies, therapeutic effect size increased linearly with serum valproate concentrations (Allen et al. 2006). In acute mania studies of the adjunctive second-generation antipsychotics risperidone, olanzapine, and quetiapine, target serum valproate concentrations have ranged from 50 to 125 µg/mL, and mean serum valproate concentrations have ranged between 64 and 70 µg/mL (Sachs et al. 2002; Tohen et al. 2002b; Yatham et al. 2004). In a divalproex delayed-release versus lithium versus placebo maintenance study, serum trough valproate concentrations were maintained at 71–125 µg/mL, with a mean of 85 µg/mL at day 30 of randomized treatment (Bowden et al. 2000).

Clinical and Laboratory Monitoring

Patients taking valproate need to be advised of adverse effects and drug interactions. Clinical assessments with valproate therapy include a baseline physical examination, as well as routine querying of patients regarding hepatic and hematological disorders and adverse effects at baseline and during treatment. Laboratory monitoring during valproate therapy commonly includes a baseline complete blood count, differential, platelets, and hepatic indices, followed by reevaluation every 6–12 months and as clinically indicated (American Psychiatric Association 2002). As with carbamazepine, most of the concerning hematological reactions occur in the first 3 months of therapy (Tohen et al. 1995). Serum valproate concentrations are typically assessed 12 hours after dosing at steady state, which occurs 2–3 days after a change in dosage, and then as clinically indicated by inefficacy or adverse effects.

Carbamazepine

Pharmacokinetics and Drug Interactions

Carbamazepine has erratic absorption and a bioavailability of about 80% (Bertilsson 1978; Bertilsson and Tomson 1986; Graves et al. 1998). It is about 75% bound to plasma proteins and has a moderate volume of distribution of about 1 L/kg. Carbamazepine is extensively metabolized, with approximately 1% excreted unchanged in the urine. Before autoinduction of the epoxide pathway (presumably via induction of CYP3A3/4), the half-life of carbamazepine is about 24 hours, and the clearance is about 25 mL/min. However, after autoinduction (2–4 weeks into therapy), the half-life falls to about 8 hours, and clearance rises to about 75 mL/min. This may require dosage adjustment to maintain adequate blood levels and therapeutic effects. The active carbamazepine-10,11-epoxide metabolite has a half-life of about 6 hours. Two sustained-release carbamazepine formulations have been approved for the treatment of epilepsy in the United States. These formulations given twice a day yield steady-state carbamazepine levels similar to those seen with the immediate-release formulation given four times a day (Garnett et al. 1998; Thakker et al. 1992) and potentially fewer adverse effects in view of lower peak serum concentrations (Aldenkamp et al. 1987; Persson et al. 1990). One of these, an extended-release capsule formulation, has been approved for the treatment of acute mania in the United States (Weisler et al. 2004a, 2005).

The pharmacokinetic properties of carbamazepine are atypical among medications prescribed by psychiatrists and necessitate special care when treating patients concurrently with other medications (Ketter et al. 1991a, 1991b). Carbamazepine is extensively metabolized, with only approximately 1% being excreted unchanged in the urine (Bertilsson 1978; Bertilsson and Tomson 1986). The main metabolic pathway of carbamazepine (to its active 10,11-epoxide) appears to be mediated primarily by CYP3A3/4, with a minor contribution by CYP2C8 (Kerr et al. 1994). This epoxide pathway accounts for about 40% of carbamazepine disposition, and even more in patients with induced epoxide pathway metabolism (presumably via CYP3A3/4 induction) (Faigle and Feldmann 1995). Although a genetic polymorphism has been observed for CYP2C8 (Wrighton and Stevens 1992), this probably does not account for the variability observed in carbamazepine disposition, in view of the minor role of this isoform. The frequency distribution of carbamazepine kinetic parameters is unimodal, consistent with CYP3A3/4 (which lacks genetic polymorphism) being the crucial isoform. With enzyme induction (of the epoxide pathway, presumably via CYP3A3/4 induction), formation of carbamazepine-epoxide triples, its subsequent transformation to the inactive diol doubles, and thus the carbamazepine-epoxide/carbamazepine ratio increases (Eichelbaum et al. 1985). Other pathways include aromatic hydroxylation (25%), which is apparently mediated by CYP1A2 and not induced concurrently with the epoxide pathway, and glucuronide conjugation of the carbamoyl side chain (15%) by UGT, presumably primarily by UGT2B7 (Staines et al. 2004). These other pathways yield inactive metabolites.

Carbamazepine induces not only CYP3A3/4 and conjugation but also presumably other cytochrome P450 isoforms (which remain to be characterized).

Thus, carbamazepine decreases the serum levels of not only carbamazepine itself (autoinduction) but also many other medications (heteroinduction) (Table 13–8). Carbamazepine-induced decreases in serum levels of certain concurrent medications can render them ineffective. Moreover, if carbamazepine is discontinued, serum levels of these other medications can rise, leading to toxic effects from these agents (Denbow and Fraser 1990). Also, carbamazepine metabolism can be inhibited by CYP3A3/4 inhibitors, yielding increased serum carbamazepine levels and intoxication (Table 13–9).

The active carbamazepine-epoxide metabolite can yield therapeutic and adverse effects similar to those of carbamazepine but is not detected in conventional carbamazepine assays. The unwary clinician may misinterpret the significance of therapeutic or adverse effects associated with low or moderate serum carbamazepine levels. In addition, valproate displaces carbamazepine from plasma proteins, yielding an increase in free carbamazepine, which, in combination with valproate-induced increases in carbamazepine-epoxide, can yield toxicity when carbamazepine plus valproate combination therapy is utilized.

Carbamazepine has a wide variety of drug-drug interactions (Tables 13–8 and 13–9), in excess of those seen with lithium or valproate, because of carbamazepine's constellation of pharmacokinetic properties. Knowledge of carbamazepine drug-drug interactions and strategies for treating refractory symptoms is crucial in effective management. Carbamazepine drug-drug interactions are predominantly mediated by pharmacokinetic mechanisms. Advances in molecular pharmacology have characterized the specific cytochrome P450 isoforms responsible for metabolism of various medications (Ketter et al. 1991a), which may allow clinicians to anticipate and avoid pharmacokinetic drug-drug interactions and thus provide more effective pharmacotherapy combinations. The reader interested in detailed reviews of carbamazepine drug-drug interactions may find these in other articles (Ketter et al. 1991a, 1991b).

Carbamazepine and lithium are frequently combined in treating bipolar disorder and may provide additive or synergistic antimanic, antidepressant, and mood-stabilizing effects (Denicoff et al. 1997; Kramlinger and Post 1989). A few case reports suggest that some individuals may experience neurotoxicity with the carbamazepine plus lithium combination, presumably related to a pharmacodynamic interaction, despite having serum concentrations of both drugs within the therapeutic range (Chaudhry and Waters 1983; Ghose 1980; Reynolds 1975; Shukla et al. 1984). Nevertheless, the carbamazepine plus lithium combination is generally well tolerated, with merely additive neurotoxicity, which can be minimized by gradual dosage escalation.

TABLE 13–8. Selected drugs with increased clearance with carbamazepine

Alprazolam (?)	Ethosuximide	Oxcarbazepine
Amitriptyline	Felbamate	Oxiracetam (?)
Aripiprazole	Felodipine	Pancuronium
Bupropion	Fentanyl (?)	Phenytoin
Chlorpromazine (?)	Fluphenazine (?)	Praziquantel
Citalopram	Glucocorticoids	Prednisolone
Clobazam	Haloperidol	Primidone
Clonazepam	Hormonal contraceptives	Quetiapine
Clozapine	Imipramine	Risperidone
Cyclosporine (?)	Indinavir	Sertraline
Delavirdine	Itraconazole	Theophylline (?)
Desipramine	Lamotrigine	Thiothixene (?)
Dexamethasone	Levetiracetam (?)	Tiagabine
Diazepam	Levothyroxine	Topiramate
Dicumarol (?)	Methadone	Valproate
Doxacurium	Midazolam	Vecuronium
Doxepin	Mirtazapine	Warfarin
Doxycycline	Nortriptyline	Ziprasidone (?)
Escitalopram	Olanzapine	Zonisamide

Note. (?) = limited data.

TABLE 13–9. Selected drugs that decrease clearance of carbamazepine

Acetazolamide	Fluvoxamine	Ponsinomycin
Cimetidine	Grapefruit juice	Propoxyphene
Clarithromycin	Isoniazid	Quetiapine ($\uparrow$ CBZ-E) (?)
Danazol	Itraconazole	Quinine
Dextropropoxyphene	Josamycin	Ritonavir
Diltiazem	Ketoconazole	Troleandomycin
Erythromycin	Nefazodone	Valproate ($\uparrow$ CBZ-E)
Fluoxetine	Nelfinavir	Verapamil
Flurithromycin	Nicotinamide	Viloxazine

Note. CBZ-E = carbamazepine-10,11-epoxide; (?) = limited data.

The carbamazepine plus valproate combination not only appears to be tolerated but may show psychotropic synergy (Ketter et al. 1992). Carbamazepine induces valproate metabolism, yielding decreased serum valproate concentrations (Jann et al. 1988; Levy et al. 1982). Valproate inhibits epoxide hydrolase, increasing the serum carbamazepine-epoxide levels (Pisani et al. 1990), at times without altering total serum carbamazepine levels. These interactions can potentially confound clinicians because patients can have neurotoxicity due to elevated carbamazepine-epoxide or free carbamazepine concentrations in spite of therapeutic total carbamazepine levels. Thus, in view of increased carbamazepine-epoxide levels, carbamazepine levels as low as about one-half of those seen without valproate may be required. Carbamazepine decreases serum valproate levels, and discontinuation of carbamazepine can yield increased serum valproate levels and toxicity. As a general rule, clinicians should carefully monitor patients on the carbamazepine plus valproate combination for side effects and consider decreasing the carbamazepine dosage in advance (because of the expected displacement of carbamazepine from plasma proteins and increase in carbamazepine-epoxide) and ultimately increasing the valproate dosage (because of expected carbamazepine-induced decrements in valproate).

Carbamazepine induces lamotrigine metabolism (May et al. 1996), so that, as described in the "Lamotrigine" section below, lamotrigine therapy in the presence of carbamazepine requires higher dosages of lamotrigine. Although lamotrigine does not yield clinically significant changes in serum carbamazepine concentrations (Grasela et al. 1999), lamotrigine appears to enhance carbamazepine neurotoxicity, probably by a pharmacodynamic interaction (Besag et al. 1998).

Carbamazepine increases metabolism of haloperidol (Arana et al. 1986; Hesslinger et al. 1999; Iwahashi et al. 1995; Jann et al. 1985; Kahn et al. 1990; Kidron et al. 1985; Raitasuo et al. 1994; Yasui-Furukori et al. 2003) and possibly other first-generation antipsychotics, such as chlorpromazine (Raitasuo et al. 1994), fluphenazine (Jann et al. 1989), and thiothixene (Ereshefsky et al. 1986). Some patients may have improvement or no deterioration in psychiatric status or fewer neuroleptic side effects during combination treatment (Jann et al. 1985; Kahn et al. 1990; Yasui-Furukori et al. 2003), whereas others may have deterioration in psychiatric status (Arana et al. 1986; Cohen and Diemont 2002; Hesslinger et al. 1999; Kahn et al. 1990). Haloperidol may increase carbamazepine levels (Iwahashi et al. 1995), whereas loxapine and the amoxapine plus chlorpromazine combination may increase carbamazepine-epoxide levels (Pitterle and Collins 1988).

Carbamazepine induces clozapine metabolism (Jerling et al. 1994b; Raitasuo et al. 1993, 1994; Tiihonen et al. 1995), and this combination is not recommended in view of possible (but not proven) synergistic bone marrow suppression (Junghan et al. 1993). Carbamazepine also increases metabolism of olanzapine (Linnet and Olesen 2002; Lucas et al. 1998), risperidone (Ono et al. 2002; Spina et al. 2000a; Yatham et al. 2003), quetiapine (Grimm et al. 2006), aripiprazole (*Physicians' Desk Reference* 2008), and ziprasidone (Miceli et al. 2000a). Although the clinical significance of carbamazepine-induced decreases in ziprasidone serum concentrations remains to be determined, carbamazepine interactions with other second-generation antipsychotics can be clinically significant. For example, in an acute mania combination therapy study, carbamazepine decreased serum risperidone plus active metabolite concentrations by 40%, interfering with efficacy (Yatham et al. 2003). In another combination therapy study, carbamazepine yielded lower than expected blood olanzapine concentrations, and even though this was addressed in part by more aggressive olanzapine dosage, the efficacy of the olanzapine plus carbamazepine combination was still not significantly better than that of carbamazepine monotherapy in the treatment of acute mania (Tohen et al. 2008). In two patients, quetiapine appeared to increase carbamazepine-epoxide levels (Fitzgerald and Okos 2002).

Carbamazepine appears to induce metabolism of tricyclic antidepressants (Brøsen and Kragh-Sørensen 1993; Brown et al. 1990; Jerling et al. 1994a; Leinonen et al. 1991; Spina et al. 1995; Szymura-Oleksiak et al. 2001), bupropion (Ketter et al. 1995a), citalopram (Steinacher et al. 2002), mirtazapine (Sitsen et al. 2001), mianserin (Eap et al. 1999), sertraline (Khan et al. 2000; Pihlsgard and Eliasson 2002), and to some extent trazodone (Otani et al. 1996). Carbamazepine may increase rather than decrease serum levels of transdermal selegiline and its metabolites (*Physicians' Desk Reference* 2008). Theoretical grounds have been stated for concern about combining carbamazepine with monoamine oxidase inhibitors. However, preliminary data suggest that the addition of phenelzine or tranylcypromine to carbamazepine may be well tolerated, does not affect carbamazepine levels, and may provide relief of refractory depressive symptoms in some patients (Ketter et al. 1995b). The CYP3A3/4 inhibitors fluoxetine (Grimsley et al. 1991; Pearson 1990), fluvoxamine (Bonnet et al. 1992; Fritze et al. 1991; Martinelli et al. 1993), and nefazodone (Ashton and Wolin 1996) have been reported to inhibit carbamazepine metabolism, yielding increased carbamazepine levels and toxicity (see Table 13–9).

Carbamazepine is commonly administered along with benzodiazepines in patients with bipolar disorders, with merely additive central nervous system adverse effects (e.g., sedation, ataxia). Indeed, contemporary controlled carbamazepine trials routinely permit some adjunctive benzodiazepine (e.g., lorazepam) administration (Weisler et al. 2004a, 2005). However, carbamazepine may decrease serum levels of clonazepam (Lai et al. 1978; Yukawa et al. 2001), alprazolam (Arana et al. 1988; Furukori et al. 1998), clobazam (Levy et al. 1983), and midazolam (Backman et al. 1996), potentially decreasing the efficacy of these agents. The newer hypnotics eszopiclone and zolpidem may have drug interactions with carbamazepine, because these agents appear more susceptible than zaleplon to drugs that induce CYP3A4 (Drover 2004).

Carbamazepine induces the metabolism of multiple other anticonvulsants, including topiramate (Sachdeo et al. 1996), tiagabine (Samara et al. 1998), oxcarbazepine (McKee et al. 1994), zonisamide (Ojemann et al. 1986), and possibly levetiracetam (May et al. 2003), but not gabapentin (Radulovic et al. 1994) or pregabalin (Brodie et al. 2005). Phenytoin, phenobarbital, primidone, felbamate, and methsuximide decrease serum carbamazepine levels. In addition, carbamazepine may have a pharmacodynamic interaction with levetiracetam (Sisodiya et al. 2002).

The commonly used calcium channel blockers verapamil (Price and DiMarzio 1988) and diltiazem (Brodie and MacPhee 1986) can increase carbamazepine levels and cause clinical toxicity, but this does not occur with the dihydropyridines nifedipine (Brodie and MacPhee 1986) and nimodipine (T. A. Ketter and R. M. Post, unpublished observations). Also, enzyme-inducing anticonvulsants like carbamazepine appear to decrease nimodipine (Tartara et al. 1991) and felodipine (Capewell et al. 1988) levels.

Carbamazepine decreases L-thyroxine (T_4), free T_4 index, and less consistently liothyronine (T_3) concentrations. In contrast, thyroid-binding globulin, reverse T_3, and basal plasma TSH concentrations, and basal metabolic rates, are not substantially changed with carbamazepine therapy.

Drug-drug interactions between carbamazepine and other (nonpsychotropic) drugs are also of substantial clinical importance. Carbamazepine induces metabolism of diverse medications (see Table 13–8), raising the possibility of its undermining the efficacy of steroids such as hormonal contraceptives (Crawford et al. 1990; Doose et al. 2003b). In women taking carbamazepine, oral contraceptive preparations need to contain at least 50 µg of ethinyl estradiol, levonorgestrel implants are contraindicated because of cases of contraceptive failure, and medroxyprogesterone injections need to be given every 10 rather than 12 weeks (Crawford 2002). Carbamazepine also induces metabolism of prednisolone and methylprednisolone; the methylxanthines theophylline and aminophylline; the antibiotic doxycycline; the neuromuscular blockers pancuronium, vecuronium, and doxacurium; the anticoagulant warfarin; and possibly the anticoagulant dicumarol. Coadministration of carbamazepine and delavirdine may lead to delavirdine inefficacy (Tran et al. 2001).

Similarly, a variety of medications can increase serum carbamazepine levels and potentially yield clinical toxicity (see Table 13–9), including nicotinamide (Bourgeois et al. 1982); the antibiotics erythromycin (Steketee et al. 1988), triacetyloleandomycin (Mesdjian et al. 1980), clarithromycin (Albani et al. 1993), and isoniazid (Wright et al. 1982); the protease inhibitors ritonavir (Kato et al. 2000) and nelfinavir (Bates and Herman 2006); and the carbonic anhydrase inhibitor acetazolamide (Forsythe et al. 1981). In addition, other medications such as cisplatin and doxorubicin may decrease serum carbamazepine levels, potentially yielding inefficacy (Neef and de Voogd-van der Straaten 1988).

Adverse Effects

Carbamazepine therapy is associated with common benign adverse events, as well as rare serious adverse events. The most common dosage-related adverse effects with carbamazepine involve problems with the central nervous system (diplopia, blurred vision, fatigue, sedation, dizziness, and ataxia) or gastrointestinal system (nausea, vomiting) (Pellock 1987). Carbamazepine central nervous system adverse effects tend to occur early in therapy, before autoinduction and the development of some tolerance to carbamazepine's central adverse effects. Gradual initial dosing and careful attention to potential drug-drug interactions can help attenuate such problems. Carbamazepine-induced gastrointestinal disturbance can be approached in a fashion similar to that described for lithium.

The U.S. prescribing information for carbamazepine includes boxed warnings regarding the risks of serious dermatological reactions and the HLA-B*1502 allele, as well as aplastic anemia (16/million patient-years) and agranulocytosis (48/million patient-years). Other warnings in the prescribing information include the risks of teratogenicity, as well as increased intraocular pressure due to mild anticholinergic activity. Thus, carbamazepine can yield hematological (benign leukopenia, benign thrombocytopenia), dermatological (benign rash), electrolyte (asymptomatic hyponatremia), and hepatic (benign transaminase elevations) problems. Much less commonly, carbamazepine can yield analogous serious problems. For example, mild leukopenia and benign rash occur in as many as 1 in 10 patients, with the slight possibility that these usually benign phenomena are heralding malignant aplastic anemia, seen in approximately 1 in 100,000 patients, and Stevens-Johnson syndrome or toxic epidermal necrolysis, seen in 1–6 in 10,000 patients (Kramlinger et al. 1994; Tohen et al. 1995). Recent evidence indicates that the risk of serious rash may be 10 times as high in some Asian countries and strongly linked to the HLA-B*1502 allele (Hung et al. 2006). Thus, the U.S. prescribing information states that Asians ought to be genetically tested, and if they are found to be HLA-B*1502 positive, they should not be treated with carbamazepine unless the benefit clearly outweighs the risk. Hematological monitoring needs to be intensified in patients with low or marginal leukocyte counts, and carbamazepine is generally discontinued if the leukocyte count falls below 3,000/μL or the granulocyte count below 1,000/μL. Rash presenting with systemic illness, or involvement of the eyes, mouth, or bladder (dysuria) constitutes a medical emergency, and carbamazepine ought to be immediately discontinued and the patient assessed emergently. For more benign presentations, immediate dermatological consultation is required, to assess the risks of continuing therapy. In carefully selected cases, with the collaboration of dermatology, it may be safe to attempt desensitization by decreasing dosage and adding antihistamine or prednisone. Carbamazepine, like valproate, can rarely cause clinically significant hepatic problems, and generally needs to be discontinued if hepatic indices rise above three times the upper limit of normal (Martínez et al. 1993).

In 2008, the FDA released an alert regarding increased risk of suicidality (suicidal behavior or ideation) in patients with epilepsy or with psychiatric disorders for 11 anticonvulsants (including carbamazepine). In the FDA's analysis, anticonvulsants compared with placebo yielded approximately twice the risk of suicidality (0.43% vs. 0.22%). The relative risk for suicidality was higher in the patients with epilepsy than in the patients with psychiatric disorders.

Although carbamazepine can cause modest TSH increases, frank hypothyroidism is very uncommon (Joffe et al. 1984). Like other agents with tricyclic structures and sodium-blocking properties, carbamazepine may affect cardiac conduction and should be used with caution in patients with cardiac disorders (Boesen et al. 1983). A baseline electrocardiogram is worth consideration if there is any indication of cardiac problems.

Carbamazepine appears less likely than lithium (Coxhead et al. 1992) or valproate (Mattson et al. 1992) to yield weight gain (Ketter et al. 2004). For this reason, carbamazepine may provide an important alternative to other mood stabilizers for patients who struggle with this problem. Carbamazepine-induced hyponatremia is often tolerated in young physically well individuals, but can yield obtundation and other serious sequelae in medically frail older adult patients (Yassa et al. 1988).

Carbamazepine, like the other mood stabilizers, is a teratogen (FDA pregnancy category D) (Gentile 2006). Thus, carbamazepine can yield minor anomalies (craniofacial malformations and digital hypoplasia) in up to 20% of cases (Jones et al. 1989) and spina bifida in about 1% of cases (Rosa 1991). For the latter, folate supplementation may attenuate the risk, and ultrasound may allow early detection. Recent data suggest that overall rates of major congenital malformations with carbamazepine exposure could be comparable to rates with lamotrigine or no anticonvulsant exposure, and lower than rates with valproate exposure (Cunnington and Tennis 2005; Morrow et al. 2006; Vajda et al. 2007; Wyszynski et al. 2005). The issue of carbamazepine therapy in pregnancy can be approached in a fashion similar to that described above in the section on lithium. Although carbamazepine concentrations in breast milk are variable and there is very little evidence of adverse effects in newborns exposed to carbamazepine via breast milk, the FDA recommends that the mother discontinue nursing or discontinue taking the drug, depending on the importance of the drug to the mother.

Administration

In acute care settings, such as the inpatient treatment of mania, carbamazepine therapy is commonly initiated at 200–400 mg/day and increased, as necessary and tolerated, by 200 mg/day every 2–4 days. In controlled studies, a beaded extended-release capsule formulation was started at 200 mg twice a day and titrated by daily increments of 200 mg to final dosages as high as 1,600 mg/day (Weisler et al. 2004a, 2005) (Table 13–6). In a report of open extension therapy after these controlled acute mania studies, beaded extended-release capsule carbamazepine was started at 200 mg twice a day and titrated by increments of 200 mg every 3 days (vs. every day in the acute studies) to final dosages as high as 1,600 mg/day (Ketter et al. 2004). This approach decreased the incidence of central nervous system (dizziness, somnolence, ataxia), digestive (nausea, vomiting), and dermatological (pruritus) adverse effects by about 50%. Euthymic or depressed patients tend to tolerate aggressive initiation less well than do manic patients. Thus, in less acute situations, such as the initiation of prophylaxis or adjunctive use, carbamazepine is often started at 100–200 mg/day and increased, as necessary and tolerated, by 200 mg/day every 4–7 days. Even this gradual initiation may cause adverse effects. Thus, starting with 50 mg (half of a chewable 100-mg tablet) at bedtime and increasing by 50 mg every 4 days can yield a better-tolerated initiation. Because of autoinduction, dosages after 2–4 weeks of therapy may need to be twice as high as in the first week to yield comparable serum levels. Target dosages are commonly between 600 and 1,600 mg/day, yielding serum levels from 6 to 12 μg/mL (20–60 μmol/L), with the higher portion of the range used acutely and lower dosages used in prophylaxis or adjunctive therapy. In a carbamazepine versus lithium maintenance study, serum trough carbamazepine concentrations were maintained at 4–12 μg/mL, with a mean of 6.4 μg/mL (Greil et al. 1997). In another carbamazepine versus lithium maintenance study, serum trough carbamazepine concentrations were maintained at 4–12 μg/mL, with a mean of 7.7 μg/mL (Denicoff et al. 1997).

Clinical and Laboratory Monitoring

Patients taking carbamazepine need to be advised of adverse effects and drug interactions. Clinical assessments with carbamazepine therapy include a baseline physical examination and routinely querying patients regarding hepatic and hematological disorders and adverse effects at baseline and during treatment. In the past, recommended laboratory monitoring during carbamazepine therapy has included a baseline complete blood count, differential, platelets, hepatic indices, and serum sodium, with reevaluation at 2, 4, 6, and 8 weeks, and then every 3 months and as clinically indicated (American Psychiatric Association 2002). Most of the dangerous hematological reactions occur in the first 3 months of therapy (Tohen et al. 1995). In contemporary clinical practice, somewhat less focus is placed on scheduled monitoring, whereas clinically indicated monitoring (e.g., when a patient becomes ill with a fever) is emphasized. Patients who have abnormal or marginal indices at any point merit careful scheduled and clinically indicated monitoring. The U.S. prescribing information for the beaded extended-release capsule carbamazepine formulation that was recently approved for the treatment of acute mania includes monitoring baseline complete blood count, platelets, possibly reticulocytes, and serum iron, and hepatic function tests; closely monitoring patients with low or decreased white blood cell count or platelets; and considering discontinuation of carbamazepine if evidence indicates bone marrow depression (*Physicians' Desk Reference* 2008). Serum carbamazepine concentrations are typically assessed 12 hours after dosing at steady state, which occurs 2–5 days after a dosing change (depending on the degree of autoinduction), and then as indicated by inefficacy or adverse effects.

Lamotrigine

Pharmacokinetics and Drug Interactions

Lamotrigine has a bioavailability of about 98%. It is 55% bound to plasma proteins and has a moderate volume of distribution of approximately 1 L/kg and a linear dosage-to-plasma concentration relationship (Mikati et al. 1989). In monotherapy, its half-life is about 28 hours and clearance is about 40 mL/min. Lamotrigine is extensively metabolized, mostly by glucuronidation, primarily by UTG1A4 and UGT2B7 (Rowland et al. 2006), with only 10% excreted unchanged in the urine. Lamotrigine does not yield clinically significant induction or inhibition of CYP450 isoforms (Posner et al. 1991) and is thus more a target of than an instigator of drug interactions. When lamotrigine is combined with the enzyme inducer carbamazepine, lamotrigine's half-life falls 50% to about 14 hours and clearance doubles to about 80 mL/min. When lamotrigine is combined with the enzyme inhibitor valproate, lamotrigine's half-life doubles to about 56 hours and clearance falls 50% to about 20 mL/min.

Thus, approximately 85% of lamotrigine is conjugated to yield inactive glucuronide metabolites, while about 10% is excreted unchanged in the urine (Cohen et al. 1987). Enzyme inducers such as carbamazepine decrease serum lamotrigine concentrations (May et al. 1996), presumably mediated by induction of glucuronidation, whereas valproate (Anderson et al. 1996; Rambeck and Wolf 1993) increases lamotrigine levels, presumably mediated by inhibition of UGT2B7 (Rowland et al. 2006). In contrast, lamotrigine does not yield clinically significant changes in serum carbamazepine concentrations (Grasela et al. 1999), and lamotrigine may yield only modest (25%), clinically insignificant decreases in valproate levels (Anderson et al. 1996). However, lamotrigine appears to enhance carbamazepine neurotoxicity, probably by a pharmacodynamic interaction (Besag et al. 1998). Lamotrigine does not appear to have clinically significant pharmacokinetic interactions with lithium (Chen et al. 2000).

Lamotrigine does not generally have clinically significant pharmacointeractions with clozapine, risperidone, or olanzapine (Castberg and Spigset 2006; Sidhu et al. 2006a; Spina et al. 2006; Tiihonen et al. 2003). However, single cases of increased clozapine (Kossen et al. 2001) and risperidone (Bienentreu and Kronmüller 2005) concentrations with lamotrigine have been reported. Aripiprazole does not appear to have clinically significant effects on lamotrigine pharmacokinetics (Schiebar et al. 2007). Assessments from a therapeutic drug monitoring service suggested that chlorpromazine, clozapine, haloperidol, perphenazine, and quetiapine may not generally alter lamotrigine serum concentration/dosage ratios (Reimers et al. 2005).

Lamotrigine is commonly combined with antidepressants in patients with mood disorders with apparently good tolerability. Bupropion does not appear to yield clinically significant changes in lamotrigine pharmacokinetics (Odishaw and Chen 2000). In controlled clinical trials, lamotrigine did not appear to have pharmacokinetic interactions with paroxetine or fluoxetine. Assessments

from a therapeutic drug monitoring service suggested that citalopram, mirtazapine, nefazodone, venlafaxine, paroxetine, and sertraline may not generally
alter lamotrigine serum concentration/dosage ratios and, unexpectedly, that
fluoxetine may decrease lamotrigine serum concentration/dosage ratios (Reimers et al. 2005). Results from in vitro experiments suggest that fluoxetine,
phenelzine, and trazodone do not affect lamotrigine metabolism and that amitriptyline and bupropion minimally affect lamotrigine metabolism (*Physicians'
Desk Reference* 2008). However, problems may occur with some individuals, because case reports suggest that sertraline may increase serum lamotrigine levels
in some patients (Kaufman and Gerner 1998), that lamotrigine combined with
escitalopram could yield myoclonus (Rosenhagen et al. 2006), and that seizures,
ventricular tachycardia, and rhabdomyolysis may occur after an overdose of
venlafaxine and lamotrigine (Peano et al. 1997).

Lamotrigine is commonly administered along with benzodiazepines in patients with bipolar disorders, with merely additive central nervous system adverse effects (e.g., sedation, ataxia). Indeed, contemporary controlled lamotrigine trials routinely permit some adjunctive benzodiazepine (e.g., lorazepam)
administration (Bowden et al. 2003; Calabrese et al. 1999, 2000, 2003). Assessments from a therapeutic drug monitoring service suggested that clonazepam,
diazepam, oxazepam, and zopiclone may not generally alter lamotrigine serum
concentration/dosage ratios (Reimers et al. 2005). Results from in vitro experiments suggest that clonazepam and lorazepam minimally affect lamotrigine metabolism (*Physicians' Desk Reference* 2008).

Lamotrigine does not appear to have clinically significant pharmacokinetic
interactions with topiramate (Berry et al. 2002; Doose et al. 2003a), levetiracetam (Gidal et al. 2005; Perucca et al. 2003), zonisamide (Levy et al. 2005), or
pregabalin (Brodie et al. 2005). Oxcarbazepine may decrease serum lamotrigine
concentrations (May et al. 1999), but the clinical significance of this interaction
remains to be established and could vary across patients (Theis et al. 2005),
whereas lamotrigine does not appear to alter oxcarbazepine pharmacokinetics
(Theis et al. 2005). A possible pharmacodynamic interaction has been reported
with oxcarbazepine and lamotrigine (Sabers and Gram 2000).

Lamotrigine has interactions with some nonpsychotropic medications.
Rifampin increases lamotrigine clearance. Although lamotrigine does not appear to yield clinically significant changes in the pharmacokinetics of hormonal
contraceptives (Sidhu et al. 2006b), hormonal contraceptives cause clinically
significant decreases in serum lamotrigine concentrations (Christensen et al.
2007; Sabers et al. 2003; Sidhu et al. 2006b).

Adverse Effects

Lamotrigine is generally well tolerated, particularly in comparison to other treatment options for patients with bipolar disorders. The most common adverse events in patients with bipolar disorders in clinical trials were headache, benign rash, dizziness, diarrhea, dream abnormality, and pruritus.

The U.S. prescribing information for lamotrigine includes a boxed warning regarding the risk of serious rashes requiring hospitalization, which have included Stevens-Johnson syndrome, in 0.8% and 0.3% of pediatric and adult epilepsy patients receiving adjunctive therapy, respectively, and in 0.08% and 0.13% of adult mood disorder patients receiving monotherapy and adjunctive therapy, respectively. The risk of rash is higher in patients under age 16 years and may be higher with coadministration with valproate, with lamotrigine dosage that exceeds the recommended initial dosage, and with lamotrigine dosage escalation that exceeds the recommended escalation. Benign rash may be seen in 10% of patients, but because any rash is potentially serious, rashes require discontinuation of lamotrigine, unless they are clearly not drug related. Nearly all cases of life-threatening rashes have occurred within 2–8 weeks of starting lamotrigine. Other warnings in the prescribing information include the risks of hypersensitivity reactions (with fever and lymphadenopathy, but not necessarily rash), acute multiorgan failure (fatalities observed in about 1 in 400 pediatric and 1 in 1,800 adult patients with epilepsy, but not in patients with bipolar disorders), blood dyscrasia, and possibly withdrawal seizures in patients with bipolar disorders, so that unless safety concerns demand abrupt discontinuation, lamotrigine should be tapered over 2 weeks.

In 2008, the FDA released an alert regarding increased risk of suicidality (suicidal behavior or ideation) in patients with epilepsy or psychiatric disorders for 11 anticonvulsants (including lamotrigine). In the FDA's analysis, anticonvulsants compared with placebo yielded approximately twice the risk of suicidality (0.43% vs. 0.22%). The relative risk for suicidality was higher in the patients with epilepsy than in those with psychiatric disorders.

Lamotrigine can adversely affect the central nervous system (headache, somnolence, insomnia, dizziness, tremor) and gastrointestinal system (nausea, diarrhea) (Bowden et al. 2003; Calabrese et al. 1999, 2000, 2003). In most instances, these problems attenuate or resolve with time or lamotrigine dosage adjustment, but occasional patients may require lamotrigine discontinuation. Unlike other mood stabilizers, lamotrigine has not been associated with weight gain (Bowden et al. 2006a; Sachs et al. 2006a). Also of clinical importance, lamotrigine may be less likely than selective serotonin reuptake inhibitors or other anticonvulsants to cause sexual dysfunction (Carwile et al. 1997).

Lamotrigine, like the other mood stabilizers, is a teratogen (FDA pregnancy category C) (Gentile 2006). Recent data suggest that overall rates of major congenital malformations with lamotrigine exposure could be comparable to rates with carbamazepine or no anticonvulsant exposure, and lower than rates with valproate exposure (Cunnington and Tennis 2005; Morrow et al. 2006; Vajda et al. 2007; Wyszynski et al. 2005). Nevertheless, lamotrigine may increase the risk of subtypes of malformation, namely cleft lip and cleft palate. Lamotrigine concentrations in breast milk are variable but in some instances may approach "therapeutic ranges." Despite the lack of evidence of adverse effects in newborns exposed to lamotrigine via breast milk, the FDA has taken a conservative stance, considering lamotrigine administration "not recommended" during lactation.

Administration

Lamotrigine dosage is initially titrated very slowly to decrease the risk of rash. When lamotrigine is given without valproate, the prescribing information recommends starting lamotrigine at 25 mg/day for 2 weeks, then increasing to 50 mg/day for the next 2 weeks, then increasing to 100 mg/day for 1 week, and then increasing to 200 mg/day in a single daily dose, with dosages exceeding 200 mg/day not recommended unless concurrent hormonal contraceptives (which decrease serum lamotrigine concentrations) are administered (*Physicians' Desk Reference* 2008) (Table 13–6). Nevertheless, even in the absence of hormonal contraceptives, selected patients may benefit from further gradual lamotrigine titration, to final dosages as high as 400–500 mg/day. Even more gradual titration, starting with 25 mg/day for 2 weeks, then increasing to 50 mg/day for the next 2 weeks, and then increasing weekly by 25 mg/day, as necessary and tolerated, may further decrease the risk of rash (Ketter et al. 2005a).

When lamotrigine is added to valproate, recommended dosages are halved, so lamotrigine is started at 25 mg every other day (although 12.5 mg/day may be worth considering) for 2 weeks, then increased to 25 mg/day for the next 2 weeks, then increased to 50 mg/day for 1 week, and then increased to 100 mg/day in a single daily dose, with dosages exceeding 100 mg/day not recommended unless concurrent hormonal contraceptives (which decrease serum lamotrigine concentrations) are administered (*Physicians' Desk Reference* 2008). Nevertheless, even in the absence of hormonal contraceptives, selected patients concurrently taking valproate may benefit from further gradual lamotrigine titration to final dosages as high as 250 mg/day.

When lamotrigine is given with carbamazepine, lamotrigine dosages may be doubled, so lamotrigine may be started at 50 mg/day for 2 weeks, then increased to 100 mg/day for the next 2 weeks, then increased to 300 mg/day for 1 week, and then increased to 400 mg/day in divided doses, with dosages exceeding 400 mg/day not recommended unless concurrent hormonal contraceptives (which decrease serum lamotrigine concentrations) are administered (*Physicians' Desk Reference* 2008). Nevertheless, even in the absence of hormonal contraceptives, selected patients concurrently taking carbamazepine may benefit from further gradual lamotrigine titration to final dosages as high as 800 mg/day.

Patients should be advised that if they fail to take lamotrigine for five half-lives (e.g., approximately 5 days in the absence of carbamazepine, or 3 days in the presence of carbamazepine), gradual reintroduction as described above will be necessary, because rashes have been reported with rapid reintroduction.

Clinical and Laboratory Monitoring

Patients taking lamotrigine need to be advised of adverse effects and drug interactions. Clinical assessments with lamotrigine therapy include a baseline physical examination and routinely querying patients regarding rash at baseline and during treatment. Lamotrigine is generally well tolerated, and serum concentrations have not been related to therapeutic effects in patients with bipolar disorders, so therapeutic drug monitoring with lamotrigine is not generally performed. Nevertheless, in patients taking higher dosages (e.g., 400 mg/day without valproate, 200 mg/day with valproate, or 800 mg/day with carbamazepine) with inadequate therapeutic response and good tolerability, assessing serum lamotrigine concentrations may be worthwhile, to provide an assessment of adherence and/or metabolic abnormalities. In epilepsy patients, serum lamotrigine concentrations range from approximately 3 to 15 μg/mL (10–60 μmol/L) (Johannessen et al. 2003). Thus, in a patient with bipolar disorder who is taking higher dosages with inadequate therapeutic response, a serum lamotrigine concentration of less than 3 μg/mL or in excess of 15 μg/mL may suggest adherence or nonresponse problems, respectively. Serum lamotrigine concentrations are typically assessed 12 hours after dosing at steady state, which occurs 5 days after a dosage change in the absence of valproate and carbamazepine (10 days if valproate is present, and 3 days if carbamazepine is present).

Antipsychotics

Bipolar disorder patients with acute major depressive episodes may have psychotic features. Mood stabilizers may fail to provide adequate efficacy in such circumstances. Patients with acute manic or mixed episodes with profound agitation may require intramuscular medication, and patients with poor adherence may benefit from depot formulations. Unfortunately, mood stabilizers are not available in intramuscular or depot formulations. However, such formulations of antipsychotics are available. Thus, because of both efficacy and formulation availability limitations of mood stabilizers, adjunctive antipsychotics are commonly used in the treatment of patients with bipolar disorders.

First-Generation Antipsychotics

Pharmacokinetics and Drug Interactions

First-generation antipsychotics are generally well absorbed, with variable (20%–80%) bioavailability, high (80%–95%) protein binding, and variable volumes of distribution (10–40 L/kg), half-lives (12–24 hours), and clearances (70–600 mL/min) (Javaid 1994). These agents have varying and in some cases complex metabolism, which may be susceptible to induction by carbamazepine, phenobarbital, phenytoin, rifampin, and tobacco smoking. Several first-generation antipsychotics (including haloperidol, perphenazine, and thioridazine) are CYP2D6 substrates (Eap et al. 1996; Kudo and Ishizaki 1999; Olesen and Linnet 2000; Otani and Aoshima 2000; Pan and Belpaire 1999; Roh et al. 2001; Wojcikowski et al. 2006; Yoshii et al. 2000) and hence are susceptible to inhibition of metabolism. Thus, tricyclics, fluoxetine, beta-blockers, and cimetidine can increase serum concentrations of some first-generation antipsychotics. Some first-generation antipsychotics (including perphenazine, thioridazine, chlorpromazine, haloperidol, and fluphenazine) are themselves CYP2D6 inhibitors (Daniel et al. 2005; Kudo et al. 1999; Otani et al. 2000; Shin et al. 1999) and may thus increase serum levels of tricyclic antidepressants (Ghaemi and Kirkwood 1998; Mulsant et al. 1997) and risperidone (Nakagami et al. 2005). Several first-generation antipsychotics (including chlorpromazine, haloperidol, perphenazine, and thioridazine) are CYP3A4 substrates (Cashman et al. 1993; Fang et al. 2001; Kalgutkar et al. 2003; Kudo and Ishizaki 1999; Olesen and Linnet 2000; Pan and Belpaire 1999; Wojcikowski et al. 2006) and hence are susceptible to inhibition of metabolism by nefazodone (Barbhaiya et al. 1996) or induction of metabolism by carbamazepine (Iwahashi et al. 1995; Jann et al. 1985, 1989).

Oxcarbazepine compared with carbamazepine appears to have less of an effect on serum levels of haloperidol and chlorpromazine (Raitasuo et al. 1994). Tobacco smoking induces the metabolism of the first-generation antipsychotics chlorpromazine and haloperidol, as well as the second-generation antipsychotics clozapine and olanzapine (Zevin and Benowitz 1999).

Case reports have raised concerns regarding development of an encephalopathic syndrome (weakness, lethargy, fever, tremulousness, confusion, extrapyramidal symptoms, leukocytosis, elevated serum enzymes, blood urea nitrogen, and fasting blood sugar) followed by irreversible brain damage when first-generation antipsychotics (most notably haloperidol) are combined with lithium (Addonizio 1985; Cohen and Cohen 1974; Jeffries et al. 1984; Keitner and Rahman 1984; Mann et al. 1983; Miller et al. 1986; Murphy et al. 1989; Nemes et al. 1986; Prakash et al. 1982; Smith and Helms 1982; Spring and Frankel 1981; Yassa 1986). However, systematic assessments (Baastrup et al. 1976; Goldney and Spence 1986; Juhl et al. 1977; Krishna et al. 1978) and clinical trials (Biederman et al. 1979; Sachs et al. 2002; Wilson 1993) suggest that combining lithium with first-generation antipsychotics generally yields no more than merely additive adverse effects. Sporadic cases in which problems occur during such combination therapy may be due to pharmacodynamic interactions (Goldman 1996).

In view of several controlled trials confirming the efficacy of haloperidol in acute mania (McIntyre et al. 2005; Sachs et al. 2002; Tohen et al. 2003a; Vieta et al. 2005), potential drug interactions with this agent are considered in additional detail. Haloperidol is commonly administered with lithium and valproate with adequate tolerability (Sachs et al. 2002). However, case reports have raised concerns that occasional patients treated with haloperidol combined with lithium may experience serious adverse effects, possibly because of a pharmacodynamic interaction (Addonizio 1985; Cohen and Cohen 1974; Keitner and Rahman 1984; Mann et al. 1983; Miller et al. 1986; Nemes et al. 1986; Prakash et al. 1982; Spring and Frankel 1981). Haloperidol and valproate do not appear to have clinically significant pharmacokinetic interactions (Hesslinger et al. 1999; Ishizaki et al. 1984). In contrast, carbamazepine increases metabolism of haloperidol (Arana et al. 1986; Hesslinger et al. 1999; Iwahashi et al. 1995; Jann et al. 1985; Kahn et al. 1990; Kidron et al. 1985; Raitasuo et al. 1994; Yasui-Furukori et al. 2003), and haloperidol may increase carbamazepine levels (Iwahashi et al. 1995).

Fluoxetine may modestly increase serum concentrations for oral haloperidol (Avenoso et al. 1997; Goff et al. 1991, 1995) but also may more than double serum concentrations with haloperidol decanoate (Viala et al. 1996). Fluvoxamine may modestly (23%; Vandel et al. 1995) increase serum haloperidol concentrations. Venlafaxine may substantially increase (70%) serum haloperidol concentrations (*Physicians' Desk Reference* 2008). Nefazodone may modestly (36%) increase serum haloperidol concentrations (Barbhaiya et al. 1996).

Haloperidol is commonly administered along with benzodiazepines in patients with bipolar disorders, with merely additive central nervous system (e.g., sedation, ataxia) adverse effects. Indeed, contemporary controlled haloperidol acute mania trials routinely permit some adjunctive benzodiazepine (e.g., lorazepam) administration (McIntyre et al. 2005; Sachs et al. 2002; Tohen et al. 2003a; Vieta et al. 2005), and fast-acting injectable intramuscular haloperidol combined with lorazepam is commonly used to manage acute agitation (Battaglia et al. 1997). Alprazolam may modestly (23%) increase serum haloperidol concentrations (Douyon et al. 1989).

Adverse Effects

The role of first-generation antipsychotics in the management of bipolar disorders is limited, because of concerns over acute extrapyramidal symptoms (Nasrallah et al. 1988), tardive dyskinesia (Kane and Smith 1982), and induction of dysphoria (Ahlfors et al. 1981) (Table 13–10). Thus, attempts are often made to taper and discontinue these drugs after resolution of acute episodes. Nevertheless, a substantial number of patients with bipolar disorders may be maintained on antipsychotics on a chronic basis (Sernyak et al. 1997), during which these neurological adverse effects, as well as sedation and weight gain, are major concerns. High-potency agents such as haloperidol may offer less sedation but more extrapyramidal symptoms, whereas molindone may cause less weight gain (Allison et al. 1999). Concerns have been raised around QTc prolongation with agents such as thioridazine, mesoridazine, and haloperidol.

The U.S. prescribing information for haloperidol and other first-generation antipsychotics was revised to include a boxed warning that these agents (like second-generation antipsychotics) may increase mortality in older adults with dementia-related psychosis. Other warnings in the haloperidol prescribing information include the risks of cardiovascular effects (sudden death, QTc prolongation, and torsades de pointes), tardive dyskinesia, neuroleptic malignant syndrome, teratogenicity, bronchopneumonia, and (as described above) an encephalopathic syndrome followed by irreversible brain damage when haloperidol (most notably, but also with other neuroleptics) is combined with lithium. In a recent epidemiological study, current use of first- and second-generation antipsychotics was associated with dose-related increases in rates of sudden cardiac death (1.99 and 2.26, respectively) (Ray et al. 2009).

TABLE 13–10. Common and serious adverse effects of antipsychotics

First-generation	Second-generation
Depression	Weight gain
Akathisia	Sedation
Acute dystonia	Hyperglycemia, diabetes[b]
Tardive dyskinesia[a]	*Suicidality in age ≤ 24 years[c]*
Weight gain	Akathisia
Sedation	Hyperprolactinemia
Anticholinergic	Cerebrovascular in older adults[d]
Cardiac, orthostasis	Cardiac, orthostasis
Hyperprolactinemia	Tardive dyskinesia[a]
Neuroleptic malignant syndrome[a]	Neuroleptic malignant syndrome[a]
Cardiac/pneumonia in older adults[a]	*Cardiac/pneumonia in older adults[a]*

Note. Bold italics indicate adverse effects that have a boxed warning in the U.S. prescribing information.
[a]Antipsychotic class warning.
[b]Second-generation antipsychotic class warning.
[c]Aripiprazole, quetiapine, olanzapine+fluoxetine combination (antidepressant class warning).
[d]Risperidone, olanzapine, aripiprazole.

Second-Generation Antipsychotics

Second-generation antipsychotics vary with respect to both therapeutic and adverse effects. (Adverse effects are presented in Table 13–11.) These medications may be broadly subdivided into two subgroups based on adverse effect profiles: 1) agents with more sedation and weight gain, but less akathisia (clozapine, olanzapine, quetiapine, and risperidone), and 2) agents with less sedation and weight gain, but more akathisia (aripiprazole and ziprasidone). These agents are discussed individually in detail below.

Clozapine

Pharmacokinetics and drug interactions. Clozapine is well absorbed, with 70% bioavailability, 97% protein binding, a moderately large volume of distribution of 5 L/kg, a linear dosage–to–serum concentration relationship, a half-life of 12 hours, and clearance of 750 mL/min (Ackenheil 1989; Byerly and DeVane 1996; Fitton and Heel 1990; Jann et al. 1993). Clozapine is extensively metabolized, with only trace amounts excreted unchanged in the urine. N-demethylation and N-oxidation are the predominant metabolic routes, yielding active *N*-desmethylclozapine (norclozapine) and inactive *N*-oxide metabo-

TABLE 13–11. Differential adverse effects of second-generation antipsychotics

Medication	Sedation	Weight, metabolic	Akathisia	EPS	Prolactin	Orthostasis	Anticholinergic
Higher metabolic risk							
Clozapine	+++	+++	±	±	±	+++	+++
Olanzapine	+++	+++	+	+	+	+	++
Intermediate metabolic risk							
Risperidone	++	++	+	++	+++	+	+
Quetiapine	+++	++	±	±	+	++	+
Lower metabolic risk							
Aripiprazole	+	+	++	+	±	±	±
Ziprasidone	±	±	++	+	+	±	±

Note. EPS=extrapyramidal symptoms. Risk: ±=minimal/none; +=low; ++=intermediate; +++=high.
Source. Adapted from American Diabetes Association et al. 2004; Lehman et al. 2004.

lites (Dain et al. 1997). Clozapine is a CYP1A2 and to a lesser extent a CYP3A4 substrate (Eiermann et al. 1997; Tugnait et al. 1999). Clozapine does not appear to induce or inhibit most CYP450 isozymes, and thus is more of a target of than an instigator of drug interactions (Shin et al. 1999).

Case reports suggest that sporadic individuals may develop serious adverse effects, such as neuroleptic malignant syndrome, when clozapine is combined with lithium (Pope et al. 1986). However, clinical data suggest that this combination does not generally yield more than merely additive adverse effects (Bender et al. 2004; Kelly et al. 2006; Small et al. 2003). Valproate does not appear to generally yield clinically significant changes in serum clozapine concentrations (Centorrino et al. 1994; Facciola et al. 1999), although limited data suggest that valproate may decrease clozapine levels in some patients (Costello and Suppes 1995; Finley and Warner 1994; Longo and Salzman 1995). Clozapine metabolism is increased with carbamazepine (Jerling et al. 1994b; Raitasuo et al. 1993; Tiihonen et al. 1995), and coadministration of clozapine with carbamazepine is not recommended in view of possible (but not proven) synergistic bone marrow suppression (Junghan et al. 1993). Clozapine does not appear to generally have clinically significant pharmacokinetic interactions with lamotrigine (Reimers et al. 2005; Spina et al. 2006; Tiihonen et al. 2003), although a single case of increased serum clozapine with lamotrigine has been reported (Kossen et al. 2001).

Studies suggest that risperidone does not generally alter serum clozapine concentrations (Henderson and Goff 1996; Honer et al. 2006; Raaska et al. 2002). However, case studies have been reported of risperidone-related increases in serum clozapine concentrations (Koreen et al. 1995; Tyson et al. 1995); a neurotoxic syndrome, characterized as mild neuroleptic malignant syndrome, after clozapine was added to risperidone (Kontaxakis et al. 2002); and clozapine-related increases in serum risperidone concentrations (*Physicians' Desk Reference* 2008).

Clinically significant increases in serum clozapine concentrations occur with the CYP1A2 inhibitor fluvoxamine (Alfaro et al. 2001; DuMortier et al. 1996; Fabrazzo et al. 2000; Hiemke et al. 1994; Jerling et al. 1994b; Koponen et al. 1996; Lammers et al. 1999; Lu et al. 2000; Szegedi et al. 1995, 1999; Wang et al. 2004; Wetzel et al. 1998) and with fluoxetine (Centorrino et al. 1994, 1996; Spina et al. 1998). Although paroxetine may also yield increases in serum clozapine concentrations (Joos et al. 1997), the clinical significance of this interaction remains to be established (Centorrino et al. 1996; Spina et al. 2000b; Wetzel et al. 1998). Pharmacokinetic studies suggest that sertraline does not generally yield clinically significant increases in serum clozapine concentrations (Centorrino et al. 1996; Spina et al. 2000b), but case reports suggest that this could occur in some individuals (Chong et al. 1997; Pinninti and de Leon 1997). Citalopram does not appear to generally yield clinically significant increases in serum clozapine concentrations (Taylor et al. 1998), but a case report suggests that this could occur in some individuals (Borba and Henderson 2000). Nefazodone may increase serum concentrations of clozapine (Khan and Preskorn 2001), but the clinical significance of this interaction has been questioned (Taylor et al. 1999). Clozapine may modestly inhibit CYP2C9 and CYP2D6, and thus might increase serum nortriptyline concentrations (Smith and Riskin 1994).

Caution needs to be exercised when combining clozapine with benzodiazepines because some patients may develop respiratory depression or even arrest (Klimke and Klieser 1994).

Oxcarbazepine compared with carbamazepine appears to have less of an effect on serum levels of clozapine (Raitasuo et al. 1994).

The CYP1A2 inducer omeprazole (Nousbaum et al. 1994) may modestly decrease serum clozapine concentrations in nonsmokers (Mookhoek and Loonen 2004), but this interaction might be clinically significant in some patients (Frick et al. 2003). The CYP3A4 inhibitors ketoconazole (Lane et al. 2001) and erythromycin (Hagg et al. 1999) do not appear to generally yield clinically significant increases in serum clozapine concentrations, but case reports suggest that some individuals may experience toxicity with the clozapine plus erythromycin combination (Cohen et al. 1996; Funderburg et al. 1994). A single case report suggested that hormonal contraceptives could increase serum clozapine concentrations (Gabbay et al. 2002).

Tobacco smoking induces CYP1A2 (Zevin and Benowitz 1999), apparently decreasing serum concentrations of clozapine in several (Haring et al. 1990; McCarthy 1994; Meyer 2001; Seppala et al. 1999) but not all (Hasegawa et al. 1993) studies. In contrast, caffeine in excess of 400 mg/day modestly increases serum clozapine concentrations, presumably by inhibition of CYP1A2 (Carrillo et al. 1998; Hagg et al. 2000; Raaska et al. 2004; Vainer and Chouinard 1994), but this increase could be clinically significant in some patients (Vainer and Chouinard 1994).

Adverse effects.　　Clozapine generally has a challenging adverse effect profile compared with other treatment options (Baldessarini and Frankenburg 1991; Marinkovic et al. 1994; Miller 2000; Young et al. 1998). Hence, this agent tends to be held in reserve for patients with treatment-resistant bipolar disorders

(Suppes et al. 1999). The most common adverse effects associated with clozapine discontinuation include central nervous system (sedation, seizures, dizziness), cardiovascular (tachycardia, hypotension, syncope, electrocardiogram changes), gastrointestinal (nausea, vomiting), and hematological (leukopenia, granulocytopenia, agranulocytosis) problems, as well as fever (Iqbal et al. 2003).

The U.S. prescribing information for clozapine includes boxed warnings regarding the risks of 1) agranulocytosis; 2) seizures; 3) myocarditis; 4) other adverse cardiovascular and respiratory effects; and 5) increased mortality (primarily cardiovascular or infectious) in older adults with dementia-related psychosis (an antipsychotic class warning). A serious adverse effect with major clinical implications is agranulocytosis, seen in 1.3% of patients, which requires ongoing hematological monitoring (Grohmann et al. 1989). Seizures occur in 2% of patients taking less than 300 mg/day, 4% taking 300–600 mg/day, and 5% taking 600–900 mg/day. Thus, combining clozapine with an anticonvulsant mood stabilizer could be desirable. Because of pharmacokinetic interactions (Jerling et al. 1994b; Raitasuo et al. 1993; Tiihonen et al. 1995) and concerns regarding potential synergy of marrow toxicity (Junghan et al. 1993) with carbamazepine, combining clozapine with other anticonvulsants such as valproate or lamotrigine is preferred. Myocarditis may occur at a rate of 0.3/100,000 patient-years. Other adverse cardiovascular and respiratory effects include orthostatic hypotension, syncope, respiratory/cardiac arrest (in 1/3,000 patients), tachycardia, and electrocardiogram repolarization changes.

Increasing concerns have been raised regarding the risks of hyperglycemia and diabetes mellitus with clozapine and other second-generation antipsychotics. Indeed, the FDA stipulated changes in the prescribing information not only for clozapine but also for olanzapine, risperidone, quetiapine, ziprasidone, and aripiprazole, to include a warning of these risks, suggesting a second-generation antipsychotic class effect for such problems (*Physicians' Desk Reference* 2008). Clozapine, olanzapine, risperidone, and quetiapine can also cause weight gain and cholesterol and triglyceride elevations. The report of a consensus development conference on antipsychotics and obesity, diabetes, and hyperlipidemia emphasized differences between second-generation antipsychotics, with clozapine and olanzapine being the most implicated, risperidone and quetiapine being less implicated, and ziprasidone and aripiprazole being the least implicated (American Diabetes Association et al. 2004).

Thus, clinical and (as indicated) laboratory monitoring for obesity, diabetes, and hyperlipidemia are recommended for patients taking clozapine and other second-generation antipsychotics (Tables 13–1 and 13–12). Because such

TABLE 13–12. Monitoring protocol for patients taking second-generation antipsychotics[a]

Assessment	Abnormal	Baseline	4 weeks	8 weeks	12 weeks	Quarterly	Yearly	Every 5 years
Personal/family history	Positive	X					X	
Body mass index	>25 kg/m^2	X	X	X	X	X		
Waist circumference	>40 in. male; >35 in. female	X					X	
Blood pressure	>130/85 mm Hg	X			X		X	
Fasting plasma glucose	>110 mg/dL	X			X		X	
Fasting lipid profile	HDL<40 mg/dL TC>200 mg/dL TG>175 mg/dL	X			X			X

Note. HDL=high-density lipoprotein cholesterol; TC=total cholesterol; TG=triglycerides.
[a]More frequent assessments may be warranted by clinical status.
Source. Adapted from American Diabetes Association et al. 2004.

monitoring is complex and interacts with lifestyle measures to control weight and minimize metabolic problems, a collaborative approach involving both caregivers and patients is crucial. Table 13–13 lists Internet resources intended to help caregivers and patients facilitate such efforts.

Other warnings in the prescribing information include the risks of eosinophilia, neuroleptic malignant syndrome, and tardive dyskinesia. Clozapine appears to be the least likely antipsychotic to yield extrapyramidal adverse effects.

Other adverse effects from taking clozapine include cardiomyopathy (8.9/100,000 patient-years), fever, pulmonary embolism (fatal in 1/3,450 patient-years), increased transaminases, hepatitis, anticholinergic symptoms (constipation, urinary retention), hypersalivation, and headache. To date, clozapine has not been associated with congenital malformations in humans (FDA pregnancy category B).

Administration. Clozapine is commonly initiated at 25 mg/day and increased by 25–50 mg/day every 3–7 days, with 900 mg/day the maximum final dosage in schizophrenia (Table 13–6). In patients with bipolar disorders, final dosages of clozapine often range between 50 and 250 mg/day, given all or mostly at bedtime, and commonly in combination with other medications. Thus, in a controlled trial, mean dosages of adjunctive clozapine were 234 mg/day in patients with bipolar disorders and 623 mg/day in patients with schizoaffective disorder (Suppes et al. 1999).

Some data suggest that serum clozapine concentrations exceeding approximately 1.2 μmol/L (400 ng/mL) are associated with better therapeutic effects in patients with treatment-resistant schizophrenia (Hasegawa et al. 1993; Kronig

TABLE 13–13. **National Institute of Diabetes and Digestive and Kidney Diseases (NIDDK) Internet resources**

Content	Internet address
NIDDK home page	http://www2.niddk.nih.gov
Weight-control Information Network	http://win.niddk.nih.gov
Weight and waist measurement tools for adults	http://win.niddk.nih.gov/publications/ PDFs/Weightandwaist.pdf
Body mass index table	http://diabetes.niddk.nih.gov/dm/pubs/ diagnosis/bmi_tbl.pdf
National Diabetes Education Program	http://ndep.nih.gov

Note. Metabolic monitoring interacts with lifestyle measures to control weight and minimize metabolic problems. Sites accessed April 6 , 2009.

et al. 1995; Miller et al. 1994; Perry et al. 1991; Piscitelli et al. 1994; Potkin et al. 1994), whereas other data suggest that higher mean dosages (444 mg/day) used in the United States and lower mean dosages (284 mg/day) used in Europe yielded similar therapeutic effects (Fleischhacker et al. 1994). Serum clozapine concentrations exceeding 3.0 μmol/L (1,000 ng/mL) are associated with increased adverse effects (Freeman and Oyewumi 1997).

Risperidone

Pharmacokinetics and drug interactions.   Risperidone is well absorbed, with 70% bioavailability, 90% protein binding, a moderate volume of distribution of 1 L/kg, a linear dosage–to–serum concentration relationship, a clearance of 400 mL/min, and a half-life of 6 hours in extensive CYP2D6 metabolizers and 24 hours in poor CYP2D6 metabolizers (He and Richardson 1995; Mannens et al. 1993). Risperidone is substantially metabolized, with less than 30% excreted unchanged in the urine, whereas its main active 9-hydroxyrisperidone (paliperidone) metabolite is removed primarily by renal excretion. Risperidone is metabolized by CYP2D6 to (+)-9-hydroxyrisperidone, and to a lesser extent by CYP3A4 to (−)-9-hydroxyrisperidone (Fang et al. 1999; Yasui-Furukori et al. 2001). The 9-hydroxyrisperidone metabolite has activity similar to risperidone (Leysen et al. 1994), and risperidone plus 9-hydroxyrisperidone is referred to collectively as the active moiety, which has a half-life of 20 hours, and protein binding of 90% for risperidone and 70% for 9-hydroxyrisperidone. Based on pharmacokinetics related to the prominent renal excretion of the active moiety, risperidone dosage reduction and cautious dosage titration may be necessary in older adults and in patients with renal disease (Snoeck et al. 1995). Risperidone does not appear to induce or inhibit most CYP450 isozymes, and thus is more of a target of than an instigator of drug interactions (Shin et al. 1999).

Risperidone does not appear to generally yield clinically significant alterations in lithium pharmacokinetics (*Physicians' Desk Reference* 2008). Case reports suggest that sporadic individuals could develop serious adverse effects such as neuroleptic malignant syndrome when lithium is combined with risperidone (Bourgeois and Kahn 2003). However, controlled clinical trials suggest that this combination does not generally yield more than merely additive adverse effects (Sachs et al. 2002; Yatham et al. 2003). Carbamazepine yields clinically significant induction of risperidone metabolism (Ono et al. 2002; Spina et al. 2000a, 2001b; Takahashi et al. 2001; Yatham et al. 2003). Risperidone does not appear to have clinically significant pharmacokinetic interactions with valproate (Ravindran et al. 2004; Spina et al. 2000a) or with lamotrigine (Castberg and Spigset 2006; Reimers et al. 2005; Spina et al. 2006). However, a single case of increased risperidone with lamotrigine has been reported (Bienentreu and Kronmüller 2005).

Risperidone does not generally alter serum quetiapine (Potkin et al. 2002a) or clozapine concentrations (Henderson and Goff 1996; Honer et al. 2006; Raaska et al. 2002), but case studies suggest that some individuals may experience risperidone-related increases in serum clozapine concentrations (Koreen et al. 1995; Tyson et al. 1995); one patient developed a neurotoxic syndrome, characterized as mild neuroleptic malignant syndrome, after clozapine was added to risperidone (Kontaxakis et al. 2002). Some individuals may develop clozapine-related increases in serum risperidone concentrations (*Physicians' Desk Reference* 2008). The CYP2D6 inhibitor thioridazine increases risperidone serum concentrations (Nakagami et al. 2005).

CYP2D6 inhibitors such as paroxetine (Saito et al. 2005; Spina et al. 2001a) may decrease risperidone metabolism. Fluoxetine can yield clinically significant increases in serum risperidone concentrations (Bondolfi et al. 2002; Bork et al. 1999; Spina et al. 2002). Fluvoxamine can yield modest increases in serum risperidone concentrations (D'Arrigo et al. 2005), but whether or not such an interaction explains a case report of neurotoxicity with adding fluvoxamine to risperidone remains to be determined (Reeves et al. 2002). Sertraline does not appear to generally yield clinically significant increases in serum risperidone concentrations, although occasional patients may experience substantive increases (Spina et al. 2004). Although nefazodone does not appear to yield clinically significant increases in serum risperidone concentrations in general (Taylor et al. 1999), occasional patients may experience substantive increases (Khan and Preskorn 2001).

Risperidone is commonly administered along with benzodiazepines in patients with bipolar disorders, with merely additive central nervous system adverse effects (e.g., sedation, ataxia). Indeed, contemporary controlled risperidone trials routinely permit some adjunctive benzodiazepine (e.g., lorazepam) administration (Hirschfeld et al. 2004; Khanna et al. 2005; Sachs et al. 2002).

Oxcarbazepine does not yield clinically significant alterations in serum risperidone concentrations (Rosaria Muscatello et al. 2005). Topiramate does not yield clinically significant alterations in serum risperidone or 9-hydroxyrisperidone concentrations (Bialer et al. 2004; Migliardi et al. 2007).

Rifampin induces risperidone metabolism (Mahatthanatrakul et al. 2007). However, thioridazine (Nakagami et al. 2005) and ketoconazole (Fang et al. 1999) inhibit risperidone metabolism.

Adverse effects. The most common adverse events associated with risperidone discontinuation in acute mania trials were somnolence, dizziness, and extrapyramidal disorders. Dosage-related extrapyramidal symptoms are particularly evident above 6 mg/day.

The U.S. prescribing information for risperidone includes a boxed warning regarding the increased risk of mortality (primarily cardiovascular or infectious) in older adults with dementia-related psychosis (an antipsychotic class warning). The FDA has stipulated changes in the risperidone prescribing information to include a warning of the risks of hyperglycemia and diabetes mellitus (*Physicians' Desk Reference* 2008). Risperidone can also yield weight gain and elevations in cholesterol and triglycerides. The report of a consensus development conference suggests that the risks of obesity, diabetes, and hyperlipidemia with this agent are intermediate—less than with clozapine and olanzapine but more than with ziprasidone and aripiprazole (American Diabetes Association et al. 2004). Thus, clinical and (as indicated) laboratory monitoring for obesity, diabetes, and hyperlipidemia are recommended for patients taking risperidone (Tables 13–1 and 13–12). Other warnings in the prescribing information include the risks of cerebrovascular adverse events, including stroke in older adults with dementia-related psychosis (a warning shared with olanzapine and aripiprazole); neuroleptic malignant syndrome; and tardive dyskinesia.

Other adverse effects include orthostatic hypotension, tachycardia, QT prolongation, seizures (in 0.3% of patients), hyperprolactinemia, amenorrhea, galactorrhea, decreased libido and sexual function, rhinitis, constipation, and dysphagia (Conley 2000; Yen et al. 2004). Concerns have been raised regarding an increased risk of pituitary tumor with risperidone (54/77 reports with risperidone vs. 11/77 with olanzapine, 9/77 with haloperidol, 6/77 with ziprasidone, 4/77 with clozapine, 1/77 with quetiapine, and 0/77 with aripiprazole) detected in the FDA spontaneous report adverse effect database (Szarfman et al. 2006). Mania induction or exacerbation has been reported in occasional patients with risperidone, but this phenomenon occurred no more often than with placebo in controlled adjunctive trials in acute mania (Sachs et al. 2002; Yatham et al. 2003). To date, risperidone has not been associated with congenital malformations in humans (FDA pregnancy category C).

Administration. Risperidone in acute mania is commonly initiated at 2–3 mg/day and increased by 1 mg/day on a daily basis, as necessary and tolerated, with final dosages ranging between 1 and 6 mg/day, and averaging approximately 4–6 mg/day in controlled trials (Hirschfeld et al. 2004; Khanna et al.

2003; Sachs et al. 2002; Yatham et al. 2003) (Table 13–6). To limit adverse effects, risperidone in acute bipolar depression may be started at 0.25–0.5 mg/day and increased, as necessary and tolerated, every 4–7 days by 0.25–0.5 mg/day, with an initial target dosage of 1–2 mg/day. In patients with bipolar disorders, risperidone is often administered all or mostly at bedtime, and commonly in combination with other medications. Long-acting injectable risperidone in schizophrenia patients is initiated at 25 mg intramuscularly every 2 weeks, overlapping with oral risperidone or another oral antipsychotic, and increased monthly as necessary and tolerated to as high as 50 mg intramuscularly every 2 weeks. In a controlled trial in patients with a type of rapid-cycling called frequently relapsing bipolar disorder (i.e., four or more mood episodes requiring treatment in the prior year), the mean dosage of risperidone long-acting injectable added to treatment as usual was 29.7 mg every 2 weeks (MacFadden et al. 2008).

Olanzapine

Pharmacokinetics and drug interactions.   Olanzapine is well absorbed, with 80%–100% bioavailability, 93% protein binding, a large volume of distribution of 15 L/kg, a half-life of 30 hours, linear pharmacokinetics at dosages up to 20 mg, and clearance of 400 mL/min (Callaghan et al. 1999). Olanzapine is extensively (more than 80%) metabolized, primarily via glucuronidation by UGT1A4 to inactive 10-*N*-glucuronide olanzapine (Linnet 2002), as well as oxidation by CYP1A2 to inactive *N*-desmethyl olanzapine (Callaghan et al. 1999; Kassahun et al. 1997; Ring et al. 1996b). Olanzapine does not induce or inhibit CYP450 isozymes (Ring et al. 1996a), and is thus more a target of than an instigator of drug interactions.

Olanzapine does not generally have clinically significant pharmacokinetic interactions with lithium (Demmole et al. 1995). Case reports suggest that sporadic individuals could develop serious adverse effects, such as neuroleptic malignant syndrome, when lithium is combined with olanzapine (Berry et al. 2003). However, controlled clinical data suggest that this combination does not generally yield more than merely additive adverse effects (Tohen et al. 2002b). In four patients, valproate appeared to lower serum olanzapine concentrations (Bergemann et al. 2006), but the clinical significance of this possible interaction remains to be established. Carbamazepine increases metabolism of olanzapine (Licht et al. 2000; Linnet and Olesen 2002; Lucas et al. 1998; Olesen and Linnet 1999). Indeed, in a combination therapy study, carbamazepine yielded lower than expected blood olanzapine concentrations, and even though this was addressed in part by more aggressive olanzapine dosage, the efficacy of the olanzapine plus carbamazepine combination was still not significantly better than that of carbamazepine monotherapy in the treatment of acute mania (Tohen et al. 2008). Olanzapine does not appear to have clinically significant pharmacokinetic interactions with lamotrigine (Jann et al. 2006; Reimers et al. 2005; Sidhu et al. 2006a; Spina et al. 2006).

The CYP1A2 inhibitor fluvoxamine yields clinically significant increases in serum olanzapine concentrations (Albers et al. 2005; Chiu et al. 2004; de Jong et al. 2001; Hiemke et al. 2002; Mäenpää et al. 1997; Perlis et al. 2004; Wang et al. 2004; Weigmann et al. 2001).

Oxcarbazepine (Rosaria Muscatello et al. 2005) and topiramate (Migliardi et al. 2007; Tiihonen et al. 2005) do not generally yield clinically significant alterations in serum olanzapine concentrations.

Olanzapine is commonly administered along with benzodiazepines in patients with bipolar disorders, with merely additive central nervous system adverse effects (e.g., sedation, ataxia). Indeed, contemporary controlled olanzapine trials routinely permit some adjunctive benzodiazepine (e.g., lorazepam) administration (Tohen et al. 1999, 2000, 2002a, 2002b, 2003a, 2003c, 2005, 2006). Intramuscular lorazepam 1 hour after intramuscular olanzapine did not yield clinically significant pharmacokinetic interactions but was associated with additive sedation (*Physicians' Desk Reference* 2008).

CYP1A2 inducers such as omeprazole (Nousbaum et al. 1994) might decrease serum olanzapine concentrations, but whether or not such putative interactions are clinically significant needs to be definitively assessed for individual inducers. Ciprofloxacin may increase serum olanzapine concentrations (Markowitz and DeVane 1999). Tobacco smoking decreases serum olanzapine concentrations (Bergemann et al. 2004; Carrillo et al. 2003; Skogh et al. 2002), presumably by induction of CYP1A2. Indeed, tobacco smoking was associated with poorer olanzapine response in a post hoc analysis of three olanzapine acute mania studies (Berk et al. 2008). Women compared with men may have slightly (approximately 25%) decreased olanzapine clearance (Callaghan et al. 1999; Kelly et al. 1999), which in some individuals, especially if combined with other factors such as tobacco smoking, could have clinical significance.

Adverse effects. The most common adverse effects with oral olanzapine are somnolence, dry mouth, dizziness, asthenia, constipation, dyspepsia, increased appetite, and tremor. Weight gain appears to be more of a problem with olanzapine than with lithium (Tohen et al. 2003b) or valproate (Tohen et al. 2005). In a 12-month maintenance trial, the incidence of weight gain was 30% with olanzapine and 10% with lithium (Tohen et al. 2005), and in a 47-week maintenance trial, the incidence was 24% with olanzapine and 18% with valproate (Tohen et al. 2003b). Olanzapine-related weight gain can be approached in a fashion similar to that described above for lithium. Somnolence is the most common adverse effect with intramuscular olanzapine. Maximal dosing of intramuscular olanzapine may yield substantial orthostatic hypotension, so that administration of additional dosages to patients with clinically significant postural changes in systolic blood pressure is not recommended.

The U.S. prescribing information for olanzapine includes a boxed warning regarding the increased risk of mortality (primarily cardiovascular or infectious) in older adults with dementia-related psychosis (an antipsychotic class warning). The FDA has stipulated changes in the olanzapine prescribing information to include a warning of the risk of hyperglycemia and diabetes mellitus (*Physicians' Desk Reference* 2008). Olanzapine can also yield weight gain and cholesterol and triglyceride elevations. The report of a consensus development conference suggested that the risks of obesity, diabetes, and hyperlipidemia with this agent (and clozapine) are greater than with other second-generation antipsychotics (American Diabetes Association et al. 2004). Thus, clinical and (as indicated) laboratory monitoring for obesity, diabetes, and hyperlipidemia are recommended for patients taking olanzapine (Tables 13–1 and 13–12, and Figure 13–1). Other warnings in the prescribing information include the risks of cerebrovascular adverse events, including stroke, in older adults with dementia-related psychosis (a warning shared with risperidone and aripiprazole); neuroleptic malignant syndrome; and tardive dyskinesia.

Other adverse effects include orthostatic hypotension, syncope (in 0.6% of patients), seizures (in 0.9% of patients), hyperprolactinemia, and benign transaminase elevations (in 0.2% of patients) (Conley and Meltzer 2000). Mania induction or exacerbation has been occasionally reported with olanzapine, but has occurred no more often than with placebo in controlled trials. To date, olanzapine has not been associated with congenital malformations in humans (FDA pregnancy category C).

Administration.   In acute mania monotherapy, olanzapine is commonly initiated at 10–15 mg/day and increased by 5 mg daily, as necessary and tolerated, with final dosages ranging between 5 and 20 mg/day, and averaging 15–16 mg/day in controlled trials (Tohen et al. 1999, 2000) (Table 13–6). In acute mania adjunctive therapy, olanzapine is commonly initiated at 10–15 mg/day and increased by 5 mg daily, as necessary and tolerated, with final dosages ranging between 5 and 20 mg/day, and averaging 10.4 mg/day in a controlled trial (Tohen et al. 2002b). In acute bipolar I depression, olanzapine was dosed more conservatively, with a mean final dosage of 7.4 mg/day (combined with a mean final dosage of fluoxetine 39.3 mg/day) (Tohen et al. 2003c). In monotherapy maintenance treatment for bipolar I disorder, the mean final olanzapine dosage was 12.5 mg/day (Tohen et al. 2006). In patients with bipolar disorders, olanzapine is often administered all or mostly at bedtime, and commonly in combination with other medications. Mean steady-state serum olanzapine concentrations at end point in a 6-week schizophrenia trial at dosages of 5 and 15 mg/day were 10 and 31 µg/L, respectively, and were not related to clinical responses (Callaghan et al. 1999). In acute agitation, intramuscular olanzapine is started at 10 mg, with repeat doses of 10 mg as necessary and tolerated after 2 hours and 6 hours, with a maximum dosage of 30 mg in a 24-hour period. Lower dosages are recommended in older adults (5 mg intramuscularly once) or debilitated patients (2.5 mg intramuscularly once).

Quetiapine

Pharmacokinetics and drug interactions.   Quetiapine is well absorbed and 100% bioavailable, with 83% protein binding, a large volume of distribution of 10 L/kg, linear pharmacokinetics at dosages between 200 and 750 mg/day, clearance of 1,600 mL/min, and a short half-life of 6 hours (DeVane and Nemeroff 2001). Quetiapine is extensively metabolized, primarily by CYP3A4 to inactive quetiapine sulfoxide (Hasselstrom and Linnet 2006), with less than 1% excreted unchanged in the urine (DeVane and Nemeroff 2001). Quetiapine does not have clinically significant effects on CYP isozymes (DeVane and Nemeroff 2001), and is thus a target of rather than an instigator of drug interactions.

Quetiapine does not generally have clinically significant pharmacokinetic interactions with lithium (Potkin et al. 2002b). Controlled clinical trials suggest that combining quetiapine with lithium (or valproate) does not generally yield more than merely additive adverse effects (Potkin et al. 2002b; Sachs et al. 2004; Suppes et al. 2009; Vieta et al. 2008b; Yatham et al. 2004). Indeed, quetiapine combined with lithium (or valproate) is approved for the treatment of acute mania (Potkin et al. 2002b; Sachs et al. 2004; Yatham et al. 2004) and for bipolar maintenance treatment (Suppes et al. 2009; Vieta et al. 2008b). Valproate may (Aichhorn et al. 2006) or may not (*Physicians' Desk Reference* 2008) yield clinically significant increases in quetiapine serum concentrations. Quetiapine metabolism is increased with carbamazepine (Grimm et al. 2006; Hasselstrom and Linnet 2004); in two patients, quetiapine appeared to increase carbamazepine-epoxide levels (Fitzgerald and Okos 2002).

Thioridazine (but not haloperidol or risperidone) can yield clinically significant decreases in serum quetiapine concentrations (Potkin et al. 2002a). Concerns have been raised regarding the ability of quetiapine combined with ziprasidone to yield additive QTc prolongation (Minov 2004), but systematic studies are lacking to assess the clinical significance of such a putative pharmacodynamic interaction.

Quetiapine is commonly administered along with benzodiazepines in patients with bipolar disorders, with merely additive central nervous system adverse effects (e.g., sedation, ataxia). Indeed, contemporary controlled quetiapine trials routinely permit some adjunctive benzodiazepine (e.g., lorazepam) administration (Bowden et al. 2005; Calabrese et al. 2005; McIntyre et al. 2005; Thase et al. 2006; Yatham et al. 2004). Quetiapine and lorazepam do not appear to have clinically significant pharmacokinetic interactions (DeVane and Nemeroff 2001; *Physicians' Desk Reference* 2008).

Quetiapine metabolism is increased with phenytoin (Wong et al. 2001). Topiramate does not generally yield clinically significant alterations in serum quetiapine concentrations (Migliardi et al. 2007). The CYP3A4 inhibitors ketoconazole (Grimm et al. 2006) and erythromycin (Li et al. 2005) yield clinically significant increases in serum quetiapine concentrations. Tobacco smoking does not yield clinically significant decreases in serum concentrations of quetiapine, as it does with clozapine and olanzapine (DeVane and Nemeroff 2001).

Adverse effects. The most common adverse events with quetiapine are somnolence, dizziness (postural hypotension), dry mouth, constipation, increased serum glutamate pyruvate transaminase, weight gain, and dyspepsia (Adler et al. 2007).

The U.S. prescribing information for quetiapine includes boxed warnings regarding the increased risks of 1) mortality (primarily cardiovascular or infectious) in older adults with dementia-related psychosis (an antipsychotic class warning) and 2) suicidality with use of antidepressant drugs in patients up to age 24 years (based on an antidepressant class warning). The FDA has stipulated changes in the quetiapine prescribing information to include a warning of the risks of hyperglycemia and diabetes mellitus (*Physicians' Desk Reference* 2008). Quetiapine can also yield weight gain and cholesterol and triglyceride elevations. The report of a consensus development conference suggests that the risks of obesity, diabetes, and hyperlipidemia with this agent are intermediate—less than with clozapine and olanzapine but more than with ziprasidone and aripiprazole (American Diabetes Association et al. 2004). Thus, clinical and (as indicated) laboratory monitoring for obesity, diabetes, and hyperlipidemia are recommended for patients taking quetiapine (Tables 13–1 and 13–12). Other warnings in the quetiapine prescribing information include the risks of neuroleptic malignant syndrome, tardive dyskinesia, orthostatic hypotension (syncope in 1% of patients), seizures (in 0.5% of patients), hypothyroidism (rare), benign transaminse elevations (in 6% of patients), hyperprolactinemia, increased blood pressure in children and adolescents, cognitive and motor impairment, priapism (one case), body temperature regulation problems, dysphagia, cardiac problems in patients with cardiac disease, withdrawal symptoms with abrupt discontinuation, and cataracts. Concern regarding the development of cataracts in dogs has led to a recommendation of ophthalmological examinations, but the risk in humans appears to be low (Nasrallah et al. 1999). To date, quetiapine has not been associated with congenital malformations in humans (FDA pregnancy category C).

Administration. In acute mania, quetiapine immediate-release formulation is commonly initiated at 100 mg/day in two divided doses and increased daily by 100 mg, as necessary and tolerated, with final dosages ranging between 400 and 800 mg/day, and averaging approximately 500–600 mg/day in responders in controlled trials (Bowden et al. 2005; McIntyre et al. 2005; Sachs et al. 2004; Yatham et al. 2004) (Table 13–6). In acute mania, quetiapine extended-release formulation (quetiapine XR) is started at 300 mg at bedtime, increased the next day to 600 mg at bedtime, and thereafter dosed between 400 mg and 800 mg at bedtime. In acute bipolar I or II depression, quetiapine and quetiapine XR are commonly initiated at 50 mg/day at bedtime and increased daily by 100 mg, as necessary and tolerated, with final dosages ranging between 300 and 600 mg/day in controlled trials (Calabrese et al. 2005; Thase et al. 2006). Mean steady-state 12-hour trough serum quetiapine concentrations at 150 and 750 mg/day were 29 and 164 μg/L, respectively, and were not related to therapeutic effects in a 3-week trial in schizophrenia patients (DeVane and Nemeroff 2001). The U.S. prescribing information for the longer-term adjunctive use of quetiapine and quetiapine XR notes that dosages of 400–800 mg/day in divided doses were used in the registration studies, and that in the maintenance phase, patients generally continued taking the same dosage that they were taking when stabilized in the stabilization phase. However, the information also states that patients should be treated with the lowest dosage needed to maintain remission. The information does not provide recommendations for initiating quetiapine in euthymic patients. Given the risk of adverse effects, the prudent approach is to start quetiapine in euthymic patients in a gradual fashion, similar to the initiation in depressed patients rather than the rapid initiation used in manic patients.

Ziprasidone

Pharmacokinetics and drug interactions. Concurrent ingestion of food doubles ziprasidone absorption (Hamelin et al. 1998), so that ziprasidone is 60% absorbed with food and 30% unfed. Ziprasidone is 99% bound to plasma proteins, with a volume of distribution of 1.5 L/kg, a half-life of 6.6 hours, and clearance of 525 mL/min (Wilner et al. 2000). Ziprasidone is extensively metabolized, with less than 5% excreted unchanged in the urine (Prakash et al. 2000). Ziprasidone is metabolized two-thirds by aldehyde oxidase reduction to inactive *S*-methyl-dihydroziprasidone, and one-third by CYP3A4 oxidation to inactive ziprasidone sulfoxide and other inactive metabolites (Beedham et al. 2003; Prakash et al. 1997, 2000). Ziprasidone does not have clinically significant effects on CYP isozymes (Prakash et al. 2000), and is thus a target of rather than an instigator of drug interactions.

Ziprasidone does not generally affect serum concentrations of lithium (Apseloff et al. 2000). Case reports suggest that sporadic individuals could develop serious adverse effects, such as neuroleptic malignant syndrome, when lithium is combined with ziprasidone (Borovicka et al. 2006). However, clinical data suggest that this combination does not generally yield more than merely additive adverse effects (Weisler et al. 2004b). Carbamazepine decreases serum ziprasidone concentrations, but the clinical significance of this interaction remains to be determined (Miceli et al. 2000a).

Limited data are available regarding interactions between ziprasidone and other antipsychotics and antidepressants. Case reports describe blood dyscrasia with ziprasidone and quetiapine (Nair and Lippmann 2005) and a possible serotonin syndrome with citalopram following cross-titration of clozapine to ziprasidone (Kinzie and Meltzer-Brody 2005).

Concerns have been raised regarding the ability of ziprasidone to yield QTc prolongation and the possibility of exaggeration of this problem if the drug is combined with other agents with this adverse effect, such as chlorpromazine, thioridazine, pimozide, paliperidone, and quetiapine (Minov 2004). Systematic studies are lacking to assess the clinical significance of such putative pharmacodynamic interactions.

Ziprasidone is commonly administered along with benzodiazepines in patients with bipolar disorders, with merely additive central nervous system adverse effects (e.g., sedation, ataxia). Indeed, contemporary controlled ziprasidone trials routinely permit some adjunctive benzodiazepine (e.g., lorazepam) administration (Keck et al. 2003b; Potkin et al. 2005).

Ketoconazole increases serum ziprasidone concentrations, but the clinical significance of this interaction remains to be determined (Miceli et al. 2000b). Ziprasidone does not affect serum concentrations of hormonal contraceptives (Muirhead et al. 2000).

Adverse effects.   The most common adverse events associated with discontinuation of ziprasidone in acute mania were akathisia, anxiety, depression, dizziness, dystonia, rash, and vomiting (Goodnick 2001). The most common adverse events with intramuscular ziprasidone for agitation in patients with schizophrenia were somnolence, nausea, dizziness, injection site pain, and headache (Daniel et al. 2001).

Ziprasidone and aripiprazole, compared with risperidone, olanzapine, and quetiapine, yield less sedation but more akathisia. In patients with acute mania, akathisia is commonly accompanied by and at times difficult to distinguish from agitation and anxiety. These overlapping symptoms may attenuate with adjunctive benzodiazepine therapy. Indeed, a meta-analysis suggested that benzodiazepines (e.g., clonazepam 0.5–2.5 mg/day in two randomized, controlled, 1- to 2-week trials, with a total of 27 patients) can reduce symptoms of akathisia in the short term (Lima et al. 2002). Data are more limited regarding the utility of other agents for antipsychotic-related akathisia. Meta-analyses suggested that insufficient data are available to recommend beta-blockers (Barnes et al. 2004) and that no reliable evidence exists to support or refute the utility of anticholinergics (Rathbone and Soares-Weiser 2004).

The U.S. prescribing information for ziprasidone includes a boxed warning regarding the increased risk of mortality (primarily cardiovascular or infectious) in older adults with dementia-related psychosis (an antipsychotic class warning). The FDA has stipulated that the ziprasidone prescribing information include a warning of the risks of hyperglycemia and diabetes mellitus (*Physicians' Desk Reference* 2008), but the report of a consensus development conference suggests that the risks of obesity, diabetes, and hyperlipidemia with this agent are similar to those with aripiprazole and are less than those with other second-generation antipsychotics (American Diabetes Association et al. 2004). Nevertheless, clinical and (as indicated) laboratory monitoring for obesity, diabetes, and hyperlipidemia are recommended for patients taking ziprasidone

(Tables 13–1 and 13–12). Other warnings in the prescribing information include the risks of neuroleptic malignant syndrome, tardive dyskinesia, QTc prolongation, and sudden death. As noted earlier, in a recent epidemiological study, current use of first- and second-generation antipsychotics was associated with dose-related increases in rates of sudden cardiac death (1.99 and 2.26, respectively) (Ray et al. 2009). Although premarketing studies suggested that ziprasidone yielded cardiac conduction delays, postmarketing experience to date has failed to indicate clinically significant problems with cardiac conduction (Daniel 2003; Harvey and Bowie 2005).

Other adverse effects include benign rash (in 5% of patients), orthostatic hypotension, syncope (in 0.6% of patients), and seizures (in 0.4% of patients). To date, ziprasidone has not been associated with congenital malformations in humans (FDA pregnancy category C).

Administration.   In acute mania, ziprasidone is commonly initiated at 80 mg/day administered with food in two divided doses, and increased as necessary and tolerated on day 2 to 120–160 mg/day administered with food in two divided doses, with final dosages ranging between 80 and 160 mg/day, and averaging approximately 125–130 mg/day in controlled trials (Keck et al. 2003b; Potkin et al. 2005) (Table 13–6). Similar dosing was tolerated in the adjunctive treatment of major depressive disorder (Dunner et al. 2007). In clinical practice, because lower (e.g., <80 mg/day) compared with higher (e.g., ≥80 mg/day) ziprasidone dosages may increase the risk of akathisia (Oral et al. 2006), optimal titration of this agent may involve avoiding lower dosages to prevent akathisia or abruptly increasing to higher dosages if akathisia develops at lower dosages. Also, for convenience, and in view of the risk of sedation, dosing may be weighted toward dinnertime or bedtime with a snack. Although it is not recommended in the prescribing information, occasional patients may tolerate and benefit from dosages as high as 240–320 mg/day. Intramuscular ziprasidone 10 mg is administered for agitation in schizophrenia and repeated as often as every 2 hours, as necessary and tolerated, with a maximum of 40 mg/day for 3 days.

Aripiprazole

Pharmacokinetics and drug interactions.   Aripiprazole has a bioavailability of 87% and a volume of distribution of 4.9 L/kg, is 99% bound to plasma proteins, and has a long 72-hour half-life (Mallikaarjun et al. 2004). Aripiprazole is metabolized to an active dehydro-aripiprazole metabolite that has a half-life of 94 hours. Aripiprazole is extensively metabolized, primarily through oxidation by CYP2D6 and CYP3A4, with less than 1% excreted unchanged in the urine (Swainston Harrison and Perry 2004). Aripiprazole does not have clinically significant effects on CYP isozymes (Swainston Harrison and Perry 2004), and is thus a target of rather than an instigator of drug interactions. Although concerns have been raised regarding the possibility that inhibitors of CYP2D6 and CYP3A4 and inducers of CYP3A4 may affect aripiprazole pharmacokinetics, systematic data regarding such putative interactions are limited (Molden et al. 2006).

Aripiprazole does not generally have clinically significant drug interactions with lithium (*Physicians' Desk Reference* 2008). Although case reports suggest that sporadic individuals could develop serious adverse effects such as neuroleptic malignant syndrome when lithium is combined with aripiprazole (Ali et al. 2006), clinical data suggest that this combination does not generally yield more than merely additive adverse effects (Citrome et al. 2005; Vieta et al. 2008a). Indeed, aripiprazole combined with lithium (or valproate) is approved for the treatment of patients with acute manic or mixed episodes (Vieta et al. 2008a). Aripiprazole does not generally yield clinically significant drug interactions with valproate (*Physicians' Desk Reference* 2008). Carbamazepine induces aripiprazole metabolism (*Physicians' Desk Reference* 2008). Aripiprazole does not generally appear to have clinically significant effects on lamotrigine pharmacokinetics (Schiebar et al. 2007).

Few data are available regarding interactions between aripiprazole and other antipsychotics. A case of a patient with schizophrenia who experienced exacerbation of psychosis plus normalization of serum prolactin concentration when aripiprazole was added to haloperidol suggested a pharmacodynamic interaction wherein aripiprazole displaced haloperidol from dopamine D_2 receptors (Burke and Lincoln 2006).

Aripiprazole does not appear to have clinically significant effects on the pharmacokinetics of the antidepressants fluoxetine, setraline, paroxetine, escitalopram, and venlafaxine (*Physicians' Desk Reference* 2008). However, case reports of sporadic problems with aripiprazole combined with antidepressants include a possible neuroleptic malignant syndrome with the aripiprazole plus fluoxetine combination (Duggal and Kithas 2005) and urinary obstruction with the aripiprazole plus citalopram combination (Padala et al. 2006). Nevertheless, aripiprazole has been approved as adjunctive therapy to antidepressants in (unipolar) major depressive disorder.

Aripiprazole is commonly administered along with benzodiazepines in patients with bipolar disorders, with merely additive central nervous system adverse effects (e.g., sedation, ataxia). Indeed, contemporary controlled aripiprazole trials routinely permit some adjunctive benzodiazepine (e.g., lorazepam) administration (Keck et al. 2003a, 2006; Sachs et al. 2006b; Vieta et al. 2005). In healthy volunteers, intramuscular aripiprazole and intramuscular lorazepam did not have clinically significant pharmacokinetic interactions, but they did yield additive sedation and orthostatic hypotension (*Physicians' Desk Reference* 2008).

Quinidine and ketoconazole appear to increase serum aripiprazole concentrations (*Physicians' Desk Reference* 2008). Tobacco smoking does not yield clinically significant decreases in serum concentrations of aripiprazole, as it does with clozapine and olanzapine (Swainston Harrison and Perry 2004).

Adverse effects.   The most common adverse events with oral aripiprazole in acute mania trials affected the central nervous system (headache, agitation/anxiety/akathisia, insomnia, somnolence) and gastrointestinal system (nausea, dyspepsia, vomiting, constipation) (Keck et al. 2003a; Marder et al. 2003; Sachs et al. 2006b; Vieta et al. 2005). The most common adverse events with intramuscular aripiprazole in a trial in patients with acute agitation in mania also involved the central nervous system (headache, dizziness, insomnia, somnolence) and gastrointestinal system (nausea, vomiting). The most common adverse events in a longer-term trial in which bipolar disorder was treated with oral aripiprazole again involved the central nervous system (anxiety, insomnia, depression, nervousness, tremor, agitation, asthenia, headache, akathisia) and gastrointestinal system (nausea), and upper respiratory infection, vaginitis, and pain in the extremities. Aripiprazole-related akathisia may respond to benzodiazepines, as described for ziprasidone. Decreasing the dosage may attenuate akathisia with aripiprazole, unlike with ziprasidone.

Gastrointestinal adverse effects, such as nausea, dyspepsia, constipation, vomiting, and diarrhea, may be related to dopamine partial agonist effects and tend to diminish with ongoing exposure. Although aripiprazole can be dosed once daily because it has a long half-life, during the first few days of treatment, the lower maximum concentrations associated with divided doses may offer enhanced tolerability. Thus, tolerability may be enhanced in patients with gastrointestinal or other adverse effects if aripiprazole is initiated at 15 mg/day (or lower if necessary) in divided doses for a few days before increasing the dosage.

The U.S. prescribing information for aripiprazole includes boxed warnings regarding the increased risks of 1) mortality (primarily cardiovascular or infectious) in older adults with dementia-related psychosis (an antipsychotic class warning) and 2) suicidality and use of antidepressant drugs in patients up to age

24 years (based on an antidepressant class warning). The FDA has stipulated that the aripiprazole prescribing information include a warning of the risks of hyperglycemia and diabetes mellitus (*Physicians' Desk Reference* 2008). Although weight gain can occur with aripiprazole, this issue, as well as metabolic disruption, is generally less of a problem than with olanzapine (McQuade et al. 2004). Indeed, the report of a consensus development conference suggests that the risks of obesity, diabetes, and hyperlipidemia with aripiprazole are similar to those with ziprasidone and less than those with other second-generation antipsychotics (American Diabetes Association et al. 2004). Nevertheless, clinical and (as indicated) laboratory monitoring for obesity, diabetes, and hyperlipidemia are recommended for patients taking aripiprazole (Tables 13–1 and 13–12). Other warnings in the prescribing information include the risks of cerebrovascular adverse events, including stroke, in older adults with dementia-related psychosis (a warning shared with risperidone and olanzapine); neuroleptic malignant syndrome; and tardive dyskinesia.

Other adverse effects include orthostatic hypotension, syncope, seizures, and dysphagia. To date, aripiprazole has not been associated with congenital malformations in humans (FDA pregnancy category C).

When used as monotherapy or as adjunctive (added to lithium or divalproex) treatment in acute manic and mixed episodes, oral aripiprazole is recommended in the U.S. prescribing information to be initiated in adults at 15 mg once a day, which is the recommended dosage, and to be initiated in children and adolescents at 2 mg once a day and then titrated to the 10 mg/day recommended dosage. The maximum dosage is 30 mg/day for both adult and pediatric patients with acute manic or mixed episodes (Table 13–6). In early clinical trials in acute manic and mixed episodes in adults, aripiprazole was started at 30 mg/day, and approximately 15% of the patients had aripiprazole dosage decreased from 30 to 15 mg/day because of tolerability problems, yielding a mean dosage of approximately 28 mg/day (Keck et al. 2003a; Sachs et al. 2006b; Vieta et al. 2005). In monotherapy maintenance treatment for bipolar I disorder, oral aripiprazole final dosages averaged approximately 24 mg/day (Keck et al. 2006). In two negative acute bipolar I nonpsychotic depression studies, aripiprazole monotherapy was initiated at 10 mg/day and flexibly dosed within a range of 5–30 mg/day, with a pooled mean dosage of 16.5 mg/day (Thase et al. 2008). Citing high discontinuation rates, the authors speculated that this dosing may have been too aggressive for patients with acute bipolar depression. Indeed, in adjunctive (added to antidepressants) treatment of unipolar major depressive disorder, oral aripiprazole is recommended in the U.S. prescribing information to be initiated in adults at 2–5 mg once a day and titrated to a recommended dosage of 5–10 mg/day (Berman et al. 2007; Marcus et al. 2008). The latter, more conservative dosing might be better tolerated in depressed or euthymic bipolar disorder patients. Intramuscular aripiprazole is recommended to be administered as a 9.75-mg injection (or a 5.25-mg injection if clinically indicated) with additional 9.75-mg (or 5.25-mg) injections as often as every 2 hours, as necessary and tolerated, with a maximum of 30 mg/day (Zimbroff et al. 2007). The prescribing information does not recommend 15-mg intramuscular injections because of concerns regarding adverse effects, as well as the lack of additional benefit with dosages over 9.75 mg per injection in clinical trials.

Conclusion

Effective pharmacotherapy of patients with bipolar disorders requires not only familiarity with mood stabilizer and antipsychotic pharmacodynamics, dosing, pharmacokinetics, drug interactions, adverse effects, and their management as described in this chapter, but also similar knowledge of antidepressants, benzodiazepines, other anticonvulsants, and other medications, as described in Chapter 14. In the past, clinicians have relied on observational drug interaction information, but recent characterization of substrates, inhibitors, and inducers of drug metabolism now allows not only the development of mechanistic models, but also enhanced anticipation and avoidance of clinical drug-drug interactions (Table 13–14). These developments promise to yield safer and more effective therapeutics when psychotropics are combined with one another in the treatment of patients with bipolar disorders. Florida Best Practice Medication Guidelines are provided in Appendix A, and Quick Reference Medication Facts are provided in Appendix B to assist in this endeavor.

TABLE 13–14.   Substrates, inhibitors, and inducers of some important cytochrome P450 isoforms

CYP	CYP1A2	CYP2C9/10	CYP2C19[a]	CYP2D6[a]	CYP2E1	CYP3A3/4
% of all CYP[b]	13	20 (for all 2C)		2	7	30 (for all 3A)
Substrates	Duloxetine Fluvoxamine 3° amine TCAs (N-demethylation) Clozapine (major) Olanzapine Caffeine Methadone Tacrine Acetaminophen Phenacetin Propranolol Theophylline	Tetrahydrocannabinol NSAIDs Phenytoin (major) Tolbutamide S-warfarin	Citalopram (partly) Escitalopram (partly) Moclobemide 3° amine TCAs (N-demethylation) Diazepam (N-demethylation) Hexobarbital Mephobarbital Lansoprazole Omeprazole (5-hydroxylation) Rabeprazole (demethylation) Phenytoin (minor) S-Mephenytoin Nelfinavir	Duloxetine Fluoxetine (partly) Mirtazapine (partly) Paroxetine Venlafaxine (O-demethylation) 2° and 3° amine TCAs (2,8,10-hydroxylation) Aripiprazole Chlorpromazine Clozapine (minor) Haloperidol (reduction) Fluphenazine Perphenazine Risperidone Sertindole Thioridazine Codeine (hydroxylation, O-demethylation) Dextromethorphan (O-demethylation)	Ethanol Acetaminophen Chlorzoxazone Halothane Isoflurane Methoxyflurane Sevoflurane	Acetaminophen Alfentanil Codeine (demethylation) Fentanyl Sufentanil Amiodarone Disopyramide Lidocaine Propafenone Quinidine Androgens Dexamethasone Estrogens (steroids) Astemizole Loratadine Terfenadine Atorvastatin Cerivastatin Lovastatin Simvastatin (HMG-CoAR inhibitors) Carbamazepine Ethosuximide Tiagabine Zonisamide Alprazolam Diazepam (hydroxylation and N-demethylation) Midazolam Triazolam Zaleplon Zolpidem Zopiclone Buspirone Desvenlafaxine (minor) Citalopram (partly) Escitalopram (partly) Mirtazapine (partly) Nefazodone Reboxetine Sertraline 3° amine TCAs (N-demethylation)

TABLE 13–14. Substrates, inhibitors, and inducers of some important cytochrome P450 isoforms (continued)

CYP	CYP1A2	CYP2C9/10	CYP2C19[a]	CYP2D6[a]	CYP2E1	CYP3A3/4
% of all CYP[b]	13	20 (for all 2C)		2	7	30 (for all 3A)
Substrates (continued)				Hydrocodone Oxycodone Mexiletine Propafenone (1C antiarrhythmics) Beta-blockers Donepezil (partly) D- and L-fenfluramine		Trazodone Aripiprazole Chlorpromazine Sertindole Quetiapine Ziprasidone Modafinil (partly) Diltiazem Felodipine Nifedipine Nimodipine Nisoldipine Nitrendipine Verapamil Cyclophosphamide Ifosfamide Tamoxifen Vinblastine Vincristine Cyclosporine Tacrolimus Cisapride Donepezil (partly) Lovastatin Omeprazole/ rabeprazole (sulfonation) Protease inhibitors Sildenafil
Inhibitors	Fluvoxamine Moclobemide Cimetidine Fluoroquinolones (ciprofloxacin, norfloxacin)	Fluvoxamine Paroxetine Sertraline Disulfiram Cimetidine	Fluoxetine Fluvoxamine Imipramine Moclobemide Tranylcypromine Diazepam	Bupropion Duloxetine Fluoxetine Fluvoxamine (weak) Hydroxybupropion Paroxetine	Diethyldithiocarbamate (disulfiram metabolite)	Fluoxetine Fluvoxamine Nefazodone Sertraline (weak) Diltiazem Verapamil Clarithromycin Erythromycin Troleandomycin (macrolides) Fluconazole Itraconazole

TABLE 13–14. Substrates, inhibitors, and inducers of some important cytochrome P450 isoforms (*continued*)

CYP	CYP1A2	CYP2C9/10	CYP2C19[a]	CYP2D6[a]	CYP2E1	CYP3A3/4
% of all CYP[b]	13	20 (for all 2C)		2	7	30 (for all 3A)
Inhibitors (*continued*)	Naringenin (grapefruit) Ticlopidine	Amiodarone Azapropazone Fluconazole Fluvastatin Miconazole Phenylbutazone D-Propoxyphene Stiripentol Sulfaphenazole Zafirlukast	Felbamate Phenytoin Topiramate Cimetidine Omeprazole Modafinil	Sertraline (weak) Moclobemide Chlorpromazine Fluphenazine Haloperidol Perphenazine Thioridazine Amiodarone Cimetidine Methadone Quinidine Ritonavir		Dexamethasone Gestodene Ritonavir Indinavir Nelfinavir Saquinavir (protease inhibitors) Ketoconazole (azole antifungals) Amiodarone Cimetidine Mibefradil Naringenin (grapefruit)
Inducers	Tobacco Omeprazole Charbroiled meats Modafinil (modest)	Barbiturates Carbamazepine Phenytoin Rifampin	Barbiturates Carbamazepine Phenytoin Rifampin	—	Ethanol Isoniazid	Barbiturates Carbamazepine Monohydroxy derivative Phenytoin Topiramate Modafinil (modest) Dexamethasone Rifabutin Rifampin Troglitazone St. John's wort

Note. HMG-CoAR=3-hydroxy-3-methylglutaryl–coenzyme A reductase; NSAID=nonsteroidal anti-inflammatory drug; TCA=tricyclic antidepressant.
[a]Clinically significant human polymorphism reported.
[b]CYP percentages from Shimada et al. 1994.
Source. Adapted from Ketter et al. 1995a.

References

Abbott FS, Kassam J, Orr JM, et al: The effect of aspirin on valproic acid metabolism. Clin Pharmacol Ther 40:94–100, 1986

Abraham G, Owen J: Topiramate can cause lithium toxicity. J Clin Psychopharmacol 24:565–567, 2004

Ackenheil M: Clozapine: pharmacokinetic investigations and biochemical effects in man. Psychopharmacology (Berl) 99(suppl):S32–S37, 1989

Adab N, Jacoby A, Smith D, et al: Additional educational needs in children born to mothers with epilepsy. J Neurol Neurosurg Psychiatry 70:15–21, 2001

Adan-Manes J, Novalbos J, López-Rodríguez R, et al: Lithium and venlafaxine interaction: a case of serotonin syndrome. J Clin Pharm Ther 31:397–400, 2006

Addison RS, Parker-Scott SL, Eadie MJ, et al: Steady-state dispositions of valproate and diflunisal alone and coadministered to healthy volunteers. Eur J Clin Pharmacol 56:715–721, 2000a

Addison RS, Parker-Scott SL, Hooper WD, et al: Effect of naproxen co-administration on valproate disposition. Biopharm Drug Dispos 21:235–242, 2000b

Addonizio G: Rapid induction of extrapyramidal side effects with combined use of lithium and neuroleptics. J Clin Psychopharmacol 5:296–298, 1985

Adler CM, Fleck DE, Brecher M, et al: Safety and tolerability of quetiapine in the treatment of acute mania in bipolar disorder. J Affect Disord 100 (suppl 1):S15–S22, 2007

Ahlfors UG, Baastrup PC, Dencker SJ, et al: Flupenthixol decanoate in recurrent manic-depressive illness: a comparison with lithium. Acta Psychiatr Scand 64:226–237, 1981

Aichhorn W, Marksteiner J, Walch T, et al: Influence of age, gender, body weight and valproate comedication on quetiapine plasma concentrations. Int Clin Psychopharmacol 21:81–85, 2006

Albani F, Riva R, Baruzzi A: Clarithromycin-carbamazepine interaction: a case report. Epilepsia 34:161–162, 1993

Albers LJ, Ozdemir V, Marder SR, et al: Low-dose fluvoxamine as an adjunct to reduce olanzapine therapeutic dose requirements: a prospective dose-adjusted drug interaction strategy. J Clin Psychopharmacol 25:170–174, 2005

Aldenkamp AP, Alpherts WC, Moerland MC, et al: Controlled release carbamazepine: cognitive side effects in patients with epilepsy. Epilepsia 28:507–514, 1987

Alfaro CL, McClure RK, Vertrees JE, et al: Unanticipated plasma concentrations in two clozapine-treated patients. Ann Pharmacother 35:1028–1031, 2001

Ali S, Pearlman RL, Upadhyay A, et al: Neuroleptic malignant syndrome with aripiprazole and lithium: a case report. J Clin Psychopharmacol 26:434–436, 2006

Allen HM, Jackson RL, Winchester MD, et al: Indomethacin in the treatment of lithium-induced nephrogenic diabetes insipidus. Arch Intern Med 149:1123–1126, 1989

Allen MH, Hirschfeld RM, Wozniak PJ, et al: Linear relationship of valproate serum concentration to response and optimal serum levels for acute mania. Am J Psychiatry 163:272–275, 2006

Allison DB, Mentore JL, Heo M, et al: Antipsychotic-induced weight gain: a comprehensive research synthesis. Am J Psychiatry 156:1686–1696, 1999

Aly MI, Abdel-Latif AA: Studies on distribution and metabolism of valproate in rat brain, liver, and kidney. Neurochem Res 5:1231–1242, 1980

Amdisen A: Lithium and drug interactions. Drugs 24:133–139, 1982

Amdisen A, Andersen CJ: Lithium treatment and thyroid function: a survey of 237 patients in long-term lithium treatment. Pharmacopsychiatria 15:149–155, 1982

Amdisen A, Gottfries CG, Jacobsson L, et al: Grave lithium intoxication with fatal outcome. Acta Psychiatr Scand Suppl 255:25–33, 1974

American Diabetes Association, American Psychiatric Association, American Association of Clinical Endocrinologists, et al: Consensus development conference on antipsychotic drugs and obesity and diabetes. Diabetes Care 27:596–601, 2004

American Psychiatric Association: Practice guideline for the treatment of patients with bipolar disorder (revision). Am J Psychiatry 159:1–50, 2002

Anderson GD, Yau MK, Gidal BE, et al: Bidirectional interaction of valproate and lamotrigine in healthy subjects. Clin Pharmacol Ther 60:145–156, 1996

Apseloff G, Mullet D, Wilner KD, et al: The effects of ziprasidone on steady-state lithium levels and renal clearance of lithium. Br J Clin Pharmacol 49 (suppl 1):61S–64S, 2000

Arana GW, Goff DC, Friedman H, et al: Does carbamazepine-induced reduction of plasma haloperidol levels worsen psychotic symptoms? Am J Psychiatry 143:650–651, 1986

Arana GW, Epstein S, Molloy M, et al: Carbamazepine-induced reduction of plasma alprazolam concentrations: a clinical case report. J Clin Psychiatry 49:448–449, 1988

Ashton AK, Wolin RE: Nefazodone-induced carbamazepine toxicity (letter). Am J Psychiatry 153:733, 1996

Atherton JC, Green R, Hughes S, et al: Lithium clearance in man: effects of dietary salt intake, acute changes in extracellular fluid volume, amiloride and frusemide. Clin Sci (Lond) 73:645–651, 1987

Avenoso A, Spina E, Campo G, et al: Interaction between fluoxetine and haloperidol: pharmacokinetic and clinical implications. Pharmacol Res 35:335–339, 1997

Azizabadi-Farahani M, Mirazi N, Azar M, et al: The effect of concomitant use of neuroleptic drugs and lithium on the erythrocyte/plasma lithium ratio in Iranian patients with bipolar disorder. J Clin Pharm Ther 21:3–7, 1996

Baastrup PC, Hollnagel P, Sorensen R, et al: Adverse reactions in treatment with lithium carbonate and haloperidol. JAMA 236:2645–2646, 1976

Bachmann KA, Jauregui L: Use of single sample clearance estimates of cytochrome P450 substrates to characterize human hepatic CYP status in vivo. Xenobiotica 23:307–315, 1993

Backman JT, Olkkola KT, Ojala M, et al: Concentrations and effects of oral midazolam are greatly reduced in patients treated with carbamazepine or phenytoin. Epilepsia 37:253–257, 1996

Bailey CE, Stewart JT, McElroy RA: Ibuprofen-induced lithium toxicity (letter). South Med J 82:1197, 1989

Baillie TA: Metabolism of valproate to hepatotoxic intermediates. Pharm Weekbl Sci 14:122–125, 1992

Baldessarini RJ, Frankenburg FR: Clozapine: a novel antipsychotic agent. N Engl J Med 324:746–754, 1991

Baldessarini RJ, Tondo L, Faedda GL, et al: Effects of the rate of discontinuing lithium maintenance treatment in bipolar disorders. J Clin Psychiatry 57:441–448, 1996

Baptista T, Teneud L, Contreras Q, et al: Lithium and body weight gain. Pharmaco-psychiatry 28:35–44, 1995

Barbhaiya RH, Shukla UA, Greene DS, et al: Investigation of pharmacokinetic and pharmacodynamic interactions after coadministration of nefazodone and halo-peridol. J Clin Psychopharmacol 16:26–34, 1996

Barclay ML, Brownlie BE, Turner JG, et al: Lithium associated thyrotoxicosis: a report of 14 cases, with statistical analysis of incidence. Clin Endocrinol (Oxf) 40:759–764, 1994

Barnes TRE, Soares-Weiser K, Bacaltchuk J. Central action beta-blockers versus placebo for neuroleptic-induced acute akathisia. Cochrane Database Syst Rev Issue 4, Art No: CD001946. 2004 DOI: 10.1002/14651858.CD001946.pub2

Bates DE, Herman RJ: Carbamazepine toxicity induced by lopinavir/ritonavir and nel-finavir. Ann Pharmacother 40:1190–1195, 2006

Batlle DC, von Riotte AB, Gaviria M, et al: Amelioration of polyuria by amiloride in pa-tients receiving long-term lithium therapy. N Engl J Med 312:408–414, 1985

Battaglia J, Moss S, Rush J, et al: Haloperidol, lorazepam, or both for psychotic agita-tion? A multicenter, prospective, double-blind, emergency department study. Am J Emerg Med 15:335–340, 1997

Beedham C, Miceli JJ, Obach RS: Ziprasidone metabolism, aldehyde oxidase, and clin-ical implications. J Clin Psychopharmacol 23:229–232, 2003

Bell AJ, Cole A, Eccleston D, et al: Lithium neurotoxicity at normal therapeutic levels. Br J Psychiatry 162:689–692, 1993

Bender S, Linka T, Wolstein J, et al: Safety and efficacy of combined clozapine-lithium pharmacotherapy. Int J Neuropsychopharmacol 7:59–63, 2004

Bendz H: Kidney function in lithium-treated patients: a literature survey. Acta Psychi-atr Scand 68:303–324, 1983

Bendz H, Aurell M: Drug-induced diabetes insipidus: incidence, prevention and man-agement. Drug Saf 21:449–456, 1999

Bendz H, Feinberg M: Aspirin increases serum lithium ion levels. Arch Gen Psychiatry 41:310–311, 1984

Bendz H, Sjodin I, Toss G, et al: Hyperparathyroidism and long-term lithium therapy: a cross-sectional study and the effect of lithium withdrawal. J Intern Med 240:357–365, 1996

Bergemann N, Frick A, Parzer P, et al: Olanzapine plasma concentration, average daily dose, and interaction with co-medication in schizophrenic patients. Pharmacopsychiatry 37:63–68, 2004

Bergemann N, Kress KR, Abu-Tair F, et al: Valproate lowers plasma concentration of olanzapine. J Clin Psychopharmacol 26:432–434, 2006

Berigan TR, Harazin JS: A sertraline/valproic acid drug interaction. International Journal of Psychiatry in Clinical Practice 3:287–288, 1999

Berk M, Ng F, Wang WV, et al: Going up in smoke: tobacco smoking is associated with worse treatment outcomes in mania. J Affect Disord 110:126–134, 2008

Berman RM, Marcus RN, Swanink R, et al: The efficacy and safety of aripiprazole as adjunctive therapy in major depressive disorder: a multicenter, randomized, double-blind, placebo-controlled study. J Clin Psychiatry 68:843–853, 2007

Bernus I, Dickinson RG, Hooper WD, et al: The mechanism of the carbamazepine-valproate interaction in humans. Br J Clin Pharmacol 44:21–27, 1997

Berry DJ, Besag FM, Pool F, et al: Lack of an effect of topiramate on lamotrigine serum concentrations. Epilepsia 43:818–823, 2002

Berry N, Pradhan S, Sagar R, et al: Neuroleptic malignant syndrome in an adolescent receiving olanzapine-lithium combination therapy. Pharmacotherapy 23:255–259, 2003

Bertilsson L: Clinical pharmacokinetics of carbamazepine. Clin Pharmacokinet 3:128–143, 1978

Bertilsson L, Tomson T: Clinical pharmacokinetics and pharmacological effects of carbamazepine and carbamazepine-10,11-epoxide: an update. Clin Pharmacokinet 11:177–198, 1986

Bertschy G, Vandel S, Jounet JM, et al: Valpromide-amitriptyline interaction: increase in the bioavailability of amitriptyline and nortriptyline caused by valpromide [in French]. Encephale 16:43–45, 1990

Besag FM, Berry DJ, Pool F, et al: Carbamazepine toxicity with lamotrigine: pharmacokinetic or pharmacodynamic interaction? Epilepsia 39:183–187, 1998

Bialer M, Doose DR, Murthy B, et al: Pharmacokinetic interactions of topiramate. Clin Pharmacokinet 43:763–780, 2004

Biederman J, Lerner Y, Belmaker RH: Combination of lithium carbonate and haloperidol in schizo-affective disorder: a controlled study. Arch Gen Psychiatry 36:327–333, 1979

Bienentreu SD, Kronmüller KT: Increase in risperidone plasma level with lamotrigine. Am J Psychiatry 162:811–812, 2005

Bikin D, Conrad KA, Mayersohn M: Lack of influence of caffeine and aspirin on lithium elimination. Clin Res 30:249, 1982

Binder EF, Cayabyab L, Ritchie DJ, et al: Diltiazem-induced psychosis and a possible diltiazem-lithium interaction. Arch Intern Med 151:373–374, 1991

Bjornsson E: Drug-induced liver injury: Hy's rule revisited. Clin Pharmacol Ther 79:521–528, 2006

Blanche P, Raynaud E, Kerob D, et al: Lithium intoxication in an elderly patient after combined treatment with losartan (letter). Eur J Clin Pharmacol 52:501, 1997

Bocchetta A, Mossa P, Velluzzi F, et al: Ten-year follow-up of thyroid function in lithium patients. J Clin Psychopharmacol 21:594–598, 2001

Boesen F, Andersen EB, Jensen EK, et al: Cardiac conduction disturbances during carbamazepine therapy. Acta Neurol Scand 68:49–52, 1983

Bondolfi G, Eap CB, Bertschy G, et al: The effect of fluoxetine on the pharmacokinetics and safety of risperidone in psychotic patients. Pharmacopsychiatry 35:50–56, 2002

Bonnet P, Vandel S, Nezelof S, et al: Carbamazepine, fluvoxamine: is there a pharmacokinetic interaction? (letter) Therapie 47:165, 1992

Borba CP, Henderson DC: Citalopram and clozapine: potential drug interaction. J Clin Psychiatry 61:301–302, 2000

Bork JA, Rogers T, Wedlund PJ, et al: A pilot study on risperidone metabolism: the role of cytochromes P450 2D6 and 3A. J Clin Psychiatry 60:469–476, 1999

Borovicka MC, Bond LC, Gaughan KM: Ziprasidone- and lithium-induced neuroleptic malignant syndrome. Ann Pharmacother 40:139–142, 2006

Bourgeois BF: Pharmacologic interactions between valproate and other drugs. Am J Med 84:29–33, 1988

Bourgeois BF, Dodson WE, Ferrendelli JA: Interactions between primidone, carbamazepine, and nicotinamide. Neurology 32:1122–1126, 1982

Bourgeois JA, Kahn DR: Neuroleptic malignant syndrome following administration of risperidone and lithium. J Clin Psychopharmacol 23:315–317, 2003

Bowden CL, Brugger AM, Swann AC, et al: Efficacy of divalproex vs lithium and placebo in the treatment of mania. The Depakote Mania Study Group. JAMA 271:918–924, 1994

Bowden CL, Janicak PG, Orsulak P, et al: Relation of serum valproate concentration to response in mania. Am J Psychiatry 153:765–770, 1996

Bowden CL, Calabrese JR, McElroy SL, et al: A randomized, placebo-controlled 12-month trial of divalproex and lithium in treatment of outpatients with bipolar I disorder. Divalproex Maintenance Study Group. Arch Gen Psychiatry 57:481–489, 2000

Bowden CL, Calabrese JR, Sachs G, et al: A placebo-controlled 18-month trial of lamotrigine and lithium maintenance treatment in recently manic or hypomanic patients with bipolar I disorder. Arch Gen Psychiatry 60:392–400, 2003

Bowden CL, Grunze H, Mullen J, et al: A randomized, double-blind, placebo-controlled efficacy and safety study of quetiapine or lithium as monotherapy for mania in bipolar disorder. J Clin Psychiatry 66:111–121, 2005

Bowden CL, Calabrese JR, Ketter TA, et al: Impact of lamotrigine and lithium on weight in obese and nonobese patients with bipolar I disorder. Am J Psychiatry 163:1199–1201, 2006a

Bowden CL, Swann AC, Calabrese JR, et al: A randomized, placebo-controlled, multicenter study of divalproex sodium extended release in the treatment of acute mania. J Clin Psychiatry 67:1501–1510, 2006b

Bray GA, Hollander P, Klein S, et al: A 6-month randomized, placebo-controlled, dose-ranging trial of topiramate for weight loss in obesity. Obes Res 11:722–733, 2003

Brodie MJ, MacPhee GJ: Carbamazepine neurotoxicity precipitated by diltiazem. Br Med J (Clin Res Ed) 292:1170–1171, 1986

Brodie MJ, Wilson EA, Wesche DL, et al: Pregabalin drug interaction studies: lack of effect on the pharmacokinetics of carbamazepine, phenytoin, lamotrigine, and valproate in patients with partial epilepsy. Epilepsia 46:1407–1413, 2005

Brøsen K, Kragh-Sørensen P: Concomitant intake of nortriptyline and carbamazepine. Ther Drug Monit 15:258–260, 1993

Brown CS, Wells BG, Cold JA, et al: Possible influence of carbamazepine on plasma imipramine concentrations in children with attention deficit hyperactivity disorder. J Clin Psychopharmacol 10:359–362, 1990

Bruun NE, Skott P, Lonborg-Jensen H, et al: Unchanged lithium clearance during acute amiloride treatment in sodium-depleted man. Scand J Clin Lab Invest 49:259–263, 1989

Bryant AE 3rd, Dreifuss FE: Valproic acid hepatic fatalities, III: U.S. experience since 1986. Neurology 46:465–469, 1996

Burke MJ, Lincoln J: Aripiprazole and haloperidol: a clinically relevant interaction with a dopamine antagonist and partial agonist. Ann Clin Psychiatry 18:129–130, 2006

Byerly MJ, DeVane CL: Pharmacokinetics of clozapine and risperidone: a review of recent literature. J Clin Psychopharmacol 16:177–187, 1996

Calabrese JR, Bowden CL, Sachs GS, et al; Lamictal 602 Study Group: A double-blind placebo-controlled study of lamotrigine monotherapy in outpatients with bipolar I depression. J Clin Psychiatry 60:79–88, 1999

Calabrese JR, Suppes T, Bowden CL, et al; Lamictal 614 Study Group: A double-blind, placebo-controlled, prophylaxis study of lamotrigine in rapid-cycling bipolar disorder. J Clin Psychiatry 61:841–850, 2000

Calabrese JR, Bowden CL, Sachs G, et al: A placebo-controlled 18-month trial of lamotrigine and lithium maintenance treatment in recently depressed patients with bipolar I disorder. J Clin Psychiatry 64:1013–1024, 2003

Calabrese JR, Keck PE Jr, Macfadden W, et al: A randomized, double-blind, placebo-controlled trial of quetiapine in the treatment of bipolar I or II depression. Am J Psychiatry 162:1351–1360, 2005

Callaghan JT, Bergstrom RF, Ptak LR, et al: Olanzapine: pharmacokinetic and pharmacodynamic profile. Clin Pharmacokinet 37:177–193, 1999

Calvo R, Carlos R, Erill S: Differential effects of valproic acid on the serum protein binding of lorazepam and diazepam. Int J Clin Pharmacol Res 6:213–215, 1986

Capewell S, Freestone S, Critchley JA, et al: Reduced felodipine bioavailability in patients taking anticonvulsants. Lancet 2:480–482, 1988

Carrillo JA, Herraiz AG, Ramos SI, et al: Effects of caffeine withdrawal from the diet on the metabolism of clozapine in schizophrenic patients. J Clin Psychopharmacol 18:311–316, 1998

Carrillo JA, Herraiz AG, Ramos SI, et al: Role of the smoking-induced cytochrome P450 (CYP)1A2 and polymorphic CYP2D6 in steady-state concentration of olanzapine. J Clin Psychopharmacol 23:119–127, 2003

Carwile ST, Husain AM, Miller PP, et al: Lamotrigine and sexual dysfunction in male patients with epilepsy, in Annual Meeting of the American Epilepsy Society, Boston, MA, December 7–10, 1997 (abstract 5.040). Epilepsia 38 (suppl 8):180, 1997

Cashman JR, Yang Z, Yang L, et al: Stereo- and regioselective N- and S-oxidation of tertiary amines and sulfides in the presence of adult human liver microsomes. Drug Metab Dispos 21:492–501, 1993

Castberg I, Spigset O: Risperidone and lamotrigine: no evidence of a drug interaction (letter). J Clin Psychiatry 67:1159, 2006

Castrogiovanni P: A novel slow-release formulation of lithium carbonate (Carbolithium Once-a-Day) vs. standard carbolithium: a comparative pharmacokinetic study. Clin Ter 153:107–115, 2002

Centorrino F, Baldessarini RJ, Kando J, et al: Serum concentrations of clozapine and its major metabolites: effects of cotreatment with fluoxetine or valproate. Am J Psychiatry 151:123–125, 1994

Centorrino F, Baldessarini RJ, Frankenburg FR, et al: Serum levels of clozapine and norclozapine in patients treated with selective serotonin reuptake inhibitors. Am J Psychiatry 153:820–822, 1996

Chan HH, Wing Y, Su R, et al: A control study of the cutaneous side effects of chronic lithium therapy. J Affect Disord 57:107–113, 2000

Chapron DJ, Cameron IR, White LB, et al: Observations on lithium disposition in the elderly. J Am Geriatr Soc 30:651–655, 1982

Chaudhry RP, Waters BG: Lithium and carbamazepine interaction: possible neurotoxicity. J Clin Psychiatry 44:30–31, 1983

Chen C, Veronese L, Yin Y: The effects of lamotrigine on the pharmacokinetics of lithium. Br J Clin Pharmacol 50:193–195, 2000

Chiu CC, Lane HY, Huang MC, et al: Dose-dependent alternations in the pharmaco-kinetics of olanzapine during coadministration of fluvoxamine in patients with schizophrenia. J Clin Pharmacol 44:1385–1390, 2004

Chong SA, Tan CH, Lee HS: Worsening of psychosis with clozapine and selective sero-tonin reuptake inhibitor combination: two case reports. J Clin Psychopharmacol 17:68–69, 1997

Christensen J, Petrenaite V, Atterman J, et al: Oral contraceptives induce lamotrigine metabolism: evidence from a double-blind, placebo-controlled trial. Epilepsia 48:484–489, 2007

Citrome L, Josiassen R, Bark N, et al: Pharmacokinetics of aripiprazole and concomi-tant lithium and valproate. J Clin Pharmacol 45:89–93, 2005

Cohen AF, Land GS, Breimer DD, et al: Lamotrigine, a new anticonvulsant: pharmaco-kinetics in normal humans. Clin Pharmacol Ther 42:535–541, 1987

Cohen D, Diemont WL: Deterioration of schizoaffective disorder due to an interaction between haloperidol and carbamazepine [in Dutch]. Ned Tijdschr Geneeskd 146:1942–1944, 2002

Cohen LG, Chesley S, Eugenio L, et al: Erythromycin-induced clozapine toxic reaction. Arch Intern Med 156:675–677, 1996

Cohen LS, Friedman JM, Jefferson JW, et al: A reevaluation of risk of in utero exposure to lithium. JAMA 271:146–150, 1994

Cohen LS, Sichel DA, Robertson LM, et al: Postpartum prophylaxis for women with bi-polar disorder. Am J Psychiatry 152:1641–1645, 1995

Cohen WJ, Cohen NH: Lithium carbonate, haloperidol, and irreversible brain damage. JAMA 230:1283–1287, 1974

Colussi G, Rombola G, Surian M, et al: Effects of acute administration of acetazolamide and frusemide on lithium clearance in humans. Nephrol Dial Transplant 4:707–712, 1989

Conley RR: Risperidone side effects. J Clin Psychiatry 61 (suppl 8):20–23; discussion 24–25, 2000

Conley RR, Meltzer HY: Adverse events related to olanzapine. J Clin Psychiatry 61 (suppl 8):26–29; discussion 30, 2000

Coppen A, Abou-Saleh M, Milln P, et al: Decreasing lithium dosage reduces morbidity and side-effects during prophylaxis. J Affect Disord 5:353–362, 1983

Costello LE, Suppes T: A clinically significant interaction between clozapine and val-proate. J Clin Psychopharmacol 15:139–141, 1995

Coves-Orts FJ, Borras-Blasco J, Navarro-Ruiz A, et al: Acute seizures due to a probable interaction between valproic acid and meropenem. Ann Pharmacother 39:533–537, 2005

Coxhead N, Silverstone T, Cookson J: Carbamazepine versus lithium in the prophylaxis of bipolar affective disorder. Acta Psychiatr Scand 85:114–118, 1992

Crabtree BL, Mack JE, Johnson CD, et al: Comparison of the effects of hydrochlorothiazide and furosemide on lithium disposition. Am J Psychiatry 148:1060–1063, 1991

Crawford P: Interactions between antiepileptic drugs and hormonal contraception. CNS Drugs 16:263–272, 2002

Crawford P, Chadwick D, Cleland P, et al: The lack of effect of sodium valproate on the pharmacokinetics of oral contraceptive steroids. Contraception 33:23–29, 1986

Crawford P, Chadwick DJ, Martin C, et al: The interaction of phenytoin and carbamazepine with combined oral contraceptive steroids. Br J Clin Pharmacol 30:892–896, 1990

Cruz-Flores S, Hayat GR, Mirza W: Valproic toxicity with fluoxetine therapy. Mo Med 92:296–297, 1995

Cunnington M, Tennis P: Lamotrigine and the risk of malformations in pregnancy. Neurology 64:955–960, 2005

Dain JG, Nicoletti J, Ballard F: Biotransformation of clozapine in humans. Drug Metab Dispos 25:603–609, 1997

Daniel DG: Tolerability of ziprasidone: an expanding perspective. J Clin Psychiatry 64 (suppl 19):40–49, 2003

Daniel DG, Potkin SG, Reeves KR, et al: Intramuscular (IM) ziprasidone 20 mg is effective in reducing acute agitation associated with psychosis: a double-blind, randomized trial. Psychopharmacology (Berl) 155: 128–134, 2001

Daniel WA, Haduch A, Wojcikowski J: Inhibition of rat liver CYP2D in vitro and after 1-day and long-term exposure to neuroleptics in vivo: possible involvement of different mechanisms. Eur Neuropsychopharmacol 15:103–110, 2005

D'Arrigo C, Migliardi G, Santoro V, et al: Effect of fluvoxamine on plasma risperidone concentrations in patients with schizophrenia. Pharmacol Res 52:497–501, 2005

Dasgupta A, Emerson L: Interaction of valproic acid with nonsteroidal antiinflammatory drugs mefenamic acid and fenoprofen in normal and uremic sera: lack of interaction in uremic sera due to the presence of endogenous factors. Ther Drug Monit 18:654–659, 1996

Dasgupta A, Volk A: Displacement of valproic acid and carbamazepine from protein binding in normal and uremic sera by tolmetin, ibuprofen, and naproxen: presence of inhibitor in uremic serum that blocks valproic acid–naproxen interactions. Ther Drug Monit 18:284–287, 1996

DasGupta K, Jefferson JW: The use of lithium in the medically ill. Gen Hosp Psychiatry 12:83–97, 1990

DeToledo JC, Haddad H, Ramsay RE: Status epilepticus associated with the combination of valproic acid and clomipramine. Ther Drug Monit 19:71–73, 1997

Degkwitz R, Koufen H, Consbruch U, et al: Lithium balance in mania [in German]. Int Pharmacopsychiatry 14:199–212, 1979

de Jong J, Hoogenboom B, van Troostwijk LD, et al: Interaction of olanzapine with fluvoxamine. Psychopharmacology (Berl) 155:219–220, 2001

Delva NJ, Hawken ER: Preventing lithium intoxication: guide for physicians. Can Fam Physician 47:1595–1600, 2001

Demmole D, Onkelinx C, Müller-Oerlinghausen B: Interaction between olanzapine and lithium in healthy male volunteers (abstract). Therapie 50:486, 1995

Denbow CE, Fraser HS: Clinically significant hemorrhage due to warfarin-carbamazepine interaction. South Med J 83:981, 1990

Denicoff KD, Smith-Jackson EE, Disney ER, et al: Comparative prophylactic efficacy of lithium, carbamazepine, and the combination in bipolar disorder. J Clin Psychiatry 58:470–478, 1997

des Lauriers A, Lassays C, Jouvent R: Lithium and diabetes insipidus: theoretical and practical aspects. Therapeutic value of thiazide diuretics [in French]. Sem Hop 58:703–710, 1982

DeVane CL: Pharmacokinetics, drug interactions, and tolerability of valproate. Psychopharmacol Bull 37 (suppl 2):25–42, 2003

DeVane CL, Nemeroff CB: Clinical pharmacokinetics of quetiapine: an atypical antipsychotic. Clin Pharmacokinet 40:509–522, 2001

Dhillon S, Richens A: Valproic acid and diazepam interaction in vivo. Br J Clin Pharmacol 13:553–560, 1982

Doose DR, Brodie MJ, Wilson EA, et al: Topiramate and lamotrigine pharmacokinetics during repetitive monotherapy and combination therapy in epilepsy patients. Epilepsia 44:917–922, 2003a

Doose DR, Wang SS, Padmanabhan M, et al: Effect of topiramate or carbamazepine on the pharmacokinetics of an oral contraceptive containing norethindrone and ethinyl estradiol in healthy obese and nonobese female subjects. Epilepsia 44:540–549, 2003b

Douyon R, Angrist B, Peselow E, et al: Neuroleptic augmentation with alprazolam: clinical effects and pharmacokinetic correlates. Am J Psychiatry 146:231–234, 1989

Dreifuss FE, Langer DH: Side effects of valproate. Am J Med 84:34–41, 1988

Droulers A, Bodak N, Oudjhani M, et al: Decrease of valproic acid concentration in the blood when coprescribed with fluoxetine. J Clin Psychopharmacol 17:139–140, 1997

Drover DR: Comparative pharmacokinetics and pharmacodynamics of short-acting hypnosedatives: zaleplon, zolpidem and zopiclone. Clin Pharmacokinet 43:227–238, 2004

Duggal HS, Kithas J: Possible neuroleptic malignant syndrome with aripiprazole and fluoxetine. Am J Psychiatry 162:397–398, 2005

DuMortier G, Lochu A, Colen de Melo P, et al: Elevated clozapine plasma concentrations after fluvoxamine initiation. Am J Psychiatry 153:738–739, 1996

Dunner DL, Amsterdam JD, Shelton RC, et al: Efficacy and tolerability of adjunctive ziprasidone in treatment-resistant depression: a randomized, open-label, pilot study. J Clin Psychiatry 68:1071–1077, 2007

Eap CB, Guentert TW, Schaublin-Loidl M, et al: Plasma levels of the enantiomers of thioridazine, thioridazine 2-sulfoxide, thioridazine 2-sulfone, and thioridazine 5-sulfoxide in poor and extensive metabolizers of dextromethorphan and mephenytoin. Clin Pharmacol Ther 59:322–331, 1996

Eap CB, Yasui N, Kaneko S, et al: Effects of carbamazepine coadministration on plasma concentrations of the enantiomers of mianserin and of its metabolites. Ther Drug Monit 21:166–170, 1999

Eichelbaum M, Tomson T, Tybring G, et al: Carbamazepine metabolism in man: induction and pharmacogenetic aspects. Clin Pharmacokinet 10:80–90, 1985

Eiermann B, Engel G, Johansson I, et al: The involvement of CYP1A2 and CYP3A4 in the metabolism of clozapine. Br J Clin Pharmacol 44:439–446, 1997

Ereshefsky L, Jann MW, Saklad SR, et al: Bioavailability of psychotropic drugs: historical perspective and pharmacokinetic overview. J Clin Psychiatry 47:6–15, 1986

Ethell BT, Anderson GD, Burchell B: The effect of valproic acid on drug and steroid glucuronidation by expressed human UDP-glucuronosyltransferases. Biochem Pharmacol 65:1441–1449, 2003

Evans RL, Nelson MV, Melethil S, et al: Evaluation of the interaction of lithium and alprazolam. J Clin Psychopharmacol 10:355–359, 1990

Fabrazzo M, La Pia S, Monteleone P, et al: Fluvoxamine increases plasma and urinary levels of clozapine and its major metabolites in a time- and dose-dependent manner. J Clin Psychopharmacol 20:708–710, 2000

Facciola G, Avenoso A, Scordo MG, et al: Small effects of valproic acid on the plasma concentrations of clozapine and its major metabolites in patients with schizophrenic or affective disorders. Ther Drug Monit 21:341–345, 1999

Faigle JW, Feldmann KF: Carbamazepine: chemistry and biotransformation, in Antiepileptic Drugs, 4th Edition. Edited by Levy RH, Mattson RH, Meldrum BS. New York, Raven Press, 1995, pp 499–513

Fang J, Bourin M, Baker GB: Metabolism of risperidone to 9-hydroxyrisperidone by human cytochromes P450 2D6 and 3A4. Naunyn Schmiedebergs Arch Pharmacol 359:147–151, 1999

Fang J, McKay G, Song J, et al: In vitro characterization of the metabolism of haloperidol using recombinant cytochrome p450 enzymes and human liver microsomes. Drug Metab Dispos 29:1638–1643, 2001

Faught E, Morris G, Jacobson M, et al: Adding lamotrigine to valproate: incidence of rash and other adverse effects. Postmarketing Antiepileptic Drug Survey (PADS) Group. Epilepsia 40:1135–1140, 1999

Fernandez de Gatta MR, Alonso Gonzalez AC, Garcia Sanchez MJ, et al: Effect of sodium valproate on phenobarbital serum levels in children and adults. Ther Drug Monit 8:416–420, 1986

Finch CK, Kelley KW, Williams RB: Treatment of lithium-induced diabetes insipidus with amiloride. Pharmacotherapy 23:546–550, 2003

Finley P, Warner D: Potential impact of valproic acid therapy on clozapine disposition. Biol Psychiatry 36:487–488, 1994

Finley PR, Warner MD, Peabody CA: Clinical relevance of drug interactions with lithium. Clin Pharmacokinet 29:172–191, 1995

Fitton A, Heel RC: Clozapine: a review of its pharmacological properties, and therapeutic use in schizophrenia. Drugs 40:722–747, 1990

Fitzgerald BJ, Okos AJ: Elevation of carbamazepine-10,11-epoxide by quetiapine. Pharmacotherapy 22:1500–1503, 2002

Fleischhacker WW, Hummer M, Kurz M, et al: Clozapine dose in the United States and Europe: implications for therapeutic and adverse effects. J Clin Psychiatry 55 (suppl B):78–81, 1994

Flicker MR, Quigley MA, Caldwell EG: Diltiazem-lithium interaction: an opposing viewpoint. J Clin Psychiatry 49:325–326, 1988

Forsman A, Ohman R: Studies on serum protein binding of haloperidol. Curr Ther Res Clin Exp 21:245–255, 1977

Forsythe WI, Owens JR, Toothill C: Effectiveness of acetazolamide in the treatment of carbamazepine-resistant epilepsy in children. Dev Med Child Neurol 23:761–769, 1981

Freeman DJ, Oyewumi LK: Will routine therapeutic drug monitoring have a place in clozapine therapy? Clin Pharmacokinet 32:93–100, 1997

Frick A, Kopitz J, Bergemann N: Omeprazole reduces clozapine plasma concentrations: a case report. Pharmacopsychiatry 36:121–123, 2003

Fritze J, Unsorg B, Lanczik M: Interaction between carbamazepine and fluvoxamine. Acta Psychiatr Scand 84:583–584, 1991

Frölich JC, Leftwich R, Ragheb M, et al: Indomethacin increases plasma lithium. Br Med J 1:1115–1116, 1979

Frye MA, Kimbrell TA, Dunn RT, et al: Gabapentin does not alter single-dose lithium pharmacokinetics. J Clin Psychopharmacol 18:461–464, 1998

Frye MA, Denicoff KD, Bryan AL, et al: Association between lower serum free T4 and greater mood instability and depression in lithium-maintained bipolar patients. Am J Psychiatry 156:1909–1914, 1999

Fu C, Katzman M, Goldbloom DS: Valproate/nortriptyline interaction. J Clin Psychopharmacol 14:205–206, 1994

Fudio S, Carcas A, Piñana E, et al: Epileptic seizures caused by low valproic acid levels from an interaction with meropenem. J Clin Pharm Ther 31:393–396, 2006

Funderburg LG, Vertrees JE, True JE, et al: Seizure following addition of erythromycin to clozapine treatment. Am J Psychiatry 151:1840–1841, 1994

Furnell MM, Davies J: The effect of sulindac on lithium therapy. Drug Intell Clin Pharm 19:374–376, 1985

Furukori H, Otani K, Yasui N, et al: Effect of carbamazepine on the single oral dose pharmacokinetics of alprazolam. Neuropsychopharmacology 18:364–369, 1998

Gabbay V, O'Dowd MA, Mamamtavrishvili M, et al: Clozapine and oral contraceptives: a possible drug interaction. J Clin Psychopharmacol 22:621–622, 2002

Gabriel E, Karobath M, Lenz G: The extrapyramidal symptoms in the combination of lithium long-term lithium therapy with nortriptyline: a case report on the formation of a pathogenesis hypothesis [in German]. Nervenarzt 47:46–48, 1976

Gadde KM, Franciscy DM, Wagner HR 2nd, et al: Zonisamide for weight loss in obese adults: a randomized controlled trial. JAMA 289:1820–1825, 2003

Gaily E, Kantola-Sorsa E, Hiilesmaa V, et al: Normal intelligence in children with prenatal exposure to carbamazepine. Neurology 62:28–32, 2004

Garnett WR, Levy B, McLean AM, et al: Pharmacokinetic evaluation of twice-daily extended-release carbamazepine (CBZ) and four-times-daily immediate-release CBZ in patients with epilepsy. Epilepsia 39:274–279, 1998

Gelenberg AJ: Lithium efficacy and adverse effects. J Clin Psychiatry 49(suppl):8–11, 1988

Gelenberg AJ, Jefferson JW: Lithium tremor. J Clin Psychiatry 56:283–287, 1995

Gelenberg AJ, Kane JM, Keller MB, et al: Comparison of standard and low serum levels of lithium for maintenance treatment of bipolar disorder. N Engl J Med 321:1489–1493, 1989

Gentile S: Prophylactic treatment of bipolar disorder in pregnancy and breastfeeding: focus on emerging mood stabilizers. Bipolar Disord 8:207–220, 2006

Ghadirian AM, Nair NP, Schwartz G: Effect of lithium and neuroleptic combination on lithium transport, blood pressure, and weight in bipolar patients. Biol Psychiatry 26:139–144, 1989

Ghaemi SN, Kirkwood CK: Elevation of nortriptyline plasma levels after cotreatment with paroxetine and thioridazine. J Clin Psychopharmacol 18:342–343, 1998

Ghose K: Interaction between lithium and carbamazepine (letter). Br Med J 280:1122, 1980

Gidal BE, Anderson GD, Spencer NW, et al: Valproic acid (VPA) associated weight gain in monotherapy patients with epilepsy, in Annual Meeting of the American Epilepsy Society, New Orleans, LA, December 2–8, 1994 (abstract). Epilepsia 35 (suppl 8):142, 1994

Gidal BE, Baltes E, Otoul C, et al: Effect of levetiracetam on the pharmacokinetics of adjunctive antiepileptic drugs: a pooled analysis of data from randomized clinical trials. Epilepsy Res 64:1–11, 2005

Gitlin MJ, Cochran SD, Jamison KR: Maintenance lithium treatment: side effects and compliance. J Clin Psychiatry 50:127–131, 1989

Goff DC, Midha KK, Brotman AW, et al: Elevation of plasma concentrations of haloperidol after the addition of fluoxetine. Am J Psychiatry 148:790–792, 1991

Goff DC, Midha KK, Sarid-Segal O, et al: A placebo-controlled trial of fluoxetine added to neuroleptic in patients with schizophrenia. Psychopharmacology (Berl) 117:417–423, 1995

Goldman SA: Lithium and neuroleptics in combination: is there enhancement of neurotoxicity leading to permanent sequelae? J Clin Pharmacol 36:951–962, 1996

Goldney RD, Spence ND: Safety of the combination of lithium and neuroleptic drugs. Am J Psychiatry 143:882–884, 1986

Goodnick PJ: Ziprasidone: profile on safety. Expert Opin Pharmacother 2:1655–1662, 2001

Goulden KJ, Dooley JM, Camfield PR, et al: Clinical valproate toxicity induced by acetylsalicylic acid. Neurology 37:1392–1394, 1987

Granneman GR, Schneck DW, Cavanaugh JH, et al: Pharmacokinetic interactions and side effects resulting from concomitant administration of lithium and divalproex sodium. J Clin Psychiatry 57:204–206, 1996

Grasela TH, Fiedler-Kelly J, Cox E, et al: Population pharmacokinetics of lamotrigine adjunctive therapy in adults with epilepsy. J Clin Pharmacol 39:373–384, 1999

Graves NM: Neuropharmacology and drug interactions in clinical practice. Epilepsia 36 (suppl 2):S27–S33, 1995

Graves NM, Brundage RC, Wen Y, et al: Population pharmacokinetics of carbamazepine in adults with epilepsy. Pharmacotherapy 18:273–281, 1998

Greil W, Stoltzenburg MC, Mairhofer ML, et al: Lithium dosage in the elderly: a study with matched age groups. J Affect Disord 9:1–4, 1985

Greil W, Ludwig-Mayerhofer W, Erazo N, et al: Lithium versus carbamazepine in the maintenance treatment of bipolar disorders: a randomised study. J Affect Disord 43:151–161, 1997

Grimaldi R, Lecchini S, Crema F, et al: In vivo plasma protein binding interaction between valproic acid and naproxen. Eur J Drug Metab Pharmacokinet 9:359–363, 1984

Grimm SW, Richtand NM, Winter HR, et al: Effects of cytochrome P450 3A modulators ketoconazole and carbamazepine on quetiapine pharmacokinetics. Br J Clin Pharmacol 61:58–69, 2006

Grimsley SR, Jann MW, Carter JG, et al: Increased carbamazepine plasma concentrations after fluoxetine coadministration. Clin Pharmacol Ther 50:10–15, 1991

Grohmann R, Ruther E, Sassim N, et al: Adverse effects of clozapine. Psychopharmacology (Berl) 99(suppl):S101–S104, 1989

Gunja N, Graudins A, Dowsett R: Lithium toxicity: a potential interaction with celecoxib (letter). Intern Med J 32:494, 2002

Hagg S, Spigset O, Mjorndal T, et al: Absence of interaction between erythromycin and a single dose of clozapine. Eur J Clin Pharmacol 55:221–226, 1999

Hagg S, Spigset O, Mjorndal T, et al: Effect of caffeine on clozapine pharmacokinetics in healthy volunteers. Br J Clin Pharmacol 49:59–63, 2000

Hamelin BA, Allard S, Laplante L, et al: The effect of timing of a standard meal on the pharmacokinetics and pharmacodynamics of the novel atypical antipsychotic agent ziprasidone. Pharmacotherapy 18:9–15, 1998

Hansen HE, Amdisen A: Lithium intoxication (report of 23 cases and review of 100 cases from the literature). Q J Med 47:123–144, 1978

Haring C, Fleischhacker WW, Schett P, et al: Influence of patient-related variables on clozapine plasma levels. Am J Psychiatry 147:1471–1475, 1990

Harrison TM, Davies DW, Norris CM: Lithium carbonate and piroxicam. Br J Psychiatry 149:124–125, 1986

Harvey NS, Merriman S: Review of clinically important drug interactions with lithium. Drug Saf 10:455–463, 1994

Harvey PD, Bowie CR: Ziprasidone: efficacy, tolerability, and emerging data on wide-ranging effectiveness. Expert Opin Pharmacother 6:337–346, 2005

Hasegawa M, Gutierrez-Esteinou R, Way L, et al: Relationship between clinical efficacy and clozapine concentrations in plasma in schizophrenia: effect of smoking. J Clin Psychopharmacol 13:383–390, 1993

Hasselstrom J, Linnet K: Quetiapine serum concentrations in psychiatric patients: the influence of comedication. Ther Drug Monit 26:486–491, 2004

Hasselstrom J, Linnet K: In vitro studies on quetiapine metabolism using the substrate depletion approach with focus on drug-drug interactions. Drug Metabol Drug Interact 21:187–211, 2006

He H, Richardson JS: A pharmacological, pharmacokinetic and clinical overview of risperidone, a new antipsychotic that blocks serotonin $5-HT_2$ and dopamine D_2 receptors. Int Clin Psychopharmacol 10:19–30, 1995

Helmuth D, Ljaljevic Z, Ramirez L, et al: Choreoathetosis induced by verapamil and lithium treatment. J Clin Psychopharmacol 9:454–455, 1989

Henderson DC, Goff DC: Risperidone as an adjunct to clozapine therapy in chronic schizophrenics. J Clin Psychiatry 57:395–397, 1996

Henry C: Lithium side-effects and predictors of hypothyroidism in patients with bipolar disorder: sex differences. J Psychiatry Neurosci 27:104–107, 2002

Herschberg SN, Sierles FS: Indomethacin-induced lithium toxicity. Am Fam Physician 28:155–157, 1983

Hesslinger B, Normann C, Langosch JM, et al: Effects of carbamazepine and valproate on haloperidol plasma levels and on psychopathologic outcome in schizophrenic patients. J Clin Psychopharmacol 19:310–315, 1999

Hetmar O: The impact of long-term lithium treatment on renal function and structure. Acta Psychiatr Scand Suppl 345:85–89, 1988

Hewick DS, Newbury P, Hopwood S, et al: Age as a factor affecting lithium therapy. Br J Clin Pharmacol 4:201–205, 1977

Hiemke C, Weigmann H, Hartter S, et al: Elevated levels of clozapine in serum after addition of fluvoxamine. J Clin Psychopharmacol 14:279–281, 1994

Hiemke C, Peled A, Jabarin M, et al: Fluvoxamine augmentation of olanzapine in chronic schizophrenia: pharmacokinetic interactions and clinical effects. J Clin Psychopharmacol 22:502–506, 2002

Himmelhoch JM, Poust RI, Mallinger AG, et al: Adjustment of lithium dose during lith-
ium-chlorothiazide therapy. Clin Pharmacol Ther 22:225–227, 1977

Hirschfeld RM, Keck PE Jr, Kramer M, et al: Rapid antimanic effect of risperidone
monotherapy: a 3-week multicenter, double-blind, placebo-controlled trial. Am J
Psychiatry 161:1057–1065, 2004

Honer WG, Thornton AE, Chen EY, et al: Clozapine alone versus clozapine and risperidone with refractory schizophrenia. N Engl J Med 354:472–482, 2006

Honig A, Arts BM, Ponds RW, et al: Lithium induced cognitive side-effects in bipolar
disorder: a qualitative analysis and implications for daily practice. Int Clin Psychopharmacol 14:167–171, 1999

Hung SI, Chung WH, Jee SH, et al: Genetic susceptibility to carbamazepine-induced
cutaneous adverse drug reactions. Pharmacogenet Genomics 16:297–306, 2006

Iqbal MM, Rahman A, Husain Z, et al: Clozapine: a clinical review of adverse effects and
management. Ann Clin Psychiatry 15:33–48, 2003

Ishizaki T, Chiba K, Saito M, et al: The effects of neuroleptics (haloperidol and chlorpromazine) on the pharmacokinetics of valproic acid in schizophrenic patients.
J Clin Psychopharmacol 4:254–261, 1984

Isojarvi JI, Laatikainen TJ, Pakarinen AJ, et al: Polycystic ovaries and hyperandrogenism
in women taking valproate for epilepsy. N Engl J Med 329:1383–1388, 1993

Iwahashi K, Miyatake R, Suwaki H, et al: The drug-drug interaction effects of haloperidol on plasma carbamazepine levels. Clin Neuropharmacol 18:233–236, 1995

Jann MW, Ereshefsky L, Saklad SR, et al: Effects of carbamazepine on plasma haloperidol levels. J Clin Psychopharmacol 5:106–109, 1985

Jann MW, Fidone GS, Israel MK, et al: Increased valproate serum concentrations upon
carbamazepine cessation. Epilepsia 29:578–581, 1988

Jann MW, Fidone GS, Hernandez JM, et al: Clinical implications of increased antipsychotic plasma concentrations upon anticonvulsant cessation. Psychiatry Res
28:153–159, 1989

Jann MW, Grimsley SR, Gray EC, et al: Pharmacokinetics and pharmacodynamics of
clozapine. Clin Pharmacokinet 24:161–176, 1993

Jann MW, Hon YY, Shamsi SA, et al: Lack of pharmacokinetic interaction between
lamotrigine and olanzapine in healthy volunteers. Pharmacotherapy 26:627–633,
2006

Javaid JI: Clinical pharmacokinetics of antipsychotics. J Clin Pharmacol 34:286–295,
1994

Jefferson JW, Ayd FJ Jr: Combining lithium and antidepressants. J Clin Psychopharmacol 3:303–307, 1983

Jefferson JW, Kalin NH: Serum lithium levels and long-term diuretic use. JAMA
241:1134–1136, 1979

Jefferson JW, Greist JH, Baudhuin M: Lithium: interactions with other drugs. J Clin
Psychopharmacol 1:124–134, 1981

Jefferson JW, Greist JH, Clagnaz PJ, et al: Effect of strenuous exercise on serum lithium level in man. Am J Psychiatry 139:1593–1595, 1982

Jefferson JW, Greist JH, Ackerman DL, et al: Lithium Encyclopedia for Clinical Practice, 2nd Edition. Washington, DC, American Psychiatric Press, 1987

Jeffries J, Remington G, Wilkins J: The question of lithium/neuroleptic toxicity. Can J Psychiatry 29:601–604, 1984

Jerling M, Bertilsson L, Sjöqvist F: The use of therapeutic drug monitoring data to document kinetic drug interactions: an example with amitriptyline and nortriptyline. Ther Drug Monit 16:1–12, 1994a

Jerling M, Lindstrom L, Bondesson U, et al: Fluvoxamine inhibition and carbamazepine induction of the metabolism of clozapine: evidence from a therapeutic drug monitoring service. Ther Drug Monit 16:368–374, 1994b

Joffe H, Cohen LS, Suppes T, et al: Valproate is associated with new-onset oligoamenorrhea with hyperandrogenism in women with bipolar disorder. Biol Psychiatry 59:1078–1086, 2006

Joffe RT, Gold PW, Uhde TW, et al: The effects of carbamazepine on the thyrotropin response to thyrotropin-releasing hormone. Psychiatry Res 12:161–166, 1984

Johannessen SI, Battino D, Berry DJ, et al: Therapeutic drug monitoring of the newer antiepileptic drugs. Ther Drug Monit 25:347–363, 2003

Jones KL, Lacro RV, Johnson KA, et al: Pattern of malformations in the children of women treated with carbamazepine during pregnancy. N Engl J Med 320:1661–1666, 1989

Jones MT, Stoner SC: Increased lithium concentrations reported in patients treated with sulindac. J Clin Psychiatry 61:527–528, 2000

Joos AA, Konig F, Frank UG, et al: Dose-dependent pharmacokinetic interaction of clozapine and paroxetine in an extensive metabolizer. Pharmacopsychiatry 30:266–270, 1997

Joseph AB, Wroblewski BA: Potentially toxic serum concentrations of desipramine after discontinuation of valproic acid. Brain Inj 7:463–465, 1993

Juhl RP, Tsuang MT, Perry PJ: Concomitant administration of haloperidol and lithium carbonate in acute mania. Dis Nerv Syst 38:675–676, 1977

Junghan U, Albers M, Woggon B: Increased risk of hematological side-effects in psychiatric patients treated with clozapine and carbamazepine? (letter) Pharmacopsychiatry 26:262, 1993

Kahn EM, Schulz SC, Perel JM, et al: Change in haloperidol level due to carbamazepine—a complicating factor in combined medication for schizophrenia. J Clin Psychopharmacol 10:54–57, 1990

Kalgutkar AS, Taylor TJ, Venkatakrishnan K, et al: Assessment of the contributions of CYP3A4 and CYP3A5 in the metabolism of the antipsychotic agent haloperidol to its potentially neurotoxic pyridinium metabolite and effect of antidepressants on the bioactivation pathway. Drug Metab Dispos 31:243–249, 2003

Kane JM, Smith JM: Tardive dyskinesia: prevalence and risk factors, 1959 to 1979. Arch Gen Psychiatry 39:473–481, 1982

Kassahun K, Mattiuz E, Nyhart E Jr, et al: Disposition and biotransformation of the antipsychotic agent olanzapine in humans. Drug Metab Dispos 25:81–93, 1997

Kato Y, Fujii T, Mizoguchi N, et al: Potential interaction between ritonavir and carbamazepine. Pharmacotherapy 20:851–854, 2000

Kaufman KR, Gerner R: Lamotrigine toxicity secondary to sertraline. Seizure 7:163–165, 1998

Keck PE Jr, Marcus R, Tourkodimitris S, et al: A placebo-controlled, double-blind study of the efficacy and safety of aripiprazole in patients with acute bipolar mania. Am J Psychiatry 160:1651–1658, 2003a

Keck PE Jr, Versiani M, Potkin S, et al: Ziprasidone in the treatment of acute bipolar mania: a three-week, placebo-controlled, double-blind, randomized trial. Am J Psychiatry 160:741–748, 2003b

Keck PE Jr, Calabrese JR, McQuade RD, et al: A randomized, double-blind, placebo-controlled 26-week trial of aripiprazole in recently manic patients with bipolar I disorder. J Clin Psychiatry 67:626–637, 2006

Keitner GI, Rahman S: Reversible neurotoxicity with combined lithium-haloperidol administration. J Clin Psychopharmacol 4:104–105, 1984

Kelly DL, Conley RR, Tamminga CA: Differential olanzapine plasma concentrations by sex in a fixed-dose study. Schizophr Res 40:101–104, 1999

Kelly DL, Conley RR, Feldman S, et al: Adjunct divalproex or lithium to clozapine in treatment-resistant schizophrenia. Psychiatr Q 77:81–95, 2006

Kerr BM, Thummel KE, Wurden CJ, et al: Human liver carbamazepine metabolism: role of CYP3A4 and CYP2C8 in 10,11-epoxide formation. Biochem Pharmacol 47:1969–1979, 1994

Ketter TA, Post RM, Worthington K: Principles of clinically important drug interactions with carbamazepine, part I. J Clin Psychopharmacol 11:198–203, 1991a

Ketter TA, Post RM, Worthington K: Principles of clinically important drug interactions with carbamazepine, part II. J Clin Psychopharmacol 11:306–313, 1991b

Ketter TA, Pazzaglia PJ, Post RM: Synergy of carbamazepine and valproic acid in affective illness: case report and review of the literature. J Clin Psychopharmacol 12:276–281, 1992

Ketter TA, Jenkins JB, Schroeder DH, et al: Carbamazepine but not valproate induces bupropion metabolism. J Clin Psychopharmacol 15:327–333, 1995a

Ketter TA, Post RM, Parekh PI, et al: Addition of monoamine oxidase inhibitors to carbamazepine: preliminary evidence of safety and antidepressant efficacy in treatment-resistant depression. J Clin Psychiatry 56:471–475, 1995b

Ketter TA, Kalali AH, Weisler RH: A 6-month, multicenter, open-label evaluation of beaded, extended-release carbamazepine capsule monotherapy in bipolar disorder patients with manic or mixed episodes. J Clin Psychiatry 65:668–673, 2004

Ketter TA, Wang PW, Chandler RA, et al: Dermatology precautions and slower titration yield low incidence of lamotrigine treatment-emergent rash. J Clin Psychiatry 66:642–645, 2005a

Ketter TA, Wang PW, Nowakowska C, et al: Treatment of acute mania in bipolar disorder, in Advances in the Treatment of Bipolar Disorder. Edited by Ketter TA. Washington, DC, American Psychiatric Publishing, 2005b, pp 11–55

Khan AY, Preskorn SH: Increase in plasma levels of clozapine and norclozapine after administration of nefazodone. J Clin Psychiatry 62:375–376, 2001

Khan A, Shad MU, Preskorn SH: Lack of sertraline efficacy probably due to an interaction with carbamazepine. J Clin Psychiatry 61:526–527, 2000

Khanna S, Hirschfeld RMA, Karcher K, et al: Risperidone monotherapy in acute bipolar mania (NR424), in 2003 New Research Program and Abstracts, American Psychiatric Association 156th Annual Meeting, San Francisco, CA, May 17–22, 2003. Washington, DC, American Psychiatric Association, 2003, p 159

Khanna S, Vieta E, Lyons B, et al: Risperidone in the treatment of acute mania: double-blind, placebo-controlled study. Br J Psychiatry 187:229–234, 2005

Kidron R, Averbuch I, Klein E, et al: Carbamazepine-induced reduction of blood levels of haloperidol in chronic schizophrenia. Biol Psychiatry 20:219–222, 1985

Kinzie E, Meltzer-Brody S: Possible serotonin syndrome with citalopram following cross-titration of clozapine to ziprasidone. Gen Hosp Psychiatry 27:223–224, 2005

Kleiner J, Altshuler L, Hendrick V, et al: Lithium-induced subclinical hypothyroidism: review of the literature and guidelines for treatment. J Clin Psychiatry 60:249–255, 1999

Klimke A, Klieser E: Sudden death after intravenous application of lorazepam in a patient treated with clozapine (letter). Am J Psychiatry 151:780, 1994

Koczerginski D, Kennedy SH, Swinson RP: Clonazepam and lithium: a toxic combination in the treatment of mania? Int Clin Psychopharmacol 4:195–199, 1989

Kontaxakis VP, Havaki-Kontaxaki BJ, Stamouli SS, et al: Toxic interaction between risperidone and clozapine: a case report. Prog Neuropsychopharmacol Biol Psychiatry 26:407–409, 2002

Koponen HJ, Leinonen E, Lepola U: Fluvoxamine increases the clozapine serum levels significantly. Eur Neuropsychopharmacol 6:69–71, 1996

Koreen AR, Lieberman JA, Kronig M, et al: Cross-tapering clozapine and risperidone (letter). Am J Psychiatry 152:1690, 1995

Kossen M, Selten JP, Kahn RS: Elevated clozapine plasma level with lamotrigine (letter). Am J Psychiatry 158:1930, 2001

Kosten TR, Forrest JN: Treatment of severe lithium-induced polyuria with amiloride. Am J Psychiatry 143:1563–1568, 1986

Kramlinger KG, Post RM: Adding lithium carbonate to carbamazepine: antimanic efficacy in treatment-resistant mania. Acta Psychiatr Scand 79:378–385, 1989

Kramlinger KG, Phillips KA, Post RM: Rash complicating carbamazepine treatment. J Clin Psychopharmacol 14:408–413, 1994

Krishna NR, Taylor MA, Abrams R: Combined haloperidol and lithium carbonate in treating manic patients. Compr Psychiatry 19:119–120, 1978

Kristoff CA, Hayes PE, Barr WH, et al: Effect of ibuprofen on lithium plasma and red blood cell concentrations. Clin Pharm 5:51–55, 1986

Kronig MH, Munne RA, Szymanski S, et al: Plasma clozapine levels and clinical response for treatment-refractory schizophrenic patients. Am J Psychiatry 152:179–182, 1995

Kudo S, Ishizaki T: Pharmacokinetics of haloperidol: an update. Clin Pharmacokinet 37:435–456, 1999

Kukopoulos A, Reginaldi D: Variations of serum lithium concentrations correlated with the phases of manic-depressive psychosis. Agressologie 19:219–222, 1978

Kukopoulos A, Minnai G, Müller-Oerlinghausen B: The influence of mania and depression on the pharmacokinetics of lithium: a longitudinal single-case study. J Affect Disord 8:159–166, 1985

Lai AA, Levy RH, Cutler RE: Time-course of interaction between carbamazepine and clonazepam in normal man. Clin Pharmacol Ther 24:316–323, 1978

Lai ML, Huang JD: Dual effect of valproic acid on the pharmacokinetics of phenytoin. Biopharm Drug Dispos 14:365–370, 1993

Lammers CH, Deuschle M, Weigmann H, et al: Coadministration of clozapine and fluvoxamine in psychotic patients: clinical experience. Pharmacopsychiatry 32:76–77, 1999

Lane HY, Chiu CC, Kazmi Y, et al: Lack of CYP3A4 inhibition by grapefruit juice and ketoconazole upon clozapine administration in vivo. Drug Metabol Drug Interact 18:263–278, 2001

Lapierre YD: Control of lithium tremor with propranolol. Can Med Assoc J 114:619–620, 624, 1976

Lee SA, Lee JK, Heo K: Coma probably induced by lorazepam-valproate interaction. Seizure 11:124–125, 2002

Lehman AF, Lieberman JA, Dixon LB, et al: Practice guideline for the treatment of patients with schizophrenia, second edition. Am J Psychiatry 161:1–56, 2004

Leinonen E, Lillsunde P, Laukkanen V, et al: Effects of carbamazepine on serum antidepressant concentrations in psychiatric patients. J Clin Psychopharmacol 11:313–318, 1991

Lertora JJ, Rege AB, Greenspan DL, et al: Pharmacokinetic interaction between zidovudine and valproic acid in patients infected with human immunodeficiency virus. Clin Pharmacol Ther 56:272–278, 1994

Leung M, Remick RA: Potential drug interaction between lithium and valsartan. J Clin Psychopharmacol 20:392–393, 2000

Levin GM, Grum C, Eisele G: Effect of over-the-counter dosages of naproxen sodium and acetaminophen on plasma lithium concentrations in normal volunteers. J Clin Psychopharmacol 18:237–240, 1998

Levy RH, Morselli PL, Bianchetti G, et al: Interaction between valproic acid and carbamazepine in epileptic patients, in Metabolism of Antiepileptic Drugs. Edited by Levy RH, Pitlick WH, Eichelbaum M, et al. New York, Raven Press, 1982, pp 45–51

Levy RH, Lane EA, Guyot M, et al: Analysis of parent drug-metabolite relationship in the presence of an inducer: application to the carbamazepine-clobazam interaction in normal man. Drug Metab Dispos 11:286–292, 1983

Levy RH, Ragueneau-Majlessi I, Brodie MJ, et al: Lack of clinically significant pharmacokinetic interactions between zonisamide and lamotrigine at steady state in patients with epilepsy. Ther Drug Monit 27:193–198, 2005

Leysen JE, Janssen PM, Megens AA, et al: Risperidone: a novel antipsychotic with balanced serotonin-dopamine antagonism, receptor occupancy profile, and pharmacologic activity. J Clin Psychiatry 55(suppl):5–12, 1994

Li KY, Li X, Cheng ZN, et al: Effect of erythromycin on metabolism of quetiapine in Chinese suffering from schizophrenia. Eur J Clin Pharmacol 60:791–795, 2005

Licht RW, Olesen OV, Friis P, et al: Olanzapine serum concentrations lowered by concomitant treatment with carbamazepine. J Clin Psychopharmacol 20:110–112, 2000

Lima AR, Soares Weiser K, Bacaltchuk J, et al: Benzodiazepines for neuroleptic induced acute akathisia. Cochrane Database Syst Rev CD001950, 2002

Lima WJ, Dopheide JA, Kramer BA, et al: A naturalistic comparison of adverse effects between slow titration and loading of divalproex sodium in psychiatric inpatients. J Affect Disord 52:261–267, 1999

Linnet K: Glucuronidation of olanzapine by cDNA-expressed human UDP-glucuronosyltransferases and human liver microsomes. Hum Psychopharmacol 17:233–238, 2002

Linnet K, Olesen OV: Free and glucuronidated olanzapine serum concentrations in psychiatric patients: influence of carbamazepine comedication. Ther Drug Monit 24:512–517, 2002

Livingstone C, Rampes H: Lithium: a review of its metabolic adverse effects. J Psychopharmacol 20:347–355, 2006

Longo LP, Salzman C: Valproic acid effects on serum concentrations of clozapine and norclozapine (letter). Am J Psychiatry 152:650, 1995

Lu ML, Lane HY, Chen KP, et al: Fluvoxamine reduces the clozapine dosage needed in refractory schizophrenic patients. J Clin Psychiatry 61:594–599, 2000

Lucas RA, Gilfillan DJ, Bergstrom RF: A pharmacokinetic interaction between carbamazepine and olanzapine: observations on possible mechanism. Eur J Clin Pharmacol 54:639–643, 1998

Lucena MI, Blanco E, Corrales MA, et al: Interaction of fluoxetine and valproic acid (letter). Am J Psychiatry 155:575, 1998

Lundmark J, Gunnarsson T, Bengtsson F: A possible interaction between lithium and rofecoxib. Br J Clin Pharmacol 53:403–404, 2002

MacFadden W, Haskins T, Kujawa M, et al: Adjunctive risperidone long-acting inject-able is effective in delaying relapse to a mood episode in patients with frequently relapsing bipolar disorder, in 55th Annual Convention and Scientific Program of the Society of Biological Psychiatry, Washington, DC, May 1–3, 2008 (abstract 584). Biol Psychiatry 63(suppl):186S, 2008

Mäenpää J, Wrighton SA, Bergstrom RF, et al: Pharmacokinetic and pharmacodynamic interactions between fluvoxamine and olanzapine (abstract). Clin Pharmacol Ther 61:225, 1997

Mahatthanatrakul W, Nontaput T, Ridtitid W, et al: Rifampin, a cytochrome P450 3A inducer, decreases plasma concentrations of antipsychotic risperidone in healthy volunteers. J Clin Pharm Ther 32:161–167, 2007

Mallikaarjun S, Salazar DE, Bramer SL: Pharmacokinetics, tolerability, and safety of aripiprazole following multiple oral dosing in normal healthy volunteers. J Clin Pharmacol 44:179–187, 2004

Mann SC, Greenstein RA, Eilers R: Early onset of severe dyskinesia following lithium-haloperidol treatment. Am J Psychiatry 140:1385–1386, 1983

Mannens G, Huang ML, Meuldermans W, et al: Absorption, metabolism, and excretion of risperidone in humans. Drug Metab Dispos 21:1134–1141, 1993

Marchesi C, Paini M, Maggini C: Severe diurnal somnolence induced by fluvoxamine-lithium combination. Pharmacopsychiatry 38:145–146, 2005

Marcus RN, McQuade RD, Carson WH, et al: The efficacy and safety of aripiprazole as adjunctive therapy in major depressive disorder: a second multicenter, random-ized, double-blind, placebo-controlled study. J Clin Psychopharmacol 28:156–165, 2008

Marcus WL: Lithium: a review of its pharmacokinetics, health effects, and toxicology. J Environ Pathol Toxicol Oncol 13:73–79, 1994

Marder SR, McQuade RD, Stock E, et al: Aripiprazole in the treatment of schizophrenia: safety and tolerability in short-term, placebo-controlled trials. Schizophr Res 61:123–136, 2003

Marinkovic D, Timotijevic I, Babinski T, et al: The side-effects of clozapine: a four year follow-up study. Prog Neuropsychopharmacol Biol Psychiatry 18:537–544, 1994

Markowitz JS, DeVane CL: Suspected ciprofloxacin inhibition of olanzapine resulting in increased plasma concentration. J Clin Psychopharmacol 19:289–291, 1999

Martinelli V, Bocchetta A, Palmas AM, et al: An interaction between carbamazepine and fluvoxamine. Br J Clin Pharmacol 36:615–616, 1993

Martínez P, González de Etxabarri S, Ereño C, et al: Acute severe hepatic insufficiency caused by carbamazepine [in Spanish]. Rev Esp Enferm Dig 84:124–126, 1993

Mattson GF, Mattson RH, Cramer JA: Interaction between valproic acid and carbamaz-epine: an in vitro study of protein binding. Ther Drug Monit 4:181–184, 1982

Mattson RH, Cramer JA: Valproic acid and ethosuximide interaction. Ann Neurol 7:583–584, 1980

Mattson RH, Cramer JA, Collins JF: A comparison of valproate with carbamazepine for the treatment of complex partial seizures and secondarily generalized tonic-clonic seizures in adults. The Department of Veterans Affairs Epilepsy Cooperative Study No. 264 Group. N Engl J Med 327:765–771, 1992

May TW, Rambeck B, Jurgens U: Serum concentrations of lamotrigine in epileptic patients: the influence of dose and comedication. Ther Drug Monit 18:523–531, 1996

May TW, Rambeck B, Jurgens U: Influence of oxcarbazepine and methsuximide on lamotrigine concentrations in epileptic patients with and without valproic acid comedication: results of a retrospective study. Ther Drug Monit 21:175–181, 1999

May TW, Rambeck B, Jurgens U: Serum concentrations of levetiracetam in epileptic patients: the influence of dose and co-medication. Ther Drug Monit 25:690–699, 2003

McCarthy RH: Seizures following smoking cessation in a clozapine responder. Pharmacopsychiatry 27:210–211, 1994

McElroy SL, Keck PE, Stanton SP, et al: A randomized comparison of divalproex oral loading versus haloperidol in the initial treatment of acute psychotic mania. J Clin Psychiatry 57:142–146, 1996

McElroy SL, Guerdjikova A, Kotwal R, et al: Atomoxetine in the treatment of binge-eating disorder: a randomized placebo-controlled trial. J Clin Psychiatry 68:390–398, 2007

McIntyre RS, Brecher M, Paulsson B, et al: Quetiapine or haloperidol as monotherapy for bipolar mania: a 12-week, double-blind, randomised, parallel-group, placebo-controlled trial. Eur Neuropsychopharmacol 15:573–585, 2005

McKee PJ, Blacklaw J, Forrest G, et al: A double-blind, placebo-controlled interaction study between oxcarbazepine and carbamazepine, sodium valproate and phenytoin in epileptic patients. Br J Clin Pharmacol 37:27–32, 1994

McQuade RD, Stock E, Marcus R, et al: A comparison of weight change during treatment with olanzapine or aripiprazole: results from a randomized, double-blind study. J Clin Psychiatry 65 (suppl 18):47–56, 2004

Mesdjian E, Dravet C, Cenraud B, et al: Carbamazepine intoxication due to triacetyloleandomycin administration in epileptic patients. Epilepsia 21:489–496, 1980

Meyer JM: Individual changes in clozapine levels after smoking cessation: results and a predictive model. J Clin Psychopharmacol 21:569–574, 2001

Miceli JJ, Anziano RJ, Robarge L, et al: The effect of carbamazepine on the steady-state pharmacokinetics of ziprasidone in healthy volunteers. Br J Clin Pharmacol 49 (suppl 1):65S–70S, 2000a

Miceli JJ, Smith M, Robarge L, et al: The effects of ketoconazole on ziprasidone pharmacokinetics: a placebo-controlled crossover study in healthy volunteers. Br J Clin Pharmacol 49 (suppl 1):71S–76S, 2000b

Migliardi G, D'Arrigo C, Santoro V, et al: Effect of topiramate on plasma concentrations of clozapine, olanzapine, risperidone, and quetiapine in patients with psychotic disorders. Clin Neuropharmacol 30:107–113, 2007

Mikati MA, Schachter SC, Schomer DL, et al: Long-term tolerability, pharmacokinetic and preliminary efficacy study of lamotrigine in patients with resistant partial seizures. Clin Neuropharmacol 12:312–321, 1989

Miller DD: Review and management of clozapine side effects. J Clin Psychiatry 61 (suppl 8):14–17; discussion 18–19, 2000

Miller DD, Fleming F, Holman TL, et al: Plasma clozapine concentrations as a predictor of clinical response: a follow-up study. J Clin Psychiatry 55 (suppl B):117–121, 1994

Miller F, Menninger J, Whitcup SM: Lithium-neuroleptic neurotoxicity in the elderly bipolar patient. J Clin Psychopharmacol 6:176–178, 1986

Miller LG, Bowman RC, Bakht F: Sparing effect of sulindac on lithium levels. J Fam Pract 28:592–593, 1989

Minov C: Risk of QTc prolongation due to combination of ziprasidone and quetiapine [in German]. Psychiatr Prax 31 (suppl 1):S142–S144, 2004

Mitchell JE, Mackenzie TB: Cardiac effects of lithium therapy in man: a review. J Clin Psychiatry 43:47–51, 1982

Molden E, Lunde H, Lunder N, et al: Pharmacokinetic variability of aripiprazole and the active metabolite dehydroaripiprazole in psychiatric patients. Ther Drug Monit 28:744–749, 2006

Monji A, Maekawa T, Miura T, et al: Interactions between lithium and non-steroidal anti-inflammatory drugs. Clin Neuropharmacol 25:241–242, 2002

Mookhoek EJ, Loonen AJ: Retrospective evaluation of the effect of omeprazole on clozapine metabolism. Pharm World Sci 26:180–182, 2004

Morrow J, Russell A, Guthrie E, et al: Malformation risks of antiepileptic drugs in pregnancy: a prospective study from the UK Epilepsy and Pregnancy Register. J Neurol Neurosurg Psychiatry 77:193–198, 2006

Muirhead GJ, Harness J, Holt PR, et al: Ziprasidone and the pharmacokinetics of a combined oral contraceptive. Br J Clin Pharmacol 49 (suppl 1):49S–56S, 2000

Mulsant BH, Foglia JP, Sweet RA, et al: The effects of perphenazine on the concentration of nortriptyline and its hydroxymetabolites in older patients. J Clin Psychopharmacol 17:318–321, 1997

Murphy DJ, Gannon MA, Hartman ML: Extrapyramidal symptoms with addition of lithium to neuroleptics (letter). J Nerv Ment Dis 177:708, 1989

Nacarkucuk E, Saglam H, Okan M: Meropenem decreases serum level of valproic acid. Pediatr Neurol 31:232–234, 2004

Nair P, Lippmann S: Blood dyscrasia with quetiapine and ziprasidone. Psychosomatics 46:89–90, 2005

Nakagami T, Yasui-Furukori N, Saito M, et al: Thioridazine inhibits risperidone metabolism: a clinically relevant drug interaction. J Clin Psychopharmacol 25:89–91, 2005

Nasrallah HA, Churchill CM, Hamdan-Allan GA: Higher frequency of neuroleptic-induced dystonia in mania than in schizophrenia. Am J Psychiatry 145:1455–1456, 1988

Nasrallah HA, Dev V, Rak I, et al: Safety update on quetiapine and lenticular examinations: experience with 300,000 patients (abstract 109), in 38th Annual Meeting of the American College of Neuropsychopharmacology, Acapulco, Mexico, December 13–17, 1999. Nashville, TN, American College of Neuropsychopharmacology, 1999, p 279

Neef C, de Voogd-van der Straaten I: An interaction between cytostatic and anticonvulsant drugs. Clin Pharmacol Ther 43:372–375, 1988

Nemeroff CB, Evans DL, Gyulai L, et al: Double-blind, placebo-controlled comparison of imipramine and paroxetine in the treatment of bipolar depression. Am J Psychiatry 158:906–912, 2001

Nemes ZC, Volavka J, Cooper TB, et al: Lithium and haloperidol. Biol Psychiatry 21:568–569, 1986

Nierenberg AA, Fava M, Trivedi MH, et al: A comparison of lithium and T_3 augmentation following two failed medication treatments for depression: a STAR*D report. Am J Psychiatry 163:1519–1530; quiz 1665, 2006

Noormohamed FH, Lant AF: Renal handling of lithium and the effects of mannitol and arginine vasopressin in man. Clin Sci (Lond) 89:27–36, 1995

Nordenstrom J, Elvius M, Bagedahl-Strindlund M, et al: Biochemical hyperparathyroidism and bone mineral status in patients treated long-term with lithium. Metabolism 43:1563–1567, 1994

Norman TR, Walker RG, Burrows GD: Renal function related changes in lithium kinetics. Clin Pharmacokinet 9:349–353, 1984

Nousbaum JB, Berthou F, Carlhant D, et al: Four-week treatment with omeprazole increases the metabolism of caffeine. Am J Gastroenterol 89:371–375, 1994

Obach R, Borja J, Prunonosa J, et al: Lack of correlation between lithium pharmacokinetic parameters obtained from plasma and saliva. Ther Drug Monit 10:265–268, 1988

Odishaw J, Chen C: Effects of steady-state bupropion on the pharmacokinetics of lamotrigine in healthy subjects. Pharmacotherapy 20:1448–1453, 2000

Ojemann LM, Shastri RA, Wilensky AJ, et al: Comparative pharmacokinetics of zonisamide (CI-912) in epileptic patients on carbamazepine or phenytoin monotherapy. Ther Drug Monit 8:293–296, 1986

Olesen OV, Linnet K: Olanzapine serum concentrations in psychiatric patients given standard doses: the influence of comedication. Ther Drug Monit 21:87–90, 1999

Olesen OV, Linnet K: Identification of the human cytochrome P450 isoforms mediating in vitro N-dealkylation of perphenazine. Br J Clin Pharmacol 50:563–571, 2000

Ono S, Mihara K, Suzuki A, et al: Significant pharmacokinetic interaction between risperidone and carbamazepine: its relationship with CYP2D6 genotypes. Psychopharmacology (Berl) 162:50–54, 2002

Oral ET, Altinbas K, Demirkiran S: Sudden akathisia after a ziprasidone dose reduction (letter). Am J Psychiatry 163:546, 2006

Orr JM, Abbott FS, Farrell K, et al: Interaction between valproic acid and aspirin in epileptic children: serum protein binding and metabolic effects. Clin Pharmacol Ther 31:642–649, 1982

Otani K, Aoshima T: Pharmacogenetics of classical and new antipsychotic drugs. Ther Drug Monit 22:118–121, 2000

Otani K, Ishida M, Kaneko S, et al: Effects of carbamazepine coadministration on plasma concentrations of trazodone and its active metabolite, m-chlorophenylpiperazine. Ther Drug Monit 18:164–167, 1996

Padala PR, Sadiq HJ, Padala KP: Urinary obstruction with citalopram and aripiprazole combination in an elderly patient. J Clin Psychopharmacol 26:667–668, 2006

Pan L, Belpaire FM: In vitro study on the involvement of CYP1A2, CYP2D6 and CYP3A4 in the metabolism of haloperidol and reduced haloperidol. Eur J Clin Pharmacol 55:599–604, 1999

Pandey GN, Goel I, Davis JM: Effect of neuroleptic drugs on lithium uptake by the human erythrocyte. Clin Pharmacol Ther 26:96–102, 1979

Panjehshahin MR, Bowmer CJ, Yates MS: Effect of valproic acid, its unsaturated metabolites and some structurally related fatty acids on the binding of warfarin and dansylsarcosine to human albumin. Biochem Pharmacol 41:1227–1233, 1991

Peano C, Leikin JB, Hanashiro PK: Seizures, ventricular tachycardia, and rhabdomyolysis as a result of ingestion of venlafaxine and lamotrigine. Ann Emerg Med 30:704–708, 1997

Pearson HJ: Interaction of fluoxetine with carbamazepine. J Clin Psychiatry 51:126, 1990

Pellock JM: Carbamazepine side effects in children and adults. Epilepsia 28 (suppl 3): S64–S70, 1987

Perlis RH, Miyahara S, Marangell LB, et al: Long-term implications of early onset in bipolar disorder: data from the first 1000 participants in the Systematic Treatment Enhancement Program for Bipolar Disorder (STEP-BD). Biol Psychiatry 55:875–881, 2004

Perry PJ, Miller DD, Arndt SV, et al: Clozapine and norclozapine plasma concentrations and clinical response of treatment-refractory schizophrenic patients. Am J Psychiatry 148:231–235, 1991

Persson LI, Ben-Menachem E, Bengtsson E, et al: Differences in side effects between a conventional carbamazepine preparation and a slow-release preparation of carbamazepine. Epilepsy Res 6:134–140, 1990

Perucca E, Gidal BE, Baltes E: Effects of antiepileptic comedication on levetiracetam pharmacokinetics: a pooled analysis of data from randomized adjunctive therapy trials. Epilepsy Res 53:47–56, 2003

Peselow ED, Dunner DL, Fieve RR, et al: Lithium carbonate and weight gain. J Affect Disord 2:303–310, 1980

Phelan KM, Mosholder AD, Lu S: Lithium interaction with the cyclooxygenase 2 inhibitors rofecoxib and celecoxib and other nonsteroidal anti-inflammatory drugs. J Clin Psychiatry 64:1328–1334, 2003

Physicians' Desk Reference, 62nd Edition. Montvale, NJ, Thomson Healthcare, 2008

Pihlsgard M, Eliasson E: Significant reduction of sertraline plasma levels by carbamazepine and phenytoin. Eur J Clin Pharmacol 57:915–916, 2002

Pinkofsky HB, Sabu R, Reeves RR: A nifedipine-induced inhibition of lithium clearance. Psychosomatics 38:400–401, 1997

Pinninti NR, de Leon J: Interaction of sertraline with clozapine. J Clin Psychopharmacol 17:119–120, 1997

Pinninti NR, Zelinski G: Does topiramate elevate serum lithium levels? (letter) J Clin Psychopharmacol 22:340, 2002

Pisani F, Narbone MC, Trunfio C, et al: Valproic acid–ethosuximide interaction: a pharmacokinetic study. Epilepsia 25:229–233, 1984

Pisani F, Caputo M, Fazio A, et al: Interaction of carbamazepine-10,11-epoxide, an active metabolite of carbamazepine, with valproate: a pharmacokinetic study. Epilepsia 31:339–342, 1990

Piscitelli SC, Frazier JA, McKenna K, et al: Plasma clozapine and haloperidol concentrations in adolescents with childhood-onset schizophrenia: association with response. J Clin Psychiatry 55 (suppl B):94–97, 1994

Pitterle ME, Collins DM: Carbamazepine-10,11-epoxide evaluation associated with coadministration of loxapine or amoxapine (abstract). Epilepsia 29:654, 1988

Pope HG Jr, Cole JO, Choras PT, et al: Apparent neuroleptic malignant syndrome with clozapine and lithium. J Nerv Ment Dis 174:493–495, 1986

Posner J, Webster H, Yuen WC: Investigation of the ability of lamotrigine, a novel antiepileptic drug, to induce mixed function oxygenase enzymes. Br J Clin Pharmacol 32:658P, 1991

Potkin SG, Bera R, Gulasekaram B, et al: Plasma clozapine concentrations predict clinical response in treatment-resistant schizophrenia. J Clin Psychiatry 55 (suppl B): 133–136, 1994

Potkin SG, Thyrum PT, Alva G, et al: The safety and pharmacokinetics of quetiapine when coadministered with haloperidol, risperidone, or thioridazine. J Clin Psychopharmacol 22:121–130, 2002a

Potkin SG, Thyrum PT, Bera R, et al: Open-label study of the effect of combination quetiapine/lithium therapy on lithium pharmacokinetics and tolerability. Clin Ther 24:1809–1823, 2002b

Potkin SG, Keck PE Jr, Segal S, et al: Ziprasidone in acute bipolar mania: a 21-day randomized, double-blind, placebo-controlled replication trial. J Clin Psychopharmacol 25:301–310, 2005

Prakash C, Kamel A, Gummerus J, et al: Metabolism and excretion of a new antipsychotic drug, ziprasidone, in humans. Drug Metab Dispos 25:863–872, 1997

Prakash C, Kamel A, Cui D, et al: Identification of the major human liver cytochrome P450 isoform(s) responsible for the formation of the primary metabolites of ziprasidone and prediction of possible drug interactions. Br J Clin Pharmacol 49 (suppl 1):35S–42S, 2000

Prakash R, Kelwala S, Ban TA: Neurotoxicity with combined administration of lithium and a neuroleptic. Compr Psychiatry 23:567–571, 1982

Price WA, DiMarzio LR: Verapamil-carbamazepine neurotoxicity (letter). J Clin Psychiatry 49:80, 1988

Price WA, Giannini AJ: Neurotoxicity caused by lithium-verapamil synergism. J Clin Pharmacol 26:717–719, 1986

Price WA, Shalley JE: Lithium-verapamil toxicity in the elderly. J Am Geriatr Soc 35:177–178, 1987

Raaska K, Raitasuo V, Neuvonen PJ: Therapeutic drug monitoring data: risperidone does not increase serum clozapine concentration. Eur J Clin Pharmacol 58:587–591, 2002

Raaska K, Raitasuo V, Laitila J, et al: Effect of caffeine-containing versus decaffeinated coffee on serum clozapine concentrations in hospitalised patients. Basic Clin Pharmacol Toxicol 94:13–18, 2004

Radulovic LL, Wilder BJ, Leppik IE, et al: Lack of interaction of gabapentin with carbamazepine or valproate. Epilepsia 35:155–161, 1994

Ragheb MA: Aspirin does not significantly affect patients' serum lithium levels (letter). J Clin Psychiatry 48:425, 1987a

Ragheb M: Ibuprofen can increase serum lithium level in lithium-treated patients. J Clin Psychiatry 48:161–163, 1987b

Ragheb M: The clinical significance of lithium-nonsteroidal anti-inflammatory drug interactions. J Clin Psychopharmacol 10:350–354, 1990

Ragheb MA, Powell AL: Failure of sulindac to increase serum lithium levels. J Clin Psychiatry 47:33–34, 1986a

Ragheb M, Powell AL: Lithium interaction with sulindac and naproxen. J Clin Psychopharmacol 6:150–154, 1986b

Ragheb M, Ban TA, Buchanan D, et al: Interaction of indomethacin and ibuprofen with lithium in manic patients under a steady-state lithium level. J Clin Psychiatry 41:397–398, 1980

Raitasuo V, Lehtovaara R, Huttunen MO: Carbamazepine and plasma levels of clozapine (letter). Am J Psychiatry 150:169, 1993

Raitasuo V, Lehtovaara R, Huttunen MO: Effect of switching carbamazepine to oxcarbazepine on the plasma levels of neuroleptics: a case report. Psychopharmacology (Berl) 116:115–116, 1994

Rambeck B, Wolf P: Lamotrigine clinical pharmacokinetics. Clin Pharmacokinet 25:433–443, 1993

Rasgon N: The relationship between polycystic ovary syndrome and antiepileptic drugs: a review of the evidence. J Clin Psychopharmacol 24:322–334, 2004

Rasgon NL, Altshuler LL, Fairbanks L, et al: Reproductive function and risk for PCOS in women treated for bipolar disorder. Bipolar Disord 7:246–259, 2005

Rathbone J, Soares-Weiser K: Anticholinergics for neuroleptic-induced acute akathisia. Cochrane Database Syst Rev CD003727, 2004

Ratz Bravo AE, Egger SS, Crespo S, et al: Lithium intoxication as a result of an interaction with rofecoxib. Ann Pharmacother 38:1189–1193, 2004

Ravindran A, Silverstone P, Lacroix D, et al: Risperidone does not affect steady-state pharmacokinetics of divalproex sodium in patients with bipolar disorder. Clin Pharmacokinet 43:733–740, 2004

Ray WA, Chung CP, Murray KT, et al: Atypical antipsychotic drugs and the risk of sudden cardiac death. N Engl J Med 360:225–235, 2009

Reeves RR, Mack JE, Beddingfield JJ: Neurotoxic syndrome associated with risperidone and fluvoxamine. Ann Pharmacother 36:440–443, 2002

Reimann IW, Frölich JC: Effects of diclofenac on lithium kinetics. Clin Pharmacol Ther 30:348–352, 1981

Reimann IW, Diener U, Frölich JC: Indomethacin but not aspirin increases plasma lithium ion levels. Arch Gen Psychiatry 40:283–286, 1983

Reimann IW, Golbs E, Fischer C, et al: Influence of intravenous acetylsalicylic acid and sodium salicylate on human renal function and lithium clearance. Eur J Clin Pharmacol 29:435–441, 1985

Reimers A, Skogvoll E, Sund JK, et al: Drug interactions between lamotrigine and psychoactive drugs: evidence from a therapeutic drug monitoring service. J Clin Psychopharmacol 25:342–348, 2005

Reynolds EH: Neurotoxicity of carbamazepine. Adv Neurol 11:345–353, 1975

Ring BJ, Binkley SN, Vandenbranden M, et al: In vitro interaction of the antipsychotic agent olanzapine with human cytochromes P450 CYP2C9, CYP2C19, CYP2D6 and CYP3A. Br J Clin Pharmacol 41:181–186, 1996a

Ring BJ, Catlow J, Lindsay TJ, et al: Identification of the human cytochromes P450 responsible for the in vitro formation of the major oxidative metabolites of the antipsychotic agent olanzapine. J Pharmacol Exp Ther 276:658–666, 1996b

Rivera-Calimlim L, Kerzner B, Karch FE: Effect of lithium on plasma chlorpromazine levels. Clin Pharmacol Ther 23:451–455, 1978

Rogers MP, Whybrow PC: Clinical hypothyroidism occurring during lithium treatment: two case histories and a review of thyroid function in 19 patients. Am J Psychiatry 128:158–163, 1971

Roh HK, Chung JY, Oh DY, et al: Plasma concentrations of haloperidol are related to CYP2D6 genotype at low, but not high doses of haloperidol in Korean schizophrenic patients. Br J Clin Pharmacol 52:265–271, 2001

Roose SP, Nurnberger JI, Dunner DL, et al: Cardiac sinus node dysfunction during lithium treatment. Am J Psychiatry 136:804–806, 1979

Rosa FW: Spina bifida in infants of women treated with carbamazepine during pregnancy. N Engl J Med 324:674–677, 1991

Rosaria Muscatello M, Pacetti M, Cacciola M, et al: Plasma concentrations of risperidone and olanzapine during coadministration with oxcarbazepine. Epilepsia 46:771–774, 2005

Rosenhagen MC, Schmidt U, Weber F, et al: Combination therapy of lamotrigine and escitalopram may cause myoclonus. J Clin Psychopharmacol 26:346–347, 2006

Rowland A, Elliot DJ, Williams JA, et al: In vitro characterization of lamotrigine N_2-glucuronidation and the lamotrigine-valproic acid interaction. Drug Metab Dispos 34:1055–1062, 2006

Sabers A, Gram L: Newer anticonvulsants: comparative review of drug interactions and adverse effects. Drugs 60:23–33, 2000

Sabers A, Ohman I, Christensen J, et al: Oral contraceptives reduce lamotrigine plasma levels. Neurology 61:570–571, 2003

Sachdeo RC, Sachdeo SK, Walker SA, et al: Steady-state pharmacokinetics of topiramate and carbamazepine in patients with epilepsy during monotherapy and concomitant therapy. Epilepsia 37:774–780, 1996

Sachs GS, Grossman F, Ghaemi SN, et al: Combination of a mood stabilizer with risperidone or haloperidol for treatment of acute mania: a double-blind, placebo-controlled comparison of efficacy and safety. Am J Psychiatry 159:1146–1154, 2002

Sachs G, Chengappa KN, Suppes T, et al: Quetiapine with lithium or divalproex for the treatment of bipolar mania: a randomized, double-blind, placebo-controlled study. Bipolar Disord 6:213–223, 2004

Sachs G, Bowden C, Calabrese JR, et al: Effects of lamotrigine and lithium on body weight during maintenance treatment of bipolar I disorder. Bipolar Disord 8:175–181, 2006a

Sachs G, Sanchez R, Marcus R, et al: Aripiprazole in the treatment of acute manic or mixed episodes in patients with bipolar I disorder: a 3-week placebo-controlled study. J Psychopharmacol 20:536–546, 2006b

Sachs GS, Nierenberg AA, Calabrese JR, et al: Effectiveness of adjunctive antidepressant treatment for bipolar depression. N Engl J Med 356:1711–1722, 2007

Sackellares JC, Sato S, Dreifuss FE, et al: Reduction of steady-state valproate levels by other antiepileptic drugs. Epilepsia 22:437–441, 1981

Saito M, Yasui-Furukori N, Nakagami T, et al: Dose-dependent interaction of paroxetine with risperidone in schizophrenic patients. J Clin Psychopharmacol 25:527–532, 2005

Salama AA, Shafey M: A case of severe lithium toxicity induced by combined fluoxetine and lithium carbonate (letter). Am J Psychiatry 146:278, 1989

Samara EE, Granneman RG, Witt GF, et al: Effect of valproate on the pharmacokinetics and pharmacodynamics of lorazepam. J Clin Pharmacol 37:442–450, 1997

Samara EE, Gustavson LE, El-Shourbagy T, et al: Population analysis of the pharmacokinetics of tiagabine in patients with epilepsy. Epilepsia 39:868–873, 1998

Sandson NB, Marcucci C, Bourke DL, et al: An interaction between aspirin and valproate: the relevance of plasma protein displacement drug-drug interactions. Am J Psychiatry 163:1891–1896, 2006

Sattar SP, Ramaswamy S, Bhatia SC, et al: Somnambulism due to probable interaction of valproic acid and zolpidem. Ann Pharmacother 37:1429–1433, 2003

Schaffer CB, Batra K, Garvey MJ, et al: The effect of haloperidol on serum levels of lithium in adult manic patients. Biol Psychiatry 19:1495–1499, 1984

Schiebar F, Boulton DW, Benson J, et al: No meaningful effect of aripiprazole on the steady-state pharmacokinetics of lamotrigine in subjects with bipolar I disorder (abstract P-477E), in 42nd American Society of Health-System Pharmacists Midyear Clinical Meeting, Las Vegas, NV, December 2–6, 2007. Bethesda, MD, American Society of Health-System Pharmacists, 2007

Schmidt D: Adverse effects of valproate. Epilepsia 25 (suppl 1):S44–S49, 1984

Schou M, Weinstein MR: Problems of lithium maintenance treatment during pregnancy, delivery and lactation. Agressologie 21:7–9, 1980

Seppala NH, Leinonen EV, Lehtonen ML, et al: Clozapine serum concentrations are lower in smoking than in non-smoking schizophrenic patients. Pharmacol Toxicol 85:244–246, 1999

Sernyak MJ, Godleski LS, Griffin RA, et al: Chronic neuroleptic exposure in bipolar outpatients. J Clin Psychiatry 58:193–195, 1997

Shelley RK: Lithium toxicity and mefenamic acid: a possible interaction and the role of prostaglandin inhibition. Br J Psychiatry 151:847–848, 1987

Shimada T, Yamazaki H, Mimura M, et al: Interindividual variations in human liver cytochrome P-450 enzymes involved in the oxidation of drugs, carcinogens and toxic chemicals: studies with liver microsomes of 30 Japanese and 30 Caucasians. J Pharmacol Exp Ther 270:414–423, 1994

Shin JG, Soukhova N, Flockhart DA: Effect of antipsychotic drugs on human liver cytochrome P-450 (CYP) isoforms in vitro: preferential inhibition of CYP2D6. Drug Metab Dispos 27:1078–1084, 1999

Shukla S, Godwin CD, Long LE, et al: Lithium-carbamazepine neurotoxicity and risk factors. Am J Psychiatry 141:1604–1606, 1984

Shulman KI, Mackenzie S, Hardy B: The clinical use of lithium carbonate in old age: a review. Prog Neuropsychopharmacol Biol Psychiatry 11:159–164, 1987

Sidhu J, Job S, Bullman J, et al: Pharmacokinetics and tolerability of lamotrigine and olanzapine coadministered to healthy subjects. Br J Clin Pharmacol 61:420–426, 2006a

Sidhu J, Job S, Singh S, et al: The pharmacokinetic and pharmacodynamic consequences of the co-administration of lamotrigine and a combined oral contraceptive in healthy female subjects. Br J Clin Pharmacol 61:191–199, 2006b

Singer L, Imbs JL, Danion JM, et al: Risk of lithium poisoning during combination with non steroid anti-inflammatory drugs [in French]. Therapie 36:323–326, 1981

Sisodiya SM, Sander JW, Patsalos PN: Carbamazepine toxicity during combination therapy with levetiracetam: a pharmacodynamic interaction. Epilepsy Res 48:217–219, 2002

Sitsen J, Maris F, Timmer C: Drug-drug interaction studies with mirtazapine and carbamazepine in healthy male subjects. Eur J Drug Metab Pharmacokinet 26:109–121, 2001

Skogh E, Reis M, Dahl ML, et al: Therapeutic drug monitoring data on olanzapine and its N-demethyl metabolite in the naturalistic clinical setting. Ther Drug Monit 24:518–526, 2002

Sletten I, Pichardo J, Korol B, et al: The effect of chlorpromazine on lithium excretion in psychiatric subjects. Curr Ther Res Clin Exp 8:441–446, 1966

Slordal L, Samstad S, Bathen J, et al: A life-threatening interaction between lithium and celecoxib. Br J Clin Pharmacol 55:413–414, 2003

Small JG, Klapper MH, Malloy FW, et al: Tolerability and efficacy of clozapine combined with lithium in schizophrenia and schizoaffective disorder. J Clin Psychopharmacol 23:223–228, 2003

Smith MC, Centorrino F, Welge JA, et al: Clinical comparison of extended-release divalproex versus delayed-release divalproex: pooled data analyses from nine trials. Epilepsy Behav 5:746–751, 2004

Smith RE, Helms PM: Adverse effects of lithium therapy in the acutely ill elderly patient. J Clin Psychiatry 43:94–99, 1982

Smith T, Riskin J: Effect of clozapine on plasma nortriptyline concentration. Pharmacopsychiatry 27:41–42, 1994

Snoeck E, Van Peer A, Sack M, et al: Influence of age, renal and liver impairment on the pharmacokinetics of risperidone in man. Psychopharmacology (Berl) 122:223–229, 1995

Sobanski T, Bagli M, Laux G, et al: Serotonin syndrome after lithium add-on medication to paroxetine. Pharmacopsychiatry 30:106–107, 1997

Solomon JG: Seizures during lithium-amitriptyline therapy. Postgrad Med 66:145–146, 148, 1979

Sovner R, Davis JM: A potential drug interaction between fluoxetine and valproic acid (letter). J Clin Psychopharmacol 11:389, 1991

Spina E, Avenoso A, Campo GM, et al: The effect of carbamazepine on the 2-hydroxylation of desipramine. Psychopharmacology (Berl) 117:413–416, 1995

Spina E, Avenoso A, Facciola G, et al: Effect of fluoxetine on the plasma concentrations of clozapine and its major metabolites in patients with schizophrenia. Int Clin Psychopharmacol 13:141–145, 1998

Spina E, Avenoso A, Facciola G, et al: Plasma concentrations of risperidone and 9-hydroxyrisperidone: effect of comedication with carbamazepine or valproate. Ther Drug Monit 22:481–485, 2000a

Spina E, Avenoso A, Salemi M, et al: Plasma concentrations of clozapine and its major metabolites during combined treatment with paroxetine or sertraline. Pharmacopsychiatry 33:213–217, 2000b

Spina E, Avenoso A, Facciola G, et al: Plasma concentrations of risperidone and 9-hydroxyrisperidone during combined treatment with paroxetine. Ther Drug Monit 23:223–227, 2001a

Spina E, Scordo MG, Avenoso A, et al: Adverse drug interaction between risperidone and carbamazepine in a patient with chronic schizophrenia and deficient CYP2D6 activity. J Clin Psychopharmacol 21:108–109, 2001b

Spina E, Avenoso A, Scordo MG, et al: Inhibition of risperidone metabolism by fluoxetine in patients with schizophrenia: a clinically relevant pharmacokinetic drug interaction. J Clin Psychopharmacol 22:419–423, 2002

Spina E, D'Arrigo C, Migliardi G, et al: Plasma risperidone concentrations during combined treatment with sertraline. Ther Drug Monit 26:386–390, 2004

Spina E, D'Arrigo C, Migliardi G, et al: Effect of adjunctive lamotrigine treatment on the plasma concentrations of clozapine, risperidone and olanzapine in patients with schizophrenia or bipolar disorder. Ther Drug Monit 28:599–602, 2006

Spring G, Frankel M: New data on lithium and haloperidol incompatibility. Am J Psychiatry 138:818–821, 1981

Sproule B: Lithium in bipolar disorder: can drug concentrations predict therapeutic effect? Clin Pharmacokinet 41:639–660, 2002

Staines AG, Coughtrie MW, Burchell B: N-glucuronidation of carbamazepine in human tissues is mediated by UGT2B7. J Pharmacol Exp Ther 311:1131–1137, 2004

Steinacher L, Vandel P, Zullino DF, et al: Carbamazepine augmentation in depressive patients non-responding to citalopram: a pharmacokinetic and clinical pilot study. Eur Neuropsychopharmacol 12:255–260, 2002

Steketee RW, Wassilak SG, Adkins WN Jr, et al: Evidence for a high attack rate and efficacy of erythromycin prophylaxis in a pertusis outbreak in a facility for the developmentally disabled. J Infect Dis 157:434–440, 1988

Stockley IH: Interactions between lithium and NSAIDs. CMAJ 152:152–153, 1995

Su YP, Chang CJ, Hwang TJ: Lithium intoxication after valsartan treatment (letter). Psychiatry Clin Neurosci 61:204, 2007

Suppes T, Webb A, Paul B, et al: Clinical outcome in a randomized 1-year trial of clozapine versus treatment as usual for patients with treatment-resistant illness and a history of mania. Am J Psychiatry 156:1164–1169, 1999

Suppes T, Vieta E, Liu S, et al: Maintenance treatment for patients with bipolar I disorder: results from a North American study of quetiapine in combination with lithium or divalproex (trial 127). Am J Psychiatry 166:476–488, 2009

Svinarov DA, Pippenger CE: Valproic acid–carbamazepine interaction: is valproic acid a selective inhibitor of epoxide hydrolase? Ther Drug Monit 17:217–220, 1995

Swainston Harrison T, Perry CM: Aripiprazole: a review of its use in schizophrenia and schizoaffective disorder. Drugs 64:1715–1736, 2004

Swann AC, Berman N, Frazer A, et al: Lithium distribution in mania: single-dose pharmacokinetics and sympathoadrenal function. Psychiatry Res 32:71–84, 1990

Szarfman A, Tonning JM, Levine JG, et al: Atypical antipsychotics and pituitary tumors: a pharmacovigilance study. Pharmacotherapy 26:748–758, 2006

Szegedi A, Wiesner J, Hiemke C: Improved efficacy and fewer side effects under clozapine treatment after addition of fluvoxamine. J Clin Psychopharmacol 15:141–143, 1995

Szegedi A, Anghelescu I, Wiesner J, et al: Addition of low-dose fluvoxamine to low-dose clozapine monotherapy in schizophrenia: drug monitoring and tolerability data from a prospective clinical trial. Pharmacopsychiatry 32:148–153, 1999

Szymura-Oleksiak J, Wyska E, Wasieczko A: Pharmacokinetic interaction between imipramine and carbamazepine in patients with major depression. Psychopharmacology (Berl) 154:38–42, 2001

Takahashi H, Yoshida K, Higuchi H, et al: Development of parkinsonian symptoms after discontinuation of carbamazepine in patients concurrently treated with risperidone: two case reports. Clin Neuropharmacol 24:358–360, 2001

Tartara A, Galimberti CA, Manni R, et al: Differential effects of valproic acid and enzyme-inducing anticonvulsants on nimodipine pharmacokinetics in epileptic patients. Br J Clin Pharmacol 32:335–340, 1991

Taylor D, Ellison Z, Ementon Shaw L, et al: Co-administration of citalopram and clozapine: effect on plasma clozapine levels. Int Clin Psychopharmacol 13:19–21, 1998

Taylor D, Bodani M, Hubbeling A, et al: The effect of nefazodone on clozapine plasma concentrations. Int Clin Psychopharmacol 14:185–187, 1999

Terao T, Abe H, Abe K: Irreversible sinus node dysfunction induced by resumption of lithium therapy. Acta Psychiatr Scand 93:407–408, 1996

Thakker KM, Mangat S, Garnett WR, et al: Comparative bioavailability and steady state fluctuations of Tegretol commercial and carbamazepine OROS tablets in adult and pediatric epileptic patients. Biopharm Drug Dispos 13:559–569, 1992

Thase ME, Macfadden W, Weisler RH, et al: Efficacy of quetiapine monotherapy in bipolar I and II depression: a double-blind, placebo-controlled study (the BOLDER II study). J Clin Psychopharmacol 26:600–609, 2006

Thase ME, Jonas A, Khan A, et al: Aripiprazole monotherapy in nonpsychotic bipolar I depression: results of 2 randomized, placebo-controlled studies. J Clin Psychopharmacol 28:13–20, 2008

Theis JG, Sidhu J, Palmer J, et al: Lack of pharmacokinetic interaction between oxcarbazepine and lamotrigine. Neuropsychopharmacology 30:2269–2274, 2005

Thomsen K, Schou M: Renal lithium excretion in man. Am J Physiol 215:823–827, 1968

Tiihonen J, Vartiainen H, Hakola P: Carbamazepine-induced changes in plasma levels of neuroleptics. Pharmacopsychiatry 28:26–28, 1995

Tiihonen J, Hallikainen T, Ryynanen OP, et al: Lamotrigine in treatment-resistant schizophrenia: a randomized placebo-controlled crossover trial. Biol Psychiatry 54:1241–1248, 2003

Tiihonen J, Halonen P, Wahlbeck K, et al: Topiramate add-on in treatment-resistant schizophrenia: a randomized, double-blind, placebo-controlled, crossover trial. J Clin Psychiatry 66:1012–1015, 2005

Timmer RT, Sands JM: Lithium intoxication. J Am Soc Nephrol 10:666–674, 1999

Tohen M, Castillo J, Baldessarini RJ, et al: Blood dyscrasias with carbamazepine and valproate: a pharmacoepidemiological study of 2,228 patients at risk. Am J Psychiatry 152:413–418, 1995

Tohen M, Sanger TM, McElroy SL, et al: Olanzapine versus placebo in the treatment of acute mania. Olanzapine HGEH Study Group. Am J Psychiatry 156:702–709, 1999

Tohen M, Jacobs TG, Grundy SL, et al: Efficacy of olanzapine in acute bipolar mania: a double-blind, placebo-controlled study. The Olanzapine HGGW Study Group. Arch Gen Psychiatry 57:841–849, 2000

Tohen M, Baker RW, Altshuler LL, et al: Olanzapine versus divalproex in the treatment of acute mania. Am J Psychiatry 159:1011–1017, 2002a

Tohen M, Chengappa KN, Suppes T, et al: Efficacy of olanzapine in combination with valproate or lithium in the treatment of mania in patients partially nonresponsive to valproate or lithium monotherapy. Arch Gen Psychiatry 59:62–69, 2002b

Tohen M, Goldberg JF, Gonzalez-Pinto Arrillaga AM, et al: A 12-week, double-blind comparison of olanzapine vs haloperidol in the treatment of acute mania. Arch Gen Psychiatry 60:1218–1226, 2003a

Tohen M, Ketter TA, Zarate CA, et al: Olanzapine versus divalproex sodium for the treatment of acute mania and maintenance of remission: a 47-week study. Am J Psychiatry 160:1263–1271, 2003b

Tohen M, Vieta E, Calabrese J, et al: Efficacy of olanzapine and olanzapine-fluoxetine combination in the treatment of bipolar I depression. Arch Gen Psychiatry 60:1079–1088, 2003c

Tohen M, Greil W, Calabrese JR, et al: Olanzapine versus lithium in the maintenance treatment of bipolar disorder: a 12-month, randomized, double-blind, controlled clinical trial. Am J Psychiatry 162:1281–1290, 2005

Tohen M, Calabrese JR, Sachs GS, et al: Randomized, placebo-controlled trial of olanzapine as maintenance therapy in patients with bipolar I disorder responding to acute treatment with olanzapine. Am J Psychiatry 163:247–256, 2006

Tohen M, Bowden CL, Smulevich AB, et al: Olanzapine plus carbamazepine v. carbamazepine alone in treating manic episodes. Br J Psychiatry 192:135–143, 2008

Tran JQ, Gerber JG, Kerr BM: Delavirdine: clinical pharmacokinetics and drug interactions. Clin Pharmacokinet 40:207–226, 2001

Tugnait M, Hawes EM, McKay G, et al: Characterization of the human hepatic cytochromes P450 involved in the in vitro oxidation of clozapine. Chem Biol Interact 118:171–189, 1999

Turck D, Heinzel G, Luik G: Steady-state pharmacokinetics of lithium in healthy volunteers receiving concomitant meloxicam. Br J Clin Pharmacol 50:197–204, 2000

Tyson SC, Devane CL, Risch SC: Pharmacokinetic interaction between risperidone and clozapine (letter). Am J Psychiatry 152:1401–1402, 1995

Vainer JL, Chouinard G: Interaction between caffeine and clozapine. J Clin Psychopharmacol 14:284–285, 1994

Vajda FJ, Hitchcock A, Graham J, et al: The Australian Register of Antiepileptic Drugs in Pregnancy: the first 1002 pregnancies. Aust N Z J Obstet Gynaecol 47:468–474, 2007

Valdiserri EV: A possible interaction between lithium and diltiazem: case report. J Clin Psychiatry 46:540–541, 1985

Vandel S, Bertschy G, Baumann P, et al: Fluvoxamine and fluoxetine: interaction studies with amitriptyline, clomipramine and neuroleptics in phenotyped patients. Pharmacol Res 31:347–353, 1995

Vendsborg PB, Bech P, Rafaelsen OJ: Lithium treatment and weight gain. Acta Psychiatr Scand 53:139–147, 1976

Verdoux H, Bourgeois ML: A case of lithium neurotoxicity with irreversible cerebellar syndrome. J Nerv Ment Dis 178:761–762, 1990

Vestergaard P, Amdisen A: Lithium treatment and kidney function: a follow-up study of 237 patients in long-term treatment. Acta Psychiatr Scand 63:333–345, 1981

Vestergaard P, Schou M: The effect of age on lithium dosage requirements. Pharmacopsychiatry 17:199–201, 1984

Vestergaard P, Amdisen A, Hansen HE, et al: Lithium treatment and kidney function: a survey of 237 patients in long-term treatment. Acta Psychiatr Scand 60:504–520, 1979

Vestergaard P, Amdisen A, Schou M: Clinically significant side effects of lithium treatment: a survey of 237 patients in long-term treatment. Acta Psychiatr Scand 62:193–200, 1980

Viala A, Aymard N, Leyris A, et al: Pharmaco-clinical correlations during fluoxetine administration in patients with depressive schizophrenia treated with haloperidol decanoate [in French]. Therapie 51:19–25, 1996

Vieta E, Bourin M, Sanchez R, et al: Effectiveness of aripiprazole v. haloperidol in acute bipolar mania: double-blind, randomised, comparative 12-week trial. Br J Psychiatry 187:235–242, 2005

Vieta E, T'Joen C, McQuade RD, et al: Efficacy of adjunctive aripiprazole to either valproate or lithium in bipolar mania patients partially nonresponsive to valproate/

lithium monotherapy: a placebo-controlled study. Am J Psychiatry 165: 1316–1325, 2008a

Vieta E, Suppes T, Eggens I, et al: Efficacy and safety of quetiapine in combination with lithium or divalproex for maintenance of patients with bipolar I disorder (international trial 126). J Affect Disord 109:251–263, 2008b

Viguera AC, Newport DJ, Ritchie J, et al: Lithium in breast milk and nursing infants: clinical implications. Am J Psychiatry 164:342–345, 2007

von Knorring L, Smigan L, Perris C, et al: Lithium and neuroleptic drugs in combination: effect on lithium RBC/plasma ratio. Int Pharmacopsychiatry 17:287–292, 1982

Wagner ML, Graves NM, Marienau K, et al: Discontinuation of phenytoin and carbamazepine in patients receiving felbamate. Epilepsia 32:398–406, 1991

Walbridge DG, Bazire SR: An interaction between lithium carbonate and piroxicam presenting as lithium toxicity. Br J Psychiatry 147:206–207, 1985

Wang CY, Zhang ZJ, Li WB, et al: The differential effects of steady-state fluvoxamine on the pharmacokinetics of olanzapine and clozapine in healthy volunteers. J Clin Pharmacol 44:785–792, 2004

Ward ME, Musa MN, Bailey L: Clinical pharmacokinetics of lithium. J Clin Pharmacol 34:280–285, 1994

Watson B: Absence status and the concurrent administration of clonazepam and valproate sodium (letter). Am J Hosp Pharm 36:887, 1979

Weigmann H, Gerek S, Zeisig A, et al: Fluvoxamine but not sertraline inhibits the metabolism of olanzapine: evidence from a therapeutic drug monitoring service. Ther Drug Monit 23:410–413, 2001

Weisler RH, Kalali AH, Ketter TA: A multicenter, randomized, double-blind, placebo-controlled trial of extended-release carbamazepine capsules as monotherapy for bipolar disorder patients with manic or mixed episodes. J Clin Psychiatry 65:478–484, 2004a

Weisler RH, Warrington L, Dunn J, et al: Adjunctive ziprasidone in bipolar mania: short-term and long-term data (NR358), in 2004 New Research Program and Abstracts, American Psychiatric Association 157th Annual Meeting, New York, May 1–6, 2004. Washington, DC, American Psychiatric Association, 2004b, pp 132–133

Weisler RH, Keck PE Jr, Swann AC, et al: Extended-release carbamazepine capsules as monotherapy for acute mania in bipolar disorder: a multicenter, randomized, double-blind, placebo-controlled trial. J Clin Psychiatry 66:323–330, 2005

Wen X, Wang JS, Kivisto KT, et al: In vitro evaluation of valproic acid as an inhibitor of human cytochrome P450 isoforms: preferential inhibition of cytochrome P450 2C9 (CYP2C9). Br J Clin Pharmacol 52:547–553, 2001

Werstiuk ES, Grof P, Rotstein E, et al: Effect of combined haloperidol-lithium treatment on vitro RBC lithium uptake in patients with affective disorders. Prog Neuropsychopharmacol Biol Psychiatry 7:831–834, 1983

Wetzel H, Anghelescu I, Szegedi A, et al: Pharmacokinetic interactions of clozapine with selective serotonin reuptake inhibitors: differential effects of fluvoxamine and paroxetine in a prospective study. J Clin Psychopharmacol 18:2–9, 1998

Wilner KD, Tensfeldt TG, Baris B, et al: Single- and multiple-dose pharmacokinetics of ziprasidone in healthy young and elderly volunteers. Br J Clin Pharmacol 49 (suppl 1):15S–20S, 2000

Wilson WH: Addition of lithium to haloperidol in non-affective, antipsychotic non-responsive schizophrenia: a double blind, placebo controlled, parallel design clinical trial. Psychopharmacology (Berl) 111:359–366, 1993

Winsberg ME, DeGolia SG, Strong CM, et al: Divalproex therapy in medication-naive and mood-stabilizer-naive bipolar II depression. J Affect Disord 67:207–212, 2001

Wojcikowski J, Maurel P, Daniel WA: Characterization of human cytochrome p450 enzymes involved in the metabolism of the piperidine-type phenothiazine neuroleptic thioridazine. Drug Metab Dispos 34:471–476, 2006

Wong SL, Cavanaugh J, Shi H, et al: Effects of divalproex sodium on amitriptyline and nortriptyline pharmacokinetics. Clin Pharmacol Ther 60:48–53, 1996

Wong YW, Yeh C, Thyrum PT: The effects of concomitant phenytoin administration on the steady-state pharmacokinetics of quetiapine. J Clin Psychopharmacol 21:89–93, 2001

Wright BA, Jarrett DB: Lithium and calcium channel blockers: possible neurotoxicity. Biol Psychiatry 30:635–636, 1991

Wright JM, Stokes EF, Sweeney VP: Isoniazid-induced carbamazepine toxicity and vice versa: a double drug interaction. N Engl J Med 307:1325–1327, 1982

Wrighton SA, Stevens JC: The human hepatic cytochromes P450 involved in drug metabolism. Crit Rev Toxicol 22:1–21, 1992

Wyszynski DF, Nambisan M, Surve T, et al: Increased rate of major malformations in offspring exposed to valproate during pregnancy. Neurology 64:961–965, 2005

Yassa R: A case of lithium-chlorpromazine interaction. J Clin Psychiatry 47:90–91, 1986

Yassa R, Iskandar H, Nastase C, et al: Carbamazepine and hyponatremia in patients with affective disorder. Am J Psychiatry 145:339–342, 1988

Yasui-Furukori N, Hidestrand M, Spina E, et al: Different enantioselective 9-hydroxylation of risperidone by the two human CYP2D6 and CYP3A4 enzymes. Drug Metab Dispos 29:1263–1268, 2001

Yasui-Furukori N, Kondo T, Mihara K, et al: Significant dose effect of carbamazepine on reduction of steady-state plasma concentration of haloperidol in schizophrenic patients. J Clin Psychopharmacol 23:435–440, 2003

Yatham LN, Grossman F, Augustyns I, et al: Mood stabilisers plus risperidone or placebo in the treatment of acute mania: international, double-blind, randomised controlled trial. Br J Psychiatry 182:141–147, 2003

Yatham LN, Paulsson B, Mullen J, et al: Quetiapine versus placebo in combination with lithium or divalproex for the treatment of bipolar mania. J Clin Psychopharmacol 24:599–606, 2004

Yen YC, Lung FW, Chong MY: Adverse effects of risperidone and haloperidol treatment in schizophrenia. Prog Neuropsychopharmacol Biol Psychiatry 28:285–290, 2004

Yeung CK, Chan HH: Cutaneous adverse effects of lithium: epidemiology and management. Am J Clin Dermatol 5:3–8, 2004

Yoshii K, Kobayashi K, Tsumuji M, et al: Identification of human cytochrome P450 isoforms involved in the 7-hydroxylation of chlorpromazine by human liver microsomes. Life Sci 67:175–184, 2000

Young CR, Bowers MB Jr, Mazure CM: Management of the adverse effects of clozapine. Schizophr Bull 24:381–390, 1998

Yukawa E, Nonaka T, Yukawa M, et al: Pharmacoepidemiologic investigation of a clonazepam-carbamazepine interaction by mixed effect modeling using routine clinical pharmacokinetic data in Japanese patients. J Clin Psychopharmacol 21:588–593, 2001

Yukawa E, Nonaka T, Yukawa M, et al: Pharmacoepidemiologic investigation of a clonazepam valproic acid interaction by mixed effect modeling using routine clinical pharmacokinetic data in Japanese patients. J Clin Pharm Ther 28:497–504, 2003

Zajecka JM, Weisler R, Sachs G, et al: A comparison of the efficacy, safety, and tolerability of divalproex sodium and olanzapine in the treatment of bipolar disorder. J Clin Psychiatry 63:1148–1155, 2002

Zarate CA Jr, Tohen M, Narendran R, et al: The adverse effect profile and efficacy of divalproex sodium compared with valproic acid: a pharmacoepidemiology study. J Clin Psychiatry 60:232–236, 1999

Zevin S, Benowitz NL: Drug interactions with tobacco smoking: an update. Clin Pharmacokinet 36:425–438, 1999

Zimbroff DL, Marcus RN, Manos G, et al: Management of acute agitation in patients with bipolar disorder: efficacy and safety of intramuscular aripiprazole. J Clin Psychopharmacol 27:171–176, 2007

Zwanzger P, Marcuse A, Boerner RJ, et al: Lithium intoxication after administration of AT1 blockers. J Clin Psychiatry 62:208–209, 2001

CHAPTER 14

Antidepressants, Anxiolytics/ Hypnotics, and Other Medications

Pharmacokinetics, Drug Interactions, Adverse Effects, and Administration

Terence A. Ketter, M.D.

Po W. Wang, M.D.

Patients with bipolar disorders commonly have inadequate efficacy or tolerability with the mood stabilizers and antipsychotics that we discussed in the previous chapter. In particular, bipolar depression and comorbid anxiety and substance use disorders often require additional pharmacotherapy in clinical settings. In this chapter, we describe the varying pharmacokinetics, drug-drug interactions, and adverse effects of antidepressants, anxiolytics/hypnotics, and other medications, to permit clinicians to more effectively administer these diverse agents along with the mood stabilizers and antipsychotics described in the preceding chapter, in efforts to provide safe, effective, state-of-the-art pharmacotherapy for patients with bipolar disorders. Florida Best Practice Medication Guidelines are provided in Appendix A, and Quick Reference Medication Facts are provided in Appendix B to assist in this endeavor.

Adjunctive Antidepressants

The mood stabilizers lithium, valproate, and carbamazepine appear to offer more robust antimanic than antidepressant effects, and adjunctive antidepressant therapy is commonly used in treating patients with bipolar disorders (Sharma et al. 1997). However, systematic data to support the practice are limited, and controversy exists regarding efficacy, with some evidence suggesting benefit (Gijsman et al. 2004; Tohen et al. 2003) and other data suggesting lack of benefit (Nemeroff et al. 2001; Sachs et al. 2007). Adjunctive antidepressants need to be administered with care, and in many cases for relatively brief periods, because these agents can induce mania, hypomania, mixed states, and cycle acceleration (Altshuler et al. 1995). The U.S. Food and Drug Administration (FDA) has stipulated that the prescribing information for antidepressants include a boxed warning regarding the risk of increased suicidal ideation and behavior in children and adolescents with antidepressants (4%) compared with placebo (2%) (Licinio and Wong 2005), as well as warnings of similar problems in adults (Lenzer 2005), and the need to screen depressed patients for bipolar disorder (Hirschfeld et al. 2000). However, in at least some (perhaps 15%) patients with bipolar disorders, antidepressants combined with mood stabilizers or second-generation antipsychotics administered longer term may yield benefits (Altshuler et al. 2003). To date, the only antidepressant with FDA approval for bipolar depression is fluoxetine in combination with olanzapine (Tohen et al. 2003).

Selective Serotonin Reuptake Inhibitors

Selective serotonin reuptake inhibitors (SSRIs) are generally well absorbed, with variable (fluvoxamine 53% to citalopram 80%) bioavailability, high (fluvoxamine 80% to sertraline 98%) protein binding, and variable volumes of distribution (citalopram 12 L/kg to fluoxetine up to 45 L/kg), half-lives (fluvoxamine 16 hours to fluoxetine 4 days), metabolite half-lives (norfluoxetine up to 7 days), and clearance (fluoxetine 300 mL/min to fluvoxamine 1,600 mL/min) (Baumann 1992).

Manufacturers have emphasized pharmacokinetic and drug interaction differences among these agents (Baker et al. 1998). SSRIs are metabolized by varying cytochrome P450 (CYP) isoforms, including CYP2D6 (fluoxetine, paroxetine) and CYP3A3/4 (sertraline, citalopram), and they can inhibit CYP2D6 (fluoxetine, paroxetine, and to a lesser extent sertraline), CYP3A3/4 (fluoxetine, fluvoxamine), CYP2C19 (fluvoxamine), CYP1A2 (fluvoxamine), and CYP2C9 (fluoxetine, fluvoxamine) (Baumann 1992). Fluvoxamine inhibits CYP1A2 to a greater extent than CYP2D6 and CYP3A4 (Olesen and Linnet 2000). SSRIs can thus be instigators as well as targets of CYP-mediated drug interactions. The most prominent clinical concerns have been raised with agents that inhibit CYP2D6 and CYP3A3/4, thus increasing serum levels of substrates of these isoforms. Administration of monoamine oxidase inhibitors (MAOIs) and SSRIs within 2 weeks of one another is avoided (in the case of fluoxetine, a 5-week wait is needed before starting MAOIs) because of potentially fatal pharmacodynamic interactions, possibly related to induction of hyperserotonergic states. The sections on mood stabilizers and antipsychotics in Chapter 13 ("Mood Stabilizers and Antipsychotics") describe interactions between these agents and SSRIs.

Decreased libido and sexual function are common with SSRIs (Masand and Gupta 2002; Vanderkooy et al. 2002), and various strategies may be attempted to treat these problems in patients with unipolar major depressive disorder (Hirschfeld 1999; Keltner et al. 2002). Other adverse effects vary across individual agents. For example, patients treated chronically with some of these medications can experience sedation, gastrointestinal disturbance, or weight gain (Blackwell 1981b; Ferguson 2001; Kusturica et al. 2002; Masand and Gupta 2002; Vanderkooy et al. 2002). SSRI calming effects may be welcome in anxious patients but oversedating in anergic patients. SSRI initiation and titration vary across agents, as do the maximum recommended doses (across all indications): fluoxetine (up to 80 mg/day), sertraline (up to 200 mg/day), paroxetine (up to 60 mg/day), controlled-release paroxetine (up to 75 mg/day), fluvoxamine (up to 300 mg/day), citalopram (up to 60 mg/day), and escitalopram (up to 20 mg/day). Mania induction can occur with SSRIs but may be less of an issue than with tricyclic antidepressants (TCAs) (Peet 1994; Stoll et al. 1994) or the serotonin-norepinephrine reuptake inhibitor (SNRI) venlafaxine (Post et al. 2006; Vieta et al. 2002).

Serotonin-Norepinephrine Reuptake Inhibitors

SNRIs act primarily by dual blockade of synaptic serotonin and norepinephrine uptake (Horst and Preskorn 1998; Kasamo et al. 1996). In view of the serotonin uptake blockade, SNRI therapeutic effects (e.g., antidepressant, anxiolytic) and adverse effects (e.g., sexual dysfunction) overlap those of SSRIs. As with SSRIs, administration within 2 weeks of MAOIs should be avoided. The added norepinephrine uptake blockade may confer upon SNRIs additional therapeutic effects (e.g., analgesic) and adverse effects (e.g., hypertension, increased switching into mania) compared with SSRIs.

Venlafaxine is an SNRI that may be effective in bipolar depression (Amsterdam 1998; Post et al. 2006; Vieta et al. 2002). Venlafaxine is only 27% protein bound and has a volume of distribution of 8 L/kg, a half-life of 5 hours, and a clearance of 1,400 mL/min (Taft et al. 1997). The extended-release formulation is preferred in view of the brief half-life of immediate-release venlafaxine, which can result in withdrawal symptoms (Fava et al. 1997). Venlafaxine is metabolized by CYP2D6, and it has minimal effects on CYP450 isoforms, decreasing the risk of drug interactions (Ereshefsky and Dugan 2000). Adverse effects include abnormal ejaculation, gastrointestinal complaints (nausea, dry mouth, and anorexia), central nervous system complaints (dizziness, somnolence, and abnormal dreams), and sweating (Masand and Gupta 2002; Vanderkooy et al. 2002). Venlafaxine is commonly started at 37.5–75 mg/day to avoid early nausea and then increased, as necessary and tolerated, every 4–7 days by 75 mg/day, with recommended final dosages ranging between 375 mg/day for immediate-release and 225 mg/day for extended-release formulations, although clinicians occasionally utilize dosages as high as 450 mg/day of either formulation. In the higher part of the dosage range, venlafaxine can increase blood pressure. Experience with this agent in patients with bipolar depression suggests that mania induction can occur, perhaps at a rate higher than that seen with SSRIs (such as sertraline and paroxetine) and bupropion (Post et al. 2006; Vieta et al. 2002).

Desvenlafaxine is an SNRI that is the major active metabolite of venlafaxine (Yang and Plosker 2008). Desvenlafaxine has bioavailability of 80%, is only 30% protein bound, has a volume of distribution of 3.4 L/kg, a half-life of 11 hours, linear pharmacokinetics in a dosage range of 100–600 mg/day, and is manufactured in an extended-release formulation. Desvenlafaxine is 45% excreted unchanged in the urine, and is metabolized primarily by conjugation, and to a minor extent by CYP3A4 oxidation, and has minimal effects on CYP450 isoforms, decreasing the risk of drug interactions (Yang and Plosker 2008). Adverse effects include nausea, dizziness, insomnia, hyperhidrosis, constipation, somnolence, decreased appetite, anxiety, and sexual dysfunction. As with venlafaxine, desvenlafaxine can increase blood pressure. Desvenlafaxine is started at 50 mg/day. In clinical trials in major depressive disorder, dosages as high as 400 mg/day were more effective than placebo, but no more effective than 50 mg/day, and higher doses yielded more adverse effects. Gradual discontinuation is recommended whenever possible to attenuate the risk of discontinuation symptoms. As it is a relatively new medication, experience with desvenlafaxine in bipolar disorder is very limited.

Duloxetine is a newer SNRI with antidepressant and analgesic effects. Duloxetine is 90% protein bound, has a volume of distribution of 23 L/kg, and has a half-life of 12 hours (Lantz et al. 2003). Duloxetine is metabolized by CYP1A2 and CYP2D6; in view of the former, smoking may reduce and fluvoxamine may increase serum duloxetine concentrations. Duloxetine has minimal effects on CYP450 isoforms, decreasing the risk of hepatically mediated drug interactions. Adverse effects include sexual dysfunction, nausea, dry mouth, constipation, decreased appetite, fatigue, somnolence, and increased sweating. Duloxetine is commonly started at 30 mg/day to avoid early nausea and then increased, as necessary and tolerated, every 4–7 days by 30 mg/day, with final dosages ranging between 60 mg/day for depression and 120 mg/day for diabetic neuropathy. In the higher part of the dosage range, duloxetine can increase blood pressure. Because duloxetine is a newer drug, few data have been published regarding the effects of this agent in patients with bipolar disorder. To date, insufficient data are available to assess the risk of mood elevation with duloxetine compared with other agents such as SSRIs (Vîktrup et al. 2004).

Bupropion and Atypical Antidepressants

A variety of other antidepressants with diverse mechanisms of action have been introduced. In general, these agents have favorable adverse effect profiles compared with TCAs, and some do not cause the sexual difficulties encountered with SSRIs.

Bupropion has nonserotonergic, presumably dopaminergic/noradrenergic, mechanism(s) (Horst and Preskorn 1998). Bupropion is well absorbed, is 85% protein bound, and has a large volume of distribution of 20 L/kg, a half-life of 21 hours, and a clearance of 2,300 mL/min (Goodnick 1991). Immediate-release, sustained-release, and extended-release formulations are available. Bupropion is metabolized by CYP2B6 (Hesse et al. 2000) and can inhibit CYP2D6 (Kotlyar et al. 2005), suggesting potential drug interactions mediated by these isoforms. Carbamazepine (but not valproate) dramatically decreases bupropion and increases (active) metabolite levels (Ketter et al. 1995a). Administration of bupropion within 2 weeks of MAOIs should be avoided. Bupropion is generally well tolerated; lacks the sexual, weight gain, and sedation problems seen with at least some SSRIs (Masand and Gupta 2002); and has energizing effects that may be welcome in anergic patients but overstimulating in anxious patients, but it can cause seizures (Van Wyck Fleet et al. 1983). Adverse effects include abdominal pain, agitation, anxiety, dizziness, dry mouth, insomnia, myalgia, nausea, palpitations, pharyngitis, sweating, tinnitus, and increased urinary frequency (Vanderkooy et al. 2002). The sustained-release and extended-release formulations of bupropion are preferred, because they lower peak serum levels, attenuating the risk of seizures. For example, sustained-release bupropion given in divided doses of up to 300 mg/day decreases the risk of seizures to 0.1%. Adjunctive bupropion is commonly used in treating bipolar depression (Post et al. 2006; Sachs et al. 1994, 2007) and has the advantage of helping with smoking cessation (Tønnesen et al. 2003). Bupropion appears less likely than TCAs (Sachs et al. 1994) and venlafaxine (Post et al. 2006) to cause switches into mania.

Trazodone blocks serotonin receptors 5-HT_1 and 5-HT_2 and α_2 receptors (Marek et al. 1992) and has more prominent sedative than antidepressant properties. Therefore, it is commonly used as an adjunctive hypnotic agent in unipolar major depressive disorder and in bipolar disorder, despite concerns regarding the limited systematic data to support this practice (Mendelson 2005). Trazodone is well absorbed and has 80% bioavailability, 90% protein binding, a moderate volume of distribution of 1 L/kg, a half-life of 4 hours, and a clearance of 120–200 mL/min (Nilsen et al. 1993). Trazodone has relatively few metabolic drug-drug interactions. It is typically given in dosages of 50–200 mg at bedtime, but some patients may tolerate dosages as high as 600 mg/day. The main adverse effects are sedation, dizziness, and psychomotor impairment (Mendelson 2005). Priapism can occur but is rare (Warner et al. 1987). Trazodone has been reported to induce mania (Lennhoff 1987), but limited experience precludes assessment of this risk relative to other agents. However, perhaps because of its rather modest antidepressant effects, the practice of low-dose adjunctive trazodone does not appear clinically to yield much risk of inducing manic switches, but this issue has not been systematically explored.

Nefazodone blocks 5-HT_1, 5-HT_2, and α_2 receptors and serotonin uptake (Horst and Preskorn 1998). It is well absorbed but has only 20% bioavailability, and it has 99% protein binding, a low volume of distribution of 0.5 L/kg, a short half-life of 3 hours, and a clearance of 500–2,000 mL/min (Greene and Barbhaiya 1997). Because nefazodone is a CYP3A3/4 substrate and inhibitor, it can increase serum levels of CYP3A3/4 substrates such as alprazolam, triazolam, and carbamazepine. Nefazodone may increase serum concentrations of clozapine (Khan and Preskorn 2001), but the clinical significance of this interaction has been questioned (Taylor et al. 1999).

Nefazodone labeling includes contraindications to combination with terfenadine, astemizole, cisapride, and pimozide out of concern that elevated levels of these CYP3A3/4 substrates will yield potentially fatal cardiac adverse events. Nefazodone should not be administered within 2 weeks of MAOIs. Nefazodone is typically given in dosages of 300–600 mg, with the bulk of the dosage at bedtime. Nefazodone does not cause sexual problems, and initially its most prominent adverse effects were considered to be sedation, dry mouth, and gastrointestinal disturbance (Khouzam 2000; Masand and Gupta 2002). However, serious hepatotoxicity has markedly decreased the utilization of this agent (Stewart 2002). Few data have been reported regarding nefazodone use in patients with bipolar disorders. Mania induction has been reported with nefazodone (Dubin et al. 1997; Jeffries and al-Jeshi 1995; Zaphiris et al. 1996), but limited experience precludes assessment of this risk relative to other agents.

Mirtazapine blocks α_2, 5-HT$_2$, 5-HT$_3$, and H$_1$ receptors (Gillman 2006). It has only 50% bioavailability and is 85% protein bound, with a volume of distribution of 4 L/kg, a half-life of 30 hours, and a clearance of 500 mL/min (Timmer et al. 2000). Mirtazapine is a CYP2D6, more than CYP1A2 or CYP3A4, substrate and is not a clinically significant enzyme inhibitor. Carbamazepine induces the metabolism of mirtazapine (Sitsen et al. 2001), and TCAs and mirtazapine inhibit metabolism of one another (Sennef et al. 2003), but lithium and mirtazapine do not alter the pharmacokinetics of one another (Sitsen et al. 2000). Administration within 2 weeks of MAOIs should be avoided. Adverse effects include sedation, dizziness, weight gain, cholesterol increases, agranulocytosis (in 0.1% of patients), and transaminase elevation above three times the upper limit of normal (in 2% of patients) (Masand and Gupta 2002; Nutt 1997; Wells and Gelenberg 1981). Few data have been published regarding mirtazapine in patients with bipolar disorders. Mania induction with mirtazapine has been reported (Bhanji et al. 2002; De Leon et al. 1999; Ng 2002), but limited experience precludes assessment of this risk relative to other agents.

Monoamine Oxidase Inhibitors

Monoamine oxidase inhibitors (MAOIs) block the metabolism of serotonin, norepinephrine, and dopamine (Goodman and Charney 1985). Older agents such as phenelzine, tranylcypromine, and isocarboxazid inhibit both monoamine oxidase A (MAO-A) and monoamine oxidase B (MAO-B) irreversibly and are thus called irreversible MAOIs, whereas some newer agents such as moclobemide are reversible inhibitors of monoamine oxidase A (RIMAs).

Irreversible MAOIs are potent antidepressants, effective in treating refractory depression and bipolar depression (Thase et al. 1992). They have brief half-lives that are not directly related to their clinical effects, presumably because of the irreversible nature of their MAO inhibition, which provides an MAO deficit until a sufficient amount of new enzyme is produced (in about 2 weeks) (Mallinger and Smith 1991). Thus, foods and drugs that are incompatible with MAOIs must not be ingested within 2 weeks of discontinuing MAOIs. In addition, MAOIs should not be initiated within about five (parent or metabolite, whichever is greater) half-lives after discontinuing incompatible medications. For most drugs, this means waiting about 2 weeks. However, after discontinuing drugs with long half-lives, or metabolite half-lives, such as fluoxetine, up to 5 weeks should elapse prior to starting MAOIs. Irreversible MAOIs have complex and incompletely characterized metabolism, which has a "suicide" inhibition component, whereby they are inactivated by covalently bonding to MAO. Older irreversible MAOIs have serious and potentially fatal interactions with a variety of high-tyramine foods, such as aged meats, cheese, Chianti wine, and fava beans (Gardner et al. 1996), and with drugs such as SSRIs, clomipramine, venlafaxine, stimulants, decongestants, and opiates (Livingston and Livingston 1996). They appear compatible with lithium, valproate, antipsychotics, trazodone, and anxiolytics. Although concerns have been raised around combining these agents with carbamazepine, limited evidence suggests that this combination may be tolerated and confers benefit in some treatment-refractory bipolar disorder patients (Ketter et al. 1995b). Irreversible MAOIs can cause sedation, sleep fragmentation, orthostasis, gastrointestinal disturbance, urinary retention, and decreased libido and sexual function (Blackwell 1981a; Pollack and Rosenbaum 1987; Rabkin et al. 1984). Irreversible MAOIs, compared with TCAs, may be more effective in bipolar depression and less likely to trigger severe manic switches (Himmelhoch et al. 1991; Thase et al. 1992).

RIMAs, such as moclobemide, may have more modest antidepressant effects than reversible MAOIs but may have utility in bipolar depression (Angst and Stabl 1992; Silverstone 2001). Moclobemide is a benzamide derivative that inhibits MAO-A for about 24 hours (Cesura et al. 1992). It is well absorbed, with 90% bioavailability, and it has low (50%) protein binding, a moderate volume of distribution of 1 L/kg, and a short half-life of 2 hours, which increases with escalating dosages (Mayersohn and Guentert 1995). Moclobemide is a CYP2C19 substrate and inhibits CYP1A2, CYP2C19, and CYP2D6. Unlike irreversible MAOIs, moclobemide lacks serious interactions with high-tyramine foods. However, caution is still necessary with respect to some of the drug-drug interactions described for irreversible MAOIs. Coadministration with SSRIs, SNRIs, or other MAOIs should be avoided. Moclobemide can cause dry mouth, headache, sedation, gastrointestinal disturbance, and sleep fragmentation, but not sexual problems or orthostasis (Vanderkooy et al. 2002). Mania induction has been reported, and may be less frequent than with TCAs (Silverstone 2001), but limited experience precludes assessment of this risk relative to other agents.

Recently, a transdermal formulation of the irreversible MAOI selegiline has been approved for the treatment of unipolar major depressive disorder in the United States. This formulation has a bioavailability of 30%, so that a 20 mg/20 cm^2 patch yields the equivalent of 6 mg of selegiline per 24 hours. Absorption is independent of dosage, which ranges from 6 to 12 mg per 24 hours (Rohatagi et al. 1997). Selegiline is 90% bound to plasma proteins and has a half-life of 24 hours and a clearance of 1,400 mL/min. The transdermal formulation has no first-pass effect, and is metabolized by *N*-dealkylation to *N*-desmethylselegiline, and by N-depropargylation to *R*(−) methamphetamine. This formulation avoids the high gastrointestinal exposure seen with oral MAOIs, so that dietary tyramine ingestion is *not* restricted for the lowest dosage of 6 mg per 24 hours. Insufficient data are available to ascertain the need for dietary restrictions with dosages of 9 or 12 mg per 24 hours. Like oral MAOIs, multiple concurrent medications (such as antidepressants, carbamazepine, oxcarbazepine, opiates, and sympathomimetics) are contraindicated within 2 weeks because of the potential for pharmacodynamic interactions. Carbamazepine may increase rather than decrease serum levels of transdermal selegiline and its metabolites (*Physicians' Desk Reference* 2008). Because transdermal selegiline is a relatively new treatment, limited data have been published regarding its use in patients with bipolar disorder.

Tricyclic Antidepressants

TCAs block reuptake of serotonin and norepinephrine to varying degrees (Goodman and Charney 1985) and in the past were first-line agents in the treatment of unipolar major depressive disorder. TCAs are generally well absorbed and have variable (20%–70%) bioavailability, high (90%) protein binding, half-lives around 24 hours, and variable volumes of distribution (10–30 L/kg) and clearances (300–1,700 mL/min) (Gram 1980). Hydroxylation by CYP2D6 is the rate-limiting metabolic step, and thus serum TCA levels rise with CYP2D6 inhibitors such as fluoxetine, sertraline, paroxetine, haloperidol, methadone, propafenone, and quinidine. TCA serum levels can also rise with methylphenidate, disulfiram, acute ethanol, hormonal contraceptives, cimetidine, chloramphenicol, and possibly valproate and azole antifungals, although the mechanism(s) of these phenomena are less clear. TCA levels fall with carbamazepine, phenobarbital, phenytoin, chronic ethanol, tobacco smoking, and possibly rifampin. Administration within 2 weeks of MAOIs is generally avoided.

TCAs can yield tremor, sedation, orthostasis, and anticholinergic adverse effects (dry mouth, tachycardia, blurred vision) (Beaumont 1988; Kusturica et al. 2002; Pollack and Rosenbaum 1987; Rabkin et al. 1984). Although TCAs may be well tolerated by some individuals, safety and tolerability problems with these agents have generally led them to be replaced by newer antidepressants (Blackwell 1981a; Kusturica et al. 2002). Thus, therapy with TCAs is generally considered a low-priority strategy in treating bipolar depression, because of adverse effects and danger in overdose, and because TCAs are the antidepressants most implicated in causing manic switches (Altshuler et al. 1995; Peet 1994; Sachs et al. 1994; Silverstone 2001; Stoll et al. 1994).

Benzodiazepines and Mechanistically Related Drugs

Benzodiazepines and mechanistically related compounds (such as zaleplon, zolpidem, and eszopiclone) modulate γ-aminobutyric acid (GABA) type A receptor (GABA$_A$) function and produce anxiolytic and hypnotic effects. Patients with bipolar disorders commonly have comorbid anxiety disorders, and may need more anxiolytic and sedative effects than those obtained with mood stabilizers. Thus, adjunctive benzodiazepines and mechanistically related drugs are commonly used in the management of bipolar disorders. Indeed, benzodiazepines are commonly administered along with mood stabilizers and antipsychotics in patients with bipolar disorder, with merely additive central nervous system adverse effects (e.g., sedation, ataxia).

Benzodiazepines and mechanistically related compounds are generally well absorbed, tend to be extensively (95%) protein bound, have moderate volumes of distribution around 1 L/kg, and have half-lives that are short (<6 hours with triazolam, clorazepate, flurazepam, zaleplon, zolpidem, and eszopiclone), intermediate (6–20 hours with alprazolam, lorazepam, oxazepam, and temazepam), and long (>20 hours with diazepam and clonazepam).

The 2-keto-benzodiazepines clorazepate, diazepam, and flurazepam are metabolized by CYP2C19 and CYP3A3/4. Serum levels of these agents are decreased by tobacco smoking, barbiturates, and rifampin, and increased by fluoxetine, fluvoxamine, disulfiram, hormonal contraceptives, ketoconazole, cimetidine, isoniazid, omeprazole, and propranolol. The triazolobenzo-diazepines alprazolam and triazolam have substantial CYP3A3/4 metabolic components. Serum levels of these agents are to varying degrees decreased by carbamazepine, and increased by fluoxetine, fluvoxamine, nefazodone, diltiazem, hormonal contraceptives, ketoconazole, cimetidine, erythromycin, and propoxyphene. In addition, eszopiclone and zolpidem appear susceptible to agents that induce CYP3A4, more so than zaleplon. Also, eszopiclone appears susceptible to agents that inhibit CYP3A4, more so than zaleplon and zolpidem. The 7-nitro-benzodiazepines clonazepam and nitrazepam and the 3-hydroxy-benzodiazepines lorazepam, oxazepam, and temazepam are metabolized by robust N-reduction and conjugation reactions, respectively.

Benzodiazepines and mechanistically related drugs are commonly administered along with mood stabilizers, antipsychotics, and antidepressants in patients with bipolar disorder, in most cases with merely additive central nervous system adverse effects (e.g., sedation, ataxia). Indeed, contemporary controlled acute mania trials of mood stabilizers and antipsychotics routinely permit some adjunctive benzodiazepine (e.g., lorazepam) administration. However, limited data suggest that for at least some patients, caution is indicated with such combinations. Interactions between benzodiazepines and individual mood stabilizers and antipsychotics are described in Chapter 13.

Benzodiazepines and mechanistically related drugs are generally safe and well tolerated in acute treatment, with sedation, memory problems, incoordination, and occasional disinhibition being the main adverse effects. However, chronic use concerns include abuse, tolerance, and withdrawal (Vgontzas et al. 1995). Thus, efforts are made to limit patient exposure to benzodiazepines and mechanistically related drugs and to find alternative agents such as trazodone for insomnia or gabapentin for anxiety. In some patients, very low-dose olanzapine (0.625–2.5 mg) or quetiapine (6.25–25 mg) may allow tapering or discontinuation of benzodiazepines and mechanistically related drugs. Nevertheless, some patients with comorbid anxiety disorders and persistent insomnia may need, tolerate, and responsibly use adjunctive benzodiazepines and mechanistically related drugs on a chronic basis. Benzodiazepines and mechanistically related drugs do not commonly trigger manic switches, although concern has been raised in case reports of patients taking alprazolam, in view of its putative modest antidepressant effects.

Newer Anticonvulsants

A series of newer anticonvulsants have been marketed over the last decade (LaRoche and Helmers 2004), and more are in development (Bialer 2006). Compared with older anticonvulsants, several of the new medications have enhanced tolerability, simpler kinetics, and fewer drug-drug interactions. These drugs have a variety of mechanisms, including enhancing neural inhibition by increasing GABAergic function and/or decreasing neural excitation by decreasing glutamatergic function (Ketter et al. 2003; Macdonald and Kelly 1995). Such agents could yield psychotropic effects because these amino acid neurotransmitters have been implicated in psychiatric disorders (Carlsson et al. 2001; Coyle 2004; Kendell et al. 2005; Ketter and Wang 2003; Ketter et al. 2003; Lloyd et al. 1989; Petty 1995). The psychotropic profiles of these new anticonvulsants have not yet been fully characterized, but important kinetic differences between them have already emerged.

In 2008, the FDA released an alert regarding increased risk of suicidality (suicidal behavior or ideation) in patients with epilepsy or psychiatric disorders for 11 anticonvulsants: carbamazepine, felbamate, gabapentin, lamotrigine, levetiracetam, oxcarbazepine, pregabalin, tiagabine, topiramate, valproate, and zonisamide. In the FDA's analysis, anticonvulsants compared with placebo yielded approximately twice the risk of suicidality (0.43% vs. 0.22%). The relative risk for suicidality was higher in the patients with epilepsy than in those with psychiatric disorders.

Felbamate

The use of felbamate is restricted to patients with refractory epilepsy because of its associations with aplastic anemia and fatal hepatitis (Leppik 1995a; Pennell et al. 1995). Felbamate appears to possess a novel stimulant-like psychotropic profile in epilepsy patients (Ketter et al. 1996).

Gabapentin

Gabapentin and the related anticonvulsant pregabalin have structures similar to GABA but do not appear to be direct functional analogs of GABA. These agents have selective inhibitory effects on voltage-gated calcium channels containing the $\alpha_2\delta$ subunit (Gee et al. 1996; Taylor et al. 1993, 2007) and decreased release of glutamate (Dooley et al. 2000b) and noradrenaline (Dooley et al. 2000a, 2002). Gabapentin increases nonsynaptic GABA release from glia, and is also a substrate and a competitive inhibitor of the large (L) neutral amino acid carrier system (Thurlow et al. 1993) and may modulate (but does not directly block) sodium channels (Taylor 1995; Wamil and McLean 1994).

Gabapentin has an anxiolytic preclinical profile. Emerging data suggested that open gabapentin augmentation was well tolerated and could help some patients with mood disorders (McElroy et al. 1997; Ryback et al. 1997; Schaffer and Schaffer 1997; Young et al. 1997, 1999). Controlled data have suggested efficacy in patients with social phobia (Pande et al. 1999) or panic disorder (Pande et al. 2000b), neuropathic pain (Serpell 2002), chronic daily headache (Spira and Beran 2003), or postherpetic neuralgia (Rowbotham et al. 1998), but have been less encouraging in patients with acute mania (Pande et al. 2000a) or treatment-refractory (primarily rapid-cycling bipolar) mood disorder (Frye et al. 2000).

Although gabapentin has generally favorable pharmacokinetic properties, it has saturable (sublinear) absorption (Stewart et al. 1993) and a bioavailability of 60%, which declines further if individual doses are greater than 900 mg (McLean 1994). Thus, many patients may need to take divided doses of gabapentin. Also, aluminum/magnesium hydroxide antacids modestly decrease gabapentin bioavailability. Like lithium, gabapentin is not bound to plasma proteins, has a moderate volume of distribution of about 1 L/kg, is not metabolized, and is more than 95% excreted unchanged in the urine. Gabapentin has a half-life of about 6 hours and a clearance similar to that of creatinine (120 mL/min, similar to the glomerular filtration rate), so that in a fashion similar to lithium, decreased renal function decreases gabapentin clearance (and dosage may need to be decreased in patients with decreased renal function), and physical activity may increase gabapentin clearance (Borchert 1996). Thus, gabapentin levels could fall with the increase in activity seen in hypomania or mania.

Because gabapentin is excreted unchanged in the urine and lacks effects on hepatic metabolism, it appears to lack hepatically mediated drug-drug interactions (Richens 1993). Thus, gabapentin lacks pharmacokinetic drug interactions with carbamazepine and valproate (Radulovic et al. 1994) and with pregabalin (*Physicians' Desk Reference* 2008) in patients with epilepsy. Also, gabapentin fails to alter lithium kinetics in patients with mood disorders who have normal renal function (Frye et al. 1998). Gabapentin does not yield clinically significant changes in the kinetics of hormonal contraceptives (Eldon et al. 1998).

Gabapentin is generally well tolerated but can cause sedation, dizziness, ataxia, fatigue, and weight gain (Goa and Sorkin 1993). Some evidence suggests that gabapentin can cause behavioral deterioration in some pediatric patients with epilepsy who also suffer from cognitive or behavioral disorders (Lee et al.

1996). Gabapentin can be initiated rapidly in epilepsy patients, with 300 mg, 600 mg, and 900 mg on the first, second, and third days. Final gabapentin dosages usually range between 900 mg/day and an approved maximum of 3,600 mg/day in three or four divided doses (*Physicians' Desk Reference* 2008), which yield serum concentrations of approximately 12–20 μg/mL (70–120 μmol/L) (Johannessen et al. 2003). In controlled trials, final gabapentin dosages ranged between 600 and 3,600 mg/day in an adjunctive acute mania study (Pande et al. 2000a), and the mean final gabapentin dosage was approximately 4,000 mg/day as monotherapy in patients with treatment-resistant (primarily rapid-cycling bipolar) mood disorder (Frye et al. 2000). Lower dosages have been reported to benefit some patients with bipolar disorders (Schaffer and Schaffer 1997). In other controlled trials, final gabapentin dosages ranged between 900 and 3,600 mg/day in social phobia (Pande et al. 1999), 600 and 3,600 mg/day in panic disorder (Pande et al. 2000b), 900 and 2,400 mg/day in neuropathic pain (Serpell 2002), and 1,200 and 3,600 mg/day in postherpetic neuralgia (Rowbotham et al. 1998), and had a mean of 2,400 mg/day in chronic daily headache (Spira and Beran 2003).

Topiramate

Topiramate is a fructopyranose sulfamate that blocks sodium channels (Zona et al. 1997) and AMPA/kainate-gated ion channels (Poulsen et al. 2004). Topiramate also positively modulates $GABA_A$ receptors (Gordey et al. 2000; White et al. 2000) and inhibits carbonic anhydrase (Shank et al. 1994). Although early open reports of topiramate in treating bipolar disorders were encouraging, later multicenter, randomized, double-blind, placebo-controlled studies were discouraging. In several trials, topiramate proved no better or worse than placebo in adults with acute mania (Kushner et al. 2006). However, topiramate appeared effective in several comorbid conditions seen in patients with bipolar disorders, with randomized, double-blind, placebo-controlled trails demonstrating efficacy in eating disorders such as bulimia (Hoopes et al. 2003), binge-eating disorder with obesity (McElroy et al. 2003), and obesity (Bray et al. 2003); alcohol dependence (Johnson et al. 2003); and the prevention of migraine headaches (Brandes et al. 2004). Weight loss has been consistently observed in controlled trials with topiramate, not only in patients with eating disorders, as noted above, but also in manic (Kushner et al. 2006) and depressed (McIntyre et al. 2002) patients with bipolar disorders.

Topiramate has a bioavailability of 80%; absorption independent of food; low (15%) binding to plasma proteins; saturable binding to erythrocytes (which contain carbonic anhydrase), which correlates with hematocrit (Gidal and Lensmeyer 1999); and a moderate volume of distribution of about 0.8 L/kg (Bourgeois 1999). Topiramate has a half-life of about 24 hours, a clearance of about 25 mL/min, and a linear elimination kinetics between dosages of 100 and 800 mg/day. During monotherapy, topiramate is 70% excreted unchanged in the urine; however, when topiramate is combined with enzyme inducers, this figure falls to about 50% (Bialer et al. 2004).

The large renal component of topiramate disposition yields this medication resistant to effects of enzyme inhibitors, yet the limited monotherapy hepatic metabolism component makes it susceptible to enzyme inducers. For example, in epilepsy patients, carbamazepine yields clinically significant decreases in topiramate serum concentrations, but topiramate does not yield clinically significant changes in carbamazepine serum concentrations (Mimrod et al. 2005; Sachdeo et al. 1996). In contrast, valproate (Mimrod et al. 2005; Rosenfeld et al. 1997b) and lamotrigine (Berry et al. 2002) do not appear to have clinically significant pharmacokinetic interactions with topiramate in patients with epilepsy. In an unpublished study, topiramate yielded clinically insignificant decreases in serum lithium concentrations in healthy volunteers (*Physicians' Desk Reference* 2008), but case reports have raised the possibility that topiramate can cause clinically significant increases in serum lithium concentrations in some individuals (Abraham and Owen 2004; Pinninti and Zelinski 2002).

Although levetiracetam does not alter topiramate concentrations, the combination may yield adverse effects through a pharmacodynamic interaction (Glauser et al. 2002). In addition, combination of topiramate with other carbonic anhydrase inhibitors, such as acetazolamide and zonisamide, is not recommended because of concerns about increasing the risk of nephrolithiasis or heat-related problems (oligohydrosis and hyperthermia). Topiramate is a mild enzyme inducer and can decrease blood concentrations of hormonal contraceptives, potentially compromising their efficacy (Rosenfeld et al. 1997a). This effect may be less problematic at dosages of 200 mg/day or less (Doose et al. 2003).

Topiramate does not generally yield clinically significant alterations in serum haloperidol (Bialer et al. 2004), clozapine (Migliardi et al. 2007), risperidone (Bialer et al. 2004; Migliardi et al. 2007), olanzapine (Migliardi et al. 2007; Tiihonen et al. 2005), or quetiapine (Migliardi et al. 2007) concentrations. Administration of topiramate with amitriptyline did not yield clinically significant changes in plasma amitriptyline or nortriptyline concentrations, but the combination might modestly decrease topiramate clearance or increase topiramate bioavailability (Bialer et al. 2004). Oxcarbazepine might modestly decrease serum concentrations of topiramate (May et al. 2002).

Topiramate can cause impaired concentration, weight loss, dizziness, speech problems, somnolence, ataxia, and paresthesias (Fröscher et al. 2005). Topiramate appears associated with renal calculi in 1%–2% of epilepsy patients, presumably because of carbonic anhydrase inhibition (Shorvon 1996). Topiramate has been associated with dosage-related hyperchloremic, non–anion gap, metabolic acidosis; with oligohydrosis and hyperthermia; and rarely with acute myopia with secondary angle closure glaucoma. Affective disturbance, psychosis, aggression, and irritability have occasionally been seen in topiramate-treated patients with epilepsy (Mula et al. 2003a).

In patients with epilepsy, topiramate is started at 50 mg/day and increased by 50 mg/day each week, with a recommended maximum dosage of 400 mg/day in two divided doses (*Physicians' Desk Reference* 2008), which yields serum concentrations of approximately 5–20 µg/mL (15–60 µmol/L) (Johannessen et al. 2003). In epilepsy studies, dosages up to 1,000 mg/day did not improve responses compared with those seen with dosages of 400 mg/day. In patients with migraine, topiramate initiation, titration, and final dosages are about half the amounts used in epilepsy. In controlled trials, final topiramate dosages were between 200 and 600 mg/day in acute mania (Kushner et al. 2006), between 50 and 200 mg/day in migraine (Brandes et al. 2004), between 64 and 384 mg/day in obesity (Bray et al. 2003), approximately 200 mg/day for obesity with binge eating (McElroy et al. 2003) and alcohol dependence (Johnson et al. 2003), and 100 mg/day for bulimia (Hoopes et al. 2003).

Tiagabine

Tiagabine is a nipecotic acid derivative that inhibits GABA reuptake in neurons and glial cells (Suzdak and Jansen 1995). No controlled studies of tiagabine use in treatment of bipolar disorders have been reported. Although some experience with open low-dose tiagabine in bipolar disorders was encouraging (Schaffer et al. 2002), other open reports suggested problems with both efficacy and tolerability. For example, rapid loading of open, primarily adjunctive tiagabine, starting at 20 mg/day (five times the recommended starting dosage), in eight inpatients with acute mania not only was ineffective but also yielded unacceptable adverse effects, with one patient having a seizure (Grunze et al. 1999). These results suggest not only that tiagabine is ineffective in mania, but also that loading or rapid dosage escalation should be avoided and that caution should be exercised in using tiagabine, particularly in the initial titration phase.

However, even more gradual initiation may be problematic: open, primarily adjunctive tiagabine initiated at 4 mg/day and increased weekly as tolerated by 4 mg/day (mean dosage 8.7 mg/day, mean duration 38 days) in outpatients with treatment-refractory bipolar disorder had limited efficacy, and raised tolerability concerns, as 2 of 13 (15%) patients had seizures, which were attributed as likely due to the medication (Suppes et al. 2002). Thus, open studies have raised both efficacy and tolerability concerns regarding tiagabine in treating bipolar disorders. In contrast, small controlled trials have reported that low-dose (≤16 mg/day) tiagabine was generally well tolerated and yielded benefit in generalized anxiety disorder (Rosenthal 2003) and primary insomnia (Roth and Walsh 2004).

Tiagabine is well absorbed, with a bioavailability of about 90%; is extensively (96%) bound to plasma proteins; and has linear kinetics at dosages between 2 and 24 mg/day (Brodie 1995; Gustavson and Mengel 1995). In monotherapy, tiagabine has a half-life of about 8 hours and clearance of about 110 mL/min; with enzyme inducers, the half-life falls to about 4 hours and clearance doubles to about 220 mL/min. Tiagabine is a CYP3A substrate, and is extensively transformed into inactive 5-oxo-tiagabine and glucuronide metabolites, with only 2% being excreted unchanged in the urine (Brodie 1995). The remainder is excreted as metabolites in the feces (65%) and the urine (25%).

Tiagabine neither induces nor inhibits hepatic enzymes and hence is a target rather than an instigator of pharmacokinetic drug interactions. Enzyme inducers such as carbamazepine can yield clinically significant decreases in serum tiagabine concentrations (Samara et al. 1998; So et al. 1995), possibly by induction of CYP3A, whereas tiagabine does not yield clinically significant changes in the pharmacokinetics of carbamazepine, phenytoin (Gustavson et al. 1998a), or valproate (Gustavson et al. 1998b). Valproate does not yield clinically significant changes in serum total tiagabine concentrations (Samara et al. 1998) but appears to displace tiagabine from protein binding sites, yielding an increase in free tiagabine (*Physicians' Desk Reference* 2008). Tiagabine does not yield clinically significant changes in the kinetics of hormonal contraceptives (Mengel et al. 1994).

Tiagabine can cause dizziness, fatigue, sedation, tremor, weakness, and gastrointestinal disturbance (Leppik 1995b). In epilepsy patients also taking enzyme inducers, tiagabine is typically initiated at 4 mg/day and increased weekly by 4–8 mg/day as tolerated, with an approved maximum dosage of 56 mg/day in two to four divided doses (*Physicians' Desk Reference* 2008), which yields serum concentrations of approximately 20–100 ng/mL (50–250 nmol/L) (Johannessen et al. 2003). A 50% decrease in these dosages may be required in patients not taking concurrent enzyme inducers. As noted above, rapid loading of open, primarily adjunctive tiagabine, starting at 20 mg/day, yielded unacceptable adverse effects in patients with acute mania, with one patient having a seizure (Grunze et al. 1999). Furthermore, even more gradual initiation in outpatients with bipolar disorders, with the tiagabine started at 4 mg/day and increased weekly as tolerated by 4 mg/day (mean final dosage 8.7 mg/day), raised tolerability concerns, with 2 of 13 patients having seizures (Suppes et al. 2002).

Oxcarbazepine

Oxcarbazepine, the 10-keto analog of carbamazepine, has both structural and mechanistic similarities to carbamazepine (Ambrósio et al. 2002; McLean et al. 1994). Oxcarbazepine's structural similarity to carbamazepine suggests that oxcarbazepine could have psychotropic effects that overlap those of carbamazepine. As noted below, compared with carbamazepine, oxcarbazepine has more favorable adverse effect and drug interaction profiles. Unfortunately, very little controlled evidence of efficacy has been reported for oxcarbazepine in bipolar disorders, far less than for carbamazepine. Specifically, to date, no large double-blind, placebo-controlled trial has demonstrated oxcarbazepine efficacy in patients with bipolar disorder. Although small, multicenter, active-comparator studies failed to find differences between oxcarbazepine and haloperidol or between oxcarbazepine and lithium in adults with acute mania, insufficient statistical power precludes making conclusions regarding the efficacy of oxcarbazepine in acute mania (Emrich 1990). A more recent, somewhat larger study in pediatric acute mania failed to demonstrate an overall advantage of oxcarbazepine compared with placebo; however, post hoc analyses demonstrated an advantage in children but not in adolescents (Wagner et al. 2006).

Oxcarbazepine has more than 95% absorption, with no clinically significant effect of food on absorption, and may be considered a prodrug that is rapidly and extensively metabolized by cytosol arylketone reductase to its active 10-monohydroxy derivative (MHD), which appears to be the primary component responsible for clinical effects (May et al. 2003a). Oxcarbazepine and MHD have half-lives of 2 and 9 hours, respectively; protein binding of 60% and 40%, respectively; linear elimination kinetics; and no autoinduction of metabolism. MHD has a volume of distribution of 0.5 L/kg, with clearance of 20 mL/min, which is primarily by renal excretion, so that oxcarbazepine dosage may need to be decreased in patients with renal impairment (Rouan et al. 1994).

In contrast to carbamazepine, oxcarbazepine has no autoinduction and less heteroinduction, yielding fewer drug interactions (Baruzzi et al. 1994). Thus, oxcarbazepine does not yield clinically significant alterations in serum concentrations of carbamazepine or valproate (McKee et al. 1994), and compared with carbamazepine, oxcarbazepine yields less robust decreases in serum lamotrigine concentrations (May et al. 1999; Theis et al. 2005). Although oxcarbazepine may decrease serum lamotrigine concentrations (May et al. 1999), the clinical significance of this interaction remains to be established and could vary across patients (Theis et al. 2005). Lamotrigine does not appear to alter oxcarbazepine pharmacokinetics (Theis et al. 2005), although a possible pharmacodynamic interaction has been reported with oxcarbazepine and lamotrigine (Sabers and Gram 2000). Valproate (McKee et al. 1994) and lamotrigine (Theis et al. 2005) do not yield clinically significant changes in serum oxcarbazepine concentrations. In contrast, carbamazepine induces oxcarbazepine metabolism, yielding decreased serum MHD concentrations (McKee et al. 1994).

Oxcarbazepine does not yield clinically significant alterations in serum olanzapine or risperidone concentrations (Rosaria Muscatello et al. 2005). Replacing carbamazepine with oxcarbazepine may increase serum concentrations of citalopram (Leinonen et al. 1996), as well as haloperidol, chlorpromazine, and clozapine (Raitasuo et al. 1994). Oxcarbazepine may modestly decrease serum concentrations of topiramate (May et al. 2002) and levetiracetam (May et al. 2003b).

Like carbamazepine, oxcarbazepine yields clinically significant (about 50%) decreases in serum concentrations of ethinyl estradiol and levonorgestrel derived from hormonal contraceptives, presumably related to CYP3A4 induction (Fattore et al. 1999; Klosterskov Jensen et al. 1992). Oxcarbazepine also yields decreases in serum concentrations of the dihydropyridine calcium channel blocker felodipine, which is also a CYP3A4 substrate (Zaccara et al. 1993). The CYP3A4 inhibitor erythromycin (Keranen et al. 1992) and the antidepressant viloxazine (Pisani et al. 1994) do not yield clinically significant increases in serum oxcarbazepine concentrations, as they do in serum carbamazepine concentrations.

Adverse effects of oxcarbazepine most often involve the central nervous system and include dizziness, sedation, and fatigue (Friis et al. 1993). Oxcarbazepine appears to yield less neurotoxicity and rash than carbamazepine and, unlike carbamazepine, has not been associated with blood dyscrasias (Dam et al. 1989; Reinikainen et al. 1987). Cross-allergy between oxcarbazepine and carbamazepine occurs in about 25% of patients (Van Parys and Meinardi 1994). Hyponatremia occurs with oxcarbazepine (Friis et al. 1993) and may be the main adverse effect that occurs more commonly than with carbamazepine. Adverse effects with oxcarbazepine therapy appear related to serum MHD concentrations, which if over 30 μg/mL indicate increased risk (Striano et al. 2006).

In patients with epilepsy, oxcarbazepine is commonly started at 600 mg/day and increased weekly by 600 mg/day, with final dosages commonly ranging between 900 and 2,400 mg/day in two divided doses (*Physicians' Desk Reference* 2008), which yield serum concentrations of approximately 13–35 μg/mL (50–140 μmol/L) (Johannessen et al. 2003). In an early, small, double-blind, on-off-on acute mania trial, the mean oxcarbazepine dosage was 1,886 mg/day (range 1,800–2,100 mg/day) (Emrich et al. 1983). In small, multicenter, active-comparator acute mania studies, mean oxcarbazepine dosages were 2,400 mg/day and 1,400 mg/day when compared with haloperidol and lithium, respectively (Emrich 1990). In a recent study of acute mania in pediatric patients, oxcarbazepine was increased every 2 days by 300 mg/day to a maximum of 900–2,400 mg/day, with mean dosages of 1,200 mg/day and 2,040 mg/day in children and adolescents, respectively (Wagner et al. 2006).

Levetiracetam

Levetiracetam is the S-enantiomer of the ethyl analog of the nootropic agent piracetam (Shorvon 2001) and has GABAergic (Loscher et al. 1996) and anti-kindling (Loscher et al. 1998) effects, reduces voltage-dependent potassium currents (Madeja et al. 2003), and binds to the synaptic vesicle protein SV2A (Lynch et al. 2004), and thus could have effects on release of neurotransmitters from synaptic vesicles. Open studies suggest that levetiracetam may have efficacy in patients with bipolar disorder (Bersani 2004; Braunig and Kruger 2003; Goldberg and Burdick 2002; Grunze et al. 2003; Kaufman 2004; Kyomen 2006; Post et al. 2005), although reports have also been published of levetiracetam-related depression (Wier et al. 2006) and aggressive behavior (Mula et al. 2004). In controlled pilot studies, levetiracetam was no better than placebo in patients with social anxiety disorder (Zhang et al. 2005), autism (Wasserman et al. 2006), or essential tremor (Handforth and Martin 2004). Levetiracetam was effective in an animal model of mania (Lamberty et al. 2001), and a series of uncontrolled case reports (Braunig and Kruger 2003; Goldberg and Burdick 2002; Kaufman 2004) and case series (Bersani 2004; Grunze et al. 2003; Kyomen 2006; Post et al. 2005) have been encouraging. Controlled studies are needed to assess the effects of levetiracetam in patients with bipolar disorder.

Levetiracetam has a favorable pharmacokinetic profile, with absorption that is not related to food, bioavailability of more than 95%, less than 10% binding to plasma proteins, a moderate volume of distribution of about 0.6 L/kg, linear elimination pharmacokinetics at clinically relevant dosages (between 500 and 5,000 mg/day), a half-life of 8 hours, and clearance of 40 mL/min (Patsalos 2000). Levetiracetam is 66% excreted unchanged in the urine and is 24% hydrolyzed (in blood rather than in liver) to an inactive metabolite (Coupez et al. 2003). In view of the substantive renal clearance, levetiracetam dosage may need to be decreased in patients with impaired renal function. Because the minor metabolic component of levetiracetam disposition involves hydrolysis rather than oxidation or glucuronidation (Patsalos 2004) and levetiracetam does not yield clinically significant changes in hepatic oxidation or glucuronidation (Nicolas et al. 1999), these properties yield a low potential for pharmacokinetic drug interactions (Patsalos 2004).

Levetiracetam does not appear to have clinically significant pharmacokinetic interactions with valproate (Coupez et al. 2003; Gidal et al. 2005; May et al. 2003b; Perucca et al. 2003) or lamotrigine (Gidal et al. 2005; May et al. 2003b; Perucca et al. 2003) in patients with epilepsy. Carbamazepine appears to decrease serum levetiracetam concentrations, but assessments of the potential clinical significance of this interaction vary (Contin et al. 2004; May et al. 2003b; Perucca et al. 2003). Although levetiracetam does not yield clinically significant alterations in serum concentrations of carbamazepine or carbamazepine-epoxide in epilepsy patients (Gidal et al. 2005), levetiracetam plus carbamazepine may yield adverse effects through a pharmacodynamic interaction (Sisodiya et al. 2002).

Levetiracetam does not appear to have clinically significant pharmacokinetic interactions with gabapentin (Gidal et al. 2005; Perucca et al. 2003) or topiramate (May et al. 2003b) in patients with epilepsy, although the levetiracetam plus topiramate combination may yield adverse effects through a pharmacodynamic interaction (Glauser et al. 2002). Levetiracetam does not yield clinically significant alterations in serum concentrations of phenytoin, phenobarbital, or primidone in patients with epilepsy (Gidal et al. 2005). Oxcarbazepine may modestly decrease serum concentrations of levetiracetam (May et al. 2003b). Levetiracetam does not yield clinically significant changes in the metabolism of hormonal contraceptives (Ragueneau-Majlessi et al. 2002).

Levetiracetam is generally well tolerated but can cause somnolence, asthenia, dizziness, coordination problems, and mood/anxiety/behavioral problems (Harden 2001; Mula et al. 2003b, 2004). In patients with epilepsy, the latter occur in 13.3% of adults (vs. 6.2% with placebo) and in 37.6% of children (vs. 18.6% with placebo) (*Physicians' Desk Reference* 2008). Levetiracetam-related behavioral problems appeared to be more common in patients with epilepsy than in patients with cognitive or anxiety disorders (Cramer et al. 2003).

In epilepsy patients, levetiracetam is commonly started at 500–1,000 mg/day and increased, as necessary and tolerated, every 2 weeks by 1,000 mg/day up to 3,000 mg/day in two divided doses (*Physicians' Desk Reference* 2008), yielding serum concentrations of approximately 6–20 µg/mL (35–120 µmol/L) (Johannessen et al. 2003).

Zonisamide

Zonisamide is a sulfonamide that blocks sodium channels (Schauf 1987), reduces T-type calcium currents (Kito et al. 1996), facilitates dopaminergic and serotonergic neurotransmission (Kaneko et al. 1993), and is a weak carbonic anhydrase inhibitor (Masuda and Karasawa 1993). Although zonisamide binds to the GABA/benzodiazepine receptor complex (Mimaki et al. 1990), it does not alter chloride currents and does not appear to have major GABAergic activity. In controlled trials, zonisamide yielded weight loss in obesity patients as monotherapy (Gadde et al. 2003) or combined with bupropion (Gadde et al. 2007), and provided benefit in binge eating disorder with obesity (McElroy et al. 2006). Open studies suggest that zonisamide may have efficacy in patients with bipolar disorder (Anand et al. 2005; Baldassano et al. 2004; Ghaemi et al. 2006; Kanba et al. 1994; McElroy et al. 2005; Wilson and Findling 2007), although other reports have been published of zonisamide-related affective disturbance (Charles et al. 1990; Ozawa et al. 2004; Sullivan et al. 2006). Controlled studies are needed to assess the effects of zonisamide in patients with bipolar disorder.

Zonisamide has generally favorable pharmacokinetic properties, with good (close to 100%) bioavailability, only 40%–60% binding to plasma proteins (but extensive binding to erythrocytes), a clearance of 20 mL/min, and a moderate volume of distribution of 1.5 L/kg (Leppik 2004; Sills and Brodie 2007). Zonisamide has linear pharmacokinetics between 200 and 400 mg/day, but has disproportionate serum concentrations at 800 mg, presumably related to saturable binding to carbonic anhydrase in erythrocytes. As monotherapy, zonisamide has a half-life of 60 hours, which falls to 30 hours if the drug is administered with enzyme inducers. Zonisamide is reduced to 2-sulfamoylacetylphenol, primarily by CYP3A4, and is only 30% excreted unchanged in the urine (Nakasa et al. 1993; Stiff et al. 1992). Zonisamide does not inhibit CYP450 isoenzymes, does not induce its own metabolism, and is a target rather than an instigator of drug interactions.

Carbamazepine decreases serum zonisamide concentrations (Ojemann et al. 1986), whereas zonisamide does not appear to yield clinically significant changes in carbamazepine pharmacokinetics (Ragueneau-Majlessi et al. 2004). Zonisamide and valproate (Ragueneau-Majlessi et al. 2005; Tasaki et al. 1995) and zonisamide and lamotrigine (Levy et al. 2005) do have clinically significant pharmacokinetic interactions in patients with epilepsy.

Phenytoin and phenobarbital decrease serum zonisamide concentrations (Ojemann et al. 1986). A combination of zonisamide with other carbonic anhydrase inhibitors, such as acetazolamide and topiramate, is not recommended because of concerns about increasing the risk of nephrolithiasis or heat-related problems (oligohydrosis and hyperthermia). Zonisamide does not alter hormonal contraceptive pharmacokinetics (Griffith and Dai 2004).

Zonisamide is generally well tolerated, but can cause somnolence, anorexia, dizziness, headache, nausea, and agitation/irritability (Faught 2004; Peters and Sorkin 1993). Zonisamide has been associated with nephrolithiasis in approximately 4% of patients (but only symptomatic in approximately 1% of patients) (*Physicians' Desk Reference* 2008), presumably because of carbonic anhydrase inhibition. In patients with epilepsy, zonisamide is started at 100 mg/day and increased every 2 weeks, as necessary and tolerated, by 100 mg/day, with final dosages commonly ranging between 300 and 600 mg/day in two divided doses (*Physicians' Desk Reference* 2008), yielding serum concentrations of approximately 10–38 µg/mL (45–180 µmol/L) (Johannessen et al. 2003). In a controlled study in obesity, the mean final zonisamide dosage was 427 mg/day (Gadde et al. 2003).

Pregabalin

Pregabalin, or *S*-(+)-3-isobutylgaba, has a structure and mechanisms that overlap those of gabapentin (Ben-Menachem 2004; Sills 2006; Taylor et al. 2007). Both pregabalin and gabapentin are structural but not direct functional analogs of GABA that have selective inhibitory effects on voltage-gated calcium channels containing the $\alpha_2\delta$ subunit (Gee et al. 1996; Taylor et al. 1993, 2007), reducing depolarization-induced calcium influx at nerve terminals (Fink et al. 2002), thus resulting in decreased release of excitatory neurotransmitters such as glutamate (Dooley et al. 2000b) and noradrenaline (Dooley et al. 2000a, 2002).

In controlled trials, pregabalin appeared effective for generalized anxiety disorder (Feltner et al. 2003; Montgomery et al. 2006; Pande et al. 2003; Pohl et al. 2005; Rickels et al. 2005), social anxiety disorder (Pande et al. 2004), neuropathic pain associated with postherpetic neuralgia (Dworkin et al. 2003; Freynhagen et al. 2005; Sabatowski et al. 2004), diabetic peripheral neuropathy (Freynhagen et al. 2005; Richter et al. 2005; Rosenstock et al. 2004), and spinal cord injury (Siddall et al. 2006), as well as for relief of pain, disturbed sleep, and fatigue in fibromyalgia syndrome (Crofford et al. 2005). Because pregabalin is a newer medicine, its effects in patients with bipolar disorder remain to be assessed.

Pregabalin appears to have generally favorable pharmacokinetic properties (Ben-Menachem 2004). Similar to gabapentin, pregabalin is not bound to plasma proteins, has a moderate volume of distribution of 0.5 L/kg, has a half-life of 6 hours (requiring dosing three times a day), is not metabolized, is more than 95% excreted unchanged in urine, and has a clearance of 80 mL/min that varies with creatinine clearance. Thus, decreased renal function decreases gabapentin clearance, and dosage reduction may be necessary in patients with decreased renal function (Randinitis et al. 2003). Pregabalin lacks hepatic metabolism, does not induce or inhibit hepatic metabolism, and lacks metabolic drug interactions. Unlike gabapentin, pregabalin has higher (>90%) bioavailability and absorption that is proportional to dosage. Food has no clinically relevant effect on pregabalin absorption.

Like gabapentin, in view of the absence of hepatic metabolism, pregabalin lacks metabolic drug interactions. Thus, in patients with epilepsy, pregabalin lacks clinically significant pharmacokinetic drug interactions with carbamazepine, valproate, and lamotrigine (Brodie et al. 2005).

In patients with epilepsy, pregabalin lacks clinically significant pharmacokinetic drug interactions with gabapentin and topiramate (*Physicians' Desk Reference* 2008). Although tiagabine does not affect pregabalin pharmacokinetics, the presence or absence of a pregabalin effect on tiagabine pharmacokinetics remains to be established.

Pregabalin does not yield clinically significant changes in the kinetics of hormonal contraceptives (Ben-Menachem 2004).

Pregabalin is generally well tolerated but can cause dizziness, somnolence, dry mouth, edema, blurred vision, weight gain, and problems with concentration/attention (Montgomery 2006). In pain syndromes, pregabalin is started at 150 mg/day and increased to 300 mg/day over 1 week, with a maximum recommended dosage of 600 mg in three divided doses. In controlled trials, dosages have ranged from 150 to 600 mg/day in generalized anxiety disorder (Feltner et al. 2003; Montgomery et al. 2006; Pande et al. 2003; Pohl et al. 2005; Rickels et al. 2005) and social anxiety disorder (Pande et al. 2004). Weighting the dose toward bedtime or administering all at bedtime may enhance tolerability in patients with mood disorders.

Other Medications

Older and emerging evidence suggests the utility of other medications in the management of patients with bipolar disorders. Thyroid hormones, modafinil, and pramipexole are of particular interest, because controlled trials have suggested that they may be useful adjuncts in the management of bipolar disorders.

Thyroid Hormones

L-thyroxine (T_4) and triiodothyronine (T_3, also referred to as liothyronine) are used not only in the treatment of hypothyroidism, which is common in patients with mood disorders, but also as adjuncts in the management of primary mood disorders. T_3 has been used primarily in physiological dosages in addition to other agents (most often antidepressants) to accelerate treatment response in nonrefractory depression and to enhance treatment response in treatment-resistant depression. T_4 in supraphysiological dosages has been used to a more limited extent, primarily in the management of treatment-resistant rapid-cycling bipolar disorder.

T_4 and T_3 diffuse into cell nuclei and bind to thyroid receptors on deoxyribonucleic acid (DNA), and thus are believed to affect DNA transcription and protein synthesis to influence normal growth and development of the central nervous system and bone. The thyroid gland produces T_4 and T_3 in a ratio of approximately 7:1, but the majority (approximately 80%) of T_3 is formed by peripheral deiodination of T_4 to T_3. T_3 has approximately four times the biological potency of T_4 and more rapid onset and offset of action, potentially yielding increased and more dynamic therapeutic and adverse effects, unless dosed accordingly.

T_4 is 40%–80% absorbed and is more than 99% bound to plasma proteins, with a higher protein binding affinity than T_3, and hence a smaller volume of distribution of 0.2 L/kg and a longer half-life of approximately 7 days. T_3 is rapidly (within 4 hours) almost totally (95%) absorbed and has greater than 99% binding to plasma proteins, but has a lower protein binding affinity than T_4 and hence a larger volume of distribution of 0.7 L/kg, and a shorter half-life of approximately 2 days. T_4 and T_3 are metabolized primarily in the liver, by deiodination, conjugation, and sulfation, with primarily renal excretion, but there is a minor bile and gut excretion/enterohepatic circulation excretory component.

The U.S. prescribing information for T_4 and T_3 includes boxed warnings advising not to use thyroid hormones either alone or combined with other agents for the treatment of obesity, because therapeutic dosages are ineffective and larger dosages can yield serious or even life-threatening toxicity, particularly when administered with sympathomimetic amines for weight loss. Other warnings and precautions in the prescribing information include the risks of cardiovascular complications of thyrotoxicosis and bone demineralization. Thyroid hormones may yield cardiac (palpitations, tachycardia, angina, hypertension, arrhythmias), central nervous system (anxiety, insomnia, tremor, headache), and gastrointestinal (nausea, diarrhea, weight loss) adverse effects, as well as diaphoresis. In spite of the above, with appropriate titration, thyroid hormones are generally very well tolerated. Limited studies suggest that long-term administration of supraphysiological dosages of T_4 does not appear to alter bone mineral density in women with mood disorders in general (Bauer et al. 2004; Gyulai et al. 2001), but this may occur in sporadic individuals (Bauer et al. 2004). Thus, it may be prudent to recommend concurrent calcium and vitamin D in patients at risk for bone demineralization.

Drug interactions relevant to the management of bipolar disorder include carbamazepine induction of thyroid hormone metabolism (usually without affecting serum thyrotropin concentrations), increased pharmacodynamic sensitivity to therapeutic and toxic effects of thyroid hormones when administered with antidepressants, and more clinically problematic lithium suppression of thyroid hormone secretion. Also, thyroid hormones and sympathomimetic amines may increase the actions of one another.

The U.S. prescribing information recommends starting T_3 in younger adults at 25 µg/day and increasing by 25 µg/day every 1–2 weeks, as indicated by clinical response and serum T_3 and/or thyrotropin concentrations, with final dosages of 25–75 µg/day. The recommended T_3 starting dosage in elderly patients is 5 µg/day, with increases by 5 µg/day every 1–2 weeks, as indicated by clinical response and/or serum T_3 and thyrotropin concentrations, to final dosages of 25–37.5 µg/day.

A conservative approach, more like the above dosage for elderly patients, may be better tolerated by patients with mood disorder who may be at increased risk for central nervous system adverse effects such as anxiety and tremor and may also be taking antidepressants or other medications that potentiate the effects of T_3. In such patients, tolerability may be enhanced by starting T_3 at 5 µg/day taken in the morning, increasing weekly by 5 μg/day as indicated by clinical response and/or serum T_3 and thyrotropin concentrations, pausing for 2 weeks at 25 μg/day to assess efficacy and tolerability, and then increasing weekly by 5 μg/day, as necessary and tolerated and as indicated by clinical response and/or serum T_3 and thyrotropin concentrations, to as high as 50 μg/day. Mean dosages in mood disorder studies have commonly ranged from approximately 25 to 50 μg/day.

The U.S. prescribing information recommends starting T_4 at 25–50 μg/day in patients over age 50 years (or under age 50 years in patients with cardiac disease), increasing by 25–50 μg/day every 6–8 weeks, as indicated by clinical response and serum T_4 and/or thyrotropin concentrations, to as high as 1.7 μg/kg/day (i.e., 100–125 μg/day for a 70-kg adult), with maximum dosage of 250–300 μg/day. Elderly patients with cardiac disease may require 50% lower dosages.

Supraphysiological T_4 in mood disorder studies has been started at 50 μg/day and increased, as necessary and tolerated, every 3–7 days by 50 μg/day to as high as 500 μg/day (approximately twice the U.S. prescribing information recommended dosage), with the aim of suppressing thyrotropin and increasing free T_4 by at least 50% compared with baseline (Bauer et al. 2002). Mean dosages in such studies have commonly ranged from approximately 300 to 500 μg/day. Supraphysiological dosages of T_4 compared with physiological dosages of T_3 have not been used as extensively in patients with mood disorder, and considerable caution is warranted regarding the careful selection of patients who are considered medically appropriate (particularly with respect to cardiac and bone health).

Modafinil

Modafinil, or 2-[(diphenylmethyl)sulfinyl]acetamide, is a novel agent that promotes wakefulness, with mechanisms of action that remain to be established but that appear to differ from those of amphetamine and related compounds. Modafinil binds to the dopamine reuptake site and increases extracellular dopamine, but does not increase dopamine release. Modafinil's mechanisms may also be related to increasing adrenergic, histaminergic, glutamatergic, and hypocretin neurotransmission and decreasing GABA neurotransmission. Modafinil appears to lack direct actions at norepinephrine, serotonin, dopamine, GABA, adenosine, histamine H_3, melatonin, and benzodiazepine receptors.

Modafinil is approved for the treatment of narcolepsy and shift-work sleep disorder, and as adjunctive treatment for obstructive sleep apnea–hypopnea syndrome. Varying data have been reported regarding its ability to relieve fatigue in patients with multiple sclerosis, chronic fatigue syndrome, HIV, or fibromyalgia, and regarding its utility in children with attention-deficit/hyperactivity disorder. In a multicenter, placebo-controlled, 8-week trial in 311 major depressive disorder SSRI partial responders with persistent fatigue and sleepiness, modafinil 200 mg/day augmentation compared with placebo improved overall clinical condition (Clinical Global Impression—Improvement Scale scores) and tended to yield greater reductions in sleepiness and depression ratings (Fava et al. 2005). A multicenter, placebo-controlled, 6-week trial studied 85 patients who had bipolar I or II disorder with depression and who were sleeping at least 6 hours per night and lacked any history of stimulant-induced mania. In these patients, whose depression was inadequately responsive to a mood stabilizer with or without a concomitant antidepressant, adjunctive modafinil (mean dosage of 177 mg/day) yielded greater improvement in depressive symptoms than did placebo (Frye et al. 2007).

Modafinil has somewhat complex but linear pharmacokinetics (Robertson and Hellriegel 2003). It is a racemic mixture of two optical isomers with different kinetics, in that the S-isomer has a half-life approximately three times that of the R-isomer (armodafinil, which is currently under development), yielding three times greater total exposure of the S-isomer at steady state. The effective elimination half-life at steady state is approximately 15 hours, which reflects primarily that of the S-isomer. The absolute bioavailability has not been established but is not affected overall by food. Modafinil has a moderate 0.9 L/kg volume of distribution, is 60% bound to plasma proteins, and is extensively (approximately 90%) metabolized by deamidation, S-oxidation, aromatic ring hydroxylation, and glucuronidation to inactive metabolites. Modafinil modestly induces CYP3A4, CYP2B6, and CYP1A2; inhibits CYP2C19; and suppresses CYP2C9. Because modafinil induces CYP3A4, and is also in part metabolized by this isoform, there appears to be some autoinduction. In view of its hepatic metabolism, modafinil dosages may need to be adjusted in patients with hepatic impairment.

Modafinil decreases serum concentrations of triazolam by approximately 60% and of ethinyl estradiol by approximately 20%, and may decrease serum concentrations of cyclosporine by approximately 50%. The modest induction of CYP3A4, CYP2B6, and CYP1A2 by modafinil may yield decreased levels of substrates of these isoforms. Modafinil inhibition of CYP2C19 could yield increased levels of drugs that are primarily substrates of this isoform, such as diazepam, as well as increased tricyclic antidepressant levels in individuals deficient in CYP2D6. Because modafinil is in part metabolized by CYP3A4, potent inducers (e.g., carbamazepine) and inhibitors (e.g., fluoxetine, fluvoxamine, nefazodone) of that isoform could decrease or increase modafinil levels, respectively.

Modafinil is a Schedule IV controlled substance because it has clinical (psychoactive and euphoric) effects resembling those of stimulants. In clinical trials for sleep disorders, modafinil was generally well tolerated, with 8% adverse effect discontinuations (vs. 3% with placebo). The most common adverse effects with modafinil were headache, nausea, nervousness, rhinitis, diarrhea, back pain, anxiety, insomnia, dizziness, and dyspepsia. In patients with major depressive disorder, the most common adverse effects with adjunctive modafinil were nausea and feeling jittery. In patients with bipolar depression, the most common adverse effects with adjunctive modafinil were headache and insomnia, and no difference was found between groups in treatment-emergent hypomania or mania (six patients taking modafinil and five taking placebo) or hospitalization for mania (one patient from each group).

The U.S. prescribing information includes a warning of the risk of serious rash, including Stevens-Johnson syndrome. In pediatric clinical trials, 13 of 1,585 (0.8%) patients discontinued modafinil because of rash, including one case of possible Stevens-Johnson syndrome, one case of apparent multiorgan hypersensitivity reaction, and several cases with systemic involvement (e.g., fever, leukopenia). No serious rashes were reported in 4,264 patients in adult clinical trials. In postmarketing experience, Stevens-Johnson syndrome, toxic epidermal necrolysis, and drug rash with eosinophilia and systemic symptoms have been reported in both adults and children, in excess of the expected general population rate of 1–2/million person-years. Rashes with modafinil tend to occur during the first 3 months of therapy. Although benign rashes occur with modafinil, it is not possible to predict which rashes will become serious; therefore, modafinil should be discontinued at the first sign of rash, unless the rash is clearly not drug related. Other warnings in the prescribing information include angioedema and anaphylactoid reactions, multiorgan hypersensitivity reactions, persistent sleepiness (i.e., resistance to modafinil), and psychiatric symptoms, including mania, delusions, hallucinations, and suicidal ideation.

In clinical trials, three patients with left ventricular hypertrophy or mitral valve prolapse experienced chest pain, palpitations, dyspnea, and transient ischemic electrocardigraphic T-wave changes. Thus, modafinil should not be taken by patients with left ventricular hypertrophy or by patients with mitral valve prolapse who experienced the mitral valve prolapse syndrome when previously taking stimulants. Modafinil compared with placebo did not increase blood pressure in short-term (<3 months) clinical trials but was associated with more patients having new or increased use of antihypertensive agents (in 2.4% vs. 0.7% with placebo).

Modafinil causes reproductive problems in rats and rabbits (FDA pregnancy category C). Because it is not known whether modafinil is excreted in breast milk, the prescribing information recommends that caution be exercised when administering modafinil to nursing women.

In sleep disorders, the recommended modafinil dosage is 200 mg in the morning. Although dosages up to 400 mg/day given as a single dose have been well tolerated, they did not appear to be more efficacious than 200 mg/day. In patients with severe hepatic impairment, the dosage should be decreased by 50%. In patients with major depressive disorder, adjunctive modafinil was started at 100 mg/day and increased after 3 days to 200 mg/day.

In a controlled study of patients with bipolar depression, adjunctive modafinil was started at 100 mg each morning and increased after 1 week to 100 mg twice a day (morning and noon so as not to interfere with sleep), with the mean final dosage being 177 mg/day. Occasional patients may tolerate and benefit from further increasing by 100 mg weekly to as high as 400 mg/day. Some patients may prefer a single daily dose in the morning.

Pramipexole

Pramipexole is a synthetic aminothiazole (nonergot) agonist at dopamine D_3 and D_2 receptors that has neurotrophic properties. It has been approved for the treatment of Parkinson's disease and restless legs syndrome. Antidepressant effects have been observed with pramipexole in animal models and in uncontrolled reports on patients with unipolar or bipolar depression (Aiken 2007). Randomized controlled trials suggested efficacy as monotherapy in 174 depressed patients with nonpsychotic unipolar major depressive disorder (Corrigan et al. 2000), and as adjunctive therapy (added to mood stabilizers) in 22 depressed patients with nonpsychotic bipolar I and II disorders (Goldberg et al. 2004), as well as 21 depressed patients with bipolar II disorder (Zarate et al. 2004).

Pramipexole appears to have generally favorable pharmacokinetic properties, with bioavailability of 90%, extent of absorption not affected by food, and minimal first-pass effect. Pramipexole has a large volume of distribution of approximately 7 L/kg and is only approximately 15% bound to plasma proteins, but distributes into red blood cells with an erythrocyte-to-plasma ratio of 2:1. Pramipexole has linear pharmacokinetics, with minimal metabolism, and is 90% renally excreted (presumably by the organic cation transport system), with renal clearance of 400 mL/min (approximately three times the glomerular filtration rate). Renal clearance decreases 75% in patients with severe renal impairment (creatinine clearance 20 mL/min) and 60% in those with moderate renal impairment (creatinine clearance 40 mL/min). Thus, pramipexole dosage may need adjustment in patients with renal insufficiency. The terminal half-life is 8 hours in younger and 12 hours in elderly healthy volunteers.

Pramipexole generally lacks pharmacokinetic drug interactions, although medications secreted by the renal cation transport system, such as cimetidine, ranitidine, diltiazem, triamterene, verapamil, quinidine, and quinine, may yield modest to moderate (20% in general, perhaps more with cimetidine) decreases in pramipexole clearance.

The most common adverse effects with pramipexole in patients with early Parkinson's disease were nausea, dizziness, somnolence, insomnia, constipation, asthenia, and hallucinations, and in patients with restless legs syndrome were nausea and somnolence. In more challenging patients with advanced Parkinson's disease, the most common adverse effects with pramipexole were orthostatic hypotension, dyskinesia, extrapyramidal syndrome, insomnia, dizziness, hallucinations, accidental injury, dream abnormalities, confusion, constipation, asthenia, somnolence, dystonia, gait abnormality, hypertonia, dry mouth, amnesia, and increased urinary frequency. Gradual initiation may decrease the risks of orthostatic hypotension and nausea, with the latter also being reduced by taking pramipexole with food. Warnings in the U.S. prescribing information include the risks of orthostatic hypotension, hallucinations, and falling asleep during activities of daily living. Postmarketing experience suggests that pramipexole may yield impulse control disorders, such as pathological gambling, hypersexuality, and binge eating.

In depressed patients with nonpsychotic bipolar I or II disorder, adjunctive pramipexole was generally well tolerated, with nausea, sedation, and headache being the most common adverse effects; one patient taking adjunctive pramipexole had early discontinuation due to psychotic mania (Goldberg et al. 2004). In depressed patients with bipolar II disorder, adjunctive pramipexole was generally well tolerated, with no early discontinuations due to adverse effects, and insomnia, nausea/vomiting, and tremor being the most common adverse effects; one subject taking adjunctive pramipexole (compared with two taking placebo) developed hypomanic symptoms (Zarate et al. 2004).

Pramipexole causes reproductive problems in rats (FDA pregnancy category C). Because it is not known whether pramipexole is excreted in breast milk, the prescribing information recommends that a decision be made as to whether to discontinue nursing or discontinue the drug, taking into account the importance of the drug to the mother.

In Parkinson's disease, pramipexole is started at 0.125 mg three times a day, increased after 1 week to 0.25 mg three times a day, and thereafter increased weekly by 0.25 mg three times a day to a maximum of 1.5 mg three times a day (4.5 mg/day). These dosages are reduced by 33% in patients with moderate renal impairment (creatinine clearance 35–59 mL/min) and 67% in patients with severe renal impairment (creatinine clearance 15–34 mL/min). In restless legs syndrome, pramipexole is started at 0.125 mg 2–3 hours before bedtime and increased, if necessary, to 0.25 mg 4–7 days later and to 0.5 mg after another 4–7 days.

In a controlled trial in depressed patients with bipolar I or II disorder, adjunctive pramipexole was started at 0.125 mg twice a day and increased every 3–5 days by 0.25 mg/day to a target range of 1.0–2.5 mg/day, with a maximum of 5 mg/day and a mean peak dosage of 1.7 mg/day (Goldberg et al. 2004). In a controlled trial in depressed patients with bipolar II disorder, adjunctive pramipexole was started at 0.125 mg three times a day and increased every 5–7 days by 0.125 mg three times a day to a target range of 1.0–3.0 mg/day, with a maximum of 4.5 mg/day and a mean final dosage of 1.7 mg/day (Zarate et al. 2004).

More gradual initiation may enhance tolerability, so that it may be prudent to start pramipexole at 0.125 mg/day and increase, as necessary and tolerated, by 0.125 mg/day every 4 days to a target range of 1.0–2.0 mg/day, with a maximum of 4.5 mg/day. Because pramipexole may be sedating, a single daily dose at bedtime may be preferred, providing the patient does not experience nausea.

Conclusion

Effective pharmacotherapy of patients with bipolar disorder requires familiarity with pharmacodynamics, dosing, pharmacokinetics, drug interactions, adverse effects, and their management, not only for mood stabilizers and antipsychotics, as described in Chapter 13, but also for antidepressants, benzodiazepines, and other medications, as described in this chapter. In the past, clinicians have relied on observational drug interaction information, but recent characterization of substrates, inhibitors, and inducers of drug metabolism allows not only the development of mechanistic models, but also enhanced anticipation and avoidance of clinical drug-drug interactions (Table 13–14 in Chapter 13). These developments promise to yield safer and more effective therapeutics when psychotropics are combined with one another in the treatment of patients with bipolar disorders. Florida Best Practice Medication Guidelines are provided in Appendix A, and Quick Reference Medication Facts are provided in Appendix B to assist in this endeavor.

References

Abraham G, Owen J: Topiramate can cause lithium toxicity. J Clin Psychopharmacol 24:565–567, 2004

Aiken CB: Pramipexole in psychiatry: a systematic review of the literature. J Clin Psychiatry 68:1230–1236, 2007

Altshuler LL, Post RM, Leverich GS, et al: Antidepressant-induced mania and cycle acceleration: a controversy revisited. Am J Psychiatry 152:1130–1138, 1995

Altshuler L, Suppes T, Black D, et al: Impact of antidepressant discontinuation after acute bipolar depression remission on rates of depressive relapse at 1-year follow-up. Am J Psychiatry 160:1252–1262, 2003

Ambrósio AF, Soares Da-Silva P, Carvalho CM, et al: Mechanisms of action of carbamazepine and its derivatives, oxcarbazepine, BIA 2-093, and BIA 2-024. Neurochem Res 27:121–130, 2002

Amsterdam J: Efficacy and safety of venlafaxine in the treatment of bipolar II major depressive episode. J Clin Psychopharmacol 18:414–417, 1998

Anand A, Bukhari L, Jennings SA, et al: A preliminary open-label study of zonisamide treatment for bipolar depression in 10 patients. J Clin Psychiatry 66:195–198, 2005

Angst J, Stabl M: Efficacy of moclobemide in different patient groups: a meta-analysis of studies. Psychopharmacology (Berl) 106(suppl):S109–S113, 1992

Baker GB, Fang J, Sinha S, et al: Metabolic drug interactions with selective serotonin reuptake inhibitor (SSRI) antidepressants. Neurosci Biobehav Rev 22:325–333, 1998

Baldassano CF, Ghaemi SN, Chang A, et al: Acute treatment of bipolar depression with adjunctive zonisamide: a retrospective chart review. Bipolar Disord 6:432–434, 2004

Baruzzi A, Albani F, Riva R: Oxcarbazepine: pharmacokinetic interactions and their clinical relevance. Epilepsia 35 (suppl 3):S14–S19, 1994

Bauer M, Berghofer A, Bschor T, et al: Supraphysiological doses of L-thyroxine in the maintenance treatment of prophylaxis-resistant affective disorders. Neuropsychopharmacology 27:620–628, 2002

Bauer M, Fairbanks L, Berghofer A, et al: Bone mineral density during maintenance treatment with supraphysiological doses of levothyroxine in affective disorders: a longitudinal study. J Affect Disord 83:183–190, 2004

Baumann P: Clinical pharmacokinetics of citalopram and other selective serotonergic reuptake inhibitors (SSRI). Int Clin Psychopharmacol 6 (suppl 5):13–20, 1992

Beaumont G: Adverse effects of tricyclic and non-tricyclic antidepressants. Int Clin Psychopharmacol 3 (suppl 2):55–61, 1988

Ben-Menachem E: Pregabalin pharmacology and its relevance to clinical practice. Epilepsia 45 (suppl 6):13–18, 2004

Berry DJ, Besag FM, Pool F, et al: Lack of an effect of topiramate on lamotrigine serum concentrations. Epilepsia 43:818–823, 2002

Bersani G: Levetiracetam in bipolar spectrum disorders: first evidence of efficacy in an open, add-on study. Hum Psychopharmacol 19:355–356, 2004

Bhanji NH, Margolese HC, Saint-Laurent M, et al: Dysphoric mania induced by high-dose mirtazapine: a case for "norepinephrine syndrome"? Int Clin Psychopharmacol 17:319–322, 2002

Bialer M: New antiepileptic drugs that are second generation to existing antiepileptic drugs. Expert Opin Investig Drugs 15:637–647, 2006

Bialer M, Doose DR, Murthy B, et al: Pharmacokinetic interactions of topiramate. Clin Pharmacokinet 43:763–780, 2004

Blackwell B: Adverse effects of antidepressant drugs, part 1: monoamine oxidase inhibitors and tricyclics. Drugs 21:201–219, 1981a

Blackwell B: Adverse effects of antidepressant drugs, part 2: "Second generation" antidepressants and rational decision making in antidepressant therapy. Drugs 21:273–282, 1981b

Borchert LD: Exercise-induced exacerbation of partial seizures due to enhanced gabapentin clearance (abstract 6.26). Epilepsia 37 (suppl 5):158, 1996

Bourgeois BF: Pharmacokinetics and metabolism of topiramate. Drugs Today (Barc) 35:43–48, 1999

Brandes JL, Saper JR, Diamond M, et al: Topiramate for migraine prevention: a randomized controlled trial. JAMA 291:965–973, 2004

Braunig P, Kruger S: Levetiracetam in the treatment of rapid cycling bipolar disorder. J Psychopharmacol 17:239–241, 2003

Bray GA, Hollander P, Klein S, et al: A 6-month randomized, placebo-controlled, dose-ranging trial of topiramate for weight loss in obesity. Obes Res 11:722–733, 2003

Brodie MJ: Tiagabine pharmacology in profile. Epilepsia 36 (suppl 6):S7–S9, 1995

Brodie MJ, Wilson EA, Wesche DL, et al: Pregabalin drug interaction studies: lack of effect on the pharmacokinetics of carbamazepine, phenytoin, lamotrigine, and valproate in patients with partial epilepsy. Epilepsia 46:1407–1413, 2005

Carlsson A, Waters N, Holm-Waters S, et al: Interactions between monoamines, glutamate, and GABA in schizophrenia: new evidence. Annu Rev Pharmacol Toxicol 41:237–260, 2001

Cesura AM, Kettler R, Imhof R, et al: Mode of action and characteristics of monoamine oxidase-A inhibition by moclobemide. Psychopharmacology (Berl) 106(suppl):S15–S16, 1992

Charles CL, Stoesz L, Tollefson G: Zonisamide-induced mania. Psychosomatics 31:214–217, 1990

Contin M, Albani F, Riva R, et al: Levetiracetam therapeutic monitoring in patients with epilepsy: effect of concomitant antiepileptic drugs. Ther Drug Monit 26:375–379, 2004

Corrigan MH, Denahan AQ, Wright CE, et al: Comparison of pramipexole, fluoxetine, and placebo in patients with major depression. Depress Anxiety 11:58–65, 2000

Coupez R, Nicolas JM, Browne TR: Levetiracetam, a new antiepileptic agent: lack of in vitro and in vivo pharmacokinetic interaction with valproic acid. Epilepsia 44:171–178, 2003

Coyle JT: The GABA-glutamate connection in schizophrenia: which is the proximate cause? Biochem Pharmacol 68:1507–1514, 2004

Cramer JA, De Rue K, Devinsky O, et al: A systematic review of the behavioral effects of levetiracetam in adults with epilepsy, cognitive disorders, or an anxiety disorder during clinical trials. Epilepsy Behav 4:124–132, 2003

Crofford LJ, Rowbotham MC, Mease PJ, et al: Pregabalin for the treatment of fibromyalgia syndrome: results of a randomized, double-blind, placebo-controlled trial. Arthritis Rheum 52:1264–1273, 2005

Dam M, Ekberg R, Loyning Y, et al: A double-blind study comparing oxcarbazepine and carbamazepine in patients with newly diagnosed, previously untreated epilepsy. Epilepsy Res 3:70–76, 1989

De Leon OA, Furmaga KM, Kaltsounis J: Mirtazapine induced mania in a case of post-stroke depression. J Neuropsychiatry Clin Neurosci 11:115–116, 1999

Dooley DJ, Donovan CM, Pugsley TA: Stimulus-dependent modulation of [(3)H]nor-epinephrine release from rat neocortical slices by gabapentin and pregabalin. J Pharmacol Exp Ther 295:1086–1093, 2000a

Dooley DJ, Mieske CA, Borosky SA: Inhibition of K(+)-evoked glutamate release from rat neocortical and hippocampal slices by gabapentin. Neurosci Lett 280:107–110, 2000b

Dooley DJ, Donovan CM, Meder WP, et al: Preferential action of gabapentin and pregabalin at P/Q-type voltage-sensitive calcium channels: inhibition of K+-evoked [3H]-norepinephrine release from rat neocortical slices. Synapse 45:171–190, 2002

Doose DR, Wang SS, Padmanabhan M, et al: Effect of topiramate or carbamazepine on the pharmacokinetics of an oral contraceptive containing norethindrone and ethinyl estradiol in healthy obese and nonobese female subjects. Epilepsia 44:540–549, 2003

Dubin H, Spier S, Giannandrea P: Nefazodone-induced mania. Am J Psychiatry 154:578–579, 1997

Dworkin RH, Corbin AE, Young JP Jr, et al: Pregabalin for the treatment of postherpetic neuralgia: a randomized, placebo-controlled trial. Neurology 60:1274–1283, 2003

Eldon MA, Underwood BA, Randinitis EJ, et al: Gabapentin does not interact with a contraceptive regimen of norethindrone acetate and ethinyl estradiol. Neurology 50:1146–1148, 1998

Emrich HM: Studies with oxcarbazepine (Trileptal) in acute mania. Int Clin Psychopharmacol 5 (suppl 1):83–88, 1990

Emrich HM, Altmann H, Dose M, et al: Therapeutic effects of GABA-ergic drugs in affective disorders: a preliminary report. Pharmacol Biochem Behav 19:369–372, 1983

Ereshefsky L, Dugan D: Review of the pharmacokinetics, pharmacogenetics, and drug interaction potential of antidepressants: focus on venlafaxine. Depress Anxiety 12 (suppl 1):30–44, 2000

Fattore C, Cipolla G, Gatti G, et al: Induction of ethinylestradiol and levonorgestrel metabolism by oxcarbazepine in healthy women. Epilepsia 40:783–787, 1999

Faught E: Review of United States and European clinical trials of zonisamide in the treatment of refractory partial-onset seizures. Seizure 13 (suppl 1):S59–S65; discussion S71–S72, 2004

Fava M, Mulroy R, Alpert J, et al: Emergence of adverse events following discontinuation of treatment with extended-release venlafaxine. Am J Psychiatry 154:1760–1762, 1997

Fava M, Thase ME, DeBattista C: A multicenter, placebo-controlled study of modafinil augmentation in partial responders to selective serotonin reuptake inhibitors with persistent fatigue and sleepiness. J Clin Psychiatry 66:85–93, 2005

Feltner DE, Crockatt JG, Dubovsky SJ, et al: A randomized, double-blind, placebo-controlled, fixed-dose, multicenter study of pregabalin in patients with generalized anxiety disorder. J Clin Psychopharmacol 23:240–249, 2003

Ferguson JM: SSRI antidepressant medications: adverse effects and tolerability. Prim Care Companion J Clin Psychiatry 3:22–27, 2001

Fink K, Dooley DJ, Meder WP, et al: Inhibition of neuronal Ca(2+) influx by gabapentin and pregabalin in the human neocortex. Neuropharmacology 42:229–236, 2002

Freynhagen R, Strojek K, Griesing T, et al: Efficacy of pregabalin in neuropathic pain evaluated in a 12-week, randomised, double-blind, multicentre, placebo-controlled trial of flexible- and fixed-dose regimens. Pain 115:254–263, 2005

Friis ML, Kristensen O, Boas J, et al: Therapeutic experiences with 947 epileptic outpatients in oxcarbazepine treatment. Acta Neurol Scand 87:224–227, 1993

Fröscher W, Schier KR, Hoffmann M, et al: Topiramate: a prospective study on the relationship between concentration, dosage and adverse events in epileptic patients on combination therapy. Epileptic Disord 7:237–248, 2005

Frye MA, Kimbrell TA, Dunn RT, et al: Gabapentin does not alter single-dose lithium pharmacokinetics. J Clin Psychopharmacol 18:461–464, 1998

Frye MA, Ketter TA, Kimbrell TA, et al: A placebo-controlled study of lamotrigine and gabapentin monotherapy in refractory mood disorders. J Clin Psychopharmacol 20:607–614, 2000

Frye MA, Grunze H, Suppes T, et al: A placebo-controlled evaluation of adjunctive modafinil in the treatment of bipolar depression. Am J Psychiatry 164:1242–1249, 2007

Gadde KM, Franciscy DM, Wagner HR 2nd, et al: Zonisamide for weight loss in obese adults: a randomized controlled trial. JAMA 289:1820–1825, 2003

Gadde KM, Yonish GM, Foust MS, et al: Combination therapy of zonisamide and bupropion for weight reduction in obese women: a preliminary, randomized, open-label study. J Clin Psychiatry 68:1226–1229, 2007

Gardner DM, Shulman KI, Walker SE, et al: The making of a user friendly MAOI diet. J Clin Psychiatry 57:99–104, 1996

Gee NS, Brown JP, Dissanayake VU, et al: The novel anticonvulsant drug, gabapentin (Neurontin), binds to the alpha2delta subunit of a calcium channel. J Biol Chem 271:5768–5776, 1996

Ghaemi SN, Zablotsky B, Filkowski MM, et al: An open prospective study of zonisamide in acute bipolar depression. J Clin Psychopharmacol 26:385–388, 2006

Gidal BE, Lensmeyer GL: Therapeutic monitoring of topiramate: evaluation of the saturable distribution between erythrocytes and plasma of whole blood using an optimized high-pressure liquid chromatography method. Ther Drug Monit 21:567–576, 1999

Gidal BE, Baltes E, Otoul C, et al: Effect of levetiracetam on the pharmacokinetics of adjunctive antiepileptic drugs: a pooled analysis of data from randomized clinical trials. Epilepsy Res 64:1–11, 2005

Gijsman HJ, Geddes JR, Rendell IM, et al: Antidepressants for bipolar depression: a systematic review of randomized, controlled trials. Am J Psychiatry 161:1537–1547, 2004

Gillman PK: A systematic review of the serotonergic effects of mirtazapine in humans: implications for its dual action status. Hum Psychopharmacol 21:117–125, 2006

Glauser TA, Pellock JM, Bebin EM, et al: Efficacy and safety of levetiracetam in children with partial seizures: an open-label trial. Epilepsia 43:518–524, 2002

Goa KL, Sorkin EM: Gabapentin: a review of its pharmacological properties and clinical potential in epilepsy. Drugs 46:409–427, 1993

Goldberg JF, Burdick KE: Levetiracetam for acute mania. Am J Psychiatry 159:148, 2002

Goldberg JF, Burdick KE, Endick CJ: Preliminary randomized, double-blind, placebo-controlled trial of pramipexole added to mood stabilizers for treatment-resistant bipolar depression. Am J Psychiatry 161:564–566, 2004

Goodman WK, Charney DS: Therapeutic applications and mechanisms of action of monoamine oxidase inhibitor and heterocyclic antidepressant drugs. J Clin Psychiatry 46:6–24, 1985

Goodnick PJ: Pharmacokinetics of second generation antidepressants: bupropion. Psychopharmacol Bull 27:513–519, 1991

Gordey M, DeLorey TM, Olsen RW: Differential sensitivity of recombinant GABA(A) receptors expressed in Xenopus oocytes to modulation by topiramate. Epilepsia 41 (suppl 1):S25–S29, 2000

Gram LF: Pharmacokinetics and clinical response to tricyclic antidepressants. Acta Psychiatr Scand Suppl 280:169–180, 1980

Greene DS, Barbhaiya RH: Clinical pharmacokinetics of nefazodone. Clin Pharmacokinet 33:260–275, 1997

Griffith SG, Dai Y: Effect of zonisamide on the pharmacokinetics and pharmacodynamics of a combination ethinyl estradiol–norethindrone oral contraceptive in healthy women. Clin Ther 26:2056–2065, 2004

Grunze H, Erfurth A, Marcuse A, et al: Tiagabine appears not to be efficacious in the treatment of acute mania. J Clin Psychiatry 60:759–762, 1999

Grunze H, Langosch J, Born C, et al: Levetiracetam in the treatment of acute mania: an open add-on study with an on-off-on design. J Clin Psychiatry 64:781–784, 2003

Gustavson LE, Mengel HB: Pharmacokinetics of tiagabine, a gamma-aminobutyric acid–uptake inhibitor, in healthy subjects after single and multiple doses. Epilepsia 36:605–611, 1995

Gustavson LE, Cato A 3rd, Boellner SW, et al: Lack of pharmacokinetic drug interactions between tiagabine and carbamazepine or phenytoin. Am J Ther 5:9–16, 1998a

Gustavson LE, Sommerville KW, Boellner SW, et al: Lack of a clinically significant pharmacokinetic drug interaction between tiagabine and valproate. Am J Ther 5:73–79, 1998b

Gyulai L, Bauer M, Garcia-Espana F, et al: Bone mineral density in pre-and post-menopausal women with affective disorder treated with long-term L-thyroxine augmentation. J Affect Disord 66:185–191, 2001

Handforth A, Martin FC: Pilot efficacy and tolerability: a randomized, placebo-controlled trial of levetiracetam for essential tremor. Mov Disord 19:1215–1221, 2004

Harden C: Safety profile of levetiracetam. Epilepsia 42 (suppl 4):36–39, 2001

Hesse LM, Venkatakrishnan K, Court MH, et al: CYP2B6 mediates the in vitro hydroxylation of bupropion: potential drug interactions with other antidepressants. Drug Metab Dispos 28:1176–1183, 2000

Himmelhoch JM, Thase ME, Mallinger AG, et al: Tranylcypromine versus imipramine in anergic bipolar depression. Am J Psychiatry 148:910–916, 1991

Hirschfeld RM: Management of sexual side effects of antidepressant therapy. J Clin Psychiatry 60 (suppl 14):27–30; discussion 31–35, 1999

Hirschfeld RM, Williams JB, Spitzer RL, et al: Development and validation of a screening instrument for bipolar spectrum disorder: the Mood Disorder Questionnaire. Am J Psychiatry 157:1873–1875, 2000

Hoopes SP, Reimherr FW, Hedges DW, et al: Treatment of bulimia nervosa with topiramate in a randomized, double-blind, placebo-controlled trial, part 1: improvement in binge and purge measures. J Clin Psychiatry 64:1335–1341, 2003

Horst WD, Preskorn SH: Mechanisms of action and clinical characteristics of three atypical antidepressants: venlafaxine, nefazodone, bupropion. J Affect Disord 51:237–254, 1998

Jeffries JJ, al-Jeshi A: Nefazodone-induced mania. Can J Psychiatry 40:218, 1995

Johannessen SI, Battino D, Berry DJ, et al: Therapeutic drug monitoring of the newer antiepileptic drugs. Ther Drug Monit 25:347–363, 2003

Johnson BA, Ait-Daoud N, Bowden CL, et al: Oral topiramate for treatment of alcohol dependence: a randomised controlled trial. Lancet 361:1677–1685, 2003

Kanba S, Yagi G, Kamijima K, et al: The first open study of zonisamide, a novel anticonvulsant, shows efficacy in mania. Prog Neuropsychopharmacol Biol Psychiatry 18:707–715, 1994

Kaneko S, Okada M, Hirano T, et al: Carbamazepine and zonisamide increase extracellular dopamine and serotonin levels in vivo, and carbamazepine does not antagonize adenosine effect in vitro: mechanisms of blockade of seizure spread. Jpn J Psychiatry Neurol 47:371–373, 1993

Kasamo K, Blier P, De Montigny C: Blockade of the serotonin and norepinephrine uptake processes by duloxetine: in vitro and in vivo studies in the rat brain. J Pharmacol Exp Ther 277:278–286, 1996

Kaufman KR: Monotherapy treatment of bipolar disorder with levetiracetam. Epilepsy Behav 5:1017–1020, 2004

Keltner NL, McAfee KM, Taylor CL: Mechanisms and treatments of SSRI-induced sexual dysfunction. Perspect Psychiatr Care 38:111–116, 2002

Kendell SF, Krystal JH, Sanacora G: GABA and glutamate systems as therapeutic targets in depression and mood disorders. Expert Opin Ther Targets 9:153–168, 2005

Keranen T, Jolkkonen J, Jensen PK, et al: Absence of interaction between oxcarbazepine and erythromycin. Acta Neurol Scand 86:120–123, 1992

Ketter TA, Wang PW: The emerging differential roles of GABAergic and antiglutamatergic agents in bipolar disorders. J Clin Psychiatry 64:15–20, 2003

Ketter TA, Jenkins JB, Schroeder DH, et al: Carbamazepine but not valproate induces bupropion metabolism. J Clin Psychopharmacol 15:327–333, 1995a

Ketter TA, Post RM, Parekh PI, et al: Addition of monoamine oxidase inhibitors to carbamazepine: preliminary evidence of safety and antidepressant efficacy in treatment-resistant depression. J Clin Psychiatry 56:471–475, 1995b

Ketter TA, Malow BA, Flamini R, et al: Felbamate monotherapy has stimulant-like effects in patients with epilepsy. Epilepsy Res 23:129–137, 1996

Ketter TA, Wang PW, Becker OV, et al: The diverse roles of anticonvulsants in bipolar disorders. Ann Clin Psychiatry 15:95–108, 2003

Khan AY, Preskorn SH: Increase in plasma levels of clozapine and norclozapine after administration of nefazodone. J Clin Psychiatry 62:375–376, 2001

Khouzam HR: The antidepressant nefazodone: a review of its pharmacology, clinical efficacy, adverse effects, dosage, and administration. J Psychosoc Nurs Ment Health Serv 38:20–25, 2000

Kito M, Maehara M, Watanabe K: Mechanisms of T-type calcium channel blockade by zonisamide. Seizure 5:115–119, 1996

Klosterskov Jensen P, Saano V, Haring P, et al: Possible interaction between oxcarbazepine and an oral contraceptive. Epilepsia 33:1149–1152, 1992

Kotlyar M, Brauer LH, Tracy TS, et al: Inhibition of CYP2D6 activity by bupropion. J Clin Psychopharmacol 25:226–229, 2005

Kushner SF, Khan A, Lane R, et al: Topiramate monotherapy in the management of acute mania: results of four double-blind placebo-controlled trials. Bipolar Disord 8:15–27, 2006

Kusturica J, Zulic I, Loga-Zec S, et al: Frequency and characteristics of side effects associated with antidepressant drugs. Bosn J Basic Med Sci 2:5–11, 2002

Kyomen HH: The use of levetiracetam to decrease mania in elderly bipolar patients. Am J Geriatr Psychiatry 14:985, 2006

Lamberty Y, Margineanu DG, Klitgaard H: Effect of the new antiepileptic drug levetiracetam in an animal model of mania. Epilepsy Behav 2:454–459, 2001

Lantz RJ, Gillespie TA, Rash TJ, et al: Metabolism, excretion, and pharmacokinetics of duloxetine in healthy human subjects. Drug Metab Dispos 31:1142–1150, 2003

LaRoche SM, Helmers SL: The new antiepileptic drugs: scientific review. JAMA 291:605–614, 2004

Lee DO, Steingard RJ, Cesena M, et al: Behavioral side effects of gabapentin in children. Epilepsia 37:87–90, 1996

Leinonen E, Lepola U, Koponen H: Substituting carbamazepine with oxcarbazepine increases citalopram levels: a report on two cases. Pharmacopsychiatry 29:156–158, 1996

Lennhoff M: Trazodone-induced mania. J Clin Psychiatry 48:423–424, 1987

Lenzer J: FDA warns that antidepressants may increase suicidality in adults. BMJ 331:70, 2005

Leppik IE: Felbamate. Epilepsia 36 (suppl 2):S66–S72, 1995a

Leppik IE: Tiagabine: the safety landscape. Epilepsia 36 (suppl 6):S10–S13, 1995b

Leppik IE: Zonisamide: chemistry, mechanism of action, and pharmacokinetics. Seizure 13 (suppl 1):S5–S9; discussion S10, 2004

Levy RH, Ragueneau-Majlessi I, Brodie MJ, et al: Lack of clinically significant pharmacokinetic interactions between zonisamide and lamotrigine at steady state in patients with epilepsy. Ther Drug Monit 27:193–198, 2005

Licinio J, Wong ML: Depression, antidepressants and suicidality: a critical appraisal. Nat Rev Drug Discov 4:165–171, 2005

Livingston MG, Livingston HM: Monoamine oxidase inhibitors: an update on drug interactions. Drug Saf 14:219–227, 1996

Lloyd KG, Zivkovic B, Scatton B, et al: The gabaergic hypothesis of depression. Prog Neuropsychopharmacol Biol Psychiatry 13:341–351, 1989

Loscher W, Honack D, Bloms-Funke P: The novel antiepileptic drug levetiracetam (ucb L059) induces alterations in GABA metabolism and turnover in discrete areas of rat brain and reduces neuronal activity in substantia nigra pars reticulata. Brain Res 735:208–216, 1996

Loscher W, Honack D, Rundfeldt C: Antiepileptogenic effects of the novel anticonvulsant levetiracetam (ucb L059) in the kindling model of temporal lobe epilepsy. J Pharmacol Exp Ther 284:474–479, 1998

Lynch BA, Lambeng N, Nocka K, et al: The synaptic vesicle protein SV2A is the binding site for the antiepileptic drug levetiracetam. Proc Natl Acad Sci U S A 101:9861–9866, 2004

Macdonald RL, Kelly KM: Antiepileptic drug mechanisms of action. Epilepsia 36 (suppl 2):S2–S12, 1995

Madeja M, Margineanu DG, Gorji A, et al: Reduction of voltage-operated potassium currents by levetiracetam: a novel antiepileptic mechanism of action? Neuropharmacology 45:661–671, 2003

Mallinger AG, Smith E: Pharmacokinetics of monoamine oxidase inhibitors. Psychopharmacol Bull 27:493–502, 1991

Marek GJ, McDougle CJ, Price LH, et al: A comparison of trazodone and fluoxetine: implications for a serotonergic mechanism of antidepressant action. Psychopharmacology (Berl) 109:2–11, 1992

Masand PS, Gupta S: Long-term side effects of newer-generation antidepressants: SSRIS, venlafaxine, nefazodone, bupropion, and mirtazapine. Ann Clin Psychiatry 14:175–182, 2002

Masuda Y, Karasawa T: Inhibitory effect of zonisamide on human carbonic anhydrase in vitro. Arzneimittelforschung 43:416–418, 1993

May TW, Rambeck B, Jurgens U: Influence of oxcarbazepine and methsuximide on lamotrigine concentrations in epileptic patients with and without valproic acid comedication: results of a retrospective study. Ther Drug Monit 21:175–181, 1999

May TW, Rambeck B, Jurgens U: Serum concentrations of topiramate in patients with epilepsy: influence of dose, age, and comedication. Ther Drug Monit 24:366–374, 2002

May TW, Korn-Merker E, Rambeck B: Clinical pharmacokinetics of oxcarbazepine. Clin Pharmacokinet 42:1023–1042, 2003a

May TW, Rambeck B, Jurgens U: Serum concentrations of levetiracetam in epileptic patients: the influence of dose and co-medication. Ther Drug Monit 25:690–699, 2003b

Mayersohn M, Guentert TW: Clinical pharmacokinetics of the monoamine oxidase-A inhibitor moclobemide. Clin Pharmacokinet 29:292–332, 1995

McElroy SL, Soutullo CA, Keck PE Jr, et al: A pilot trial of adjunctive gabapentin in the treatment of bipolar disorder. Ann Clin Psychiatry 9:99–103, 1997

McElroy SL, Arnold LM, Shapira NA, et al: Topiramate in the treatment of binge eating disorder associated with obesity: a randomized, placebo-controlled trial. Am J Psychiatry 160:255–261, 2003

McElroy SL, Suppes T, Keck PE Jr, et al: Open-label adjunctive zonisamide in the treatment of bipolar disorders: a prospective trial. J Clin Psychiatry 66:617–624, 2005

McElroy SL, Kotwal R, Guerdjikova AI, et al: Zonisamide in the treatment of binge eating disorder with obesity: a randomized controlled trial. J Clin Psychiatry 67:1897–1906, 2006

McIntyre RS, Mancini DA, McCann S, et al: Topiramate versus bupropion SR when added to mood stabilizer therapy for the depressive phase of bipolar disorder: a preliminary single-blind study. Bipolar Disord 4:207–213, 2002

McKee PJ, Blacklaw J, Forrest G, et al: A double-blind, placebo-controlled interaction study between oxcarbazepine and carbamazepine, sodium valproate and phenytoin in epileptic patients. Br J Clin Pharmacol 37:27–32, 1994

McLean MJ: Clinical pharmacokinetics of gabapentin. Neurology 44 (suppl 5):S17–S22; discussion S31–S32, 1994

McLean MJ, Schmutz M, Wamil AW, et al: Oxcarbazepine: mechanisms of action. Epilepsia 35 (suppl 3):S5–S9, 1994

Mendelson WB: A review of the evidence for the efficacy and safety of trazodone in insomnia. J Clin Psychiatry 66:469–476, 2005

Mengel HB, Houston A, Back DJ: An evaluation of the interaction between tiagabine and oral contraceptives in female volunteers. Journal of Pharmaceutical Medicine 4:141–150, 1994

Migliardi G, D'Arrigo C, Santoro V, et al: Effect of topiramate on plasma concentrations of clozapine, olanzapine, risperidone, and quetiapine in patients with psychotic disorders. Clin Neuropharmacol 30:107–113, 2007

Mimaki T, Suzuki Y, Tagawa T, et al: Interaction of zonisamide with benzodiazepine and GABA receptors in rat brain. Med J Osaka Univ 39:13–17, 1990

Mimrod D, Specchio LM, Britzi M, et al: A comparative study of the effect of carbamazepine and valproic acid on the pharmacokinetics and metabolic profile of topiramate at steady state in patients with epilepsy. Epilepsia 46:1046–1054, 2005

Montgomery SA: Pregabalin for the treatment of generalised anxiety disorder. Expert Opin Pharmacother 7:2139–2154, 2006

Montgomery SA, Tobias K, Zornberg GL, et al: Efficacy and safety of pregabalin in the treatment of generalized anxiety disorder: a 6-week, multicenter, randomized, double-blind, placebo-controlled comparison of pregabalin and venlafaxine. J Clin Psychiatry 67:771–782, 2006

Mula M, Trimble MR, Lhatoo SD, et al: Topiramate and psychiatric adverse events in patients with epilepsy. Epilepsia 44:659–663, 2003a

Mula M, Trimble MR, Yuen A, et al: Psychiatric adverse events during levetiracetam therapy. Neurology 61:704–706, 2003b

Mula M, Trimble MR, Sander JW: Psychiatric adverse events in patients with epilepsy and learning disabilities taking levetiracetam. Seizure 13:55–57, 2004

Nakasa H, Komiya M, Ohmori S, et al: Characterization of human liver microsomal cytochrome P450 involved in the reductive metabolism of zonisamide. Mol Pharmacol 44:216–221, 1993

Nemeroff CB, Evans DL, Gyulai L, et al: Double-blind, placebo-controlled comparison of imipramine and paroxetine in the treatment of bipolar depression. Am J Psychiatry 158:906–912, 2001

Ng B: Mania associated with mirtazapine augmentation of fluoxetine. Depress Anxiety 15:46–47, 2002

Nicolas JM, Collart P, Gerin B, et al: In vitro evaluation of potential drug interactions with levetiracetam, a new antiepileptic agent. Drug Metab Dispos 27:250–254, 1999

Nilsen OG, Dale O, Husebo B: Pharmacokinetics of trazodone during multiple dosing to psychiatric patients. Pharmacol Toxicol 72:286–289, 1993

Nutt D: Mirtazapine: pharmacology in relation to adverse effects. Acta Psychiatr Scand Suppl 391:31–37, 1997

Ojemann LM, Shastri RA, Wilensky AJ, et al: Comparative pharmacokinetics of zonisamide (CI-912) in epileptic patients on carbamazepine or phenytoin monotherapy. Ther Drug Monit 8:293–296, 1986

Olesen OV, Linnet K: Fluvoxamine-clozapine drug interaction: inhibition in vitro of five cytochrome P450 isoforms involved in clozapine metabolism. J Clin Psychopharmacol 20:35–42, 2000

Ozawa K, Kobayashi K, Noda S, et al: Zonisamide-induced depression and mania in patients with epilepsy. J Clin Psychopharmacol 24:110–111, 2004

Pande AC, Davidson JR, Jefferson JW, et al: Treatment of social phobia with gabapentin: a placebo-controlled study. J Clin Psychopharmacol 19:341–348, 1999

Pande AC, Crockatt J, Janney CA, et al; Gabapentin Bipolar Disorder Study Group: Gabapentin in bipolar disorder: a placebo-controlled trial of adjunctive therapy. Bipolar Disord 2:249–255, 2000a

Pande AC, Pollack MH, Crockatt J, et al: Placebo-controlled study of gabapentin treatment of panic disorder. J Clin Psychopharmacol 20:467–471, 2000b

Pande AC, Crockatt JG, Feltner DE, et al: Pregabalin in generalized anxiety disorder: a placebo-controlled trial. Am J Psychiatry 160:533–540, 2003

Pande AC, Feltner DE, Jefferson JW, et al: Efficacy of the novel anxiolytic pregabalin in social anxiety disorder: a placebo-controlled, multicenter study. J Clin Psychopharmacol 24:141–149, 2004

Patsalos PN: Pharmacokinetic profile of levetiracetam: toward ideal characteristics. Pharmacol Ther 85:77–85, 2000

Patsalos PN: Clinical pharmacokinetics of levetiracetam. Clin Pharmacokinet 43:707–724, 2004

Peet M: Induction of mania with selective serotonin re-uptake inhibitors and tricyclic antidepressants. Br J Psychiatry 164:549–550, 1994

Pennell PB, Ogaily MS, Macdonald RL: Aplastic anemia in a patient receiving felbamate for complex partial seizures. Neurology 45:456–460, 1995

Perucca E, Gidal BE, Baltes E: Effects of antiepileptic comedication on levetiracetam pharmacokinetics: a pooled analysis of data from randomized adjunctive therapy trials. Epilepsy Res 53:47–56, 2003

Peters DH, Sorkin EM: Zonisamide: a review of its pharmacodynamic and pharmacokinetic properties, and therapeutic potential in epilepsy. Drugs 45:760–787, 1993

Petty F: GABA and mood disorders: a brief review and hypothesis. J Affect Disord 34:275–281, 1995

Physicians' Desk Reference, 62nd Edition. Montvale, NJ, Thomson Healthcare, 2008

Pinninti NR, Zelinski G: Does topiramate elevate serum lithium levels? J Clin Psychopharmacol 22:340, 2002

Pisani F, Fazio A, Oteri G, et al: Effects of the antidepressant drug viloxazine on oxcarbazepine and its hydroxylated metabolites in patients with epilepsy. Acta Neurol Scand 90:130–132, 1994

Pohl RB, Feltner DE, Fieve RR, et al: Efficacy of pregabalin in the treatment of generalized anxiety disorder: double-blind, placebo-controlled comparison of BID versus TID dosing. J Clin Psychopharmacol 25:151–158, 2005

Pollack MH, Rosenbaum JF: Management of antidepressant-induced side effects: a practical guide for the clinician. J Clin Psychiatry 48:3–8, 1987

Post RM, Altshuler LL, Frye MA, et al: Preliminary observations on the effectiveness of levetiracetam in the open adjunctive treatment of refractory bipolar disorder. J Clin Psychiatry 66:370–374, 2005

Post RM, Altshuler LL, Leverich GS, et al: Mood switch in bipolar depression: comparison of adjunctive venlafaxine, bupropion and sertraline. Br J Psychiatry 189:124–131, 2006

Poulsen CF, Simeone TA, Maar TE, et al: Modulation by topiramate of AMPA and kainate mediated calcium influx in cultured cerebral cortical, hippocampal and cerebellar neurons. Neurochem Res 29:275–282, 2004

Rabkin J, Quitkin F, Harrison W, et al: Adverse reactions to monoamine oxidase inhibitors, part I: a comparative study. J Clin Psychopharmacol 4:270–278, 1984

Radulovic LL, Wilder BJ, Leppik IE, et al: Lack of interaction of gabapentin with carbamazepine or valproate. Epilepsia 35:155–161, 1994

Ragueneau-Majlessi I, Levy RH, Janik F: Levetiracetam does not alter the pharmacokinetics of an oral contraceptive in healthy women. Epilepsia 43:697–702, 2002

Ragueneau-Majlessi I, Levy RH, Bergen D, et al: Carbamazepine pharmacokinetics are not affected by zonisamide: in vitro mechanistic study and in vivo clinical study in epileptic patients. Epilepsy Res 62:1–11, 2004

Ragueneau-Majlessi I, Levy RH, Brodie M, et al: Lack of pharmacokinetic interactions between steady-state zonisamide and valproic acid in patients with epilepsy. Clin Pharmacokinet 44:517–523, 2005

Raitasuo V, Lehtovaara R, Huttunen MO: Effect of switching carbamazepine to oxcarbazepine on the plasma levels of neuroleptics: a case report. Psychopharmacology (Berl) 116:115–116, 1994

Randinitis EJ, Posvar EL, Alvey CW, et al: Pharmacokinetics of pregabalin in subjects with various degrees of renal function. J Clin Pharmacol 43:277–283, 2003

Reinikainen KJ, Keranen T, Halonen T, et al: Comparison of oxcarbazepine and carbamazepine: a double-blind study. Epilepsy Res 1:284–289, 1987

Richens A: Clinical pharmacokinetics of gabapentin, in New Trends in Epilepsy Management: The Role of Gabapentin. Edited by Chadwick D. London, Royal Society of Medicine Services, 1993, pp 41–46

Richter RW, Portenoy R, Sharma U, et al: Relief of painful diabetic peripheral neuropathy with pregabalin: a randomized, placebo-controlled trial. J Pain 6:253–260, 2005

Rickels K, Pollack MH, Feltner DE, et al: Pregabalin for treatment of generalized anxiety disorder: a 4-week, multicenter, double-blind, placebo-controlled trial of pregabalin and alprazolam. Arch Gen Psychiatry 62:1022–1030, 2005

Robertson P Jr, Hellriegel ET: Clinical pharmacokinetic profile of modafinil. Clin Pharmacokinet 42:123–137, 2003

Rohatagi S, Barrett JS, DeWitt KE, et al: Integrated pharmacokinetic and metabolic modeling of selegiline and metabolites after transdermal administration. Biopharm Drug Dispos 18:567–584, 1997

Rosaria Muscatello M, Pacetti M, Cacciola M, et al: Plasma concentrations of risperidone and olanzapine during coadministration with oxcarbazepine. Epilepsia 46:771–774, 2005

Rosenfeld WE, Doose DR, Walker SA, et al: Effect of topiramate on the pharmacokinetics of an oral contraceptive containing norethindrone and ethinyl estradiol in patients with epilepsy. Epilepsia 38:317–323, 1997a

Rosenfeld WE, Liao S, Kramer LD, et al: Comparison of the steady-state pharmacokinetics of topiramate and valproate in patients with epilepsy during monotherapy and concomitant therapy. Epilepsia 38:324–333, 1997b

Rosenstock J, Tuchman M, LaMoreaux L, et al: Pregabalin for the treatment of painful diabetic peripheral neuropathy: a double-blind, placebo-controlled trial. Pain 110:628–638, 2004

Rosenthal M: Tiagabine for the treatment of generalized anxiety disorder: a randomized, open-label, clinical trial with paroxetine as a positive control. J Clin Psychiatry 64:1245–1249, 2003

Roth T, Walsh JK: Sleep-consolidating effects of tiagabine in patients with primary insomnia (abstract NR839), in 2004 New Research Program and Abstracts, American Psychiatric Association 157th Annual Meeting, New York, May 1–6, 2004. Washington, DC, American Psychiatric Association, 2004, pp 315–316

Rouan MC, Lecaillon JB, Godbillon J, et al: The effect of renal impairment on the pharmacokinetics of oxcarbazepine and its metabolites. Eur J Clin Pharmacol 47:161–167, 1994

Rowbotham M, Harden N, Stacey B, et al: Gabapentin for the treatment of postherpetic neuralgia: a randomized controlled trial. JAMA 280:1837–1842, 1998

Ryback RS, Brodsky L, Munasifi F: Gabapentin in bipolar disorder (letter). J Neuropsychiatry Clin Neurosci 9:301, 1997

Sabatowski R, Galvez R, Cherry DA, et al: Pregabalin reduces pain and improves sleep and mood disturbances in patients with post-herpetic neuralgia: results of a randomised, placebo-controlled clinical trial. Pain 109:26–35, 2004

Sabers A, Gram L: Newer anticonvulsants: comparative review of drug interactions and adverse effects. Drugs 60:23–33, 2000

Sachdeo RC, Sachdeo SK, Walker SA, et al: Steady-state pharmacokinetics of topiramate and carbamazepine in patients with epilepsy during monotherapy and concomitant therapy. Epilepsia 37:774–780, 1996

Sachs GS, Lafer B, Stoll AL, et al: A double-blind trial of bupropion versus desipramine for bipolar depression. J Clin Psychiatry 55:391–393, 1994

Sachs GS, Nierenberg AA, Calabrese JR, et al: Effectiveness of adjunctive antidepressant treatment for bipolar depression. N Engl J Med 356:1711–1722, 2007

Samara EE, Gustavson LE, El-Shourbagy T, et al: Population analysis of the pharmacokinetics of tiagabine in patients with epilepsy. Epilepsia 39:868–873, 1998

Schaffer CB, Schaffer LC: Gabapentin in the treatment of bipolar disorder (letter). Am J Psychiatry 154:291–292, 1997

Schaffer L, Schaffer C, Howe J: An open case series on the utility of tiagabine as an augmentation in refractory bipolar outpatients. J Affect Disord 71:259, 2002

Schauf CL: Zonisamide enhances slow sodium inactivation in Myxicola. Brain Res 413:185–188, 1987

Sennef C, Timmer CJ, Sitsen JM: Mirtazapine in combination with amitriptyline: a drug-drug interaction study in healthy subjects. Hum Psychopharmacol 18:91–101, 2003

Serpell MG: Gabapentin in neuropathic pain syndromes: a randomised, double-blind, placebo-controlled trial. Pain 99:557–566, 2002

Shank RP, Gardocki JF, Vaught JL, et al: Topiramate: preclinical evaluation of structurally novel anticonvulsant. Epilepsia 35:450–460, 1994

Sharma V, Mazmanian DS, Persad E, et al: Treatment of bipolar depression: a survey of Canadian psychiatrists. Can J Psychiatry 42:298–302, 1997

Shorvon SD: Safety of topiramate: adverse events and relationships to dosing. Epilepsia 37 (suppl 2):S18–S22, 1996

Shorvon S: Pyrrolidone derivatives. Lancet 358:1885–1892, 2001

Siddall PJ, Cousins MJ, Otte A, et al: Pregabalin in central neuropathic pain associated with spinal cord injury: a placebo-controlled trial. Neurology 67:1792–1800, 2006

Sills GJ: The mechanisms of action of gabapentin and pregabalin. Curr Opin Pharmacol 6:108–113, 2006

Sills GJ, Brodie MJ: Pharmacokinetics and drug interactions with zonisamide. Epilepsia 48:435–441, 2007

Silverstone T: Moclobemide vs. imipramine in bipolar depression: a multicentre double-blind clinical trial. Acta Psychiatr Scand 104:104–109, 2001

Sisodiya SM, Sander JW, Patsalos PN: Carbamazepine toxicity during combination therapy with levetiracetam: a pharmacodynamic interaction. Epilepsy Res 48:217–219, 2002

Sitsen JM, Voortman G, Timmer CJ: Pharmacokinetics of mirtazapine and lithium in healthy male subjects. J Psychopharmacol 14:172–176, 2000

Sitsen J, Maris F, Timmer C: Drug-drug interaction studies with mirtazapine and carbamazepine in healthy male subjects. Eur J Drug Metab Pharmacokinet 26:109–121, 2001

So EL, Wolff D, Graves NM, et al: Pharmacokinetics of tiagabine as add-on therapy in patients taking enzyme-inducing antiepilepsy drugs. Epilepsy Res 22:221–226, 1995

Spira PJ, Beran RG: Gabapentin in the prophylaxis of chronic daily headache: a randomized, placebo-controlled study. Neurology 61:1753–1759, 2003

Stewart BH, Kugler AR, Thompson PR, et al: A saturable transport mechanism in the intestinal absorption of gabapentin is the underlying cause of the lack of proportionality between increasing dose and drug levels in plasma. Pharm Res 10:276–281, 1993

Stewart DE: Hepatic adverse reactions associated with nefazodone. Can J Psychiatry 47:375–377, 2002

Stiff DD, Robicheau JT, Zemaitis MA: Reductive metabolism of the anticonvulsant agent zonisamide, a 1,2-benzisoxazole derivative. Xenobiotica 22:1–11, 1992

Stoll AL, Mayer PV, Kolbrener M, et al: Antidepressant-associated mania: a controlled comparison with spontaneous mania. Am J Psychiatry 151:1642–1645, 1994

Striano S, Striano P, Di Nocera P, et al: Relationship between serum mono-hydroxycarbazepine concentrations and adverse effects in patients with epilepsy on high-dose oxcarbazepine therapy. Epilepsy Res 69:170–176, 2006

Sullivan KL, Ward CL, Zesiewicz TA: Zonisamide-induced mania in an essential tremor patient. J Clin Psychopharmacol 26:439–440, 2006

Suppes T, Chisholm KA, Dhavale D, et al: Tiagabine in treatment refractory bipolar disorder: a clinical case series. Bipolar Disord 4:283–289, 2002

Suzdak PD, Jansen JA: A review of the preclinical pharmacology of tiagabine: a potent and selective anticonvulsant GABA uptake inhibitor. Epilepsia 36:612–626, 1995

Taft DR, Iyer GR, Behar L, et al: Application of a first-pass effect model to characterize the pharmacokinetic disposition of venlafaxine after oral administration to human subjects. Drug Metab Dispos 25:1215–1218, 1997

Tasaki K, Minami T, Ieiri I, et al: Drug interactions of zonisamide with phenytoin and sodium valproate: serum concentrations and protein binding. Brain Dev 17:182–185, 1995

Taylor CP: Gabapentin: mechanisms of action, in Antiepileptic Drugs, 4th Edition. Edited by Levy RH, Mattson RH, Meldrum BS. New York, Raven Press, 1995, pp 829–841

Taylor CP, Vartanian MG, Yuen PW, et al: Potent and stereospecific anticonvulsant activity of 3-isobutyl GABA relates to in vitro binding at a novel site labeled by tritiated gabapentin. Epilepsy Res 14:11–15, 1993

Taylor CP, Angelotti T, Fauman E: Pharmacology and mechanism of action of pregabalin: the calcium channel alpha2-delta (alpha2-delta) subunit as a target for antiepileptic drug discovery. Epilepsy Res 73:137–150, 2007

Taylor D, Bodani M, Hubbeling A, et al: The effect of nefazodone on clozapine plasma concentrations. Int Clin Psychopharmacol 14:185–187, 1999

Thase ME, Mallinger AG, McKnight D, et al: Treatment of imipramine-resistant recurrent depression, IV: a double-blind crossover study of tranylcypromine for anergic bipolar depression. Am J Psychiatry 149:195–198, 1992

Theis JG, Sidhu J, Palmer J, et al: Lack of pharmacokinetic interaction between oxcarbazepine and lamotrigine. Neuropsychopharmacology 30:2269–2274, 2005

Thurlow RJ, Brown JP, Gee NS, et al: [3H]Gabapentin may label a system-L-like neutral amino acid carrier in brain. Eur J Pharmacol 247:341–345, 1993

Tiihonen J, Halonen P, Wahlbeck K, et al: Topiramate add-on in treatment-resistant schizophrenia: a randomized, double-blind, placebo-controlled, crossover trial. J Clin Psychiatry 66:1012–1015, 2005

Timmer CJ, Sitsen JM, Delbressine LP: Clinical pharmacokinetics of mirtazapine. Clin Pharmacokinet 38:461–474, 2000

Tohen M, Vieta E, Calabrese J, et al: Efficacy of olanzapine and olanzapine-fluoxetine combination in the treatment of bipolar I depression. Arch Gen Psychiatry 60:1079–1088, 2003

Tønnesen P, Tonstad S, Hjalmarson A, et al: A multicentre, randomized, double-blind, placebo-controlled, 1-year study of bupropion SR for smoking cessation. J Intern Med 254:184–192, 2003

Vanderkooy JD, Kennedy SH, Bagby RM: Antidepressant side effects in depression patients treated in a naturalistic setting: a study of bupropion, moclobemide, paroxetine, sertraline, and venlafaxine. Can J Psychiatry 47:174–180, 2002

Van Parys JA, Meinardi H: Survey of 260 epileptic patients treated with oxcarbazepine (Trileptal) on a named-patient basis. Epilepsy Res 19:79–85, 1994

Van Wyck Fleet J, Manberg PJ, Miller LL, et al: Overview of clinically significant adverse reactions to bupropion. J Clin Psychiatry 44:191–196, 1983

Vgontzas AN, Kales A, Bixler EO: Benzodiazepine side effects: role of pharmacokinetics and pharmacodynamics. Pharmacology 51:205–223, 1995

Vieta E, Martinez-Aran A, Goikolea JM, et al: A randomized trial comparing paroxetine and venlafaxine in the treatment of bipolar depressed patients taking mood stabilizers. J Clin Psychiatry 63:508–512, 2002

Viktrup L, Perahia DG, Tylee A: Duloxetine treatment of stress urinary incontinence in women does not induce mania or hypomania. Prim Care Companion J Clin Psychiatry 6:239–243, 2004

Wagner KD, Kowatch RA, Emslie GJ, et al: A double-blind, randomized, placebo-controlled trial of oxcarbazepine in the treatment of bipolar disorder in children and adolescents. Am J Psychiatry 163:1179–1186, 2006

Wamil AW, McLean MJ: Limitation by gabapentin of high frequency action potential firing by mouse central neurons in cell culture. Epilepsy Res 17:1–11, 1994

Warner MD, Peabody CA, Whiteford HA, et al: Trazodone and priapism. J Clin Psychiatry 48:244–245, 1987

Wasserman S, Iyengar R, Chaplin WF, et al: Levetiracetam versus placebo in childhood and adolescent autism: a double-blind placebo-controlled study. Int Clin Psychopharmacol 21:363–367, 2006

Wells BG, Gelenberg AJ: Chemistry, pharmacology, pharmacokinetics, adverse effects, and efficacy of the antidepressant maprotiline hydrochloride. Pharmacotherapy 1:121–139, 1981

White HS, Brown SD, Woodhead JH, et al: Topiramate modulates GABA-evoked currents in murine cortical neurons by a nonbenzodiazepine mechanism. Epilepsia 41 (suppl 1):S17–S20, 2000

Wier LM, Tavares SB, Tyrka AR, et al: Levetiracetam-induced depression in a healthy adult. J Clin Psychiatry 67:1159–1160, 2006

Wilson MS, Findling RL: Zonisamide for bipolar depression. Expert Opin Pharmacother 8:111–113, 2007

Yang LP, Plosker GL: Desvenlafaxine extended release. CNS Drugs 22:1061–1069, 2008

Young LT, Robb JC, Patelis-Siotis I, et al: Acute treatment of bipolar depression with gabapentin. Biol Psychiatry 42:851–853, 1997

Young LT, Robb JC, Hasey GM, et al: Gabapentin as an adjunctive treatment in bipolar disorder. J Affect Disord 55:73–77, 1999

Zaccara G, Gangemi PF, Bendoni L, et al: Influence of single and repeated doses of oxcarbazepine on the pharmacokinetic profile of felodipine. Ther Drug Monit 15:39–42, 1993

Zaphiris HA, Blaisdell GD, Jermain DM: Probable nefazodone-induced mania in a patient with unreported bipolar disorder. Ann Clin Psychiatry 8:207–210, 1996

Zarate CA Jr, Payne JL, Singh J, et al: Pramipexole for bipolar II depression: a placebo-controlled proof of concept study. Biol Psychiatry 56:54–60, 2004

Zhang W, Connor KM, Davidson JR: Levetiracetam in social phobia: a placebo controlled pilot study. J Psychopharmacol 19:551–553, 2005

Zona C, Ciotti MT, Avoli M: Topiramate attenuates voltage-gated sodium currents in rat cerebellar granule cells. Neurosci Lett 231:123–126, 1997

Adjunctive Psychosocial Interventions in the Management of Bipolar Disorders

Jenifer L. Culver, Ph.D.

Laura C. Pratchett, M.S.

In recent years, significant advances have occurred in pharmacotherapy for bipolar disorders. As described in the preceding chapters in this volume, new medications are emerging at an increasing pace, giving new hope for improved treatment outcomes with fewer adverse effects, and providing patients and clinicians with an ever-expanding array of somatic treatment options for managing the disorder.

Despite these recent advances, effective treatments for bipolar depression and well-tolerated maintenance treatments remain key unmet needs in this population. Thus, for many patients, pharmacotherapy is not sufficient to fully resolve symptoms and restore psychosocial functioning. Even with optimal adherence to medications, subsyndromal (particularly depressive) symptoms may persist between acute mood episodes, and many patients will experience relapse/recurrence (Gitlin et al. 1995; Judd et al. 2002; Post et al. 2003). Clearly, additional interventions are needed to provide patients with more complete and longer-lasting symptomatic recovery.

The course of bipolar disorder can be even more debilitating when patient adherence to pharmacotherapy is poor (Lew et al. 2006). Adherence to medications remains a substantial challenge in the treatment of the disorder (Keck et al. 1997; Lingam and Scott 2002; Scott and Pope 2002). Clinicians may not fully understand patients' reasons for nonadherence. In one study, the most likely reasons for patient nonadherence, according to clinicians, were "missing highs" and "felt well, saw no need to take medication," whereas patients most commonly endorsed "bothered by the idea that moods were controlled by medication," "bothered by the idea of a chronic illness," and "felt depressed" (Pope and Scott 2003). Attitudes and beliefs may be comparable in importance to adverse side effects as contributors to nonadherence (Lingam and Scott 2002; Pope and Scott 2003), suggesting an important target for psychological interventions. Indeed, medication adherence enhancement is a common goal of psychosocial therapies (Colom et al. 2003a; Frank 2005; Lam et al. 2003; Miklowitz et al. 2003) that has been achieved with intensive interventions (Colom et al. 2005; Peet and Harvey 1991).

Given the pernicious nature of mood episodes and subsyndromal symptoms despite pharmacotherapy, attention to adjunctive psychosocial interventions has grown in recent years. Unfortunately, there are still only limited data on the use of adjunctive psychosocial treatments by individuals with bipolar disorders. A retrospective study examined prior psychosocial service utilization by 500 individuals enrolled in the Systematic Treatment Enhancement Program for Bipolar Disorder (STEP-BD) and found that 54% were engaged in at least one adjunctive treatment in addition to pharmacotherapy upon entry into STEP-BD (Lembke et al. 2004). The most common type of treatment was therapy with a psychologist, followed by self-help group attendance, therapy with a social worker, and therapy with another type of provider. Greater rates of psychotherapy service utilization were found among those with comorbid conditions (personality disorders, substance abuse disorders, and anxiety disorders) and those with poorer global functioning.

A subsequent prospective 1-year study found that 60% of 1,000 STEP-BD patients receiving naturalistic treatment had at least one psychotherapy session (Miklowitz et al. 2006). Better outcomes (less severe depressive symptoms and better functioning) were associated with more frequent subsequent psychotherapy sessions among patients with severe depressive symptoms or low functioning at baseline, but with less frequent subsequent psychotherapy sessions among patients with less severe depressive symptoms or higher functioning at baseline. The authors concluded that intensive psychotherapy might be most useful to severely ill patients, whereas briefer treatments may be adequate for less severely ill individuals.

In addition to naturalistic studies, growing evidence from large, randomized controlled trials, as reviewed by Scott et al. (2007), suggests that adjunctive psychosocial interventions can substantially improve outcomes in patients with bipolar disorders. Evidence has emerged to suggest the efficacy of four specific structured manualized interventions, namely psychoeducation, family-focused therapy (FFT), cognitive-behavioral therapy (CBT), and interpersonal and social rhythm therapy (IPSRT). In this chapter, we review the key randomized controlled trials of these interventions.

The primary goals of psychosocial interventions in patients with bipolar disorder are symptom reduction, prevention of episodes, and optimizing psychosocial outcomes such as interpersonal and occupational functioning. Psychosocial treatments may approach these goals via slightly different routes and from different theoretical foundations. Scott et al. (2007) identified shared targets (see Table 15–1) of each of the primary psychosocial approaches. Each intervention emphasizes such targets to greater or lesser degrees. Effective management of bipolar disorder requires self-management, and each of these psychosocial interventions attempts to provide patients with the necessary skills, knowledge, and tools to better achieve self-management.

In addition to sharing treatment targets, the interventions discussed in this chapter share several other important characteristics. All of these interventions are structured and manualized, which makes them readily reproducible and thus subject to multiple independent evaluations in clinical trials. They are time limited, with most interventions ranging in duration from several sessions to 1 year. In addition, these interventions are evidence based, with empirically supported theoretical foundations. Finally, all of these psychosocial interventions target factors related to relapse/recurrence.

Despite the similarities of the targets of these interventions, they approach the treatment of bipolar disorder with different emphases and from different

TABLE 15–1. Shared targets of psychosocial interventions

Psychoeducation about bipolar disorder and its treatment

Enhancing lifestyle regularity (e.g., sleep-wake patterns, social rhythms)

Reducing substance misuse

Increased adherence to medications

Increased recognition of prodromal symptoms to facilitate early intervention

Source. Adapted from Scott et al. 2007.

theoretical foundations. In the following sections, we discuss these interventions individually, along with the outcome data of controlled trials.

Psychoeducation

Psychoeducational programs are typically designed to provide patients with information about bipolar disorder and its treatment. A primary goal of psychoeducation is to increase patients' understanding of the disorder to enhance treatment adherence. Some psychoeducational interventions emphasize prodromal symptom recognition and the development of coping skills to prevent relapse/recurrence. The patient plays a key role in the intervention and is encouraged to be actively engaged. Psychoeducation is frequently conducted in group settings, which might also serve to decrease stigma associated with the disorder and to facilitate informal peer support.

Controlled trials have shown that adding psychoeducation to medical management can increase patients' knowledge about their pharmacotherapy, resulting in more positive attitudes toward it (Peet and Harvey 1991). Psychoeducation has also been shown to delay manic relapse/recurrence (65 weeks vs. 17 weeks with medical management alone) and decrease the number of manic episodes by 30% (Perry et al. 1999).

More recently, Colom et al. (2003a, 2003b) provided particularly strong support for psychoeducation as part of maintenance therapy through a single-blind, randomized controlled trial of psychoeducation compared with an unstructured group (in which leaders avoided providing psychoeducation) in 120 recovered (euthymic at least 6 months) patients with bipolar I or II disorder. Psychoeducation consisted of 21 weekly sessions aimed at increasing awareness of bipolar disorder, teaching early detection of prodromal symptoms and recurrences, enhancing treatment adherence, and increasing lifestyle regularity (Colom et al. 2006). Both the psychoeducation and control arms were conducted in groups of 8–12 patients, with sessions lasting 90 minutes. The mean number of missed sessions was low and did not differ significantly between groups (3.8 and 3.4 in control and psychoeducation groups, respectively). Over 2 years, patients in the psychoeducation group compared with patients in the unstructured group had fewer recurrences (67% vs. 92%, number needed to treat [NNT]=4; Figure 15–1, leftmost graph); longer time to recurrence of depressive, manic, hypomanic, and mixed mood episodes; fewer hospitalizations per patient; and fewer days of hospitalization.

The psychoeducation group intervention improved outcomes, even in the subgroup with comorbid personality disorders; 100% of such patients in the

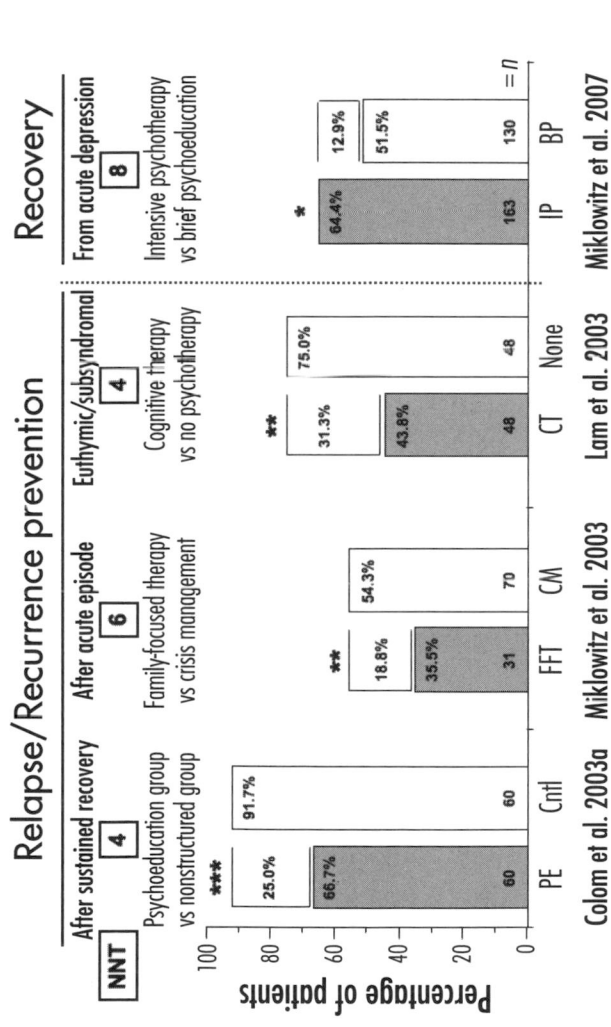

FIGURE 15–1.   Overview of adjunctive psychosocial treatment studies, numbers needed to treat (NNTs), and relapse/recurrence rates.

Adjunctive psychosocial interventions yielded single-digit NNTs, similar to those seen with approved pharmacotherapies. BP=brief psychoeducation control; CM=crisis management; Cntl=nonstructured control group; CT=cognitive therapy; FFT=family-focused therapy; IP=intensive psychotherapy (FFT, cognitive-behavioral therapy, or interpersonal and social rhythm therapy; PE=psychoeducation group. *P<0.05, **P<0.01, ***P<0.001 versus control intervention.

control group had recurrence, compared with 67% of the psychoeducation group (NNT=4) (Colom et al. 2005). Patients in the psychoeducation group also spent significantly fewer days in the hospital than did patients in the control group.

The group psychoeducational intervention appeared to be associated with more consistent lithium adherence, as evidenced by more stable serum lithium levels, suggesting one possible mechanism by which psychoeducation may confer benefits (Colom et al. 2005). In another study, enhanced treatment adherence alone did not account for the benefits of psychoeducation, as there were benefits of psychoeducation (fewer recurrences, fewer hospitalizations) in patients who were already highly adherent to medications prior to randomization (Colom et al. 2003b).

It is important to note that in these studies, benefits were obtained during maintenance of patients who were recovered (euthymic for at least 6 months) prior to the intervention (Colom et al. 2003a, 2003b, 2004). More intensive psychosocial treatment may be required in patients experiencing acute episodes or less sustained euthymia.

Family-Focused Therapy

Miklowitz and colleagues adapted FFT, which has been found to help prevent relapse/recurrence in schizophrenia (Falloon et al. 1985), for use in treating patients with bipolar disorders (Miklowitz and Goldstein 1997). FFT is based on research indicating that high levels of *expressed emotion* (characterized by family overinvolvement and criticism) among family members are associated with increased risk of relapse/recurrence and poor outcomes in patients with bipolar disorders (Miklowitz et al. 1986). The FFT approach includes 21 hour-long family therapy sessions administered over 9 months of treatment. Treatment begins with a family assessment and then focuses on psychoeducation about bipolar disorder and its treatment, training in communication skills, and training in problem solving (Miklowitz and Goldstein 1997).

Randomized controlled trials have supported the use of FFT in treating patients with bipolar disorders. Miklowitz et al. (2003) found that in 101 patients who had experienced a mood episode (14 depressed, 54 manic, 33 mixed) in the previous 3 months, FFT compared with brief crisis management (two 1-hour sessions of family education and crisis intervention sessions as needed) yielded less relapse/recurrence (35% and 54%, NNT=6; Figure 15–1, second graph from left) during the subsequent 2 years. In addition, time to relapse/recurrence was longer with FFT than with the control intervention (73.5 vs. 53.2 weeks). FFT also yielded greater decreases in affective symptom scores and better medication adherence.

In a similar study of 53 recently hospitalized patients with bipolar disorders, FFT compared with individual supportive therapy yielded fewer mood episodes during the subsequent 2-year period, as well as decreased rehospitalization (12% vs. 60% over the 2-year period, NNT=3) (Rea et al. 2003). Although this study matched treatment groups on the number of therapy sessions, FFT sessions involved more contact, with two cotherapists for 1 hour compared one therapist for 30 minutes with individual therapy sessions. Taken together, the results of these studies suggest that FFT may be a useful adjunct to pharmacotherapy for decreasing the number of relapses/recurrences and hospitalizations in patients with bipolar disorders.

Cognitive-Behavioral Therapy

CBT has demonstrated efficacy in unipolar depression (Kuyken et al. 2007), and recent studies indicate that it may be efficacious in bipolar disorders as well. CBT focuses on changing dysfunctional cognitions and maladaptive behaviors that increase vulnerability to mood episodes. In recent years, adaptations of CBT have been developed for bipolar disorder with published treatment manuals (Lam et al. 1999; Newman et al. 2002; Ramirez Basco and Rush 2005). CBT, as adapted for bipolar disorder, consists of the traditional components of this therapy with the addition of psychoeducation about bipolar disorder, as well as adaptation of cognitive-behavioral skills to increase awareness of mood, improve ability to recognize prodromal symptoms, and teach early intervention to prevent escalation into a syndromal mood episode.

Early, small controlled studies found adjunctive CBT compared with medication alone could improve clinical outcomes for individuals with bipolar disorders (Cochran 1984; Lam et al. 2000; Scott et al. 2001).

In the first large (*N*=103) controlled study of patients with bipolar disorders (who did not currently meet criteria for a mood episode), adjunctive cognitive therapy (CT) group (12–18 sessions of therapy during the first 6 months plus two booster sessions during the following 6 months) compared with medication-alone treatment yielded fewer relapses at the end of treatment and at the 12-month follow-up (44% vs. 75%, NNT=4; Figure 15–1, third graph from left), fewer mood episodes, fewer days spent in episodes, fewer hospitalizations (15% vs. 33%, NNT=6), and less time hospitalized (27 days vs. 88 days) (Lam et al. 2003). The CT group also yielded better coping with emerging manic symptoms, increased self-reported medication adherence, and better social functioning. This study involved patients with prior frequent relapses despite treatment with pharmacotherapy, making these findings even more encouraging.

Additional 18-month posttreatment follow-up (with no additional booster sessions) indicated that the effect of CT group for relapse/recurrence prevention was absent (Lam et al. 2005). The authors suggested that maintenance booster sessions may be necessary to extend the benefits of CT for relapse/recurrence prevention over time.

Although the evidence for CBT is promising, recent data suggest that not everyone may benefit similarly from brief CBT treatment. Lam and colleagues reanalyzed the results of their study (described above) to examine the role of a "sense of hyper-positive self" in predicting clinical outcome (Lam et al. 2005). They devised the Sense of Hyper-Positive Self Scale, which included a list of adjectives frequently associated with a state of being "mildly high" (e.g., *dynamic, entertaining, adorable*). In contrast to the investigators' expectation, CT group was less efficacious in patients who scored high as compared with low on the scale. Thus, for patients with high sense of hyper-positive self, targeting this attitude may be an important component in CBT.

More recently, a large multicenter trial of CBT in individuals with highly recurrent or severe bipolar disorder was discouraging (Scott et al. 2006). Sixty-four percent of patients entered the study either 1) in a current mood episode, 2) with substance abuse or dependence, 3) with another comorbid Axis I disorder, 4) with comorbid borderline or antisocial personality disorder, or 5) with a history of 30 or more previous mood episodes. This study enrolled patients with far more acute, severe, long-standing illness than have other studies. CBT (weekly for the first 15 weeks and gradually less frequently through 26 weeks, with two additional booster sessions at weeks 32 and 38) and treatment as usual (regular meetings with mental health professionals as necessary but no systematic psychotherapy for bipolar disorder) yielded similar symptom ratings, rates of recurrence, and time spent in mood episodes. A post hoc analysis indicated that the intervention may have had some benefit for individuals with fewer than 12 mood episodes. The authors suggested that CBT may be of more benefit to patients in earlier stages of illness and may not be the treatment of choice for individuals with frequently occurring episodes. The authors also reported that 40% of patients did not receive all planned components of CBT, suggesting that the intervention may not have been delivered fully for many participants. Additional research is needed to examine the role of intensive psychotherapy in individuals with severe recurrent illness, particularly given the tendency of this population to be less likely to respond to pharmacotherapy.

Although questions about the effectiveness of CBT in treatment of the most severe form of bipolar illness remain, the results of the studies discussed above provide strong evidence for the efficacy of CBT in improving clinical outcomes in general.

Interpersonal and Social Rhythm Therapy

IPSRT for bipolar disorders was adapted from interpersonal therapy by Ellen Frank and colleagues at the University of Pittsburgh (Frank 2005). IPSRT integrates psychoeducation, social rhythm therapy, and interpersonal psychotherapy components in a treatment specifically developed for the management of patients with bipolar disorders. IPSRT is based on a model proposing that individuals with this illness are genetically predisposed to abnormalities in circadian rhythms and sleep-wake cycles, which can be further disrupted by daily routines and life events. These abnormalities in circadian rhythms and sleep-wake cycles are thought to underlie recurrences of mood episodes. The goal of IPSRT is to address this link between life events, social rhythms, and mood episodes by helping patients stabilize their daily routines, reduce interpersonal problems, and increase adherence to pharmacotherapy (Frank et al. 2000).

In an early, small ($N=38$) study, adjunctive IPSRT compared with clinical status and symptom review treatment (CSSRT) in acutely ill patients with bipolar I disorder yielded no significant differences in time to remission or subsequent symptomatology during 2-year follow-up. However, IPSRT did result in greater stability of patients' social rhythms compared with CSSRT (Frank et al. 1997).

In a subsequent larger study, patients in acute episodes were stabilized with either IPSRT or intensive clinical management (ICM; 20- to 25-minute sessions that focused on providing support and education about bipolar disorder, medications, and sleep; review of symptoms and side effects; and management of side effects as necessary). Patients who had remission of their bipolar episode were reassigned to receive IPSRT or ICM for long-term preventive treatment. There were no differences between the treatments in time to remission, rate of remission (70% with IPSRT vs. 72% with ICM), or affective symptomatology (Frank et al. 1999, 2005). However, during the 2-year follow-up, those who received IPSRT during the acute treatment phase survived longer without recurrence and were less likely to have relapse/recurrence (41% with IPSRT vs. 46%

with ICM, NNT=22) (Frank et al. 2005). This effect of IPSRT appeared to be mediated by increased stability of daily routines. Also, participants who changed treatment modality (i.e., from IPSRT to ICM, or from ICM to IPSRT) had poorer outcomes compared with those who received the same treatment for stabilization and long-term prevention (Frank et al. 1999). These findings support the notion that instability of routines (and of treatment regimens in this case) can increase vulnerability to relapse/recurrence in patients with bipolar disorders.

Intensive Psychosocial Interventions

Considered collectively, intensive psychosocial treatments are beneficial. Scott and colleagues conducted a meta-analysis of eight randomized controlled trials of adjunctive CBT (Cochran 1984; Lam et al. 2000, 2003; Scott et al. 2001), prodrome identification (Perry et al. 1999), FFT (Miklowitz et al. 2000), IPSRT (Frank et al. 2005), and psychoeducation (Colom et al. 2003a) involving a total of 830 patients (Scott et al. 2007). Results revealed relapse/recurrence rates with adjunctive psychosocial treatments and standard treatments of 38.2% and 49.4%, respectively (NNT= 9). Adjunctive psychosocial therapies were more effective in patients who had been euthymic for more than a year. Patients with a dozen or more prior episodes did not show benefit with CBT (Scott et al. 2006) or psychoeducation (Scott et al. 2007).

In addition to the benefits of intensive psychotherapies for relapse/recurrence, preliminary data suggest that intensive psychotherapies may extend the protection against suicide offered by lithium or other appropriate pharmacotherapy, as demonstrated in a recent study showing that participation in adjunctive psychotherapy (either IPSRT or ICM) over 2 years was associated with a significantly reduced number of suicide attempts (Rucci et al. 2002).

In a large, multisite, randomized controlled study conducted as part of the STEP-BD, three adjunctive intensive psychotherapy interventions were compared collectively to a more limited adjunctive psychoeducational control intervention in the treatment of acute bipolar depression (Miklowitz et al. 2007). This study examined the effects of intensive (thirty 50-minute sessions over 9 months) CBT, FFT, and IPSRT, compared with a brief (three 50-minute sessions) psychoeducational control interventions in 293 outpatients with acute bipolar depression. Patients receiving an intensive psychotherapy (CBT, FFT, or IPSRT) recovered more quickly and had a higher recovery rate (64.4% vs. 51.5%, NNT = 8; Figure 15–1, rightmost graph) than did those receiving the control intervention. This study was not powered to find and did not find differences in outcomes between the three adjunctive intensive psychosocial treatments. It is worth noting that another STEP-BD randomized trial examining the use of adjunctive antidepressants (added to mood stabilizers) in acute bipolar depression failed to find benefits of adjunctive antidepressant treatment (Sachs et al. 2007), further highlighting the need for adjunctive psychosocial interventions in bipolar depression.

Treatment Implications

Randomized controlled studies confirm that four adjunctive, intensive, psychosocial interventions (psychoeducation, FFT, CBT, and IPSRT) are helpful for patients with bipolar disorders, yielding single-digit NNTs not only for relapse/recurrence prevention, but also for recovery from acute depression (see Figure 15–1). Thus, the NNTs for adjunctive intensive psychosocial interventions are comparable to those for pharmacotherapies approved for bipolar disorders by the U.S. Food and Drug Administration.

Evidence-based adjunctive psychotherapy is an important part of optimal clinical management of patients with bipolar disorder, as highlighted by recommendations for the inclusion of psychosocial interventions within bipolar disorder treatment practice guidelines (American Psychiatric Association 2002; Calabrese et al. 2004; Goodwin 2003). Unfortunately, the existence of evidence-based treatments for bipolar disorder does not equate to the widespread availability of such treatments. As indicated in Table 15–2, published manuals are available for each of these treatments; however, wider dissemination of and training in these interventions will be important in making these treatments more accessible to individuals with bipolar disorders.

Given the evidence presented in this chapter, referral for adjunctive psychosocial interventions should be routinely considered and discussed with patients

TABLE 15–2. **Treatment manuals for evidence-based psychosocial interventions**

Intervention	Resource
Psychoeducation	Colom et al. 2006
Family-focused therapy	Miklowitz and Goldstein 1997
Cognitive-behavioral therapy	Lam et al. 1999 Ramirez Basco and Rush 2005
Interpersonal and social rhythm therapy	Frank 2005

when their mood is euthymic or depressed, or when they are recovering from mood elevation. However, not all patients will accept referrals for psychotherapy or will have the resources of time and money to engage in intensive adjunctive psychotherapy. As previously noted, the few data that exist on utilization of adjunctive psychosocial treatments suggest that only about half of patients with bipolar disorders engage in psychosocial treatments (Lembke et al. 2004).

Therefore, some treatment settings (particularly within large organizations) may benefit from the development of comprehensive case management programs that incorporate psychoeducation, evidence-based pharmacotherapy, and increased access to care. For example, a randomized controlled trial found that of 441 patients with bipolar disorders in a health maintenance organization, those receiving systematic care management (structured group psychoeducation, monthly telephone monitoring, and feedback to and coordination with a mental health treatment team) provided by nurse care managers compared with those receiving treatment as usual had lower mean mania ratings over 24 months (Simon et al. 2006). In another randomized controlled trial of 306 veterans with bipolar disorders, a collaborative model for chronic care (group psychoeducation, nurse care coordinators to improve information flow and access to and continuity of care, and clinician decision support with simplified practice guidelines) compared with treatment as usual reduced weeks in (primarily manic) mood episodes, and improved social role function, mental quality of life, and treatment satisfaction over 36 months (Bauer et al. 2006a, 2006b).

In the absence of a more systemwide intervention, patients might benefit from the incorporation of brief psychosocial interventions into standard pharmacotherapy sessions. Psychopharmacologists may incorporate brief, structured psychoeducation; teach specific strategies to enhance medication adherence; encourage patients to monitor symptoms with structured mood charting to facilitate prodrome identification (Denicoff et al. 2002); and routinely develop early intervention plans should symptoms increase. Because patients have been found to be generally able to reliably identify prodromal symptoms of both manic and depressive episodes (Lam et al. 2001), the incorporation of this focus is unlikely to be an arduous task for practitioners. Lam et al. (2001) found that patients who employed behavioral strategies and early medical intervention when they recognized prodromal symptoms were less likely to experience relapses/recurrences of both depression and mania. Therefore, psychoeducation about prodromal symptoms, as well as a focus on behavioral coping strategies, is likely a simple yet potentially effective intervention to incorporate in treatment.

Conclusion

The addition of psychosocial interventions to pharmacotherapy has the potential to significantly reduce the toll of bipolar disorder on patients and their families. Adjunctive psychosocial treatments appear effective both for treatment of acute depressive episodes and as part of maintenance therapy. Although evidence supporting the efficacy of psychosocial treatments is mounting, more information is needed to determine the mechanisms of action underlying the effectiveness of these therapies. In addition, more information is needed to determine patient characteristics that may affect response to particular treatments. With such additional information, the use of evidence-based psychosocial interventions will likely become an even more important part of optimal clinical management of patients with bipolar disorders. Appendix C in this volume includes quick reference bipolar disorder resources and readings for patients and clinicians to facilitate the important task of psychoeducation.

References

American Psychiatric Association: Practice guideline for the treatment of patients with bipolar disorder (revision). Am J Psychiatry 159:1–50, 2002

Bauer MS, McBride L, Williford WO, et al: Collaborative care for bipolar disorder, part I: intervention and implementation in a randomized effectiveness trial. Psychiatr Serv 57:927–936, 2006a

Bauer MS, McBride L, Williford WO, et al: Collaborative care for bipolar disorder, part II: impact on clinical outcome, function, and costs. Psychiatr Serv 57:937–945, 2006b

Calabrese JR, Kasper S, Johnson G, et al: International Consensus Group on Bipolar I Depression Treatment Guidelines. J Clin Psychiatry 65:571–579, 2004

Cochran SD: Preventing medical noncompliance in the outpatient treatment of bipolar affective disorders. J Consult Clin Psychol 52:873–878, 1984

Colom F, Vieta E, Martinez-Aran A, et al: A randomized trial on the efficacy of group psychoeducation in the prophylaxis of recurrences in bipolar patients whose disease is in remission. Arch Gen Psychiatry 60:402–407, 2003a

Colom F, Vieta E, Reinares M, et al: Psychoeducation efficacy in bipolar disorders: beyond compliance enhancement. J Clin Psychiatry 64:1101–1105, 2003b

Colom F, Vieta E, Sanchez-Moreno J, et al: Psychoeducation in bipolar patients with comorbid personality disorders. Bipolar Disord 6:294–298, 2004

Colom F, Vieta E, Sanchez-Moreno J, et al: Stabilizing the stabilizer: group psychoeducation enhances the stability of serum lithium levels. Bipolar Disord 7 (suppl 5): 32–36, 2005

Colom F, Vieta E, Scott J: Psychoeducation Manual for Bipolar Disorder. New York, Cambridge University Press, 2006

Denicoff KD, Ali SO, Sollinger AB, et al: Utility of the daily prospective National Institute of Mental Health Life-Chart Method (NIMH-LCM-p) ratings in clinical trials of bipolar disorder. Depress Anxiety 15:1–9, 2002

Falloon IR, Boyd JL, McGill CW, et al: Family management in the prevention of morbidity of schizophrenia: clinical outcome of a two-year longitudinal study. Arch Gen Psychiatry 42:887–896, 1985

Frank E: Treating Bipolar Disorder: A Clinician's Guide to Interpersonal and Social Rhythm Therapy. New York, Guilford Press, 2005

Frank E, Hlastala S, Ritenour A, et al: Inducing lifestyle regularity in recovering bipolar disorder patients: results from the maintenance therapies in bipolar disorder protocol. Biol Psychiatry 41:1165–1173, 1997

Frank E, Swartz HA, Mallinger AG, et al: Adjunctive psychotherapy for bipolar disorder: effects of changing treatment modality. J Abnorm Psychol 108:579–587, 1999

Frank E, Swartz HA, Kupfer DJ: Interpersonal and social rhythm therapy: managing the chaos of bipolar disorder. Biol Psychiatry 48:593–604, 2000

Frank E, Kupfer DJ, Thase ME, et al: Two-year outcomes for interpersonal and social rhythm therapy in individuals with bipolar I disorder. Arch Gen Psychiatry 62:996–1004, 2005

Gitlin MJ, Swendsen J, Heller TL, et al: Relapse and impairment in bipolar disorder. Am J Psychiatry 152:1635–1640, 1995

Goodwin GM: Evidence-based guidelines for treating bipolar disorder: recommendations from the British Association for Psychopharmacology. J Psychopharmacol 17:149–173; discussion 147, 2003

Judd LL, Akiskal HS, Schettler PJ, et al: The long-term natural history of the weekly symptomatic status of bipolar I disorder. Arch Gen Psychiatry 59:530–537, 2002

Keck PE Jr, McElroy SL, Strakowski SM, et al: Compliance with maintenance treatment in bipolar disorder. Psychopharmacol Bull 33:87–91, 1997

Kuyken W, Dalgleish T, Holden ER: Advances in cognitive-behavioural therapy for unipolar depression. Can J Psychiatry 52:5–13, 2007

Lam DH, Jones SH, Hayward P, et al: Cognitive Therapy for Bipolar Disorder: A Therapist's Guide to Concepts, Methods, and Practice. Chichester, UK, Wiley, 1999

Lam DH, Bright J, Jones S, et al: Cognitive therapy for bipolar illness: a pilot study of relapse prevention. Cognit Ther Res 24:503–520, 2000

Lam D, Wong G, Sham P: Prodromes, coping strategies and course of illness in bipolar affective disorder: a naturalistic study. Psychol Med 31:1397–1402, 2001

Lam DH, Watkins ER, Hayward P, et al: A randomized controlled study of cognitive therapy for relapse prevention for bipolar affective disorder: outcome of the first year. Arch Gen Psychiatry 60:145–152, 2003

Lam DH, Hayward P, Watkins ER, et al: Relapse prevention in patients with bipolar disorder: cognitive therapy outcome after 2 years. Am J Psychiatry 162:324–329, 2005

Lembke A, Miklowitz DJ, Otto MW, et al: Psychosocial service utilization by patients with bipolar disorders: data from the first 500 participants in the Systematic Treatment Enhancement Program. J Psychiatr Pract 10:81–87, 2004

Lew KH, Chang EY, Rajagopalan K, et al: The effect of medication adherence on health care utilization in bipolar disorder. Manag Care Interface 19:41–46, 2006

Lingam R, Scott J: Treatment non-adherence in affective disorders. Acta Psychiatr Scand 105:164–172, 2002

Miklowitz DJ, Goldstein MJ: Bipolar Disorder: A Family Focused Treatment Approach. New York, Guilford Press, 1997

Miklowitz DJ, Goldstein MJ, Nuechterlein KH, et al: Expressed emotion, affective style, lithium compliance, and relapse in recent onset mania. Psychopharmacol Bull 22:628–632, 1986

Miklowitz DJ, Simoneau TL, George EL, et al: Family focused treatment of bipolar disorder: 1-year effects of a psychoeducational program in conjunction with pharmacotherapy. Biol Psychiatry 48:582–592, 2000

Miklowitz DJ, George EL, Richards JA, et al: A randomized study of family focused psychoeducation and pharmacotherapy in the outpatient management of bipolar disorder. Arch Gen Psychiatry 60:904–912, 2003

Miklowitz DJ, Otto MW, Wisniewski SR, et al: Psychotherapy, symptom outcomes, and role functioning over one year among patients with bipolar disorder. Psychiatr Serv 57:959–965, 2006

Miklowitz DJ, Otto MW, Frank E, et al: Intensive psychosocial intervention enhances functioning in patients with bipolar depression: results from a 9-month randomized controlled trial. Am J Psychiatry 164:1340–1347, 2007

Newman CF, Leahy RL, Beck AT, et al: Bipolar Disorder: A Cognitive Therapy Approach. Washington, DC, American Psychological Association, 2002

Peet M, Harvey NS: Lithium maintenance, 1: a standard education programme for patients. Br J Psychiatry 158:197–200, 1991

Perry A, Tarrier N, Morriss R, et al: Randomised controlled trial of efficacy of teaching patients with bipolar disorder to identify early symptoms of relapse and obtain treatment. BMJ 318:149–153, 1999

Pope M, Scott J: Do clinicians understand why individuals stop taking lithium? J Affect Disord 74:287–291, 2003

Post RM, Denicoff KD, Leverich GS, et al: Morbidity in 258 bipolar outpatients followed for 1 year with daily prospective ratings on the NIMH life chart method. J Clin Psychiatry 64:680–690, 2003

Ramirez Basco M, Rush A: Cognitive-Behavioral Therapy for Bipolar Disorders, 2nd Edition. New York, Guilford Press, 2005

Rea MM, Tompson MC, Miklowitz DJ, et al: Family focused treatment versus individual treatment for bipolar disorder: results of a randomized clinical trial. J Consult Clin Psychol 71:482–492, 2003

Rucci P, Frank E, Kostelnik B, et al: Suicide attempts in patients with bipolar I disorder during acute and maintenance phases of intensive treatment with pharmacotherapy and adjunctive psychotherapy. Am J Psychiatry 159:1160–1164, 2002

Sachs GS, Nierenberg AA, Calabrese JR, et al: Effectiveness of adjunctive antidepressant treatment for bipolar depression. N Engl J Med 356:1711–1722, 2007

Scott J, Pope M: Nonadherence with mood stabilizers: prevalence and predictors. J Clin Psychiatry 63:384–390, 2002

Scott J, Garland A, Moorhead S: A pilot study of cognitive therapy in bipolar disorders. Psychol Med 31:459–467, 2001

Scott J, Paykel E, Morriss R, et al: Cognitive-behavioural therapy for severe and recurrent bipolar disorders: randomised controlled trial. Br J Psychiatry 188:313–320, 2006

Scott J, Colom F, Vieta E: A meta-analysis of relapse rates with adjunctive psychological therapies compared to usual psychiatric treatment for bipolar disorders. Int J Neuropsychopharmacol 10:123–129, 2007

Simon GE, Ludman EJ, Bauer MS, et al: Long-term effectiveness and cost of a systematic care program for bipolar disorder. Arch Gen Psychiatry 63:500–508, 2006

Florida Best Practice Medication Guidelines for Bipolar Disorder

Terence A. Ketter, M.D.
Po W. Wang, M.D.

In view of the complexity of treatment of bipolar disorder, practice guidelines can be useful. As of early 2009, the revision of the American Psychiatric Association's (2002) "Practice Guideline for the Treatment of Patients With Bipolar Disorder" was 7 years old, but a second revision was in process. The Texas Implementation of Medication Algorithms' update to the algorithms for treatment of bipolar I disorder was more recently published, but was still 4 years old (Suppes et al. 2005). Canadian guidelines (Yatham et al. 2005, 2006) and European guidelines (Goodwin 2003; Grunze et al. 2002, 2003, 2004) are broadly consistent with the American Psychiatric Association's and other American guidelines, but they differ in some aspects (Keck et al. 2004; Sachs et al. 2000),

The age of guidelines and the amount of detail they provide can influence their utility for individual clinicians. This appendix provides three tables from the Florida Best Practice Medication Guidelines (University of South Florida 2007), which summarize a recent and concise approach to treating bipolar disorder. These guidelines are periodically updated and are available at http://flmedicaidbh.fmhi.usf.edu/recommended_adult_guidelines.htm. Even such guidelines may lag behind recent developments. For example, as of early 2009, the Florida guidelines had not yet incorporated recent data regarding the utility of adjunctive quetiapine (added to lithium or valproate) in longer-term bipolar treatment (Suppes et al. 2009; Vieta et al. 2008).

TABLE A–1.   Principles of practice for adults

1. Careful diagnostic evaluation
    - Bipolarity must be assessed in patients presenting with depression
    - Suicidality must be carefully assessed
    - Psychiatric and physical comorbidities must be carefully assessed
    - Substance abuse must be evaluated and addressed
2. Measurement-based care
    - Treatment targets need to be precisely defined
    - Effectiveness and safety/tolerability of medication treatment must be systematically assessed by methodical use of appropriate rating scales and side-effect assessment protocols
    - *For schizophrenia:*
      - Clinical Global Impression Scale (CGI) and
      - Brief Psychiatric Rating Scale (BPRS)
    - *For major depressive disorder:*
      - Hamilton Rating Scale for Depression (HRSD) and
      - Patient Health Questionnaire (PHQ)
      - Montgomery-Åsberg Depression Rating Scale (MADRS) as an acceptable alternative to HRSD
    - *For bipolar disorder:*
      - Young Mania Rating Scale for Bipolar Disorder (YMRS)
      - Hamilton Rating Scale for Depression (HRSD)
      - Encourage self-rating scale for depression such as
        - Beck Depression Inventory (BDI)
        - 16-Item Quick Inventory of Depression Symptomatology (QIDS-SR16)
3. Collaborative treatment decision making
    - Ongoing calibration of expected outcomes and progression toward goals

Source.   Reprinted with permission from Medicaid Drug Therapy Management Program for Behavioral Health: "Florida Best Practice Medication Guidelines: Principles of Practice for Adults." Available at http://flmedicaidbh.fmhi.usf.edu/recommended_adult_guidelines.htm. Tampa, FL, University of South Florida.

TABLE A–2.   Treatment of bipolar I disorder adult acute mania

Level 0

• Complete assessment

Level 1

If not treatment resistant and not very severe

• (May start at level 2 if treatment resistant or very severe)

  – Aripiprazole, lithium, olanzapine, quetiapine, risperidone, valproate, or ziprasidone monotherapy

  – Carbamazepine (accounting for drug interactions) is an alternative monotherapy

Level 2

If level 1 is not effective

• Two-drug combination of lithium plus valproate, or [lithium or valproate] plus level 1 second-generation antipsychotic

• Two-drug combination with carbamazepine (accounting for drug interactions) with level 1 drugs an alternative

Level 3

If levels 1 and 2 ineffective or not tolerated*

• Different two-drug combination of level 1 drugs (*but not two antipsychotics*) and may include oxcarbazepine

Level 4

If levels 1, 2, 3 ineffective or not tolerated*

• Two-drug or three-drug combinations of level 1, 2, 3 drugs, may include first-generation antipsychotic (*but not two antipsychotics*)

• Example:

  – Lithium + (valproate, carbamazepine, or oxcarbazepine) + antipsychotic

• Electroconvulsive therapy

• Clozapine

---

*Number of iterations at each level and adjunctive treatment(s) to be determined by clinician judgment and patient needs.

Source.   Reprinted with permission from Medicaid Drug Therapy Management Program for Behavioral Health: "Florida Best Practice Medication Guidelines for Treatment of Bipolar I Disorder Adult Acute Mania." Available at http://flmedicaidbh.fmhi.usf.edu/recommended_adult_guidelines.htm. Tampa, FL, University of South Florida.

TABLE A–3.   Treatment of bipolar I disorder adult acute depression

Level 0

• Comprehensive assessment

Level 1

• Olanzapine-fluoxetine combination or quetiapine monotherapy

• Two-agent combination of (bupropion or SSRI) with (carbamazepine, lithium, or valproate)

Level 2

If level 1 ineffective or not tolerated[a]

• Any combinations of level 1 treatments

  – Also combinations of (MAOI, SNRI, other antidepressant) with (lithium, valproate, second-generation antipsychotics)

  – Lamotrigine or olanzapine monotherapy

    ▪ Risperidone or ziprasidone monotherapy is an alternative

  – Antipsychotic (SGA or FGA) combined with either lamotrigine, lithium, or valproate

Level 3

If levels 1 and 2 ineffective or not tolerated[a]

• Adjunctive clozapine, inositol, pramipexole, stimulants, or thyroid hormones added to existing mood stabilizer therapy

Note.   FGA=first-generation antipsychotic; MAOI=monoamine oxidase inhibitor; SGA = second-generation antipsychotic; SNRI=serotonin-norepinephrine reuptake inhibitor; SSRI=selective serotonin reuptake inhibitor.
[a]Number of iterations at each level and adjunctive treatment(s) to be determined by clinician judgment and patient needs.

Source.   Reprinted with permission from Medicaid Drug Therapy Management Program for Behavioral Health: "Florida Best Practice Medication Guidelines for Treatment of Bipolar I Disorder Adult Acute Depression." Available at http://flmedicaidbh.fmhi.usf.edu/recommended_adult_guidelines.htm. Tampa, FL, University of South Florida.

TABLE A–4. Bipolar maintenance therapy

Level 1

• Continue effective and well-tolerated level 1 treatment for acute mania or acute depression
  - If frequent, recent or severe mania
    ▪ Aripiprazole, lithium, olanzapine, valproate
  - If frequent, recent, or severe depression
    ▪ Lamotrigine, lithium, olanzapine, valproate

Level 2

If level 1 ineffective or not tolerated

• Monotherapy with carbamazepine, quetiapine, risperidone, ziprasidone (in absence of acute response data)
• Lithium + valproate or carbamazepine or lamotrigine
• Lithium or valproate + antipsychotic (SGA or FGA)

Level 3

If levels 1 and 2 ineffective or not tolerated

• Combinations of other level 1 or 2 acute mania or depression agents
• Adjunctive clozapine, electroconvulsive therapy, oxcarbazepine

Note. ECT=electroconvulsive therapy; FGA=first-generation antipsychotic; SGA=second-generation antipsychotic.

Source. Reprinted with permission from Medicaid Drug Therapy Management Program for Behavioral Health: "Florida Best Practice Medication Guidelines for Bipolar Maintenance Therapy After Depressive Episodes." Available at http://flmedicaidbh.fmhi.usf.edu/recommended_adult_guidelines.htm. Tampa, FL, University of South Florida.

References

American Psychiatric Association: Practice guideline for the treatment of patients with bipolar disorder (revision). Am J Psychiatry 159:1–50, 2002

Goodwin GM: Evidence-based guidelines for treating bipolar disorder: recommendations from the British Association for Psychopharmacology. J Psychopharmacol 17:149–173; discussion 147, 2003

Grunze H, Kasper S, Goodwin G, et al: World Federation of Societies of Biological Psychiatry (WFSBP) guidelines for biological treatment of bipolar disorders, part I: treatment of bipolar depression. World J Biol Psychiatry 3:115–124, 2002

Grunze H, Kasper S, Goodwin G, et al: The World Federation of Societies of Biological Psychiatry (WFSBP) guidelines for the biological treatment of bipolar disorders, part II: treatment of mania. World J Biol Psychiatry 4:5–13, 2003

Grunze H, Kasper S, Goodwin G, et al: The World Federation of Societies of Biological Psychiatry (WFSBP) guidelines for the biological treatment of bipolar disorders, part III: maintenance treatment. World J Biol Psychiatry 5:120–135, 2004

Keck PE Jr, Perlis RH, Otto MW, et al: The expert consensus guideline series: medication treatment of bipolar disorder 2004. Postgrad Med (spec rep):1–120, 2004

Sachs GS, Printz DJ, Kahn DA, et al: The expert consensus guideline series: medication treatment of bipolar disorder 2000. Postgrad Med (spec rep):1–104, 2000

Suppes T, Dennehy EB, Hirschfeld RM, et al: The Texas Implementation of Medication Algorithms: update to the algorithms for treatment of bipolar I disorder. J Clin Psychiatry 66:870–886, 2005

Suppes T, Vieta E, Liu S, et al: Maintenance treatment for patients with bipolar I disorder: results from a North American study of quetiapine in combination with lithium or divalproex (trial 127). Am J Psychiatry 166:476–488, 2009

University of South Florida: Florida best practice medication adult guidelines. 2007. Available at: http://flmedicaidbh.fmhi.usf.edu/recommended_adult_guidelines.htm. Accessed April 9, 2009.

Vieta E, Suppes T, Eggens I, et al: Efficacy and safety of quetiapine in combination with lithium or divalproex for maintenance of patients with bipolar I disorder (international trial 126). J Affect Disord 109:251–263, 2008

Yatham LN, Kennedy SH, O'Donovan C, et al: Canadian Network for Mood and Anxiety Treatments (CANMAT) guidelines for the management of patients with bipolar disorder: consensus and controversies. Bipolar Disord 7:5–69, 2005

Yatham LN, Kennedy SH, O'Donovan C, et al: Canadian Network for Mood and Anxiety Treatments (CANMAT) guidelines for the management of patients with bipolar disorder: update 2007. Bipolar Disord 8:721–739, 2006

Quick Reference Medication Facts

Terence A. Ketter, M.D.

Po W. Wang, M.D.

This appendix provides a quick reference for medication facts that are important in the management of bipolar disorders, complementing the more detailed information in Chapters 13 and 14 of this volume.

General Facts

- More aggressive initiation and higher final dosages are needed and tolerated in acute manic and mixed episodes compared with other illness phases.
- Most agents are more effective at combating mood elevation compared with depressive symptoms, with the notable exceptions of lamotrigine, which does the opposite, and quetiapine, which has comparable efficacy for mood elevation and depression.
- Combination therapy is common, but only a few two-drug combinations are supported by evidence.
- Gradual titration and weighting dosage toward bedtime may help limit adverse effects.
- Most common adverse effects involve the central nervous system and gastrointestinal system.

Mood Stabilizer Facts

■ All mood stabilizers have at least one boxed safety warning.

Lithium

■ A boxed safety warning is provided regarding risk of lithium toxicity that can occur at dosages close to therapeutic levels.

■ The U.S. Food and Drug Administration (FDA) has approved lithium monotherapy for acute mania and longer-term treatment in bipolar disorder patients, but as of early 2009, not for acute mixed episodes.

■ The FDA has approved lithium for combination therapy with olanzapine, risperidone, quetiapine, or aripiprazole for acute mania, and with quetiapine for longer-term treatment.

■ Lithium is effective in pure mania and psychotic mania, but less so in mixed episodes or dysphoric mania.

■ In treating acute mania, lithium is started with low divided doses (e.g., 300 mg two or three times a day) and increased, as necessary and tolerated, by 300 mg/day every 1–4 days.

■ Gradual titration can decrease risks of central nervous system, gastrointestinal, and other adverse effects.

■ Lithium serum concentrations are classically 0.8–1.2 mEq/L in acute mania monotherapy, but mean concentrations were only 0.70–0.82 mEq/L in combination therapy acute mania trials.

Divalproex

■ Boxed safety warnings are provided for divalproex regarding risks of 1) hepatotoxicity, 2) teratogenicity, and 3) pancreatitis.

■ Monotherapy FDA indications are provided for divalproex for acute manic (delayed- or extended-release formulation) and mixed (extended-release formulation) episodes.

■ The FDA has approved divalproex for combination therapy with olanzapine, risperidone, quetiapine, and aripiprazole for acute mania, and with quetiapine for longer-term treatment.

■ As of early 2009, divalproex lacked a monotherapy FDA indication for longer-term treatment in patients with bipolar disorder, but was commonly used for longer-term treatment (often in combination with other agents).

- Divalproex has a broader efficacy spectrum than lithium, with greater benefits in mixed episodes and dysphoric mania.

- In treating acute mania, divalproex is started at 20–30 mg/kg/day (single daily dose with extended release), and the dosage is adjusted as necessary and tolerated.

- Contemporary valproate serum concentrations are 85–125 μg/mL (with more adverse effects above 100 μg/mL) for acute mania monotherapy, but mean concentrations were only 64–104 μg/mL in combination therapy acute mania trials.

Carbamazepine

- Boxed safety warnings are provided for carbamazepine regarding the risks of serious dermatological reactions and the HLA-B*1502 allele, as well as aplastic anemia (16/million patient-years) and agranulocytosis (48/million patient-years).

- Carbamazepine has received a FDA monotherapy indication for acute manic and mixed episodes.

- As of early 2009, carbamazepine lacked FDA indications for combination therapy and longer term treatment in patients with bipolar disorder.

- Carbamazepine has a broader efficacy spectrum than lithium, with greater benefits in mixed episodes and dysphoric mania.

- In treating acute mania, carbamazepine should be started with low divided doses (e.g., 200 mg twice a day) and increased, as necessary and tolerated, by 200 mg/day every 1–4 days.

- Gradual titration can decrease the risk of central nervous system and other adverse effects.

- Therapeutic acute mania serum concentrations are not yet established, so dosage should be increased gradually until efficacy is attained, adverse effects supervene, or serum concentration exceeds 12 μg/mL.

- Metabolic induction decreases concentrations of multiple medications (including carbamazepine itself, but not lithium), potentially decreasing efficacy of divalproex, lamotrigine, and second-generation antipsychotics, as well as other agents. Controlled studies failed to demonstrate additional benefit from adding risperidone or olanzapine to carbamazepine in acute mania.

- Patients should be monitored clinically (and with laboratories as indicated) for blood dyscrasia.

Lamotrigine

- A boxed safety warning is provided for lamotrigine regarding the risk of rare, serious rashes requiring hospitalization, which have included Stevens-Johnson syndrome, that require hospitalization.

- Lamotrigine has been proven ineffective in acute mania, but has a bipolar longer-term monotherapy treatment FDA indication and possible modest efficacy in acute bipolar depression.

- Gradual titration (25 mg/day for 2 weeks, 50 mg/day for 2 weeks, 100 mg/day for 1 week, and then 200 mg/day) is necessary to attenuate the risk of rash. Titration kits facilitate gradual initiation.

- The FDA-recommended lamotrigine dosage is 200 mg/day, but dosages as high as 400–500 mg/day may be tolerated and yield benefit.

- Lamotrigine dosages must be halved with divalproex and doubled with carbamazepine because of pharmacokinetic interactions.

- Final lamotrigine dosages with concurrent hormonal contraceptives, compared to without, may need to be higher because of a pharmacokinetic interaction.

Second-Generation Antipsychotic Facts

- All antipsychotics have boxed safety warnings regarding the risk of increased mortality in older adults with dementia-related psychosis.

- All second-generation antipsychotics have safety warnings regarding the risks of hyperglycemia and diabetes mellitus, and require baseline assessment and longitudinal monitoring for these problems.

Clozapine

- Boxed warnings are provided regarding risks of 1) agranulocytosis, 2) seizures, 3) myocarditis, 4) other adverse cardiovascular and respiratory effects, and 5) increased mortality in older adults with dementia-related psychosis (an antipsychotic class warning).

- Clozapine lacks an FDA indication for bipolar disorder (as of early 2009).

- Clozapine is a possible option in treatment-resistant bipolar disorder.

- In treating acute mania, clozapine should be started at a low bedtime dose (25 mg/day) and gradually increased (daily by 25 mg/day) to attenuate adverse effects.

■ Final dosages of clozapine in bipolar disorder are commonly below 300 mg/day, lower than in schizophrenia.

■ Gradual titration can decrease the risk of orthostasis and other adverse effects.

■ Adverse effects (e.g., agranulocytosis, weight gain, sedation, seizures) limit the utility of clozapine.

■ Patients taking clozapine should have clinical and blood monitoring for agranulocytosis.

Olanzapine

■ The FDA has approved olanzapine for monotherapy and adjunctive (added to lithium or valproate) treatment of acute manic and mixed episodes, and combined with fluoxetine for acute bipolar depression.

■ Olanzapine has received a monotherapy FDA indication for longer-term treatment in patients with bipolar disorder.

■ A rapid-acting intramuscular formulation of olanzapine has a FDA indication for agitation in acute mania.

■ In treating acute mania, oral olanzapine formulations should be started at 10–15 mg at bedtime and may be increased rapidly to 20 mg at bedtime.

■ Olanzapine is slightly more effective than divalproex but has slightly more acute adverse effects (e.g., sedation, weight gain).

■ Chronic olanzapine adverse effects (e.g., sedation, weight gain, metabolic problems) may ultimately require discontinuation.

Risperidone

■ The FDA has approved risperidone for monotherapy and adjunctive (added to lithium or valproate) treatment of acute manic and mixed episodes.

■ As of early 2009, risperidone lacked a FDA indication for longer-term treatment in patients with bipolar disorder.

■ As of early 2009, the long-acting injectable formulation of risperidone had FDA approval for schizophrenia but not for bipolar disorder.

■ In treating acute mania, risperidone should be started at 2–3 mg at bedtime and increased as necessary and tolerated daily by 1 mg/day to as high as 6 mg/day.

■ Higher risperidone dosages increase the risk of extrapyramidal adverse effects.

Quetiapine

■ The FDA has approved quetiapine for acute manic episodes (immediate and extended-release formulations) and acute mixed episodes (extended-release formulation), both as monotherapy and as adjunctive (added to lithium or valproate) treatment.

■ Monotherapy efficacy has been demonstrated for acute mania not only at 3 weeks (as with other agents) but also at 12 weeks.

■ Quetiapine immediate- and extended-release formulations have received FDA approval for adjunctive therapy (added to lithium or valproate) in longer-term treatment in patients with bipolar disorder.

■ In treating acute mania, quetiapine immediate-release formulation should be started at 100 mg/day (label recommends divided doses, but clinically the daily dosage is commonly taken at bedtime) and increased daily, as necessary and tolerated, by 100 mg/day to as high as 800 mg/day. In acute mania, quetiapine extended-release formulation is started at 300 mg at bedtime, increased the next day to 600 mg at bedtime, and thereafter dosed between 400 and 800 mg at bedtime.

■ In treating acute bipolar depression, quetiapine immediate- and extended-release formulations are commonly initiated at 50 mg at bedtime, and increased by 50-100 mg, as necessary and tolerated, with final dosages of 300 or 600 mg/day in controlled trials, but commonly lower in practice.

■ Gradual titration can decrease risks of sedation, orthostasis and other adverse effects.

Ziprasidone

■ The FDA has approved ziprasidone monotherapy for acute manic and mixed episodes.

■ As of early 2009, the FDA had not approved ziprasidone for combination / therapy, acute bipolar depression, and longer-term treatment in patients with bipolar disorder.

■ A rapid-acting intramuscular ziprasidone formulation has been indicated for agitation in schizophrenia but not (as of early 2009) for acute mania.

■ Ziprasidone monotherapy was ineffective in controlled trials in acute bipolar depression.

■ In treating acute mania, ziprasidone should be started with at least 80 mg/day and then abruptly increased (e.g., to 160 mg/day) to attenuate the risk of akathisia emerging on lower dosages. Some patients may benefit from dosages over the recommended 160 mg/day maximum (e.g., 240–320 mg/day). The label recommends two divided doses, but single daily doses with dinner or at bedtime with a snack may be more feasible.

- Taking ziprasidone with food is crucial, as this doubles absorption.
- Compared with olanzapine, risperidone, and quetiapine, ziprasidone has less risk of sedation and weight gain but more risk of akathisia.
- Adjunctive lorazepam may decrease problems with akathisia.

Aripiprazole

- The FDA has approved aripiprazole for monotherapy and adjunctive (added to lithium or valproate) treatment for acute manic and mixed episodes.
- Aripiprazole has received a FDA monotherapy indication for longer-term bipolar disorder treatment.
- A rapid-acting intramuscular formulation of aripiprazole has been indicated for agitation in acute manic and mixed episodes.
- Aripiprazole monotherapy was ineffective in controlled trials in acute bipolar depression.
- In treating acute mania, oral formulations of aripiprazole should be started at 15 mg once daily and, if necessary, increased to 30 mg once daily.
- Compared with olanzapine, risperidone, and quetiapine, aripiprazole has less risk of sedation and weight gain but more risk of akathisia.
- Adjunctive lorazepam may decrease problems with akathisia.

First-Generation Antipsychotic Facts

- First-generation antipsychotics have been superseded by second-generation antipsychotics, which appear better tolerated and have more evidence of efficacy in bipolar disorder.
- All antipsychotics have a boxed safety warning regarding the risk of increased mortality in older adults with dementia-related psychosis.
- The utility of chlorpromazine, the only first-generation agent with an acute mania indication, is limited by sedation and hypotension.
- Haloperidol has substantial contemporary evidence of acute antimanic efficacy when used as monotherapy or when combined with lithium or divalproex.

Newer-Anticonvulsant Facts

Oxcarbazepine

■ Although lacking any FDA bipolar disorder indications, oxcarbazepine is the only newer anticonvulsant with evidence of possible efficacy in acute mania.

Gabapentin, Topiramate, Tiagabine, Levetiracetam, Zonisamide

■ Gabapentin and topiramate monotherapy have been proven ineffective or lack evidence of efficacy in acute mania.
■ Some newer anticonvulsants may have utility in comorbid conditions (e.g., anxiety disorders, eating disorders, alcohol use disorders).

Adjunctive Antidepressant Facts

■ Adjunctive fluoxetine (combined with olanzapine) is the only antidepressant FDA-approved for acute bipolar depression, but use of this combination is complicated by sedation and weight gain.
■ No adjunctive antidepressant has FDA approval for longer-term treatment of bipolar depression.
■ Adjunctive antidepressant efficacy is controversial, and tolerability (switch risk) may be problematic, particularly with venlafaxine and tricyclic antidepressants.
■ If the optimized lithium serum concentration is less than 0.8 mEq/L, then an adjunctive antidepressant may yield benefit.

Other Medication Facts

Adjunctive Thyroid Hormones

■ The FDA has not indicated adjunctive thyroid hormones for bipolar disorder.
■ Limited data suggest that adjunctive (most often added to antidepressants) L-triiodothyronine (T_3) in physiological dosages may accelerate treatment response in nonrefractory depression and enhance treatment response in treatment-resistant depression.
■ Limited data suggest that L-thyroxine (T_4) in supraphysiological dosages may yield benefit in treatment-resistant rapid-cycling bipolar disorder.

Adjunctive Pramipexole

■ Although adjunctive pramipexole has not received a FDA bipolar indication, two small controlled trials have suggested adequate efficacy and tolerability in acute bipolar depression.

■ Pramipexole has risks of nausea and sedation, and it may destabilize mood.

■ To enhance tolerability in treating acute bipolar depression, pramipexole should be started at 0.125 mg/day at bedtime and increased every 4 days, as necessary and tolerated, by 0.125 mg/day to a target range of 1.0–2.0 mg/day, with a maximum of 4.5 mg/day.

Adjunctive Modafinil

■ Adjunctive modafinil has received no FDA bipolar indication, but a controlled trial suggested adequate efficacy and tolerability in acute bipolar depression.

■ Modafinil may cause rare serious rash; may destabilize mood; and modestly induces cytochrome P450 enzymes 3A4, 2B6, and 1A2.

■ In treating acute bipolar depression, modafinil should be started at 100 mg each morning and increased weekly, as necessary and tolerated, by 100 mg/day to as high as 200–400 mg/day.

Quick Reference Resources and Readings

This appendix provides a quick reference for useful resources and relevant readings for bipolar disorder information, to facilitate the important task of psychoeducation.

Resources for Bipolar Disorder Information

Bipolar News.org
http://www.bipolarnews.org

Bipolar Significant Others
http://www.bpso.org

Bipolar Trials Network
Phone: 617-632-1500
http://www.bipolartrials.org

Child & Adolescent Bipolar Foundation (CABF)
1000 Skolde Boulevard, Suite 570
Wilmette, IL 60091
Phone: 847-256-8525
http://www.cabf.org

Continuing Medical Education
2801 McGaw Avenue
Irvine, CA 92614-5835
Phone: 800-993-2632

Bipolar Disorders Information Center
http://www.mhsource.com/bipolar

Depression and Bipolar Support Alliance (DBSA)
730 N. Franklin Street, Suite 501
Chicago, IL 60610-7224
Phone: 800-826-3632
http://www.dbsalliance.org

Expert Consensus Guidelines
http://www.psychguides.com

Juvenile Bipolar Research Foundation (JBRF)
550 Ridgewood Road
Maplewood, NJ 07040
Phone: 866-333-5273
http://www.bpchildresearch.org

Medscape Psychiatry and Mental Health
http://www.medscape.com/psychiatry

Mood Garden
http://www.moodgarden.org

National Alliance for Research on Schizophrenia and Depression (NARSAD)
60 Cutter Mill Road, Suite 404
Great Neck, NY 11021
Phone: 800-829-8289
http://www.narsad.org

National Alliance on Mental Illness (NAMI)
Colonial Place Three
2107 Wilson Boulevard, Suite 300
Arlington, VA 22201-3042
Phone: 703-524-7600
http://www.nami.org

National Institute of Diabetes and Digestive and Kidney Diseases (NIDDK)
National Institute of Health Building 31, Room 9A06
31 Center Drive, MSC 2560
Bethesda, MD 20892-2560
Phone: 301-496-3583
http://www2.niddk.nih.gov

Weight-control Information Network (WIN)
http://win.niddk.nih.gov
Body mass index (BMI) and waist circumference fact sheet: http://win.niddk.nih.gov/publications/PDFs/Weightandwaist.pdf
BMI table: http://diabetes.niddk.nih.gov/dm/pubs/diagnosis/bmi_tbl.pdf

National Institute of Mental Health (NIMH)
Public Information and Communications Branch
6001 Executive Boulevard, Room 8184, MSC 9663
Bethesda, MD 20892-9663
Phone: 866-615-6464
http://www.nimh.nih.gov

Pendulum.org
http://pendulum.org

Screening for Mental Health
One Washington Street, Suite 304
Wellesley Hills, MA 02481
Phone: 781-239-0071
http://www.mentalhealthscreening.org

Stanley Medical Research Institute
8401 Connecticut Avenue, Suite 200
Chevy Chase, MD 20815
Phone: 301-571-0760
http://www.stanleyresearch.org

Systematic Treatment Enhancement Program for Bipolar Disorder (STEP-BD)
http://www.stepbd.org

Readings on Bipolar Disorder for Clinicians

Bauer M, McBride L: Structured Group Psychotherapy for Bipolar Disorder: The Life Goals Program. New York, Springer, 1996

Bauer M, Grof P, Müller-Oerlinghausen B: Lithium in Neuropsychiatry: The Comprehensive Guide. Oxon, UK, Informa, 2006

Colom F, Vieta E, Scott J: Psychoeducation Manual for Bipolar Disorder. New York, Cambridge University Press, 2006

Frank E: Treating Bipolar Disorder: A Clinician's Guide to Interpersonal and Social Rhythm Therapy. New York, Guilford Press, 2005

Goodwin FK, Jamison KR: Manic-Depressive Illness. New York, Oxford University Press, 1990

Goodwin FR, Jamison K: Manic-Depressive Illness: Bipolar Disorders and Recurrent Depression, 2nd Edition. New York, Oxford University Press, 2007

Jefferson JW, Greist JH, Ackerman DL, et al: Lithium Encyclopedia for Clinical Practice, 2nd Edition. Washington, DC, American Psychiatric Press, 1987

Lam DH, Jones SH, Hayward P, et al: Cognitive Therapy for Bipolar Disorder: A Therapist's Guide to Concepts, Methods, and Practice. Chichester, UK, Wiley, 1999

Ramirez Basco M, Rush A: Cognitive-Behavioral Therapy for Bipolar Disorders, 2nd Edition. New York, Guilford Press, 2005

Schatzberg AF, Cole JO, DeBattista C (eds): Manual of Clinical Psychopharmacology, 6th Edition. Washington, DC, American Psychiatric Publishing, 2007

Schatzberg AF, Nemeroff CB (eds): The American Psychiatric Publishing Textbook of Psychopharmacology, 4th Edition. Washington, DC, American Psychiatric Publishing, 2009

Readings on Bipolar Disorder for Patients and Families

Copeland ME: Living Without Depression and Manic-Depression: A Workbook for Maintaining Mood Stability. Oakland, CA, New Harbinger, 1994

Duke P, Hochman G: A Brilliant Madness: Living With Manic-Depressive Illness. New York, Bantam Books, 1992

Evans DL, Andrews LW: If Your Adolescent Has Depression or Bipolar Disorder: An Essential Resource for Parents. New York, Oxford University Press, 2005

Fieve RR: Moodswing, 2nd Edition. New York, Bantam Books, 1997

Goodwin G, Sachs G: Fast Facts: Bipolar Disorder. Oxford, UK, Health Press, 2004

Hinshaw SP: The Years of Silence Are Past: My Father's Life With Bipolar Disorder. Cambridge, MA, Cambridge University Press, 2002

Jamieson PE, with Rynn MA: Mind Race: A Firsthand Account of One Teenager's Experience With Bipolar Disorder. New York, Oxford University Press, 2006

Jamison KR: An Unquiet Mind. New York, Knopf, 1995

Jamison KR: Touched With Fire: Manic-Depressive Illness and the Artistic Temperament. New York, Free Press, 1996

Jamison KR: Night Falls Fast: Understanding Suicide. New York, Vintage Books/Random House, 1999

McManamy J: Living Well With Depression and Bipolar Disorder: What Your Doctor Doesn't Tell You. New York, Collins, 2006

Mondimore FM: Bipolar Disorder: A Guide for Patients and Families. Baltimore, MD, Johns Hopkins University Press, 1999

Papolos D, Papolos J: The Bipolar Child: The Definitive and Reassuring Guide to Childhood's Most Misunderstood Disorder, 3rd Edition. New York, Broadway Books, 2006

Phelps J: Why Am I Still Depressed? Recognizing and Managing the Ups and Downs of Bipolar II and Soft Bipolar Disorder. New York, McGraw-Hill, 2006

Raeburn P: Acquainted With the Night: A Parent's Quest to Understand Depression and Bipolar Disorder in His Children. New York, Broadway, 2004

Waltz M: Bipolar Disorders: A Guide to Helping Children and Adolescents. Sebastopol, CA, O'Reilly and Associates, 1999

Index

Page numbers printed in **boldface** *type refer to tables or figures.*